*ANNALS OF
THE NEW YORK ACADEMY
OF SCIENCES*

Volume 890

EDITORIAL STAFF

Executive Editor
BARBARA M. GOLDMAN

Managing Editor
JUSTINE CULLINAN

Associate Editor
COOK KIMBALL

*The New York Academy of Sciences
2 East 63rd Street
New York, New York 10021*

NEUROPROTECTIVE AGENTS
FOURTH INTERNATIONAL CONFERENCE

ANNALS OF THE NEW YORK ACADEMY OF SCIENCES
Volume 890

NEUROPROTECTIVE AGENTS
FOURTH INTERNATIONAL CONFERENCE

Edited by Bruce Trembly and William Slikker, Jr.

The New York Academy of Sciences
New York, New York
1999

Cover: *Scanning electron micrograph of human ADF cells. (See Abbracchio & Cattabeni, p. 85.)*

Library of Congress Cataloging-in-Publication Data

Neuroprotective agents: fourth international conference / edited by Bruce Trembly and William Slikker, Jr.

    p. cm. — (Annals of the New York Academy of Sciences, ISSN 0077-8923; v. 890)
Includes bibliographical references and index.
ISBN 1-57331-222-3 (cloth : alk. paper) — ISBN 1-57331-223-1 (paper)
    1. Nervous system—Degeneration—Chemoprevention—Congresses. 2. Brain damage—Chemoprevention—Congresses. 3. Cerebral ischemia—Chemoprevention—Congresses. I. Trembly, Bruce. II. Slikker, William. III. International Conference on Neuroprotective Agents: Clinical and Experimental Aspects (4th : 1998 : Annapolis, Md.) IV. Series
    [DNLM: 1. Cerebral Ischemia—drug therapy—Congresses. 2. Brain Injuries—drug therapy—Congresses. 3. Nerve Degeneration—prevention & control—Congresses. 4. Neurodegenerative Diseases—drug therapy—Congresses. 5. Neuroprotective Agents—therapeutic use—Congresses. 6. Spinal Cord Injuries—drug therapy—Congresses. WL 355 N4946 1999]
RC365 .N4786 1999
500 s—dc21
[616.8'0461]   99-047061

GYAT / PCP
Printed in the United States of America
ISBN 1-57331-222-3 (cloth)
ISBN 1-57331-223-1 (paper)
ISSN 0077-8923

NEUROPROTECTIVE AGENTS
FOURTH INTERNATIONAL CONFERENCE[a]

Editors and Conference Chairs

BRUCE TREMBLY AND WILLIAM SLIKKER, JR.

CONTENTS

[a]This volume contains the papers from a conference entitled *Fourth International Conference on Neuroprotective Agents: Clinical and Experimental Aspects*, which was held in Annapolis, Maryland on November 15–19, 1998.

Part VIII. Growth Factors

Part IX. Spinal Cord Injury:
Importance of Inflammatory Response

Part X. Glutamate Receptor Agents

Financial assistance was received from:

- NATIONAL CENTER FOR TOXICOLOGICAL RESEARCH/FDA, JEFFERSON, ARKANSAS
- DEPARTMENT OF VETERANS AFFAIRS MEDICAL CENTER, TOGUS, MAINE

Preface

This volume contains papers, poster presentations and abstracts from the Fourth International Conference on Neuroprotective Agents held in Annapolis, Maryland on November 15–19, 1998. Previous conferences were held in Rockland, Maine in 1991, Lake George, New York in 1994 (*Annals* Vol. 765) and Lake Como, Italy in 1996 (*Annals* Vol. 825).

It has been the aim of these conferences to bring together clinicians and basic science researchers from many disciplines and many parts of the world in a congenial, small and informal setting. The clinical focus of this fourth conference tended to be more in the direction of chronic conditions, such as Parkinson's and Alzheimer's disease as compared with acute stroke and traumatic brain injury. Indeed, in these acute conditions, hypothermia and tissue plasminogen activator may be the only modalities of significance in reducing neurologic damage, and hypothermia may even induce ischemic tolerance.

An interesting and critical session was devoted to examination of the role of glutamate excitotoxicity, questioning both the significance of measurement of extracellular glutamate and the role of glutamate receptor antagonists in reducing what may be excitotoxic neuronal damage.

Other papers emphasized the role of endogenous agents such as adenosine, nitric oxide, melatonin, L-carnitine, estrogens and glycemia in acute and chronic neural injury. The wide range of presentations, from a detailed paper on the very unique histopathology of spinal cord injury to the latest protective techniques in neurosurgery, served to illustrate the overall scientific scope of these conferences.

We are grateful to the New York Academy of Sciences for the opportunity to share these proceedings with other clinicians and scientists.

The Fifth International Conference on Neuroprotective Agents will be held at Lake Tahoe, California on September 17–21, 2000.

Bruce Trembly
William Slikker, Jr.

U.S. Food and Drug Administration: Future of New Product Strategies and FDA Priorities

B.A. SCHWETZ[a]

National Center for Toxicological Research/FDA, Jefferson, Arkansas 72079, USA

The greater benefit of efforts related to prevention rather than therapy alone has long been recognized within the public health community. The interaction between clinicians and researchers through this series of conferences on neuroprotective agents is an excellent example of using new scientific findings and understandings to improve our abilities to develop and evaluate better drugs and clinical procedures. While breakthroughs in research and clinical medicine continue to occur on a regular basis, the rate of acquisition of new knowledge is occurring faster today than ever before. We are now at a threshold of two changes that make the future more promising than ever.

First, with the more widespread understanding of biology at the cellular and molecular levels, we have a much more detailed knowledge of the physiology of all systems, including the nervous system. This translates into better understanding of the pharmacological and toxicological aspects of chemical and drug exposures. Even more promising for the future, this also translates into new strategies for drug development and therapeutic regimens, consistent with the theme of these meetings on neuroprotective drugs.

Second, the rapid change in the technology of information handling and real-time evaluation of data permits a much greater efficiency of research and clinical procedures. This also translates into greater efficiency and effectiveness of research and clinical medicine.

All this comes at a time when we are on the threshold of defining the human genome and that of animal models. These efforts enable us to use our new level of understanding of biology and physiology to target new drug development more effectively for protection of neurologic function. Research programs of tomorrow must be structured in anticipation of this new opportunity.

[a]Address for correspondence: Bernard Schwetz, DVM, Ph.D., NCTR, 3900 NCTR Road, Jefferson, AR 72079-9502. Phone, 870/543-7517; fax, 870/543-7576.
e-mail, bschwetz@nctr.fda.gov

Neuroprotection against Cerebral Ischemia

A Review of Animal Studies and Correlation with Human Trial Results

S. JONAS,[a,c] V. AYIGARI,[a] D. VIERA,[b] AND P. WATERMAN[a]

[a]Department of Neurology and [b]Medical Library, New York University School of Medicine, New York, New York 10016, USA

"Does effect of a neuroprotective agent on volume of experimental animal cerebral infarct predict effect of the agent on clinical outcome in human stroke?" We addressed this subject in a previous review bearing this title.[1] We now extend this review to include the experimental animal studies published through August 1998, and the results of human trials of 12 of these agents.

Among the 12 agents tried in humans, only thrombolytic treatment with tissue plasminogen activator (tPA) given in the first 3 hours after ischemic stroke has been accepted by the Food and Drug Administration (FDA) to be superior to placebo, based on clinical stroke outcomes in the 3-hour window National Institute of Neurological Disorders and Stroke/NIH (NINDS) trial. The FDA has not accepted any of the other 11 agents as useful for ischemic stroke.

We present graphically the animal results (FIG. 1): x-axis: time in minutes from induction of focal ischemia to first treatment (prophylactic treatments are assigned to −1 minute, and immediate postischemia treatments to +1 minute); y-axis: size of treated infarct relative to size of control infarct (0–100%; treated infarcts >control size are valued at 100%). The regression line for the nine results of the various experimental thrombolysis studies runs from approximately 20% at 0 time to approximately 50% at 6 hours (95% confidence curves are provided). For 10 agents, plus low molecular weight herapin (LMWH) used in low doses, all results of administration after 30 minutes lie in the "no-fly zone" above the upper 95% confidence curve for thrombolysis. LMWH in high doses (10 to 30 times the human trial doses) gave animal results (one study) in the thrombolysis range.

DISCUSSION

The thrombolysis results show that ischemic brain tissue in animals can be salvaged even up to 6 hours by restoration of blood flow. With the exception of high dose LMWH, there is no evidence that any so-called neuroprotective drug tested in humans can produce salvage in animals comparable to that seen with thrombolysis, if first administration is at more than 30 minutes after onset of focal ischemia.

[c]Corresponding author: Saran Jonas, M.D., Professor of Clinical Neurology, NYU School of Medicine, 550 First Avenue, New York, NY 10016. Phone, 212/263-7202; fax, 212/263-8228.

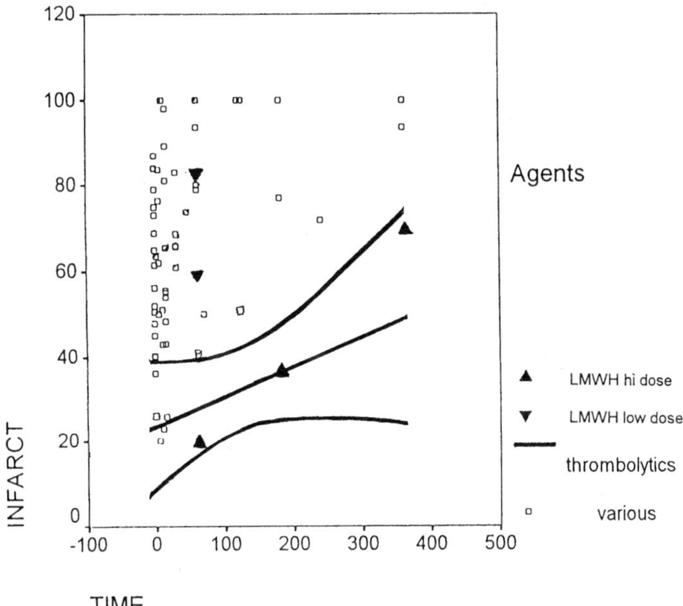

FIGURE 1. Clinically studied agents versus thrombolysis.

With regard to the predictive value of infarct size in animals for clinical outcome in human stroke patients, the implications are clear:

- None of the regimens used in human trials came close in animals to producing the results seen in animal thrombolysis studies.

- An agent with poorer animal results than thrombolysis for a given time of first treatment will fail in humans if given at that time or later.

- Of the 11 agents studied in humans and animals, only LMWH in high doses is worthy of further investigation.

REFERENCE

1. JONAS, S., A.Q. TRAN, E. EISENBERG, M. AZAM, D. VIERA & S. GRUMET. 1997. Does effect of a neuroprotective agent on volume of experimental animal cerebral infarct predict effect of the agent on clinical outcome in human stroke? Ann. N.Y. Acad. Sci. **825:** 281–287.

Questions and Answers

QUESTION FOR DR. SCHWETZ

From Dr. Palmer

My concern is neurotoxicology. There is a huge variety of new neuroprotective agents—growth factors; ICAM, stem cells, ICE, immunology, genes, BAX; etc. This is a potential minefield for neurotoxicology. Has the FDA addressed this problem or do they plan to issue guidelines for specific neurotoxicology issues for particular classes of compounds?

ANSWER (Dr. Slikker):   The two Centers of the FDA that review agents such as growth factors, genes, stem cells, etc., the Center for Biologic Evaluation and Research (CBER) and the Center for Drug Evaluation and Research (CDER) have rarely released specific guidelines concerning neurotoxicity/neuroprotection. However, within the FDA Centers and between Centers, there are internal working groups and committees that are concerned with these classes of agents. Many members of one working group, the FDA Intercenter Neurotoxicity Working Group, attended and presented at this and previous International Neuroprotective Conferences. These opportunities for information exchange serve to educate regulatory and drug development scientists alike as to the evaluation and research needs for the broad range of agents categorized as neuroprotectants.

QUESTIONS FOR DR. JONAS

COMMENT (Dr. von Lubitz):   You presented a bleak picture, Dr. Jonas. I submit that unless the climate changes, there is no hope of stroke treatment. Neither NIH nor the industry are interested in sponsoring therapeutic animal studies for whatever reason. They may have—yet both go in for extraordinarily expensive clinical testing. Unless this issue is addressed promptly, the rest will still remain in the domain of politics, dogma and unfounded hopes.

From Dr. Bowyer

Will angiogenic compound/trophic factors (endothelial trophic factor) be of any use in treating stroke/ischemia?

ANSWER: As of yet, growth factors have been of no value.

COMMENT (Dr. von Lubitz): I suggest abandoning drugs effective only in a "short window" setting may be premature. Increasing level of awareness and diagnostic stroke skills may make such early interventions extremely useful. Hence, concentrating on an agent's efficacy when given at least 3 hours past-event may eliminate a significant treatment potential. This seems to be exceedingly unwise.

From Dr. Sobotka

The direct linear relationship between clinical signs and infarct size was shown. But this was apparently established in untreated animals, i.e., without neuroprotection intervention. Thrombolytics were then shown to decrease infarct size but no specific information was presented about changes (improvement?) in clinical signs. Has the linear relationship between clinical signs and infarct size been established in animals treated with neuroprotectants such as the thrombolytics? Is this comparable to the relationship in untreated animals?

ANSWER: The data are ratios on both axes: y = (mean infarct size of treated animals)/(mean infarct size in controls); x = (mean neurologic score in treated animals)/(mean score in controls).

From Dr. Sobotka

Eliprodil-TPA provided an effective combination decreasing infarct size. Have any of the other drugs discussed by Dr. Jonas been tested in combination with TPA? With what result?

ANSWER: This is the only combination I've found.

From Dr. Marchionni

When the Phase III stroke trial for CNS 1102 (aptiganel HCl, formerly CERESTAT®) was designed, very little information was available on the duration of the period following onset of symptoms during which an acute stroke therapy could be administered and have a beneficial effect on eventual outcome of a patient. A six-hour "window" was considered practical from a patient recruitment viewpoint. A preclinical study in rats with CNS 1102 had demonstrated a reduction in infarct volume when administration of the drug was commenced one hour after the occlusion of the middle cerebral artery. Other animal studies with a variety of neuroprotective agents had shown that delaying the therapeutic intervention for some hours was possible. In a Phase II clinical trial with CNS 1102, including only patients who could be treated within 6 hours of onset of stroke symptoms, the group of patients treated with the top dose of the drug had a greater improvement in NIH Stroke Scale score, measured 3 months after the stroke, than the group of patients treated with the placebo. These findings coupled with extensive information on therapeutic plasma drug levels from animal studies, formed a strong basis for pursuing a Phase III clinical trial.

Second, work in Seth Finklestein's lab has shown a functional recovery with OP-1 treatment in a rat model, yet there was no reduction in infarct volume. What is your impression of that result?

ANSWER: First, apparently the CNS1102 data to which you refer were not published. I therefore do not have them in my database. Second, this is a very important matter suggesting that beneficial reorganization of the surviving nervous system can be promoted pharmacologically.

COMMENT (Dr. Hall): Your analysis of the preclinical stroke neuroprotective strategies vs expected clinical result points correctly to our failure to perform adequate therapeutic window studies prior to moving into clinical trials. However, other equally important deficiencies include use of varying species, inadequate dose-response analysis and definition of therapeutic pharmacokinetics as well as often total lack of definition of ideal dosing regimen (duration of dosing). These issues are also critical to address.

QUESTION: From a clinical standpoint, what is a reasonable therapeutic window within which a large number of stroke patients can be treated?

ANSWER: Patients, doctors, and EMS will not push very hard unless treatment can be safely administered to all stroke patients, and with good results. Build such a treatment and they will come if it is possible for them to do so. Three hours is feasible during the day. However, unlike a painful myocardial infarct, a stroke doesn't wake the victim from sleep, so best intentions will still lead to 11-hour delays.

From Dr. Aschner

I wish to commend you on your analysis of the neuroprotective effects of various drugs. It needs to be pointed out, nevertheless, that your meta analysis is essentially based on relatively few studies with TPA, and as you indicated the verdict is yet to be established as to whether TPA in the first place offers valuable protection in the model of focal experimental ischemia. Shouldn't it be incumbent upon the research community to unequivocally establish the effectiveness of TPA, with different dosage and time points before conclusions are drawn from the other studies?

ANSWER: The 5-hour window is being studied in the current Genintech trial, and the NIH dose rather than originally tried doses has been re-studied by the European clinical investigators.

From Dr. Meier

PARP inhibition shows a different kinetics in the induced convulsion model than it does in your animal models. PARP inhibition in our model shows a biphasic protection, which is better at 2 hours than at 5 or 40 mins post convulsions or as a pre-treatment. Are we throwing out drugs because we are using the wrong treatment regimens?

ANSWER: I cannot comment on PARP inhibition.

The Pivotal Role of Iron in NF-κB Activation and Nigrostriatal Dopaminergic Neurodegeneration

Prospects for Neuroprotection in Parkinson's Disease with Iron Chelators

M.B.H. YOUDIM,[a,b,c] E. GRÜNBLATT,[a] AND S. MANDEL[a]

[a]Technion, Faculty of Medicine, Eve Topf and US National Parkinson's Foundation Centers for Neurodegenerative Diseases, Bruce Rappaport Family Research Institute and Department of Pharmacology, Haifa, Israel

[b]Fogarty International Center, National Institute of Mental Health/NIH, Bethesda, Maryland, USA

ABSTRACT: R-Apomorphine (APO) the catechol-derived dopamine D_1-D_2 receptor agonist has been shown to be highly potent iron chelator and radical scavenger and inhibitor of membrane lipid peroxidation *in vitro*, *in vivo* and in cell culture employing PC12 cells. Its potency has been compared to the prototype iron chelator desferrioxamine (desferal), dopamine, nifedipine and dopamine D_2 receptor agonists, bromocriptine, lisuride, pergolide and pramipexole. APO also inhibits brain and mitochondrial protein oxidation. *In vivo* APO protects against MPTP (N-methyl-4-phenyl-1,2,3,6-tetrahydropyridine)-induced striatal dopaminergic neurodegeneration in C57 black mice with as low as 5 mg/kg. APO is a reversible competitive inhibitor of monoamine oxidase (MAO) A and B with IC_{50} values of 93 and 214 uM, respectively. The iron chelating and radical scavenging actions of desferal and APO explains their ability to inhibit iron and 6-hydroxydopamine (6-OHDA)-induced neurodegeneration and activation of redox-sensitive transcription factor NF-κB and the subsequent transactivation of promoters of genes involved in inflammatory cytokines. Iron is thought to play a pivotal role in neurodegeneration, and APO may be an ideal drug to investigate neuroprotection in Parkinson's disease where iron and oxidative stress have been implicated in the pathogenesis of nigrostriatal dopamine neuron degeneration.

INTRODUCTION

Abnormality of iron metabolism is associated with some of the most devastating diseases in man, including human immunodeficiency virus- tat, hepatic fibrosis, cirrhosis, hepatocellular cancer, cholestatic liver injury, cardiac diseases, diabetes, nephrotoxicity, edema and trauma, and rheumatoid arthritis (see Ref. 1). In these dis-

[c]Corresponding author: Prof. M.B.H. Youdim, B. Rappaport Family Medical Science Building, Efron Str., P.O.B. 9697, Haifa 31096, Israel. Tel, +972 4 8295271; fax, +972 4 8513145.

e-mail, youdim@tx.technion.ac.il

orders elevated cellular chelatable non-haem iron has been implicated as being directly involved in initiation of oxidative stress (OS). Until relatively recently very little attention was paid to brain iron metabolism and its role in brain function and dysfunction.[2–5] The first systematic studies to show whether brain iron could be modulated were those of Youdim *et al.*,[2–4] who showed that nutritional iron deficiency in rats can reduce brain iron in various regions, especially in the striatum and hippocampus. Dietary iron repletion restored brain iron in iron-deficient rats. However, brain iron could not be elevated beyond what normally is found in normal rat brain, suggesting a very tight regulation.[4] Earlier determination of iron in various regions of human brains from subjects with Parkinson's disease and Huntington's chorea had shown significant elevation. The suggestion was made that iron may participate in initiation of OS and neurodegeneration.[2,3,6] Since these original studies much attention has been paid to iron metabolism in neurodegenerative diseases, and consistently increases in iron have been reported in Parkinson's and Alzheimer's diseases, Haller Vorden Spatz disease, amyotrophic lateral sclerosis and other neurodegenerative disorders.

The etiology of Parkinson's disease (PD) is still elusive. A significant body of evidence from our laboratory, as supported by others, points to the presence of ongoing oxidative stress (OS) selectively in the substantia nigra pars compacta (SNPC) of Parkinsonian brains.[7–12] The evidence for OS includes proliferation of reactive microglia, activation of the redox-sensitive transcription factor, nuclear factor-κB (NF-κB) and highly significant increases in cytotoxic cytokines (tumor necrosis factor-α (TNF-α), and interleukin-1 (IL-1) and IL-6). Furthermore, not only is there significant elevation of iron in SNPC, membrane lipid peroxidation and other factors generating oxygen radical species (ORS), but radical scavenging mechanisms including depletion of reduced glutathione (GSH) are also compromized[7,10] (TABLE 1). The elevation of iron and depletion of GSH correlate with loss of SNPC dopamine (neurons) and stages of the disease.[7,8,12] Not only are iron and ferritin elevated in highly proliferated reactive microglia of SNPC,[13] but iron accumulation also occurs in the vulnerable melanin-containing dopamine neurons where iron is bound to neuromelanin.[14] Melanin has two binding sites for iron.[15,16] Whereas in the absence of iron,

TABLE 1. Mechanism of 6-hydroxydopamine-induced nigro-striatal dopaminergic neurodegeneration

1. Generation of oxygen radical species, reactive hydroxyl radical and superoxide and initiation of oxidative stress

2. Proliferation of reactive microglia

3. Inflammatory responses; activation of NF-κB, transcriptional gene expression of cytotoxic cytokines mRNA and elevation of TNF-α_1, IL-1, and IL-6

4. Increased iron and its release from ferritin

5. Depletion of reduced glutathione (GSH)

6. Inhibition of mitochondrial complex I and IV

7. Alteration of mitochondrial calcium homeostasis

8. Membrane lipid peroxidation

9. Apoptosis

TABLE 2. Neurotoxins that have been shown to release ferritin-bound iron, increase iron at the site of neurodegeneration and their neurotoxicity is prevented by iron chelators such as desferal and apomorphine

1. 6-Hydroxydopamine
2. MPTP (4-methyl-1-phenyl-1,2,3,6-tetrahydropyridine)
3. MPP$^+$ (4-methyl-1-phenyl-dihydropyridinum ion)
4. Kainate
5. Quinolate
6. TACLO (1-Trichloromethyl-1,2,3,4-tetrahydro-beta-carboline)

melanin is a cytoprotective agent with radical scavenging properties, iron-bound melanin is a highly potent radical promoter.[16,17] This feature led us to attribute the selective vulnerabilty of melanized dopamine neurons to neurodegeneration in PD, to the accumulation of iron within such neurons.

The evidence that OS may initiate the processes of dopamine neurodegeneration in PD has come from animal studies employing the neurotoxins 6-hydroxydopamine (6-OHDA) and *N*-methyl-4-phenyl-1,2,3,6-tetrahydropyridine (MPTP). Both neurotoxins induce degeneration of nigrostriatal dopamine neurons by a process involving OS.[18] The histopathological and biochemical features of OS induced by these neurotoxins in the striatum and substantia nigra of rats and mice mimics those reported for idiopathic PD, including proliferation of reactive microglia, increase of iron at the site of the lesion and depletion of GSH (TABLE 2). Indeed, a comparison of OS-initiated biochemical changes in PD and its animal models as reported shows that they are identical to what has been consistently reported for cytotoxic action of non-haem (chelatable, free) tissue iron in other diseases (e.g., cholestatic and alcohol liver injury). Free redox iron is known to directly participate in OS. Free iron and iron chelated with low molecular weight molecules, such as citrate, adenosine diphosphate (ADP), adenosine monophosphate (AMP) and histidine, can catalyze the formation of the cytotoxic hydroxyl radical through the Fenton reaction. Oxidant stress is known to release iron from ferritin, increase the size of the catalytic active pool of iron, and thereby exacerbate OS (TABLE 3). Both MPTP and 6-OHDA and other neurotoxins release iron from ferrtin *in vitro* and *in vivo*. The accumulation of iron as a consequence of 6-OHDA and MPTP-induced lesion in rodents and nonhuman primates occurs in SNPC (see Ref. 19 for review). In mice and rats radical scavengers such as vitamin E and *N*-acetylcysteine are neuroprotective against the neurotoxic action of these neurotoxins.[18–24]

The first studies to demonstrate the neuroprotective properties of iron chelators have come from Ben-Shachar *et al.*, who demonstrated that infusion of iron in rat substantia nigra induces a relatively selective lesion of dopamine neurons and that prototype iron chelator desferal (desferrioxamine) protected against iron and 6-OHDA neurotoxicity.[25,26] Confirmation has come from studies of others[72] and Chieuh *et al.*, which show that iron chelation prevents iron infusion and MPTP neurotoxicity, free radical formation and lipid peroxidation.[22,27–34] It is apparent that GSH depletion with the use of L-buthionine-(*S,R*)-sulphoximine alone in substantia nigra may enhance, but does not induce neurodegeneration.[34] The ability of iron to promote the generation of reactive hydroxyl radicals and deplete cellular GSH is in-

TABLE 3. Consequences of iron elevation in reactive microglia and dopamine neurons of substantia nigra

1. Promotion of Fenton reaction, generation of reactive hydroxyl radical (OH•) from hydrogen peroxide as a consequence of monoamine oxidase reaction, oxidative burst and dismutation of superoxide by superoxide dismutase and release of nitric oxide
2. Activation of microglia and inflammatory responses: including NF-κB activation, transcriptional gene expression of cytokines mRNA and elevation of cytotoxic cytokines, TNF-α_1, IL-1 and IL-6
3. Depletion of cellular reduced glutathione (GSH)
4. Alteration of calcium homeostasis
5. Induction of apoptosis, DNA impairment
6. Impairment of mitochondrial electron transport system
7. Release of neurotoxic agents, e.g., glutamate

dicative that it is the balance between the production and disposition of ORS that is crucial in oxidative stress and the degeneration of dopamine neurons.

Microglia in the brain are very sensitive to their microenviroment and have been assigned several properties including pathological processes such as multiple sclerosis, immunodeficiency syndrome, prion disease, Alzheimer's disease and Parkinson's disease. In addition to elaboration and secretion of cytotoxic cytokines, they have an important role in iron metabolism and the storage of iron and ferritin. With aging, they grow more numerous in numbers and richer in iron and ferritin. These features have consistently been seen in more elaborate forms in the neurodegenerative diseases of PD, Alzheimer's disease and immunodeficiency syndrome.[35] The increase of iron and OS in the reactive microglia SNPC of idiopathic PD[13] could explain the activation of the redox-sensitive transcriptional factor NF-κB, activation recently reported in SNPC of Parkinsonian brains[36] and elevation of cytokines (TNF-α, IL-1 and IL-6)[37–38] observed in the substantia nigra and striatum of Parkinsonian brains. Recent studies have shown that increased iron in macrophages and microglia, as seen in PD,[13] is linked to iron-dependent activation of NF-κB and gene regulation of IL-1, IL-6 and TNF-α.[39–44] Therefore, OS and cytokine-induced inflammatory response may act in concert to induce apoptosis-dependent progressive neurodegeneration in PD. It is worth noting that transgenic mice with overexpressed IL-6 in the brain have a constitutive blood brain barrier defect and abnormal brain iron deposition. They develop a progressive neurodegeneration,[45] and IL-6 levels in cerebrospinal fluid inversely correlate to the severity of Parkinson's disease.[46]

In line with this concept there has been a concerted attempt to look for and develop potential neuroprotective drugs with antioxidant and iron chelator activity. However, some drugs either do not cross the blood brain barrier or are ineffective and/or toxic.[47]

APOMORPHINE: AN ANTI-PARKINSON DRUG WITH POTENT IRON CHELATING, RADICAL SCAVENGING AND NEUROPROTECTIVE ACTIVITIES

(*R*)-Apomorphine (APO), the dopamine D_1-D_2 receptor agonist, is one of the most potent anti-Parkinson drugs available and is an effective replacement for L-dopa (3,4-dihydroxyphenylacetic acid) in the therapy of late stage PD. However, its rapid metabolism and pharmacokinetics have a limiting factor in therapy. This disadvantage has been overcome by the use of a continuous self-injector system.[48,49] Indications are that long-term treatment with APO can result in weaning the patient from L-dopa.[50,51] These results have been interpreted as indicating the necessity for continuous D_1-D_2 dopamine receptor stimulation and possible neuroprotection, in order to achieve a better therapeutic response.[52,53] Compounds with a catechol structure have metal chelating properties and can act as reducing agents and radical scavengers.[54] Therefore, being a catechol, with structural resemblance to dopamine, APO was considered as an inhibitor of metal-catalyzed free radical processes and as acting as a radical scavenger.[55] As a reducing agent, APO can also contribute to the generation of highly toxic OH· by maintaining iron in the ferrous state. The overall manner by which antioxidant drugs affect the level of OS depends on the balance between radical scavenging and radical activating properties.

Our previous studies showed that APO is a highly potent radical scavenger and iron chelator,[53,55] displaying IC_{50} values of 0.3–0.6 µM, making it even more potent than desferrioxamine. Similar results were also obtained with dopamine, although at higher concentrations (>50–100 µM) they acted as prooxidants. These properties are directly linked to the ability of APO to inhibit brain mitochondrial lipid peroxidation and protein oxidation (40%).[55] Cytoprotective action of APO was investigated against the actions of iron, hydrogen peroxide (H_2O_2) and 6-OHDA and compared to other dopamine receptor agonists, desferrioxamine and dopamine in PC12 cells in culture.[53]

The aim of our study was to investigate whether APO will be neuroprotective in animal models of PD with MPTP and 6-OHDA. This was considered logical, since these neurotoxins are thought to produce their dopaminergic neurotoxicity via generation of oxygen radical species,[21] liberation of ferritin iron in the substantia nigra pars compacta,[56,57] depletion of reduced glutathione (GSH)[58] and inhibition of mitochondrial complex I.[28,29,59] Furthermore, iron chelators and radical scavengers are able to protect not only against MPTP-induced neurotoxicity[22,31] but also against that induced by 6-OHDA and hydrogen peroxide by preventing inhibition of mitochondrial complex I.[20,23,25,26,30,53]

Free Radical Scavenging Property of Apomorphine

The ability of APO to inhibit lipid peroxidation and protein carbonyl formation after ascorbate/iron-induced free radical formation was examined in rat brain mitochondrial fractions. Addition of a submolecular concentration of APO to the ascorbate/iron-induced lipid peroxidation in rat brain mitochondrial fraction, induced a marked reduction in the formation of thiobarbituric acid reactive substances (TBARS) as compared with samples containing only ascorbate and iron. The effectiveness of APO inhibition was dependent on the iron concentration; the IC_{50} varied in the range between 0.1 and 1 µM. This influence could be indirect, as the overall intensity of free radical formation is also subject to changes in iron concentration. The IC_{50} values were 0.3 µM for 2.5 µM and 0.6 µM for 5 µM iron (TABLE 4). The sigmoid character of the concentration-response curve for the inhibition was stronger at the higher iron concentration, and the apparent Hill coefficient rose from 1.7

TABLE 4. Inhibition of ascorbate/iron induced lipid peroxidation by apomorphine, dopamine, and desferrioxamine

	Apomorphine		Dopamine	Desferrioxamine
FeSO$_4$ (μM)[a]	2.5	5.0	2.5	2.5
IC$_{50}$ [μM][b]	0.28 ± 0.02	0.61 ± 0.02	6.59 ± 0.2	0.78 ± 0.04
Max. inhib.[c] [%]	92 ± 1	93 ± 2	93 ± 1	75 ± 1
Hill coefficient[d]	1.7 ± 0.1	4 ± 0.3	1.0 ± 0.1	0.9 ± 0.15

[a] Concentration of ascorbate was 50 μM in all cases.
[b] Obtained from regression data (mean $\pm$ SE, $n = 6$).
[c] Maximum inhibition as determined from a triplicate experiment (mean $\pm$ SEM).
[d] Apparent values (mean $\pm$ SE, $n = 5$), as obtained from the slope of the cooperativity plot (Hill plot), log [apomorphine] vs. log (I/(I$_{max}$ − I)).

(2.5 μM FeSO$_4$) to 4.2 (5 μM FeSO$_4$) (TABLE 4). This is consistent with a multistep oxidation of APO to a melanin-like polymer as an end product.

To examine the radical scavenging action of APO, a time course of APO oxidation was monitored. During oxidation an intensive green chromophore ($\lambda_{max} = 619$ nm) is formed, which has been used to monitor the reaction, as there was little interference with other components in the assay. The color formation reflected a complicated multistep process with autoxidation of APO itself being only the initial step. The reaction is considerably slowed down by 50 μM ascorbate, but addition of 5 μM iron gave no significant change. In a system containing brain mitochondria, APO is oxidized even in the presence of ascorbate/iron. This reaction reflects the free radical scavenging effect of APO, which leads to a decrease in the formation of TBARS.

APO was compared with dopamine and desferrioxamine, a potent iron chelator that is able to inhibit iron-catalyzed lipid peroxidation. Dopamine inhibited the formation of TBARS in a similar manner as APO, while the effective concentration was twenty times higher (TABLE 4). Desferrioxamine, at the concentration used, was unable to block lipid peroxidation. At maximum inhibition, 16% of the activity remained (TABLE 4). On the basis of this data, iron chelation by APO and dopamine may be a major contribution to the observed inhibition of TBARS formation. Apomorphine also protects against oxidation of brain proteins. Measuring protein carbonyl formation is a more specific but less sensitive method to assay free radical damage in a biological system. Under conditions of OS, proline, arginine, lysine and threonine residues are converted into aldehydes and ketones, which can be labeled with specific reagents, like 1,4-dinitrophenylhydrazine. Addition of 10 μM APO, in protein oxidation assay with 250 μM ferrous iron and 15 mM ascorbic acid, gave a significant decrease of protein oxidation (40%).

Protection from Oxidative Stress in PC12 Cells by Apomorphine

The relationship between the antioxidant and prooxidant activities of APO was examined in PC12 cell culture, a well established system to study apoptotic and necrotic cell death. OS can be induced by various agents like H$_2$O$_2$, organic hydroperoxides, or 6-OHDA. We treated PC12 cells with iron citrate (data not shown) H$_2$O$_2$ and 6-OHDA and observed cell death in a concentration-dependent manner within

24 hr. There was no significant difference of the sensitivity between cells that were grown in medium containing 15% serum (1/3 fetal calf serum, 2/3 horse serum) and those that had been differentiated for six days with an additional 100 µg/ml 7S-nerve growth factor (NGF), if all the NGF had been washed out prior to the experiment. Although it takes 24 hr to observe the maximum cell death, only two hours' exposure to the toxic agent is sufficient to induce the full damage. The viability of the cells was tested by measuring the conversion of 3-(4,5-dimethylthiozol-2-yl)-2,5-diphenyltetrazolium bromide (MTT) into a colored formazane derivative and lactate dehydrogenase (LDH) leakage. EC_{50} values of 400 µM for H_2O_2 and 150 µM for 6-OHDA were necessary to kill 50% of the cultured cells. In this system, APO was tested for its ability to protect PC12 cells from the oxidative insults. At the same time, the toxicity can be monitored to obtain information about the therapeutic window of the agent. We found that APO is far more efficient as an antioxidant: only 5 µM improve the rate of survival from 50% to 85% in the presence of 400 µM H_2O_2 (FIG. 1A). The (*S*)-enantiomer of APO, which is not a dopamine agonist, showed nearly identical protective properties against H_2O_2 and 6-OHDA cell toxicity. Any protection against H_2O_2 by APO depended on the presence of the drug during the insult. Preincubation with APO and washout prior to H_2O_2 addition or addition of H_2O_2 one hour after the toxin did not improve the cell survival as compared with controls treated with the oxidant (FIG. 1A). With APO concentrations exceeding 10 µM, toxicity became increasingly dominant. APO alone induced death of PC12 cells with $EC_{50} = 100$ µM.

APO was able to provide protection against 6-OHDA cytotoxicity. The survival rate after 150 µM 6-OHDA (EC_{50}) was improved to 70% with only 1 µM apomorphine (FIG. 2A). This is the first example of a catecholamine attenuating the toxicity of 6-OHDA in cell culture (*in vivo* studies are in progress). The protective effect of APO could also be demonstrated by measuring the LDH leakage induced by H_2O_2 (0.6 mM) and 6-OHDA (150 µM). In the presence of APO (1–10 µM), the effects of both toxins were markedly attenuated. Apart from slight variations, the LDH data correlated with the findings in the MTT assay (FIGS. 1B and 2B).

THE PREVENTION OF IRON- AND 6-OHDA-INDUCED NF-κB ACTIVATION BY APOMORPHINE AND DESFERAL

In these studies the roles of iron and 6-OHDA in NF-κB and cytokine gene expression by rat brain microglia in culture and rat striatum were examined. In microglia cell cultures, iron citrate (100 µM) and bacterial lipopolysaccharide (LPS) stimulated NF-κB activation and TNF-α, IL-1 and IL-6 gene expression at the mRNA level. These were blocked by APO (10 µM) and desferal (100 µM) to the level normally seen in untreated cells. Striatum of rats injected with intraventricular (i.c.v.) 6-OHDA also showed induction of NF-κB and mRNA for TNF-α, IL-1 and IL-6, which were also blocked by pretreatment with intraperitoneal (i.p.) APO (10 mg/kg) or with desferal (15 µg/10 µl, i.c.v.) (Youdim, 1998, submitted for publication).

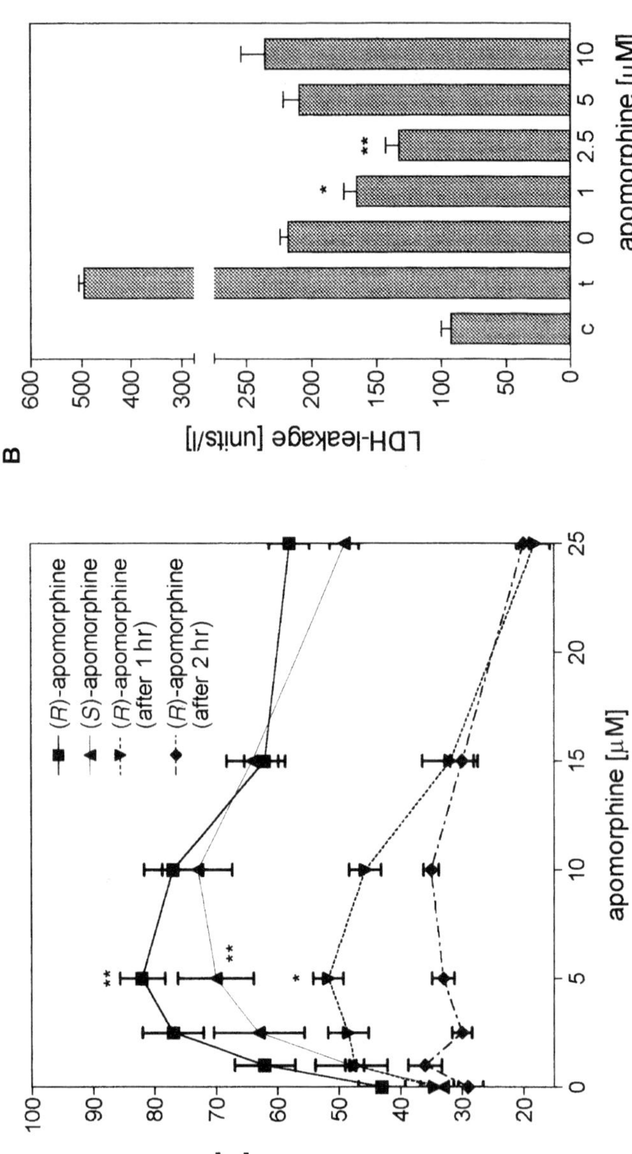

FIGURE 1. H_2O_2 toxicity in PC12 cell culture and protection by apomorphine. (**A**) Cells were treated with 0.6 µM H_2O_2 and apomorphine. Cell viability was assayed with MTT 24 hr later and expressed as percent of controls (data ± SEM, $n = 8$). The difference between (R)- and (S)-apomorphine is not significant (two-way analysis of variance (ANOVA): $p = 0.08$). (**B**) LDH leakage as determined 24 hr after treatment with H_2O_2 (0.6 mM) and apomorphine (c, controls; t, total activity after lysis of the cells, data ± SEM, $n = 5$). Peak data points were compared with controls by Mann-Whitney U-test (*, $p < 0.05$; **, $p < 0.01$).

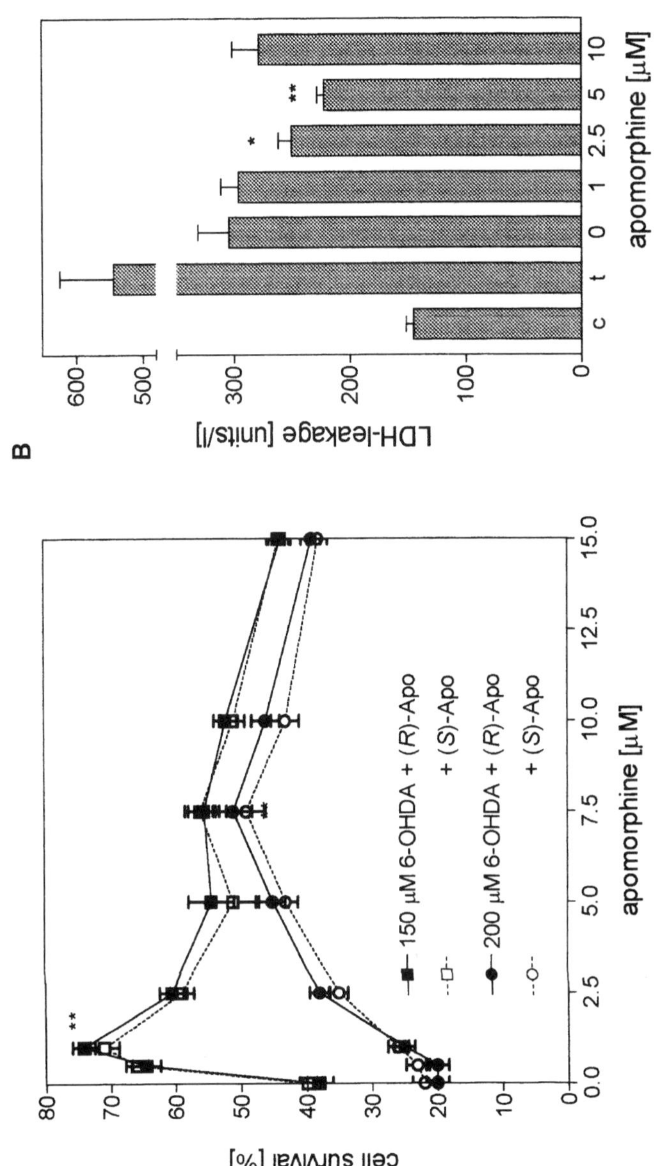

FIGURE 2. 6-Hydroxydopamine toxicity in PC12 cell culture and protection by apomorphine. (**A**) Cells were treated with 6-hydroxydopamine and apomorphine. Cell viability was assayed with MTT 24 hr later and expressed as percent of controls (data ± SEM, $n = 8$). (**B**) LDH leakage as determined 24 hr after treatment with 6-hydroxydopamine (150 μM) and apomorphine (data ± SEM, $n = 5$). Peak data points were compared with controls by Mann-Whitney U-test (*, $p < 0.05$; **, $p < 0.01$).

TABLE 5. Striatal DA and metabolites content in C57BL mice treated with APO and MPTP

Treatment	DA [pmol/ mg tissue]	DOPAC [pmol/ mg tissue]	HVA [pmol/ mg tissue]	$\dfrac{DOPAC+HVA}{DA}$	$\dfrac{HVA}{DA}$
Control	47.2 ± 3.7	2.28 ± 0.19	21.6 ± 2.1	0.50 ± 0.03	0.48 ± 0.05
APO (10 mg/kg/d)	45.6 ± 5.9	2.58 ± 0.20	14.3 ± 2.1	0.40 ± 0.04	0.31 ± 0.04
MPTP (24 mg/kg/d)	11.1 ± 1.2***[a]	0.85 ± 0.11***[a]	22.4 ± 0.7	1.73 ± 0.16	1.78 ± 0.17**[a]
APO+MPTP	34.0 ± 5.2**[b]	2.05 ± 0.14***[b]	14.9 ± 4.4	0.29 ± 0.02*[a]	0.24 ± 0.02*[a] **[b]

Mice (8–10 per treatment group) were injected once daily with APO (10 mg/kg) followed immediately by a dose of MPTP (24 mg/kg), for 5 days and sacrificed 2 days later. Controls received saline only. DA and metabolites were analyzed by HPLC.
$* p < 0.01; ** p < 0.005; ***p < 0.001$.
[a]vs. control. [b] vs. MPTP.

Neuroprotective Activity of Apomorphine in MPTP-Treated Mice

The neuroprotective effect of APO was examined *in vivo* by analyzing the striatal content of DA and its metabolites (3,4-dihydroxyphenylacetic acid (DOPAC), homovanillic acid (HVA)) by high-performance liquid chromatography (HPLC) in MPTP-treated C57 black mice. Pretreatment of mice with APO followed by MPTP resulted in partial protection of neurodegeneration as indicated by DA and DOPAC levels. With 5 mg/kg/day/5 days APO, a significant elevation to the control levels (DA to 50% and DOPAC to 60% of control) and 10 mg/kg/day/5 days APO almost completely restored the levels of DA and DOPAC to control values (82% and 90% of control, respectively) (FIGS. 3A and 3B). The ratio of (DOPAC+HVA)/DA and HVA/DA were significantly increased in MPTP-treated mice (350% and 370%, respectively), while the combination of APO (10 mg/kg) followed by MPTP resulted in reduced ratios (40% and 50%, respectively). Treatment of APO alone had no significant effect on striatal DA, DOPAC or HVA (TABLE 5).

The inhibitory effect of APO on mice striatal MAO-A and MAO-B activities were examined *in vitro* using rat brain mitochondrial preparations with serotonin and phenylethylamine. APO caused a dose-dependent inhibition of monoamine oxidase-A (MAO-A) and MAO-B activities with IC_{50} values of 93 µM and 241 µM, respectively.

In Western blot analysis for striatal tyrosine hydroxylase (TH) content, MPTP treatment markedly decreased TH levels 30% of control, while pretreatment with APO (10 mg/kg) significantly prevented loss of TH (70% of control) induced by MPTP. No significant effect on TH was observed with APO treatment alone. In addition TH activity decreased significantly in MPTP-treated mice (60%), while in APO (10 mg/kg/day/5 days)-pretreated mice only a 12% loss in TH activity was noted (FIG. 4).

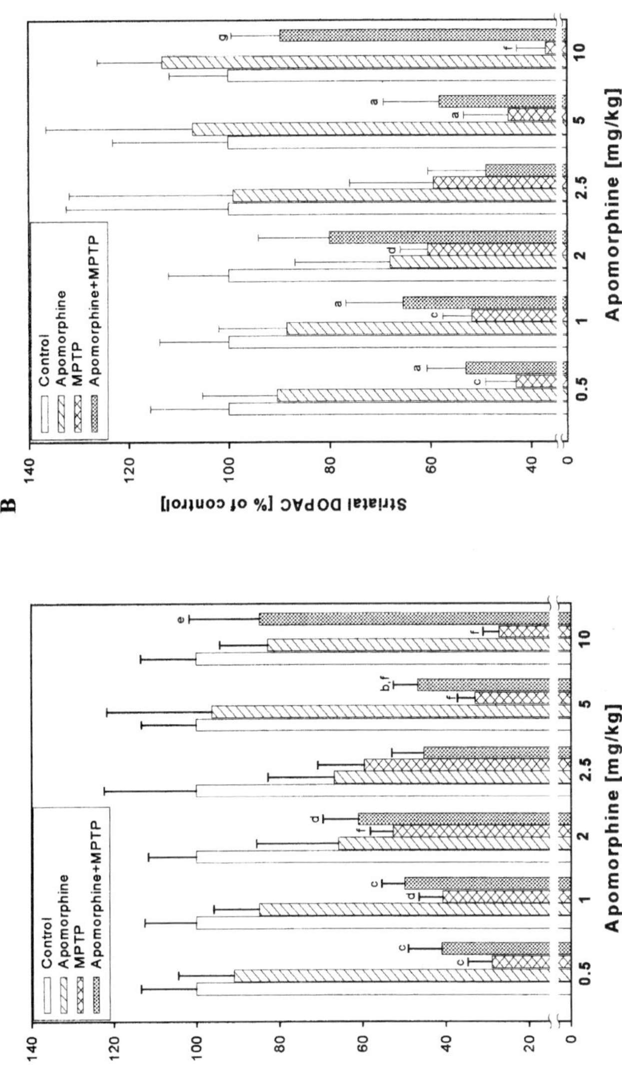

FIGURE 3. Effect of apomorphine on striatal DA (**A**) and DOPAC (**B**) content. C57-BL mice were injected with apomorphine (0.5–10 mg/kg/day/5 days) followed by a dose of MPTP (24 mg/kg/day/5 days). Controls received saline or apomorphine only. Striatal DA and DOPAC were measured by high-performance liquid chromatography (HPLC). The results represent the mean $\pm$ SEM (each group 8–10 mice). [a,b] $p < 0.05$ (vs. control/MPTP, respectively); [c] $p < 0.01$ (vs. control); [d,e] $p < 0.005$ (vs. control/MPTP, respectively); [f,g] $p < 0.001$ (vs. control/MPTP, respectively).

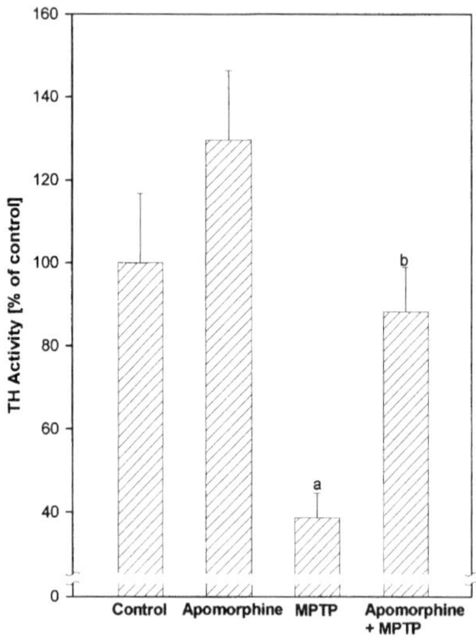

FIGURE 4. TH activity in apomorphine (10 mg/kg/day/5 days)-treated C57-BL mice. Mice were treated similarly to those in FIGURE 3 and striata were dissected. The TH activity was measured accordingly. The results represent the mean ± SEM (each group 8–10 mice). [a], $p < 0.05$ (vs. control); [b], $p < 0.005$ (vs. MPTP).

IRON, NF-κB ACTIVATION, NEURODEGENERATION: PROSPECTS FOR NEUROPROTECTION WITH IRON CHELATORS

The approaches to neuroprotection in Parkinson's disease reflect the current concepts of the etiology of the disease. Antioxidant strategies, aiming at scavenging free radicals or inhibiting their formation, have been the focus of attention. Inhibitors of MAO (e.g., L-deprenyl, L-selegiline)[60] interrupt the metabolic formation of H_2O_2, while iron chelators, such as desferrioxamine, block the formation of OH· radicals via the Fenton reaction. The protective effect of lazaroids and 21-aminosteroids had originally been attributed to radical scavenging and prevention of membrane lipid peroxidation.[61,62] Classical free radical scavengers (e.g., ascorbate, α-tocopherol) react easily with reactive oxygen species and, thus, protect biological structures from oxidation. However, promising neuroprotection obtained with L-selegiline and vitamin E in MPTP and 6-OHDA[18,20,22,58] could not be reproduced clinically to slow down the progression of Parkinson's disease.[63]

The present study has shown that APO, a dopamine D_1-D_2 receptor agonist, is a highly potent iron chelator and radical scavenger against MPTP and 6-OHDA neurotoxicity *in vitro* and *in vivo*. This protection is expressed by preventing the MPTP-induced depletion of striatal DA and TH content. Almost complete neuroprotection by apomorphine was observed at a dose as low as 5 mg/kg. This relates to the catechol-containing structure of APO, which undergoes rapid metabolism and autoxidation, since catecholamines can act both as antioxidants and prooxidants, depending on their concentration. Gassen *et al.*[53,55] demonstrated that it is the oxidized and not the reduced form of APO that initiates neuroprotection in cultured cells against iron, H_2O_2 and 6-OHDA toxicity, while the oxidation of APO itself proceeded at a much accelerated rate leading to the formation of a melanin-like polymer in a complex multistep reaction. It is well known that melanin formed from DA chelates iron and inhibits radical formation[15,16] and is accumulated within DA neurons of SNPC.[14] Furthermore, it was established that the neuroprotective actions of APO *in vitro, in vivo* and in PC12 cell culture are not related to its dopamine agonistic activity. Its optical isomer (*S*)-APO, which is inactive as a dopamine receptor agonist, is as potent as the (*R*)-enantiomer.[53,55,64,65] Other anti-Parkinson drugs or dopamine receptor agonists (lisuride, bromocriptine, pergolide or pramipexole) clinically employed do not possess the antioxidant potency of APO, nor can they exert the same neuroprotective action against iron, H_2O_2, 6-OHDA and MPTP, either in cell culture or *in vitro* or *in vivo*.

The relatively high doses of APO used to achieve neuroprotection relate to the pharmacokinetically unstable and readily oxidizable nature of APO.[49,65] The neuroprotective effect achieved by 5 and 10 mg/kg APO against the loss of neuronal TH is reflected by the increased levels of DA. This increase may result either from an increase in DA synthesis, caused by an elevation in the activity of TH, or from a decrease in the turnover of DA. We observed that APO caused an 88% elevation in TH activity in MPTP-treated mice as a result of restored TH mRNA levels by APO.[24] APO+MPTP-treated striatal DA levels were similar to those of the saline-treated group of mice, in spite of partial restoration of TH levels by APO treatment. The explanation for it can be found in the compensating mechanism proposed by Zigmond,[66] who demonstrated that DA levels are normal, so long as at least 30% of the nigrostriatal dopamine neurons remain functional. Furthermore, part of the compensating mechanism may involve the ability of APO to inhibit MAO-A and B, as observed in the *in vitro* determinations, since DA is equally metabolized by both enzymes.[67]

The neuroprotective action of APO is best explained by its iron chelating and radical scavenging properties, since both enantiomers share the same properties. 6-OHDA- and MPTP-induced neurotoxicity *in vivo* results in highly elevated contents of iron in the substantia nigra pars compacta at the site of neurodegneration.[68–71] This feature is very similar to what is observed in PD. Pretreatment with the iron chelator desferrioxamine protects rats and mice from the neurotoxicity of 6-OHDA and MPTP. The mechanism of neurotoxicity of these neurotoxins is thought to be related to their ability to release ferritin iron,[72,73] which then can participate in the Fenton chemistry-dependent generation of the highly reactive OH· radical.

The marked recruitment of reactive microglia in Parkinsonian SNPC surrounding iron melanin-containing and dying dopamine neurons can be explained by the inflammatory responses reported,[36–38] which have also been observed in MPTP- and 6-OHDA-treated animals. However, no adequate explanation has been put forward why in PD the SNPC microglia are endowed with high deposits of free chelatable iron.[13] As one possibility, altered blood brain barrier has been suggested. Whatever the cause of PD, some initial event must be responsible for the accumulation of iron. Free iron and iron chelated with low-molecular weight molecules, such as citrate, ADP and AMP, can catalyze the formation of the hydroxyl radical. It is considered that this radical propagates the process of membrane lipid peroxidation that leads to depletion of striatal GSH, which in turn results in OS-initiated reductive release of iron from ferritin, increasing the size of the catalytically active pool of iron and thereby exacerbating OS with ensuing neurodegeneration.

Increasing bodies of experimental and disease pathological evidence have indicated a direct role of OS in NF-κB activation[75] and its suppression by antioxidants[76,77] and iron chelators.[41–44,78] The neurodegeneration process is now considered to be associated with OS-dependent activation of NF-κB,[79] which has been reported to be highly activated in melanized dopamine neurons of Parkinson brains substantia nigra,[36] in the striatum of 6-OHDA-treated rats (Youdim, 1998, submitted for publication) and in mouse striatum by LPS-induced nigrostriatal dopamine neurondegeneration.[80] NF-κB, a redox-sensitive transcription factor, transactivates the promoters of numerous genes involved in inflammatory responses such as cytotoxic cytokines (TNF-α, IL-1 and IL-6)[81] resulting in their tissue elevation[37,38] and exerting direct injurious effects on the cells. Overexpression of IL-6 in mice is associated with accumulation of iron in the brain and neurodegeneration.[45] Until recently the role of iron in this process was unclear. However, the studies of Lin *et al.*[41] using liver macrophages and our own studies with rat brain microglia in cell culture and striatum from 6-OHDA-treated rats have provided evidence for direct participation of chelatable iron in NF-κB activation and its prevention with iron chelators L-1, desferal and APO. Indeed, LPS-induced nigrostriatal dopamine degeneration and NF-κB activation in mice[80] can be attributed to iron accumulation in the brain, since LPS causes the accumulation of iron in macrophages and micoglia, which can be blocked by iron chelators L-1, desferal and APO.[41] This result raises the possibility of new therapeutic approaches, which we have suggested several times before, namely, the clinical use of chelation of iron and antiinflammatory drugs (e.g., COX2 inhibitors) as neuroprotective agents in PD and other neurodegenerative diseases where iron and NF-κB are increased. This may represent a unique and effective method to suppress iron-induced oxidative stress and expression of NF-κB-responsive cytokines and consequent neurodegeneration. One study so far where desferrioxamine was used in the treatment of aceruloplasminemia, a disorder associated with progressive extrapyramidal symptoms, neurodegeneration of retina and basal ganglia, desferrioxamine was able to decrease brain iron, prevent progression of the neurological symptoms and reduce plasma lipid peroxidation.[82] These studies together with those reported for cholestatic liver injury where iron accumulates in the macrophages suggest the pivotal role of iron in NF-κB activation and subsequent pathogenetic processess, which can be alleviated with iron chelators.

APO is a unique anti-Parkinsonian drug, with a number of pharmacological features that make it superior to other so-called neuroprotective drugs, such as MAO-B inhibitors, vitamin E, iron chelators and nitric oxide synthase inhibitors. The latter drugs do not have cross-neuroprotective activity with the neurotoxins. In contrast APO has the ability to protect against the neurotoxicity of MPTP, 6-OHDA, hydrogen peroxide and iron.[24,53,55]

It is most likely that drugs with a single action will not be neuroprotective in neurodegenerative diseases where OS has been implicated. We have suggested that a cocktail of drugs may need to be employed in the therapeutic setting for PD.[32] Nevertheless, the superiority of APO pharmacological actions a) based on its radical scavenging and iron chelating properties, b) to protect against hydrogen peroxide, 6-OHDA and iron-induced neurotoxicity in PC12 cell culture, c) to prevent MPTP-induced neurotoxicity *in vivo*, d) in its ability to inhibit mitochondrial iron-induced lipid peroxidation and protein oxidation, e) its ability to prevent 6-OHDA-induced inhibition of mitochondrial complex I activity and f) its ability to inhibit MAO-A and B, makes APO an ideal drug for neuroprotective strategy in PD.

ACKNOWLEDGMENTS

The support of the National Parkinson Foundation (USA), the Golding Parkinson Research Fund (Technion, Haifa, Israel), and the Israel Ministry of Arts and Science are gratefully acknowledged. This paper was written while Moussa B.H. Youdim was a Scholar-in-Residence at the Fogarty International Center for Advanced Study in Health Sciences, National Institutes of Health, Bethesda, MD, USA.

REFERENCES

1. LAUFFER, A., Ed. 1992. Iron and Human Diseases.: 1–374. CRC Press. New York.
2. YOUDIM, M.B.H. & A.R. GREEN. 1977. Bigenic monoamine metabolism and functional activity in iron-deficient rats: behavioural correlates. Ciba Found. Symp. **51:** 201–223.
3. YOUDIM, M.B.H., D. BEN-SHACHAR & S. YEHUDA. 1989. Putative biological mechanisms of the effect of iron deficiency on brain biochemistry and behavior. Am. J. Clin. Nutr. **50:** 607–617.
4. YOUDIM, M.B.H. 1985. Brain iron metabolism: biochemical and behavioural aspects in relationship to dopaminergic neurotransmission. *In* Handbook of Neurochemistry. Vol. 10. A. Lajtha, Ed.: 731–756. Plenum Press. New York.
5. YOUDIM, M.B.H. & S. YEHUDA. 1986. Brain iron and dopamine circadian cycle. Clin. Neuropharmacol. **9:** 87–94.
6. RIEDERER, P., E. SOFIC, W.-D. RAUSCH, K. JELLINGER & M.B.H. YOUDIM. 1989. Transition metals, ferritin, glutathione and ascorbic acid in Parkinsonian brains. J. Neurochem. **52:** 515–521.
7. YOUDIM, M.B.H., D. BEN-SHACHAR & P. RIEDERER. 1993. The possible role of iron in the etiopathology of Parkinson's disease. Mov. Disord. **8:** 1–12.
8. GERLACH, M., D. BEN-SHACHAR, P. RIEDERER & M.B.H. YOUDIM. 1994. Altered brain metabolism of iron as a cause of neurodegenerative diseases? J. Neurochem. **63:** 793–806.
9. JENNER, P. & C.W. OLANOW. 1996. Pathological evidence for oxidative stress in Parkinson's disease and related degenerative disorders. *In* Neurodegeneration and Neuroprotection in Parkinson's Disease. C.W. Olanow, P. Jenner & M.B.H. Youdim, Eds.: 24–45. Academic Press. London.
10. OLANOW, C.W. & M.B.H. YOUDIM. 1996. Iron and neurodegeneration: prospects for neuroprotection. *In* Neurodegeneration and Neuroprotection in Parkinson's Disease. C.W. Olanow, P. Jenner & M.B.H. Youdim, Eds.: 50–67. Academic Press. London.
11. OLANOW, C.W. 1993. A scientific rationale for protective therapy in Parkinson's disease. J. Neural Transm. Gen. Sect. **91:** 161–180.
12. HIRSCH, E.C. & B.A. FAUCHEUX. 1998. Iron metabolism and Parkinson's disease. Mov. Disord. **13:** 39–45.
13. JELLINGER, K., W. PAULUS, I. GRUNDKE-IQBAL, P. RIEDERER & M.B.H. YOUDIM. 1990. Brain iron and ferritin in Parkinson's and Alzheimer's diseases. J. Neural Transm. Parkinson's Dis. Dementia Sect. **2:** 327–340.
14. JELLINGER, K., E. KEIZL, G. RUMPELMAIR, P. RIEDERER & M.B.H. YOUDIM. 1992. Iron melanin complex in substantia nigra of Parkinsonian brains: an X-ray microanalysis. J. Neurochem. **59:** 1168–1171.
15. BEN-SHACHAR, D., P. RIEDERER & M.B.H. YOUDIM. 1991. Iron melanin interaction: implications for Parkinson's disease. J. Neurochem. **57:** 1609–1614.
16. YOUDIM, M.B.H. 1994. The enigma of neuromelanin in Parkinsonian substantia nigra. J. Neural Transm. Suppl. **43:** 113–122.

17. YOUDIM, M.B.H., D. BEN-SHACHAR & P. RIEDERER. 1990. The role of monoamine oxidase, iron-melanin interaction, and intracellular calcium in Parkinson's disease. J. Neural Transm. Suppl. **32:** 239–248.

18. COHEN, G. & P. WERNER. 1994. Free radicals oxidative stress and neurodegeneration. *In* Neurodegenerative Disorders. D.B. Calne, Ed.: 139–162. Saunders. Philadelphia.

19. JELLINGER, K.A. 1998. The role of iron in neurodegeneration: prospects for pharmacology of Parkinson's disease. Drugs & Aging. In press.

20. CADET, J.L., M. KATZ, V. JACKSON-LEWIS & S. FAHN. 1989. Vitamin E attenuates the toxic effects of intrastriatal injection of 6-hydroxydopamine (6-OHDA) in rats: behavioral and biochemical evidence. Brain Res. **476:** 5–10.

21. EBADI, M., S.K. SRINIVASAN & M.D. BAXI. 1996. Oxidative stress and antioxidant therapy in Parkinson's disease. Prog. Neurobiol. **48:** 1–19.

22. LAN, J. & D.H. JIANG. 1997. Desferrioxamine and vitamin E protect against iron and MPTP-induced neurodegeneration in mice. J. Neural Transm. **104:** 469–481.

23. PERUMAL, A.S., V.B. GOPAL, W.K. TORDZRO, T.B. COOPER & J.L. CADET. 1992. Vitamin E attenuates the toxic effects of 6-hydroxydopamine on free radical scavenging systems in rat brain. Brain Res. Bull. **29:** 699–701.

24. GRUNBLATT, E., S. MANDEL, T. BERSUZKI & M.B.H. YOUDIM. 1998. Neuroprotective properties of apomorphine in MPTP treated mice. Mov. Disord. In press.

25. BEN-SHACHAR, D., G. ESHEL, J.P.M. FINBERG & M.B.H. YOUDIM. 1991. The iron chelator desferrioxamine (desferal) retards 6-hydroxydopamine-induced degeneration of nigrostriatal neurons. J. Neurochem. **56:** 1441–1444.

26. BEN-SHACHAR, D. & M.B.H. YOUDIM. 1991. Intranigral iron injection induces behavioral and biochemical "Parkinsonism" in rats. J. Neurochem. **57:** 2133–2138.

27. MOHANAKUMAR, K.P., A. DE BARTOLOMEIS, R.M. WU, K.J. YEH, L. STERNBERGER, S.Y. PENG, D.L. MURPHY & C.C. CHIUEH. 1999. Ferrous-citrate complex and nigral degeneration: evidence for free radical formation and lipd peroxidation. Neurobiology. In press.

28. GLINKA, Y. & M.B.H. YOUDIM. 1995. Inhibition of mitochondrial complex I and IV by 6-hydroxydopamine. Eur. J. Pharmacol. **292:** 329–332.

29. GLINKA, Y., K.F. TIPTON & M.B.H. YOUDIM. 1996. Nature of inhibition of mitochondrial respiratory complex I by 6-hydroxydopamine. J. Neurochem. **66:** 2004–2010.

30. GLINKA, Y., M. GASSEN & M.B.H. YOUDIM. 1997. Mechanism of 6-hydroxydopamine neurotoxicity. J. Neural Transm. Suppl. **50:** 55–66.

31. SANTIAGO, M., E.R. MATARREDONA, L. GRANERO, J. CANO & A. MACHADO. 1997. Neuroprotective effect of the iron chelator desferrioxamine against MPP$^+$ toxicity on striatal dopaminergic terminals. J. Neurochem. **68:** 732–738.

32. SZIRRAKI, I., K.P. MOHANAKUMAR, P. RAUHALA, H.G. KIM, J.J. YEH & C.C. CHIUEH. 1998. Manganese: a transition metal protects nigrostriatal neurons from oxidative stress in the iron-induced animal model of Parkinsonism. Neuroscience **85:** 1001–1011.

33. YOUDIM, M.B.H., G. KRISHNA & C.C. CHIUEH. 1999. Neuroprotective strategies in Parkinson's disease and Huntington chorea: MPT and #-NP induced neurodegeneration as models. *In* Mitochondrial Inhibitors and Neurodegenerative Disorders. R.R. Sandberg, H. Nishhino & C.V. Borlogan, Eds. Humana Press. New York. In press.

34. TOFFA, S., G.M. KUNIKOWSKA, B.Y. ZENG, P. JENNER & C.D. MARSDEN. 1997. Glutathione depletion in rat brain does not cause nigrostriatal pathway degeneration. J. Neural Transm. **104:** 67–75.

35. BARRON, K.D. 1995. The microglia cell. A historical review. J. Neurol. Sci. **134**(Suppl.)**:** 57–68.

36. HUNOT, S., B. BRUGG, D. RICARD, P.P. MICHEL, M.P. MURIEL, M. RUBERG, B.A. FAUCHEUX, Y. AGID & E.C. HIRSCH. 1997. Nuclear translocation of NF-κB is increased in dopaminergic neurons of patients with Parkinson's disease. Proc. Natl. Acad. Sci. USA **94:** 7531–7536.

37. MOGI, M., H. MINORU, P. RIEDERER, H. NARABAYASHI, K. FUJITA & Y. NAGATSU. 1994. Tumor necrosis factor (TNF-alpha) increases both in the brain and in the cerebrospinal fluid from Parkinsonian patients. Neurosci. Lett. **165:** 208–210.

38. MOGI, M., M. HARADA, T. KONDO, P. RIEDERER, H. INAGAKI, M. MINAMI & T. NAGATSU. 1994. Interleukin-1-beta, interleukin-6, epidermal growth factor and transforming growth factor-alpha are elevated in the brain from Parkinsonian patients. Neurosci. Lett. **180:** 147–150.

39. ROGERS, J.T., K.R. BRIDGES, G.P. DURMOWICZ, J. GLASS, P.E. AURON & H.N. MUNRO. 1990. Translational control during the acute phase response. Ferritin synthesis in response to interleukin-1. J. Biol. Chem. **265:** 14572–14578.

40. SEISER, C., S. TEIXEIRA & L.C. KUHN. 1993. Interleukin-2 dependent transcriptional and post-transcriptional regulation of transferrin receptor mRNA. J. Biol. Chem. **268:** 13074–13080.

41. SIMEONOVA, P.P. & M.I. LUSTER. 1995. Iron and reactive oxygen species in the asbestos-induced tumor necrosis factor-alpha response from alveolar macrophages. Am. J. Respir. Cell Mol. Biol. **12:** 676–683.

42. SAPPEY, C., J.R. BOELAERT, S. LEGRAND-POELS, C. FORCEILLE, A. FAVIER & J. PIETTE. 1995. Iron chelation decreases NF-κB and HIV type 1 activation due to oxidative stress. Aids Res. Hum. Retroviruses **11:** 1049–1061.

43. SHATROV, V.A., J.R. BOELAERT, D. CHOUAIB, W. DROGE & V. LEHMANN. 1997. Iron chelation decreases human immunodeficiency virus-1 Tat tumor necrosis factor-induced NF-κB activation in Jurkat cells. Eur. Cytokine Netw. **8:** 37–43.

44. LIN, M., R.A. RIPPE, O. NIEMELA, G. BRITTENHAM & H. TSUKAMOTO. 1997. Role of iron in NF-κB activation and cytokine gene expression by rat hepatic macrophages. Am. J. Physiol. **272:** G1355–G1364.

45. CASTELNAU, P.A., R.S. GARRETT, W. PALISKI, J.L. WITZTUM, I.L. CAMPBELL & H.C. PWELL. 1998. Abnormal iron deposition associated with lipid peroxidation in transgenic mice expressing interleukin-6 in the brain. J. Neuropathol. Exp. Neurol. **57:** 268–282.

46. MULLER, T., D. BLUM-DEGEN, H. PRZUNTEK & W. KUHN. 1998. Interleukin-6 levels in cerebral spinal fluid inversely correlate to severity of Parkinson's disease. Acta Neurol. Scand. **98:** 142–144.

47. GASSEN, M. & M.B.H. YOUDIM. 1998. Free radical scavengers: chemical concepts and clinical relevance. J. Neural Transm. In press.

48. GANCHER, S.T., J.G. NUTT & W.R. WOODWARD. 1995. Apomorphine infusional therapy in Parkinson's disease: clinical utility and lack of tolerance. Mov. Disord. **10:** 37–43.

49. GANCHER, S. 1995. Pharmacokinetics of apomorphine in Parkinson's disease. J. Neural Transm. Suppl. **45:** 137–141.

50. COLZI, A., K. TURNER & A.J. LEE. 1998. Continuous subcutaneous waking day apomorphine in the long term treatment of levodopa induced interdose dyskinesias in Parkinson's disease. J. Neurol. Neurosurg. Psychiatry **64:** 573–576.

51. LEES, A.J. 1996. Dopamine agonists in Parkinson's disease: a look at apomorphine. Fundam. Clin. Pharmacol. **7:** 121–128.

52. GASSEN, M., B. PINCHASI & M.B.H. YOUDIM. 1998. Apomorphine is a potent radical scavenger and protects cultured pheochromocytoma cells from 6-OHDA and hydrogen peroxide induced cell death. Adv. Pharmacol. **42:** 320–325.

53. GASSEN, M., A. GROSS & M.B.H. YOUDIM. 1998. Apomorphine enantiomers protect pheochromocytoma (PC12) cells from oxidative stress induced by hydrogen peroxide and 6-hydroxydopamine. Mov. Disord. **13:** 242–248.

54. LIU, J. & A. MORI. 1993. Monoamine metabolism provides an antioxidant defense in the brain against oxidant- and free radical-induced damage. Arch. Biochem. Biophys. **302:** 118–127.

55. GASSEN, M., Y. GLINKA, B. PINCHASI & M.B.H. YOUDIM. 1996. Apomorphine is a highly potent free radical scavenger in rat mitochondrial fraction. Eur. J. Pharmacol. **308:** 219–225.

56. YOUDIM, M.B.H. 1998. Unpublished data.

57. HALL, S., J.H. RULLEGE & T. CHALLERT. 1992. MRI brain iron and 6-hydroxydopamine experimental Parkinson's disease. J. Neurol. Sci. **113:** 198–208.

58. DI MONTE, D., M.S. SANDY & M.T. SMITH. 1987. Increase efflux rather than oxidation is the mechanism of glutathione depletion by 1-methyl-4-phenyl-1,2,3,6-tetrahydropyridine (MPTP). Biochem. Biophys. Res. Commun. **148:** 153–160.

59. SINGER, T.P., N. CASTAGNOLI, JR., R.R. RAMSAY & A.J. TREOR. 1987. Biochemical events in the development of Parkinsonism induced by 1-methyl-4-phenyl-1,2,3,6-tetrahydropyridine. J. Neurochem. **49:** 1–8.

60. HEIKKILA, R.E., L. MANZINO, F.S. CABBAT & R.C. DUVOISIN. 1984. Protection against the dopaminergic neurotoxicity of 1-methyl-4-phenyl-1,2,3,6-tetrahydropyridine by monoamine oxidase inhibitors. Nature **311:** 467–469.

61. BRAUGHLER, J.M., J.F. PREGENZER, R.L. CHASE, L.A. DUNCAN, E.J. JACOBSON & J.M. MCCALL. 1987. Novel 21-aminosteroids as potent inhibitors of iron-dependent lipid peroxidation. J. Biol. Chem. **262:** 10438–10440.

62. ZHAO, W., J.S. RICHARDSON, M.J. MOMBOURQUETTE & J.A. WEIL. 1995. An *in vitro* EPR study of the free-radical scavenging action of the lazaroid antioxidants U-74500A and U-78517F. Free Radical Biol. Med. **19:** 21–30.

63. PARKINSON STUDY GROUP. 1993. Effects of tocopherol and deprenyl on the progression of disability in early Parkinson's disease. N. Engl. J. Med. **328:** 176–183.

64. SAM, E.E. & N. VERBEKE. 1995. Free radical scavenging properties of apomorphine enantiomers and dopamine: possible implication in their mechanism of action in Parkinsonism. J. Neural Transm. Parkinson's Dis. Dementia Sect. **10:** 115–127.

65. SAM, E., A.P. JEANJEAN, J.M. MALOTEAUX & N. VERBEKE. 1995. Apomorphine pharmacokinetics in Parkinsonism after intranasal and subcutaneous application. Eur. J. Drug Metab. Pharmacokinet. **20:** 27–33.

66. ZIGMOND, M.J., T.W. BERGER, A.A. GRACE & E.M. STRICKER. 1989. Compensatory responses to nigrostriatal bundle injury. Mol. Chem. Neuropathol. **10:** 185–200.

67. O'CARROLL, A.M., C.J. FOWLER, J.P. PHILLIPS, I. TOBBIA & K.F. TIPTON. 1983. The deamination of dopamine by human brain monoamine oxidase. Specificity for the two enzyme forms in seven brain regions. Naunyn Schmiedebergs Arch. Pharmacol. **322:** 198–203.

68. MATTHEWS, R.T., L. YANG & M. BEAL. 1997. *S*-Methylthiocitrulline, a neuronal nitric oxide synthase inhibitor, protects against malonate and MPTP neurotoxicity. Exp. Neurol. **143:** 282–286.

69. TEMLETT, J.A., J.P. LANDSBERG, F. WATT & G.W. GRIME. 1994. Increased iron in the substantia nigra compacta of the MPTP-lesioned hemi-Parkinsonian African green monkey: evidence from proton microprobe element microanalysis. J. Neurochem. **62:** 134–146.

70. OESTREICHER, E., G.J. SENGSTOCK, P. RIEDERER, C.W. OLANOW, A.J. DUNN & G.W. ARENDASH. 1994. Degeneration of nigrostriatal dopaminergic neurons increases iron within the substantia nigra: a histochemical and neurochemical study. Brain Res. **660:** 8–18.

71. MOCHIZUKI, H., H. IMAI, K. ENDO, K. YOKOMIZO, Y. MURATA, N. HATTORI & Y. MIZUNO. 1994. Iron accumulation in the substantia nigra of 1-methyl-4-phenyl-1,2,3,6-tetrahydropyridine (MPTP) induced hemi-Parkinsonism in monkeys. Neurosci. Lett. **168:** 251–253.

72. MONTENIRO, H.P. & C.C. WINTERBOURN. 1989. 6-Hydroxydopamine releases iron from ferritin and promotes ferritin-dependent lipid peroxidation. Biochem. Pharmacol. **38:** 4177–4182.

73. LINERT, W., E. HERLINGER, R.F. JAMESON, E. KIENZL, K. JELLINGER & M.B.H. YOUDIM. 1996. Dopamine, 6-hydroxydopamine, iron, and dioxygen: their mutual interactions and possible implication in the development of Parkinson's disease. Biochem. Biophys. Acta **1316:** 160–168.

74. SENGSTOCK, G.J., C.W. OLANOW, A.J. DUNN, S. BARONE, JR. & G.W. ARENDASH. 1994. Progressive changes in striatal dopaminergic markers, nigral volume, and rotational behavior following iron infusion into the rat substantia nigra. Exp. Neurol. **130:** 82–94.

75. SCHRECK, R., P. RIEBER & P.A. BAEUERLE. 1991. Reactive oxygen intermediates as apparently widely used messengers in the activation of the NF-κB transcription factor and HIV-1. EMBO J. **10:** 2247–2258.

76. SCHRECK, R., D. MEIER, N. MANNEL, W. DROGE & P.D. BAEUERLE. 1992. Dithiocarbonate as potent inhibitor of nuclear factor kappa B activation in intact cells. J. Exp. Med. **175:** 1181–1194.

77. SIZUKI, Y.J. & L. PACKER. 1993. Inhibition of NF-κB activation by vitamin E derivatives. Biochem. Biophys. Res. Commun. **193:** 277–283.

78. SATRIANO, J. & D. SCHLONDORFF. 1994. Activation and attenuation of transcription factor in mouse glomerular mesangial cells in reponse to TNF-alpha. J. Clin. Invest. **94:** 1629–1636.

79. GRILLI, M., M. PIZZI, M. MEMO & P. SPANO. 1996. Neuroprotection by aspirin and sodium salicylate through blockade of NF-kappa B activation. Science **274:** 1383–1835.

80. BING, G.Y., X. LU, N.Y. ZHENG, L. JIN, C.A. STEWART, R.A. FLOYD & H.C. KIM. 1998. Microglia mediated dopaminergic cell death in the substantia nigra: a new animal model for Parkinson's disease. Soc. Neurosci. 28th Annual Meeting. 1466, Abst. 574.20.

81. SHIMIZU, P.B., K. MITOMO, T. WATANABE, S. OKAMOTO & K.I. YAMAMOTO. 1990. Involvement of a NF-κB-like transcription factor in the activation of the interleukin-6 gene by inflammatory lymphokines. Mol. Cell. Biol. **10:** 561–568.

82. MIYAJIMA, H., Y. TAKAHASHI, T. KAMATA, H. SHIMIZU, N. SAKAU & J.D. GITLIN. 1997. Use of desferrioxamine in the treatment of aceruloplasminemia. Ann. Neurol. **41:** 404–407.

Hypothermia-Induced Ischemic Tolerance

SHINSAKU NISHIO, ZONG-FU CHEN, MASATOSHI YUNOKI,
TOMIKATSU TOYODA, MATTHEW ANZIVINO, AND KEVIN S. LEE[a]

*Departments of Neuroscience and Neurosurgery, University of Virginia, Charlottesville,
Virginia 22908, USA*

ABSTRACT: Delayed resistance to ischemic injury can be induced by a variety
of conditioning stimuli. This phenomenon, known as delayed ischemic tolerance, is initiated over several hours or a day, and can persist for up to a week
or more. The present paper describes recent experiments in which transient
hypothermia was used as a conditioning stimulus to induce ischemic tolerance.
A brief period of hypothermia administered 6 to 48 hours prior to focal ischemia reduces subsequent cerebral infarction. Hypothermia-induced ischemic tolerance is reversed by 7 days postconditioning, and is blocked by the
protein synthesis inhibitor anisomycin. Electrophysiological studies utilizing *in
vitro* brain slices demonstrate that hypoxic damage to synaptic responses is reduced in slices prepared from hypothermia-preconditioned animals. Taken together, these findings indicate that transient hypothermia induces tolerance in
the brain parenchyma, and that increased expression of one or more gene
products contributes to this phenomenon. Inasmuch as hypothermia is already
an approved clinical procedure for intraischemic and postischemic therapy, it
is possible that hypothermia could provide a clinically useful conditioning
stimulus for limiting injury elicited by anticipated periods of ischemia.

INTRODUCTION

A primary complication of many types of invasive surgery is ischemic cell injury.
Common surgical procedures, such as those involving vascular clamping and/or manipulation of cardiac function, entail substantial risk for ischemic injury. The risk of
ischemic tissue damage is greatest in the nervous system, where the metabolic demands of neurons are extremely high, and very brief ischemic events can damage
vulnerable cellular populations (e.g., Ref. 1). The functional impact of ischemia during cardiovascular or cerebrovascular surgery can be profound. For instance, after
coronary artery bypass surgery, some form of cognitive deficit has been reported to
occur in the majority of patients, and late and/or persistent deficits occur in over one-
quarter of the patients.[2] The magnitude of this problem is best appreciated when one
recognizes that over 1 million cardiac surgeries are performed each year in the United States alone (American Heart Association, 1998). Consequently, efforts to develop therapeutic strategies that limit injury associated with an anticipated period of
ischemia are of considerable importance.

[a]Corresponding Author: Kevin S. Lee, Department of Neuroscience, Box 5148, MR4 Annex,
University of Virginia Health Sciences Center, Charlottesville, VA 22908. Phone, 804/924-
0262; fax, 804/982-1623.
e-mail, ksl3h@virginia.edu

Timing of Therapeutic Interventions

In general, therapeutic strategies targeting ischemic injury can be viewed from the perspective of when they are administered. *Intra*ischemic and *post*ischemic interventions have been shown to be effective in limiting functional injury in the laboratory and in the clinic. Intraischemic hypothermia, such as that used during surgical procedures, can limit ischemic damage.[3–18] Postischemic hypothermia (or resuscitative hypothermia[19]) can also limit the extent of ischemic neuronal injury (see Ref. 20 for review), and has been shown to improve the recovery of patients who suffer out-of-hospital cardiac arrest.[21] Finally, *pre*ischemic therapeutic interventions are also effective in limiting ischemic injury. For instance, a short-term form of tolerance can be induced in cardiac tissue when a brief, subinjurious period of ischemic preconditioning is given prior to an injurious ischemic challenge. This form of tolerance is induced within minutes of a brief conditioning stimulus and persists for a period of a few hours or less.[22]

Delayed Tolerance

Another potential benefit of *pre*ischemic conditioning is the induction of a delayed and more protracted form of tolerance. Delayed tolerance, which is also known as late tolerance, second window of protection, or preconditioning-induced tolerance, has a slower onset and is relatively persistent. Although the precise time course of delayed tolerance appears to vary somewhat according to the conditioning stimulus and tissue type, this phenomenon is usually initiated over a day or so, and persists for many days (e.g., Ref. 23). Perhaps the best-studied example of delayed tolerance in the brain is ischemia-induced ischemic tolerance. In this case, a brief sublethal ischemic conditioning stimulus elicits tolerance to a subsequent, and more severe, ischemic challenge.[23–26] It is noteworthy that ischemia is not the only conditioning stimulus capable of inducing delayed tolerance. Several other conditioning stimuli are also effective, including spreading depression,[27–29] hypoxia,[30] hyperthermia,[31] long-term hyperbaric oxygen,[32] toxins,[33] and cytokines.[34] The types of conditioning stimuli capable of eliciting delayed tolerance in the brain are summarized in TABLE 1.

One of the drawbacks of most preconditioning stimuli is that they are also capable of producing injury with only minor changes in their intensity or duration. In the case of ischemia-induced ischemic tolerance, the safety margin is extremely narrow. A duration of global ischemia of one minute does not induce delayed tolerance, while a duration of 2–5 minutes elicits selective neuronal death.[24,35,36] Focal ischemic preconditioning may have a wider safety margin; however, this issue remains to be resolved. Another limitation of using ischemic preconditioning to induce delayed tolerance is that it will be difficult to implement in the clinic. For instance, to achieve ischemic preconditioning in a neurosurgical setting, an invasive and/or dangerous procedure would be required a day or so prior to the actual surgery. Both of the aforementioned limitations also apply to the use of spreading depression as a preconditioning stimulus. Although other preconditioning stimuli, (i.e., hyperthermia, long-term hyperbaric oxygen, toxins and cytokines) do not require invasive procedures, these treatments have inherent dangers (e.g., toxicity) that could preclude their use in the clinical setting. Nonetheless, the need for an effective means of treat-

TABLE 1. Preconditioning-induced tolerance in neurons of the brain

Conditioning Stimulus	Test Stimulus	References
Forebrain ischemia	Forebrain ischemia or focal ischemia	Kitagawa *et al.*, 1990[24]; Kitagawa *et al.*, 1991[25]; Kirino *et al.*, 1991[26]; Kato *et al.*, 1992[54]; Kato *et al.*, 1992[55]; Kato *et al.*, 1992[35]; Liu *et al.*, 1992[56]; Aoki *et al.*, 1993a,b[57,58]; Kato *et al.*, 1993[59]; Liu *et al.*, 1993[60]; Malsuyama *et al.*, 1993[36]; Nakagomi *et al.*, 1993[61]; Nishi *et al.*, 1993[62]; Kato *et al.*, 1994[63]; Kato *et al.*, 1994[64]; Kato *et al.*, 1994[65]; Nakata *et al.*, 1994[66]; Schetinger *et al.*, 1994[67]; Shimazaki *et al.*, 1994[68]; Heurteaux *et al.*, 1995[69]; Kato *et al.*, 1995[70]; Kato *et al.*, 1995[71]; Kato *et al.*, 1995[72]; Matsushima and Hakim, 1995[73]; Sommer *et al.*, 1995[74]; Ohno and Watanabe, 1996[75]; Ohtsuki *et al.*, 1996[76]; Corbett and Crooks, 1997[77]; Katayama *et al.*, 1997[78]; Li *et al.*, 1997[79]; Sorimachi *et al.*, 1997[80]; Wada *et al.*, 1997[81]; Kawai *et al.*, 1998[82]; Nakano *et al.*, 1998[83]; Shimazaki *et al.*, 1998[50]; Tokunaga *et al.*, 1998[51]; Yoneda *et al.*, 1998[84]
Focal ischemia	Forebrain ischemia or focal ischemia	Glazier *et al.*, 1994[85]; Matsushima and Hakim, 1995[73]; Chen *et al.*, 1996[86]; Toyoda *et al.*, 1997[87]; Barone *et al.*, 1998[88]; Chimon and Wong, 1998[89]; Wang *et al.*, 1998[90]
Hypoxia/anoxia	Anoxia or ischemia/hypoxia	Gidday *et al.*, 1994[30]; Sakaki *et al.*, 1995[45]; Caprioli *et al.*, 1996[46]; Gage and Stanton, 1996[47]; Perez-Pinzon *et al.*, 1996[48]; Bergeron *et al.*, 1997[91]; Cai *et al.*, 1997[92]; Ota *et al.*, 1998[93]; Vannucci *et al.*, 1998[94]
Chemically-induced oxidative and metabolic stress	Forebrain ischemia or focal ischemia	Ohtsuki *et al.*, 1992[95]; Riepe *et al.*, 1996[96]; Bruer *et al.*, 1997[49]; Riepe *et al.*, 1997[97]
Spreading depression	Global ischemia or focal ischemia	Kobayashi *et al.*, 1995[28]; Kawahara *et al.*, 1997[98]; Plumier *et al.*, 1997[99]; Taga *et al.*, 1997[100]; Caggiano and Kraig, 1998[101]; Yanamoto *et al.*, 1998[29]
Hyperthermia	Forebrain ischemia, anoxia or excitotoxic treatment	Chopp *et al.*, 1989[31]; Caprioli *et al.*, 1996[46]
Hypothermia	Focal ischemia or hypoxia	Nishio *et al.*, 1999[102]
Platelet-derived growth factor	Focal ischemia	Sakata *et al.*, 1998[103]
Myelin basic protein	Focal ischemia	Becker *et al.*, 1997[104]
Tumor necrosis factor-alpha	Focal ischemia	Nawashiro *et al.*, 1997[34]
Lipopolysaccharide	Focal ischemia	Tasaki *et al.*, 1997[33]
Hyperbaric oxygen	Forebrain ischemia	Wada *et al.*, 1996[32]

ing anticipated periods of ischemia remains acute, and continues to stimulate the evaluation of a variety of conditioning stimuli. The ideal goal of these efforts is to identify an effective, non-invasive form of preconditioning that possesses an acceptable safety margin.

Hypothermia as a Preconditioning Stimulus

The purpose of this paper is to evaluate hypothermia as a preconditioning stimulus for inducing tolerance. Hypothermia is one of the oldest, yet most effective, *intra*ischemic treatments for limiting cellular injury. Systemic or focal cooling has been shown to provide a beneficial effect in the context of cerebrovascular, cardiovascular and other types of surgeries (e.g., Refs. 7, 14, and 18). Hypothermia has been termed the "gold standard" against which other ischemic therapies should be compared,[37,38] in the context of experimental studies using pre- and/or postischemic hypothermia to limit ischemic injury. Moreover, hypothermia is a noninvasive manipulation that exhibits a considerable safety margin (e.g., Ref. 39). The present paper provides evidence that transient hypothermia can also be protective when administered a day or more prior to an ischemic event, and provides a foundation for considering hypothermic preconditioning as a therapeutic strategy for treating anticipated periods of ischemic challenge.

MATERIALS AND METHODS

All procedures were approved by the University of Virginia Animal Research Committee. Adult Sprague-Dawley rats were subjected to a 20-minute period of conditioning hypothermia at 31–32°C (temporal muscle temperature) under halothane anesthesia. The total duration of hypothermia was actually longer than 20 minutes, because approximately 30 minutes was required to cool the animals from 37.5°C, and an additional 30 minutes was required to rewarm the animals. The interval between hypothermic preconditioning and ischemia ranged from 6 hours to 7 days. Ischemia was administered by clamping one middle cerebral artery and both carotid arteries for one hour. Twenty-four hours postischemia, animals were sacrificed by intracardial perfusion under deep anesthesia with sodium pentobarbital. Brains were removed, sectioned coronally (2 mm thick), and stained with 2% 2,3,5-triphenyltetrazolium chloride (TTC) in saline. The sections were then fixed in 4% buffered formalin. Staining with TTC allows the visualization of areas of intact and damaged tissue, and permits simple measurements of the size of the infarction. The area of infarction was measured in each section, and the volume of infarction was calculated and adjusted for swelling. Other animals received a sham preconditioning procedure that included halothane anesthesia, but no hypothermia. The interval between the sham manipulation and the ischemic challenge was 24 hours in the sham preconditioned group. A third group of animals received no preconditioning (nonpreconditioned group). All other procedures for the sham preconditioned and nonpreconditioned groups were the same as those for the hypothermia-preconditioned group.

The effects of the protein synthesis inhibitor anisomycin on hypothermia-induced tolerance were examined in two additional groups of animals. These animals received two intraperitoneal injections of anisomycin (20 mg/kg in saline per injection). In the "hypo-thermia+anisomycin" group, the first injection of anisomycin was administered immedi-ately prior to the induction of hypothermia; the second injection was given 4 hours after the first injection. This protocol of anisomycin treatment produces 80–100% inhibition of protein synthesis for approximately 2½ hours, and 40–80% inhibition for an addi-tional 1½ hours.[40] The second injection during the decay phase of inhibition rees-tablishes the 80–100% level of inhibition for a similar period.[40] Hypothermia was administered as described above. The "anisomycin-only" group received two injec-tions of anisomycin (20 mg/kg) at the same interval as in the hypothermia+anisomycin group. In the anisomycin-only group, animals were subjected to the same basic protocol as described above for the sham preconditioned group. Focal ischemia was administered 24 hours after the first injection of anisomycin in both the anisomycin-only group and the hypothermia+anisomycin group. These animals were killed 24 hours postischemia, and the volume of cerebral infarction was determined as described above.

An additional series of experiments was undertaken to examine the effects of hy-pothermic preconditioning on the vulnerability of synaptic responses to hypoxic challenge. In these experiments, two groups of animals were prepared in accordance with the non-preconditioned and hypothermia-preconditioned protocols described above. Twenty-four hours after preconditioning, animals were killed by decapitation under deep sodium pentobarbital anesthesia. *In vitro* brain slices of the rat hippoc-ampus were prepared 24 hours after hypothermic preconditioning.[41] Excitatory syn-aptic responses were recorded before, during and after a brief period of deep hypoxia. Using extracellular recording techniques, evoked potentials were recorded in stratum radiatum of CA1 in response to stimulation of the combined Schaffer col-lateral/commissural afferents. This stimulation/recording paradigm evokes excitato-ry responses known as field excitatory postsynaptic potentials (fEPSPs).[42] The slope and amplitude of the fEPSPs were measured as described previously (e.g., Ref. 43). The recovery of fEPSPs after hypoxia in hippocampal slices has been used previous-ly for the analysis of candidate therapeutic compounds for treating ischemia (e.g., Ref. 44). Evoked responses were recorded every 20 seconds during the course of each experiment. Hypoxia was achieved by exchanging the standard 95% O_2:5% CO_2 atmosphere with 95% N_2:5% CO_2. As in previous studies,[44] hypoxia elicited a generalized depolarization (hypoxic depolarization: HD) of the tissue within a few minutes. In the present study, the hypoxic challenge was terminated 2 minutes after HD, and the oxygenated atmosphere was reestablished. The posthypoxic recovery of synaptic responses was then compared between slices from preconditioned and non-preconditioned (control) animals.

RESULTS

Effects of Hypothermic Preconditioning on Focal Ischemic Injury In Vivo

Mean arterial blood pressure, temporal muscle temperature, rectal temperature, blood pH, blood pO_2 and blood pCO_2 were monitored prior to, and during, the is-chemic procedure. In general, these parameters did not differ among groups. How-ever, pO_2 values were significantly greater in the hypothermia+6 hours, anisomycin-

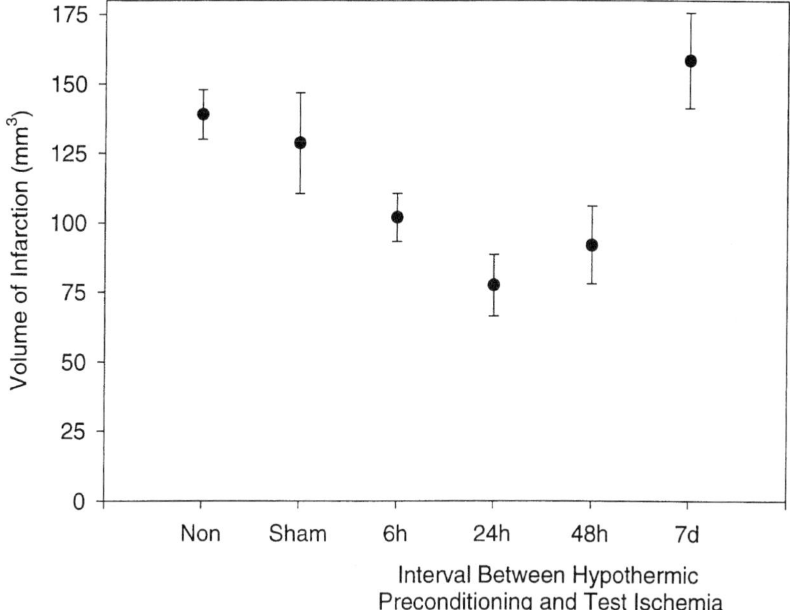

FIGURE 1. Effect of hypothermic preconditioning on ischemic infarction. The volume of ischemic infarction is shown in animals subjected to focal ischemia at 6, 24, or 48 hours or 7 days after hypothermic preconditioning. All animals were killed 24 hours after focal ischemia. Infarction volume was reduced significantly at intervals of 6, 24 and 48 hours. Statistical comparisons were performed using one-way analysis of variance and Fisher's LSD post hoc test. Levels of p <0.05 were considered significant. *Abbreviations*: non, non-preconditioned control group; sham, sham-preconditioned group.

only and hypothermia+anisomycin groups, when compared to the non-preconditioned group; these changes did not correspond to the differences in cerebral infarction observed following hypothermic preconditioning (see below).

Cerebral infarction was attenuated in hypothermia-preconditioned animals, and this effect varied as a function of the interval between preconditioning and ischemia (FIG. 1). The average infarction volumes for the 6-, 24- and 48-hour hypothermia-preconditioned groups were significantly smaller than that of the non-preconditioned group. In contrast, the volume of infarction in the 7-day group did not differ significantly from control levels. Sham preconditioning did not significantly affect the volume of cerebral infarction.

Treatment with anisomycin blocked the protective effect of hypothermic preconditioning. The average infarction volumes for the hypothermia+anisomycin ($n = 6$) and anisomycin-only ($n = 9$) groups were 132.1 ± 16.5 and 119.5 ± 12.2 mm^3 (mean ± SEM), respectively. These values did not differ significantly from one another, and neither value differed significantly from that of the non-preconditioned group.

TABLE 2. Effect of hypothermic preconditioning (*in vivo*) on hypoxic damage to synaptic responses in hippocampal slices (*in vitro*)

	Non-preconditioned ($n = 6$)	Preconditioned ($n = 6$)
Delay to hypoxic depolarization (min)	4.4 ± 1.1 min	4.9 ± 1.0 min
Post-hypoxic recovery of fEPSP (% of pre-hypoxic baseline)	49 ± 3 %	*70 ± 8 %

The delay to hypoxic depolarization did not differ significantly between the two groups. Post-hypoxic recovery of the slope of the fEPSP was significantly increased (* p <0.05, Students' *t*-test) in the slices from hypothermia-preconditioned animals. The values shown for the recovery of the fEPSP slope are percentages of the prehypoxic baseline; similar results were obtained for the amplitude of the fEPSP (data not shown).

Effects of Hypothermic Preconditioning on Hypoxic Synaptic Damage In Vitro

The effect of hypoxia on synaptic responses was examined in *in vitro* hippocampal slices prepared from hypothermia-preconditioned and non-preconditioned animals. Evoked responses in slices from preconditioned animals exhibited better recovery after hypoxia than did those from non-preconditioned animals. As shown in TABLE 2, the average recovery of fEPSPs in the "preconditioned slices" (expressed as a percentage of their prehypoxia baseline), was significantly greater than that of "non-preconditioned slices." The delay to the onset of hypoxic depolarization (HD) after the initiation of hypoxia did not differ significantly between the two groups of slices.

DISCUSSION

The findings presented here indicate that hypothermic preconditioning is capable of inducing ischemic tolerance. This phenomenon is initiated within 6 hours of preconditioning, persists for at least two days, and is completed by 7 days. The time course over which hypothermia-induced tolerance occurs, and the ability of anisomycin to block tolerance, suggest that increased expression of one or more gene products underlies this phenomenon.

Cellular Substrates of Tolerance

The cellular substrates of delayed tolerance could conceivably involve changes in neurons, glia, and/or vascular cells. Previous studies using *in vitro* brain slices and cell cultures indicate that delayed tolerance can result from direct effects on neurons.[45–51] Evidence provided here suggests that delayed tolerance induced by hypothermic preconditioning is also due to direct cellular changes in the brain parenchyma. Synaptic responses showed significantly better posthypoxic recovery in slices prepared from preconditioned animals than in slices from non-preconditioned animals. Inasmuch as systemic variables, such as blood flow and temperature, do not play a role in the slice experiments, it appears that hypothermia-induced tolerance is the result of direct effects on neurons and/or glia. It is important to stress that these findings do not rule out a protective effect resulting from changes in systemic variables in the *in vivo* setting; alterations in blood flow could occur, in addition to direct changes in neurons and glia. However, the present findings indicate that one or more cell types in the brain parenchyma become tolerant. It is noteworthy that the delay to hypoxic depolarization (HD) was not significantly affected in this study. This finding suggests that changes in metabolic factors may not be crucial to the tolerance phenomenon. For instance, if a major shift in metabolic rate had occurred in the preconditioned group, then it might be expected that the delay to HD would have been longer in the "preconditioned" slices. Because the delay to HD was unchanged, it seems more likely that hypothermic preconditioning renders neurons and/or glia more tolerant to the depolarized state.

Molecular Mechanisms of Tolerance

An important difference between hypothermia-induced tolerance and delayed tolerance induced by certain other conditioning stimuli is that the duration of hypothermia-induced tolerance is briefer. For instance, delayed tolerance induced by forebrain ischemic preconditioning can persist for a week or more (e.g., Ref. 23), while hypothermia-induced tolerance is reversed within a week. The differences in duration of tolerance in response to different types of conditioning stimuli raise the possibility that the mechanisms underlying tolerance may vary according to the inducing stimulus. On the other hand, the same types of mechanisms could be activated during the initial postconditioning stage, regardless of the type of conditioning, while more persistent or additional mechanisms are induced under conditions that elicit more prolonged tolerance. The potential mechanisms underlying delayed ischemic tolerance have been reviewed elsewhere (e.g., Ref. 52). Among the candidate mechanisms that are postulated to participate in delayed tolerance are: 1) altered levels or rates of expression of heat shock proteins, 2) enhanced antioxidant activity, 3) induction of immediate early genes, 4) altered neuromodulation by adenosine, 5) modulation of ion channel function and/or intracellular ion regulation, 6) enhanced activity of endogenous protease inhibitors, 7) induction of neurotrophic and growth factors, 8) activity of tumor necrosis factor-alpha, 9) altered second messenger function, 10) *de novo* protein synthesis, 11) enhanced interleukin-1 activity, 12) altered immune response, 13) enhanced heme-deoxygenation, 14) improved oxygen metabolism, 15) reduced lipid peroxidation, and 16) increased expression of anti-apoptotic genes (summarized in TABLE 3). It is important to stress that the precise roles of most of these mechanisms in the tolerance phenomenon have yet to be established, and many remain controversial (for review see Ref. 52). It is conceivable that temporally restricted changes in one or more of these mechanisms could contribute differentially to the early and late stages of ischemic tolerance. In the case of hypothermia-induced tolerance, it is possible that the conditioning-induced changes are restricted to those events responsible for the early stages (1–4 days) of ischemic tolerance. In contrast, more profound preconditioning that elicits longer tolerance (e.g., ischemic preconditioning) could induce additional neuroprotective mechanisms responsible for the late stages of tolerance. The issue of which cellular and molecular mechanisms are most salient to the early and late stages of tolerance is poorly understood, and is an important topic for future investigation.

TABLE 3. Mechanisms implicated in delayed neuronal tolerance

Mechanism	Reference
Altered levels or rates of expression of heat shock proteins	Kirino *et al.*, 1991[26]; Kitagawa *et al.*, 1991[25]; Aoki *et al.*, 1993a,b[57,58]; Liu *et al.*, 1993[60]; Nakata *et al.*, 1993[105]; Nishi *et al.*, 1993[62]; Ohtsuki *et al.*, 1993[106]; Glazier *et al.*, 1994[85]; Kato *et al.*, 1995[107]; Abe and Nowak, 1996[108]; Caprioli *et al.*, 1996[46]; Kitagawa *et al.*, 1996[109]; Wada *et al.*, 1996[32]; Plumier *et al.*, 1997[99]; Yenari *et al.*, 1998[110]
Enhanced antioxidant activity	Ohtsuki *et al.*, 1992[95]; Kato *et al.*, 1995[71]; Toyoda *et al.*, 1997[87]
Induction of immediate early genes	Kato *et al.*, 1995[70]; Kobayashi *et al.*, 1995[28]; Sommer *et al.*, 1995[74]; Abe and Nowak, 1996[108]; Belayev *et al.*, 1996[111]
Altered neuromodulation by adenosine	Perez-Pinzon *et al.*, 1996[48]
Modulation of ion channel function and/or intracellular ion regulation	Heurteaux *et al.*, 1995[69]; Shimazaki *et al.*, 1998[50]
Enhanced activity of endogenous protease inhibitors	Wang *et al.*, 1998[90]
Induction of neurotrophic and growth factors	Sakaki *et al.*, 1995[45]; Kawahara *et al.*, 1997[98]
Activity of tumor necrosis factor-alpha	Tasaki *et al.*, 1997[33]
Altered second messenger function	Kato *et al.*, 1992[55]
de novo protein synthesis	Barone *et al.*, 1998[88]; Yoneda *et al.*, 1998[84]; Nishio *et al.*, 1999[102]
Enhanced interleukin-1 activity	Ohtsuki *et al.*, 1996[76]; Barone *et al.*, 1998[88]
Altered immune response	Becker *et al.*, 1997[104]; Toyoda *et al.*[112]
Enhanced heme-deoxygenation	Gage and Stanton , 1996[47]
Improved oxygen metabolism	Li *et al.*, 1997[79]
Reduced lipid peroxidation	Chimon and Wong, 1998[89]
Increased expression of anti-apoptotic genes	Shimazaki *et al.*, 1994[68]; Simon *et al.*, 1995[113]

Hypothermic Preconditioning as a Therapeutic Strategy

The value of hypothermic preconditioning in the clinical setting clearly remains to be established. However, the findings presented in this chapter indicate that the clinical evaluation of hypothermic preconditioning may be warranted. In particular, hypothermia exhibits several desirable features of a candidate mechanism for inducing tolerance. First, hypothermia is a noninvasive treatment. Second, although not without side effects (e.g., Ref. 53), hypothermia exhibits a substantial safety margin with respect to neuronal injury.[39] Third, hypothermia-induced tolerance is expressed, and declines, over a manageable time course. Finally, hypothermia is already in use clinically as an intraischemic and postischemic therapy. Assuming that hypothermia proves effective as a preconditioning treatment in humans, the fact that it is already in clinical use will facilitate its approval in the context of preconditioning. Taken together, these points suggest that hypothermia could be of value as a preconditioning stimulus for inducing delayed tolerance. Implementation of this strategy could yield substantial benefit in the context of predictable ischemia, such as occurs in a wide variety of common surgical procedures.

ACKNOWLEDGMENTS

This work was supported by Grant #HL49396. We thank Natalie Harrison for assistance in preparation of this report.

REFERENCES

1. SMITH, M.L., R.N. AUER & B.K. SIESJO. 1984. The density and distribution of ischemic brain injury in the rat following 2–10 min of forebrain ischemia. Acta Neuropathol. (Berl.) **64:** 319–332.
2. MCKHANN, G.M., M.A. GOLDSBOROUGH, L.M. BOROWICZ, JR., O.A. SELNES, E.D. MELLITS, C. ENGER, S.A. QUASKEY, W.A. BAUMGARTNER, D.E. CAMERON, R.S. STUART & T.J. GARDNER. 1997. Cognitive outcome after coronary artery bypass: a one-year prospective study. Ann. Thorac. Surg. **63:** 510–515.
3. DRAKE, C., H. BARR, J. COLES & N. GERGELY. 1964. Use of extracorporal circulation and profound hypothermia in the treatment of ruptured intracranial aneurysm. J. Neurosurg. **21:** 575–581.
4. BERNTMAN, L., F.A. WELSH & J.R. HARP. 1981. Cerebral protective effect of low-grade hypothermia. Anesthesiology **55:** 495–498.
5. SILVERBERG, G.D., B.A. REITZ & A.K. REAM. 1981. Hypothermia and cardiac arrest in the treatment of giant aneurysms of the cerebral circulation and hemangioblastoma of the medulla. J. Neurosurg. **55:** 337–346.
6. ERGIN, M.A., J.V. O'CONNOR, R. GUINTO & R.B. GRIEPP. 1982. Experience with profound hypothermia and circulatory arrest in the treatment of aneurysms of the aortic arch. Aortic arch replacement for acute arch dissections. J. Thorac. Cardiovasc. Surg. **84:** 649–655.
7. THARION, J., D.C. JOHNSON, J.M. CELERMAJER, R.M. HAWKER, T.B. CARTMILL & J.H. OVERTON. 1982. Profound hypothermia with circulatory arrest: nine years' clinical experience. J. Thorac. Cardiovasc. Surg. **84:** 66–72.
8. BUSTO, R., W.D. DIETRICH, M.Y. GLOBUS, I. VALDES, P. SCHEINBERG & M.D. GINSBERG. 1987. Small differences in intraischemic brain temperature critically determine the extent of ischemic neuronal injury. J. Cereb. Blood Flow Metab. **7:** 729–738.
9. CRAWFORD, E.S., J.S. COSELLI & H.J. SAFI. 1987. Partial cardiopulmonary bypass, hypothermic circulatory arrest, and posterolateral exposure for thoracic aortic aneurysm operation. J. Thorac. Cardiovasc. Surg. **94:** 824–827.
10. SPETZLER, R.F., M.N. HADLEY, D. REGAMONTI, L.P. CARTER, P.A. RAUDZENS, S.A SHEDD & E. WILKINSON. 1998. Aneurysms of the basilar artery treated with circulatory arrest, hypothermia and barbiturate cerebral protections. J. Neurosurg. **68:** 868–879.
11. CHYATTE, D.J., J. ELEFTERIADES & B. KIM. 1989. Profound hypothermia and circulatory arrest for aneurysm surgery. Case report. J. Neurosurg. **70:** 489–491.
12. GEBHARD, M.M. 1990. Myocardial protection and ischemia tolerance of the globally ischemic heart. Thorac. Cardiovasc. Surg. **38:** 55–59.

13. ONESTI, S.T., C.J. BAKER, P.P. SUN & R.A. SOLOMON. 1991. Transient hypothermia reduces focal ischemic brain injury in the rat. Neurosurgery **29:** 369–373.

14. SOLOMON, R.A., C.R. SMITH, E.C. RAPS, W.L. YOUNG, J.G. STONE & M.E. FINK. 1991. Deep hypothermic circulatory arrest for the management of complex anterior and posterior circulation aneurysms. Neurosurgery **29:** 732–737; discussion 737–738.

15. WILLIAMS, M.D., W.G. RAINER, H.G. FIEGER, I.P. MURRAY & M.L. SANCHEZ. 1991. Cardiopulmonary bypass, profound hypothermia and circulatory arrest for neurosurgery. Ann. Thorac. Surg. **52:** 1069–1075.

16. MORIKAWA, E., M.D. GINSBERG, W.D. DIETRICH, R.C. DUNCAN, S. KRAYDIEH, M.Y. GLOBUS & R. BUSTO. 1992. The significance of brain temperature in focal cerebral ischemia: histopathological consequences of middle cerebral artery occlusion in the rat. J. Cereb. Blood Flow Metab. **12:** 380–389.

17. RIDENOUR, T.R., D.S. WARNER, M.M. TODD & A.C. MCALLISTER. 1992. Mild hypothermia reduces infarct size resulting from temporary but not permanent focal ischemia in rats. Stroke **23:** 733–738.

18. CAMBRIA, R.P., J.K. DAVISON, S. ZANNETTI, G. L'ITALIEN, D.C. BREWSTER, J.P. GERTLER, A.C. MONCURE, G.M. LAMURAGLIA & W.M. ABBOTT. 1997. Clinical experience with epidural cooling for spinal cord protection during thoracic and thoracoabdominal aneurysm repair. J. Vasc. Surg. **25:** 234–241; discussion 241–243.

19. MARION, D.W., Y. LEONOV, M. GINSBERG, L.M. KATZ, P.M. KOCHANEK, A. LECHLEUTHNER, E.M. NEMOTO, W. OBRIST, P. SAFAR, F. STERZ, S.A. TISHERMAN, R.J. WHITE, F. XIAO & H. ZAR. 1996. Resuscitative hypothermia. Crit. Care Med. **24:** S81–S89.

20. COLBOURNE, F., G. SUTHERLAND & D. CORBETT. 1997. Postischemic hypothermia: a critical appraisal with implications for clinical treatment. Mol. Neurobiol. **14:** 171–201.

21. BERNARD, S.A., B.M. JONES & M.K. HORNE. 1997. Clinical trial of induced hypothermia in comatose survivors of out-of-hospital cardiac arrest. Ann. Emerg. Med. **30:** 146–153.

22. REIMER, K.A. & R.B. JENNINGS. 1992. Preconditioning: definitions, proposed mechanisms, and implications for myocardial protection in ischemia reperfusion. *In* Myocardial Protection: The Pathophysiology of Reperfusion Injury. D.M. Yellon & R.B. Jennings, Eds. 165–183. Raven Press. New York.

23. KATO, H., Y. LIU, T. ARAKI & K. KOGURE. 1991. Temporal profile of the effects of pretreatment with brief cerebral ischemia on the neuronal damage following secondary ischemic insult in the gerbil: cumulative damage and protective effects. Brain Res. **553:** 238–242.

24. KITAGAWA, K., M. MATSUMOTO, M. TAGAYA, R. HATA, H. UEDA, M. NIINOBE, N. HANDA, R. FUKUNAGA, K. KIMURA, K. MIKOSHIBA & T. KAMADA. 1990. 'Ischemic tolerance' phenomenon found in the brain. Brain Res. **528:** 21–24.

25. KITAGAWA, K., M. MATSUMOTO, K. KUWABARA, M. TAGAYA, T. OHTSUKI, R. HATA, H. UEDA, N. HANDA, K. KIMURA & T. KAMADA. 1991. 'Ischemic tolerance' phenomenon detected in various brain regions. Brain Res. **561:** 203–211.

26. KIRINO, T., Y. TSUJITA & A. TAMURA. 1991. Induced tolerance to ischemia in gerbil hippocampal neurons. J. Cereb. Blood Flow Metab. **11:** 299–307.

27. KAWAHARA, N., C.A. RUETZLER & I. KLATZO. 1995. Protective effect of spreading depression against neuronal damage following cardiac arrest cerebral ischaemia. Neurol. Res. **17:** 9–16.

28. KOBAYASHI, S., V.A. HARRIS & F.A. WELSH. 1995. Spreading depression induces tolerance of cortical neurons to ischemia in rat brain. J. Cereb. Blood Flow Metab. **15:** 721–727.

29. YANAMOTO, H., N. HASHIMOTO, I. NAGATA & H. KIKUCHI. 1998. Infarct tolerance against temporary focal ischemia following spreading depression in rat brain. Brain Res. **784:** 239–249.

30. GIDDAY, J.M., J.C. FITZGIBBONS, A.R. SHAH & T.S. PARK. 1994. Neuroprotection from ischemic brain injury by hypoxic preconditioning in the neonatal rat. Neurosci. Lett. **168:** 221–224.

31. CHOPP, M., H. CHEN, K.L. HO, M.O. DERESKI, E. BROWN, F.W. HETZEL & K.M. WELCH. 1989. Transient hyperthermia protects against subsequent forebrain ischemic cell damage in the rat. Neurology **39:** 1396–1398.

32. WADA, K., M. ITO, T. MIYAZAWA, H. KATOH, H. NAWASHIRO, K. SHIMA & H. CHIGASAKI. 1996. Repeated hyperbaric oxygen induces ischemic tolerance in gerbil hippocampus. Brain Res. **740:** 15–20.

33. TASAKI, K., C.A. RUETZLER, T. OHTSUKI, D. MARTIN, H. NAWASHIRO & J.M. HALLENBECK. 1997. Lipopolysaccharide pre-treatment induces resistance against subsequent focal cerebral ischemic damage in spontaneously hypertensive rats. Brain Res. **748:** 267–270.

34. NAWASHIRO, H., K. TASAKI, C.A. RUETZLER & J.M. HALLENBECK. 1997. TNF-alpha pretreatment induces protective effects against focal cerebral ischemia in mice. J. Cereb. Blood Flow Metab. **17:** 483–490.

35. KATO, H., Y. LIU, T. ARAKI & K. KOGURE. 1992. MK-801, but not anisomycin, inhibits the induction of tolerance to ischemia in the gerbil hippocampus. Neurosci. Lett. **139:** 118–121.

36. MATSUYAMA, T., M. TSUCHIYAMA, H. NAKAMURA, M. MATSUMOTO & M. SUGITA. 1993. Hilar somatostatin neurons are more vulnerable to an ischemic insult than CA1 pyramidal neurons. J. Cereb. Blood Flow Metab. **13:** 229–234.

37. BUCHAN, A. 1992. Advances in cerebral ischemia: experimental approaches. Neurol. Clin. **10:** 49–61.

38. BARONE, F.C., G.Z. FEUERSTEN & R.F. WHITE. 1997. Brain cooling during transient focal ischemia provides complete neuroprotection. Neurosci. Biobehav. Rev. **21:** 31–44.

39. CHOPP, M., Y. LI, M.O. DERESKI, S.R. LEVINE, Y. YOSHIDA & J.H. GARCIA. 1992. Hypothermia reduces 72-kDa heat-shock protein induction in rat brain after transient forebrain ischemia. Stroke **23:** 104–107.

40. FLOOD, J.F., M.R. ROSENZWEIG, E.L. BENNETT & A.E. ORME. 1973. The influence of duration of protein synthesis inhibition on memory. Physiol. Behav. **10:** 555–562.

41. LEE, K.S., M. OLIVER, F. SCHOTTLER & G. LYNCH. 1981. Electron microscopic studies of brain slices: the effects of high-frequency stimulation on dendritic ultrastructure. *In* Electrophysiology of Isolated Mammalian CNS Preparations. G.A. Kerkut & H.V. Wheal, Eds. 189–211. Academic Press. London.

42. ANDERSEN, P., T.W. BLACKSTAD & T. LOMO. 1996. Location and identification of excitatory synapses on hippocampal pyramidal cells. Exp. Brain Res. **1:** 236–248.

43. CHEN, Z.-F., F. SCHOTTLER & K.S. LEE. 1996. Neuronal recovery after moderate hypoxia is improved by the calpain inhibitor MDL28170. Brain Res. **769:** 188–192.

44. ARAI, A., M. KESSLER, K.S. LEE & G. LYNCH. 1990. Calpain inhibitors improve the recovery of synaptic transmission from hypoxia in hippocampal slices. Brain Res. **532:** 63–68.

45. SAKAKI, T., K. YAMADA, H. OTSUKI, T. YUGUCHI, E. KOHMURA & T. HAYAKAWA. 1995. Brief exposure to hypoxia induces bFGF mRNA and protein and protects rat cortical neurons from prolonged hypoxic stress. Neurosci. Res. **23:** 289–296.

46. CAPRIOLI, J., S. KITANO & J.E. MORGAN. 1996. Hyperthermia and hypoxia increase tolerance of retinal ganglion cells to anoxia and excitotoxicity. Invest. Ophthalmol. Visual Sci. **37:** 2376–2381.

47. GAGE, A.T. & P.K. STANTON. 1996. Hypoxia triggers neuroprotective alterations in hippocampal gene expression via a heme-containing sensor. Brain Res. **719:** 172–178.

48. PEREZ-PINZON, M.A., P.L. MUMFORD, M. ROSENTHAL & T.J. SICK. 1996. Anoxic preconditioning in hippocampal slices: role of adenosine. Neuroscience **75:** 687–694.

49. BRUER, U., M.K. WEIH, N.K. ISAEV, A. MEISEL, K. RUSCHER, A. BERGK, G. TRENDELENBURG, F. WIEGAND, I.V. VICTOROV & U. DIRNAGL. 1997. Induction of tolerance in rat cortical neurons: hypoxic preconditioning. FEBS Lett. **414:** 117–121.

50. SHIMAZAKI, K., T. NAKAMURA, K. NAKAMURA, K. OGURO, T. MASUZAWA, Y. KUDO & N. KAWAI. 1998. Reduced calcium elevation in hippocampal CA1 neurons of ischemia-tolerant gerbils. Neuroreport **9:** 1875–1878.

51. TOKUNAGA, H., K. HIRAMATSU & T. SAKAKI. 1998. Effect of preceding *in vivo* sublethal ischemia on the evoked potentials during secondary *in vitro* hypoxia evaluated with gerbil hippocampal slices. Brain Res. **784:** 316–320.

52. CHEN, J. & R.P. SIMON. 1997. Ischemic tolerance in the brain. Neurology **48:** 306–311.

53. SCHUBERT, A. 1995. Side effects of mild hypothermia. J. Neurosurg. Anesthesiol. **7:** 139–147.

54. KATO, H., T. ARAKI & K. KOGURE. 1992. Preserved neurotransmitter receptor binding following ischemia in preconditioned gerbil brain. Brain Res. Bull. **29:** 395–400.

55. KATO, H., T. ARAKI, K. MURASE & K. KOGURE. 1992. Induction of tolerance to ischemia: alterations in second-messenger systems in the gerbil hippocampus. Brain Res. Bull. **29:** 559–565.

56. LIU, Y., H. KATO, N. NAKATA & K. KOGURE. 1992. Protection of rat hippocampus against ischemic neuronal damage by pretreatment with sublethal ischemia. Brain Res. **586:** 121–124.

57. AOKI, M., K. ABE, J. KAWAGOE, S. NAKAMURA & K. KOGURE. 1993. The preconditioned hippocampus accelerates HSP70 heat shock gene expression following transient ischemia in the gerbil. Neurosci. Lett. **155**(1): 7–10.

58. AOKI, M., K. ABE, J. KAWAGOE, S. NAKAMURA & K. KOGURE. 1993. Acceleration of HSP70 and HSC70 heat shock gene expression following transient ischemia in the preconditioned gerbil hippocampus. J. Cereb. Blood Flow Metab. **13:** 781–788.

59. KATO, H., T. CHEN, X.H. LIU, N. NAKATA & K. KOGURE. 1993. Immunohistochemical localization of ubiquitin in gerbil hippocampus with induced tolerance to ischemia. Brain Res. **619:** 339–343.

60. LIU, Y., H. KATO, N. NAKATA & K. KOGURE. 1993. Correlation between induction of ischemic tolerance and expression of heat shock protein-70 in the rat hippocampus. Brain & Nerve **45:** 157–162.

61. NAKAGOMI, T., T. KIRINO, H. KANEMITSU, Y. TSUJITA & A. TAMURA. 1993. Early recovery of protein synthesis following ischemia in hippocampal neurons with induced tolerance in the gerbil. Acta Neuropathol. (Berl.) **86:** 10–15.

62. NISHI, S., W. TAKI, Y. UEMURA, T. HIGASHI, H. KIKUCHI, H. KUDOH, M. SATOH & K. NAGATA. 1993. Ischemic tolerance due to the induction of HSP70 in a rat ischemic recirculation model. Brain Res. **615:** 281–288.

63. KATO, H., K. KOGURE, T. ARAKI & Y. ITOYAMA. 1994. Astroglial and microglial reactions in the gerbil hippocampus with induced ischemic tolerance. Brain Res. **664:** 69–76.

64. KATO, H., K. KOGURE, Y. LIU, T. ARAKI & Y. ITOYAMA. 1994. Induction of NADPH-diaphorase activity in the hippocampus in a rat model of cerebral ischemia and ischemic tolerance. Brain Res. **652:** 71–75.

65. KATO, H., Y. LIU, K. KOGURE & K. KATO. 1994. Induction of 27-kDa heat shock protein following cerebral ischemia in a rat model of ischemic tolerance. Brain Res. **634:** 235–244.

66. NAKATA, N., H. KATO & K. KOGURE. 1994. Ischemic tolerance and extracellular amino acid concentrations in gerbil hippocampus measured by intracerebral microdialysis. Brain Res. Bull. **35:** 247–251.

67. SCHETINGER, M.R., C.K. BARCELLOS, A. BARLEM, G. ZWESTCH, A. GUBERT, C. BERTUOL, N. ARTENI, R.D. DIAS, J.J. SARKIS & C.A. NETTO. 1994. Activity of synaptosomal ATP diphosphohydrolase from hippocampus of rats tolerant to forebrain ischemia. Braz. J. Med. Biol. Res. **27:** 1123–1128.

68. SHIMAZAKI, K., A. ISHIDA & N. KAWAI. 1994. Increase in bcl-2 oncoprotein and the tolerance to ischemia-induced neuronal death in the gerbil hippocampus. Neurosci. Res. **20:** 95–99.

69. HEURTEAUX, C., I. LAURITZEN, C. WIDMANN & M. LAZDUNSKI. 1995. Essential role of adenosine, adenosine A$_1$ receptors, and ATP-sensitive K$^+$ channels in cerebral ischemic preconditioning. Proc. Natl. Acad. Sci. USA **92:** 4666–4670.

70. KATO, H., K. KOGURE, T. ARAKI & Y. ITOYAMA. 1995. Induction of Jun-like immunoreactivity in gerbil hippocampus with ischemic tolerance. Neurosci. Lett. **189:** 13–16.

71. KATO, H., K. KOGURE, T. ARAKI, X.H. LIU, K. KATO & Y. ITOYAMA. 1995. Immunohistochemical localization of superoxide dismutase in the hippocampus following ischemia in a gerbil model of ischemic tolerance. J. Cereb. Blood Flow Metab. **15:** 60–70.

72. KATO, H., K. KOGURE, N. NAKATA, T. ARAKI, Y. ITOYAMA. 1995. Facilitated recovery from postischemic suppression of protein synthesis in the gerbil brain with ischemic tolerance. Brain Res. Bull. **36:** 205–208.

73. MATSUSHIMA, K. & A.M. HAKIM. 1995. Transient forebrain ischemia protects against subsequent focal cerebral ischemia without changing cerebral perfusion. Stroke **26:** 1047–1052.

74. SOMMER, C., P. GASS & M. KIESSLING. 1995. Selective c-JUN expression in CA1 neurons of the gerbil hippocampus during and after acquisition of an ischemia-tolerant state. Brain Pathol. **5:** 135–144.

75. OHNO, M. & S. WATANABE. 1996. Ischemic tolerance to memory impairment associated with hippocampal neuronal damage after transient cerebral ischemia in rats. Brain Res. Bull. **40:** 229–236.

76. OHTSUKI, T., C.A. RUETZLER, K. TASAKI & J.M. HALLENBECK. 1996. Interleukin-1 mediates induction of tolerance to global ischemia in gerbil hippocampal CA1 neurons. J. Cereb. Blood Flow Metab. **16**(6)**:** 1137–1142.

77. CORBETT, D. & P. CROOKS. 1997. Ischemic preconditioning: a long term survival study using behavioural and histological endpoints. Brain Res. **760:** 129–136.

78. KATAYAMA, Y., H. MURAMATSU, T. KAMIYA, A. MCKEE & A. TERASHI. 1997. Ischemic tolerance phenomenon from an approach of energy metabolism and the mitochondrial enzyme activity of pyruvate dehydrogenase in gerbils. Brain Res. **746:** 126–132.

79. Li, J.Y., H. Ueda, A. Seiyama, M. Nakano, M. Matsumoto & T. Yanagihara. 1997. A near-infrared spectroscopic study of cerebral ischemia and ischemic tolerance in gerbils. Stroke **28:** 1451–1456; discussion 1456–1457.

80. Sorimachi, T., S. Takeuchi, H. Abe, R. Tanaka. 1997. Effect of acquired tolerance to ischemia on focal infarction in gerbils. Neurol. Med. Chir. **37:** 236–242.

81. Wada, K., T. Miyazawa, H. Katoh, N. Nomura, A. Yano, K. Shima & H. Chigasaki. 1997. Intraischemic hypothemia during pretreatment with sublethal ischemia reduces the induction of ischemic tolerance in the gerbil hippocampus. Brain Res. **746:** 301–304.

82. Kawai, K., T. Nakagomi, T. Kirino, A. Tamura & N. Kawai. 1998. Preconditioning *in vivo* ischemia inhibits anoxic long-term potentiation and functionally protects CA1 neurons in the gerbil. J. Cereb. Blood Flow Metab. **18:** 288–296.

83. Nakano, M., H. Ueda, J.-Y. Li, M. Matsumoto & T. Yanagihara. 1998. Measurement of regional N-acetylaspartate after transient global ischemia in gerbils with and without ischemic tolerance: an index of neuronal survival. Ann. Neurol. **44:** 334–340.

84. Yoneda,Y., N. Kuramoto, Y. Azuma, K. Ogita, A. Mitani, L. Zhang, H. Yanese, S. Masuda & K. Kataoka. 1998. Possible involvement of activator protein-1 DNA binding in mechanisms underlying ischemic tolerance in the CA1 subfield of gerbil hippocampus. Neuroscience **86:** 79–97.

85. Glazier, S.S., D.M. O'Rourke, D.I. Graham & F.A. Welsh. 1994. Induction of ischemic tolerance following brief focal ischemia in rat brain. J. Cereb. Blood Flow Metab. **14:** 545–553.

86. Chen, J., S.H. Graham, R.L. Zhu & R.P. Simon. 1996. Stress proteins and tolerance to focal cerebral ischemia. J. Cereb. Blood Flow Metab. **16:** 566–577.

87. Toyoda, T., N.F. Kassell & K.S. Lee. 1997. Induction of ischemic tolerance and antioxidant activity by brief focal ischemia. Neuroreport **8:** 847–851.

88. Barone, F.C., R.F. White, P.A. Spera, J. Ellison, R.W. Currie, X. Wang & G.Z. Feuerstein. 1998. Ischemic preconditioning and brain tolerance: temporal histological and functional outcomes, protein synthesis requirement, and interleukin-1 receptor antagonist and early gene expression. Stroke **29:** 1937–1950; discussion 1950–1951.

89. Chimon, G.N. & P.T. Wong. 1998. Ischemic tolerance and lipid peroxidation in the brain. Neuroreport **9:** 2269–2272.

90. Wang, X., S. Yaish-Ohad, X. Li, F.C. Barone & G.Z. Feuerstein. 1998. Use of suppression subtractive hybridization strategy for discovery of increased tissue inhibitor of matrix metalloproteinase-1 gene expression in brain ischemic tolerance. J. Cereb. Blood Flow Metab. **18:** 1173–1177.

91. Bergeron, M., D.M. Ferriero, H.J. Vreman, D.K. Stevenson & F.R. Sharp. 1997. Hypoxia-ischemia, but not hypoxia alone, induces the expression of heme oxygenase-1 (HSP32) in newborn rat brain. J. Cereb. Blood Flow Metab. **17:** 647–658.

92. Cai, Z., J.D. Fratkin & P.G. Rhodes. 1997. Prenatal ischemia reduces neuronal injury caused by neonatal hypoxia-ischemia in rats. Neuroreport **8:** 1393–1398.

93. Ota, A., T. Ikeda, K. Abe, H. Sameshima, X.Y. Xia, & T. Ikenoue. 1998. Hypoxic-ischemic tolerance phenomenon observed in neonatal rat brain. Am. J. Obstet. Gynecol. **179:** 1075–1078.

94. Vannucci, R.C., J. Towfighi & S.J. Vannucci. 1998. Hypoxic preconditioning and hypoxic-ischemic brain damage in the immature rat: pathologic and metabolic correlates. J. Neurochem. **71:** 1215–1220.

95. Ohtsuki, T., M. Matsumoto, K. Kuwabara, K. Kitagawa, K. Suzuki, N. Taniguchi & T. Kamada. 1992. Influence of oxidative stress on induced tolerance to ischemia in gerbil hippocampal neurons. Brain Res. **599:** 246–252.

96. RIEPE, M.W., W.N. NIEMI, D. MEGOW, A.C. LUDOLPH & D.O. CARPENTER. 1996. Mitochondrial oxidation in rat hipocampus can be preconditioned by selective chemical inhibition of succinic dehydrogenase. Exp. Neurol. **138:** 15–21.

97. RIEPE, M.W. & A.C. LUDOLPH. 1997. Chemical preconditioning: a cytoprotective strategy. Mol. Cell. Biochem. **174:** 249–254.

98. KAWAHARA, N., S.D. CROLL, S.J. WIEGAND & I. KLATZO. 1997. Cortical spreading depression induces long-term alterations of BDNF levels in cortex and hippocampus distinct from lesion effects: implications for ischemic tolerance. Neurosci. Res. **29:** 37–47.

99. PLUMIER, J.-C., J.-C. DAVID, H.A. ROBERTSON & R.W. CURRIE. 1997. Cortical application of potassium chloride induces the low-molecular weight heat shock protein (Hsp27) in astrocytes. J. Cereb. Blood Flow Metab. **17:** 781–790.

100. TAGA, K., P.M. PATEL, J.C. DRUMMOND, D.J. COLE & P.J. KELLY. 1997. Transient neuronal depolarization induces tolerance to subsequent forebrain ischemia in rats. Anesthesiology **87:** 918–925.

101. CAGGIANO, A.O. & R.P. KRAIG. 1998. Neuronal nitric oxide synthase expression is induced in neocortical astrocytes after spreading depression. J. Cereb. Blood Flow Metab. **18:** 75–87.

102. NISHIO, S., M. YUNOKI, Z-F. CHEN, M. ANZIVINO & K.S. LEE. Ischemic tolerance in the rat neocortex following hypothermic preconditioning. Submitted.

103. SAKATA, M., H. YANAMOTO, N. HASHIMOTO, K. IIHARA, T. TSUKAHARA, T. TANIGUCHI & H. KIKUCHI. 1998. Induction of infarct tolerance by platelet-derived growth factor against reversible temporary focal ischemia. Brain Res. **784:** 250–255.

104. BECKER, K.J., R.M. MCCARRON, C. RUETZLER, O. LABAN, E. STERNBERG, K.C. FLANDERS & J.M. HALLENBECK. 1997. Immunologic tolerance to myelin basic protein decreases stroke size after transient focal cerebral ischemia. Proc. Natl. Acad. Sci. USA **94:** 10873–10878.

105. NAKATA, N., H. KATO & K. KOGURE. 1993. Inhibition of ischaemic tolerance in the gerbil hippocampus by quercetin and anti-heat shock protein-70 antibody. Neuroreport **4:** 695–698.

106. OHTSUKI, T., M. MATSUMOTO, K. KITAGAWA, A. TAGUCHI, Y. MAEDA, R. HATA, S. OGAWA, H. UEDA, N. HANDA & T. KAMADA. 1993. Induced resistance and susceptibility to cerebral ischemia in gerbil hippocampal neurons by prolonged but mild hypoperfusion. Brain Res. **614:** 279–284.

107. KATO, H., T. ARAKI, Y. ITOYAMA, K. KOGURE & K. KATO. 1995. An immunohistochemical study of heat shock protein-27 in the hippocampus in a gerbil model of cerebral ischemia and ischemic tolerance. Neuroscience **68:** 65–71.

108. ABE, H. & T.S. NOWAK, JR. 1996. Gene expression and induced ischemic tolerance following brief insults. Acta Neurobiol. Exp. **56:** 3–8.

109. KITAGAWA, K., M. MATSUMOTO, K. MATSUSHITA, K. MANDAI, T. MABUCHI, T. YANAGIHARA & T. KAMADA. 1996. Ischemic tolerance in moderately symptomatic gerbils after unilateral carotid occlusion. Brain Res. **716:** 39–46.

110. YENARI, M.A., S.L. FINK, G.H. SUN, L.K. CHANG, M.K. PATEL, D.M. KUNIS, D. ONLEY, D.Y. HO, R.M. SAPOLSKY & G.K.STEINBERG. 1998. Gene therapy with HSP72 is neuroprotective in rat models of stroke and epilepsy. Ann. Neurol. **44:** 584–591.

111. BELAYEV, L., M.D. GINSBERG, O.F. ALONSO, J.T. SINGER, W. ZHAO & R. BUSTO. 1996. Bilateral ischemic tolerance of rat hippocampus induced by prior unilateral focal ischemia: relationship to c-*fos* mRNA expression. Neuroreport **8:** 55–59.

112. TOYODA, T., N.F. KASSELL & K.S. LEE. Preconditioning with the endotoxin analogue, diphosphoryl lipid A, induces tolerance against ischemia/reperfusion injury in the rat brain. Submitted.

113. SIMON, R.P., J. CHEN, R.L. ZHU, J.O. LAN, D.A. GREENBERG & S.H. GRAHAM. 1995. Alteration in anti-apoptotic gene expression associated with induction of tolerance to focal ischemia. Soc. Neurosci. Abstr. **21:** 512.

A Double-Blind, Placebo-Controlled Study of the Safety, Tolerability and Pharmacokinetics of CP-101,606 in Patients with a Mild or Moderate Traumatic Brain Injury

RANDALL E. MERCHANT,[a,c] M. ROSS BULLOCK,[a] CYNTHIA A. CARMACK,[a] AJIT K. SHAH,[b] KEITH D. WILNER,[b] GRANT KO,[b] AND STEPHEN A. WILLIAMS[b]

[a]*Virginia Commonwealth University, Medical College of Virginia, Richmond, Virginia 23298-0631, USA*

[b]*Central Research Division, Pfizer Inc., Groton, Connecticut 06340, USA*

ABSTRACT: CP-101,606 is a postsynaptic antagonist of the glutamate-mediated NR2B subunit of the N-methyl-D-aspartate (NMDA) receptor. When administered intravenously (i.v.) at the time of injury, CP-101,606 is neuroprotective in animal models of traumatic brain injury (TBI) and ischemia. Minimal adverse effects have been observed in normal human volunteers given i.v. doses of up to 3 mg/kg/hr for 72 hours. The objective of the present clinical trial was to assess the safety, pharmacokinetics, and tolerability of CP-101,606 infused for various times in patients who had suffered either an acute moderate or mild TBI (Glasgow Coma Score 9–14) or hemorrhagic stroke. Patients began receiving treatment within 12 hours of brain injury. A total of 53 subjects (45 with TBI and 8 with stroke) were randomized in a double-blind fashion to receive CP-101,606 or placebo (4 drug:1 placebo). Drug/placebo was administered by i.v. infusion (0.75 mg/kg/hr) for 2 hours and then stopped ($n = 25$) or continued for 22 hours ($n = 4$) or 70 hours ($n = 24$) at a rate of 0.37 mg/kg/hr. Mean plasma drug concentrations were well above the predicted therapeutic concentration of 200 ng/ml within two hours of initiating treatment and were sustained as long as drug was infused. All the patients tolerated their drug/placebo treatment, and there were no clinically significant cardiovascular or hematological abnormalities in either group. A Neurobehavioral Rating Scale, used to detect personality changes and behavioral disturbances, indicated that all subjects showed an improvement from their postinjury, predosing baseline but did not significantly differ from each other with respect to type of head injury and/or treatment with drug or placebo. Modified Kurtzke Scoring also showed a similar pattern of improvement irrespective of type of head injury or drug/placebo treatment. This study suggests that CP-101,606, infused for up to 72 hours has no psychotropic effects and is well-tolerated in patients who have sustained a mild or moderate TBI or hemorrhagic stroke.

[c]Corresponding author: Randall E. Merchant, Ph.D., Division of Neurosurgery, Virginia Commonwealth University, Box 980631, MCV Station, Richmond, VA 23298-0631. Phone, 804/828-9528; fax, 804/828-0374.

e-mail, rmerchant@hsc.vcu.edu

INTRODUCTION

CP-101,606 is a postsynaptic *N*-methyl-D-aspartate (NMDA) antagonist with a much more restricted distribution of action than that of other antagonists in that it interacts with only receptors bearing the NR2B regulatory site. *In vitro*, it protects hippocampal neurons from toxic effects of glutamate and antagonizes NMDA-mediated responses in both hippocampal and cortical neurons.[1–3] When administered intravenously (i.v.) at a dose 0.3 mg/kg/hr at the time of injury, CP-101,606 has been shown to be neuroprotective in animal models of brain trauma and ischemia.[4–8] The drug decreased posttraumatic amnesia, neurological dysfunction, infarct size, edema, and intracranial pressure. The drug also appears to have advantages over other available NMDA antagonists in current trials in that it does not appreciably affect locomotor activity or elicit behavioral effects in animals.

Minimal adverse effects have been observed in healthy human volunteers treated i.v. with a dose of up to 3 mg/kg/hr. These subjects did not experience hallucinations, a common side effect that has been reported with other NMDA receptor antagonists.[9] In double-blind placebo-controlled trials, CP-101,606/placebo was infused i.v. for two hours at a dose of 1.5, 5.0, or 15.0 mg/kg/hr in normal male volunteers ($n = 34$). Subjects given the drug had delayed word recall tests compared to placebo, and at the two higher doses, adverse events included anterograde amnesia and memory impairment for up to 48 hours as well as hyperreflexia, dizziness, and sedation. No clinically important laboratory test abnormalities and no significant electrocardiogram (ECG) abnormalities were observed. With regard to pharmacokinetics, the mean C_{max} at the 1.5-mg/kg/hr dose, for extensive metabolizers (EMs) of dextromethorphan was 262 ng/ml, and the plasma half-life ranged from 3–6 hours. While for poor metabolizers (PMs) of dextromethorphan, the mean C_{max} at 1.5 mg/kg was 962 ng/ml and plasma half-life was 15 hours.

In another phase I trial, CP-101,606 or placebo was infused for 24 hours in six healthy volunteers (4 drug:2 placebo). All six were EMs of dextromethorphan. Over the first 15 minutes, the drug was infused at a rate of 2.5 mg/kg/hr followed by 0.3 mg/kg/hr for 23.75 hours. The adverse effects were generally mild or moderate and included dry mouth, eye tearing, floating sensation and somnolence. An additional seven volunteers (4 EMs and 3 PMs) received an i.v. infusion of 2.5 mg/kg/hr of drug for 15 minutes followed by 0.4 mg/kg/hr for 71.75 hours. Two additional EMs were given placebo. The infusions of one PM and one EM were discontinued due to anxiety and unpleasant sensation. Adverse events reported by the others included: facial numbness, nausea, headache, dizziness, spacey feeling, fatigue, amnesia, anxiety, and inflammation at the injection site. These adverse effects cleared after discontinuation of infusion. There were no clinically important laboratory test abnormalities and no significant ECG abnormalities observed. The mean C_{max} for EMs with the 72-hour infusion was 480 ng/ml and 1260 ng/ml for the two PMs.

The present dose-escalation study of CP-101,606 was performed in patients who had suffered a mild or moderate acute traumatic brain injury (TBI) or atraumatic hemorrhagic stroke. The primary objective of this clinical trial was to assess the safety and tolerability of CP-101,606 given as a two-hour i.v. infusion at a dose of 0.75 mg/kg/hr alone or immediately followed by a 22- or 70-hour infusion at 0.37 mg/kg/hr. We also measured the plasma pharmacokinetics of CP-101,606 dur-

TABLE 1. Enrollment criteria

Inclusion criteria

    Subjects between the ages of 14–75 years, inclusive.

    Enrolled within 12 hours of head injury with a GCS of 9–14.

    Positive admission CT scan.

    Females of nonchildbearing potential or negative urine pregnancy test.

    No known life-threatening disease prior to head injury.

    Stable cardiovascular and respiratory function.

    Understand, read, and write English sufficiently to complete testing.

    Legal representative present who can give Informed Consent.

Exclusion criteria

    History of severe illnesses that could affect assessment of therapy.

    Major previous cerebral damage, e.g., major stroke, severe head trauma.

    Massive, dominant hemisphere intracerebral hematoma.

    Severe multiple trauma that could affect assessment of therapy.

    Known exposure to an investigational drug within 30 days of injury.

    Gross hematuria or anuria.

    CT evidence of brainstem hemorrhage or ischemia.

    CT evidence of massive anoxia.

    Creatinine of > 2 mg/dl.

    Known diagnosis of epilepsy or history of convulsions.

ing and after its i.v. administration. Another objective was to determine if there were any trends toward improved neurological outcome compared to placebo-treated controls at three months posttreatment.

SUBJECTS

A total of 53 patients, 39 males and 14 females, ranging in age from 15–78 years who had suffered an acute TBI ($n = 45$) or hemorrhagic stroke ($n = 8$) and who met eligibility criteria (TABLE 1) participated in the study. For the patients with a TBI, their injury was further characterized using the Glasgow Coma Score (GCS). Their distribution according to baseline GCS indicated that 26 had suffered a moderate TBI (GCS 9–12) and 19 a mild TBI (GCS 13–14) (TABLE 2). Among these 45 trauma patients, 31 received their head injury as a result of a motor vehicle accident, 11 by a fall, and 3 from an assault.

Following their admission to hospital, patients were stabilized and assessed as per standard procedures. During this period, eligibility for the study was determined (TABLE 1), and informed consent was obtained from the next of kin. Relevant data particular for the study, including medical history, baseline labs and ECG, and neurological examinations were obtained (see below). In addition, in order to determine whether or not a patient was an EM or PM of dextromethorphan, a blood sample was

TABLE 2. Distribution of subjects by injury, GCS and dosing

Infusion	TBI GCS 9–12	TBI GCS 13–14	Hemorrhagic Stroke	Total Patients
2 hour*	12	6	2	20
24 hour*	2	2	0	4
72 hour*	9	6	4	19
Placebo**	3	5	2	10
Total	26	19	8	53

* Infusion of CP-101,606.
** Infusion of placebo irrespective of length of infusion.

also collected for genotyping of their cytochrome P450 2D6 status. Subjects were then randomized in a double-blind fashion to receive CP-101,606 or placebo (4 drug:1 placebo). These infusions were started within 12 hours of injury or onset of symptoms of stroke. As this was a dose-escalation study, the first series of patients had drug/placebo dosed by i.v. infusion at 0.75 mg/kg/hr for 2 hours and then stopped ($n = 25$). For the next two series of patients, after the two-hour infusion, subjects had their treatment continued at a rate of 0.37 mg/kg/hr for 22 hours ($n = 4$) or 70 hours ($n = 24$) for a total dosing time of 24 and 72 hours, respectively. Twelve different treatment categories of patients were thus defined (TABLE 2).

Over the course of infusion and up to seven days after the start of infusion, the following safety parameters were collected and recorded: mean arterial blood pressure and other vitals, laboratory tests of blood and urine, ECGs, GCS, and behavioral assessments. Plasma concentrations of CP-101,606 were determined from blood samples drawn at 0 (predose), 2, 4, 8, 12, 24, 36, 48, 72, 84, and 96 hours from the start of infusion.

A 10-item Neurobehavioral Rating Scale, was used to detect personality changes and behavioral disturbances during and/or following infusion.[10] These assessments were conducted at 0, 1, 2, 12, 24, 48, and 96 hours from the start of infusion. A Kurtzke Neurologic Status Evaluation[11] was conducted at 0, 12, 24 hours and then daily from the start of infusion for seven days or until day of discharge, whichever came sooner. At three months after injury, outcome was assessed using the Galveston Orientation and Amnesia Test (GOAT), National Institutes of Health (NIH) Stroke Scale, and a battery of nine neuropsychological tests.

RESULTS AND DISCUSSION

A total of 53 patients who met eligibility criteria were randomized in a double-blind fashion to receive CP-101,606 or placebo and began receiving their i.v. infusion of drug/placebo within 12 hours of injury. In the United States, the majority of TBI cases occur in the younger half of the male population as the result of a motor vehicle accident. This trend was evident in our patient population, where 31/45 (69%) of the subjects suffered their mild or moderate TBI as a result of a car accident. Males outnumbered females by a ratio of roughly 3 to 1. The majority (36/53) of the patients were forty years of age or younger, with the 14–20-year-old group having the greatest number represented (18/53) of any decade. The nature of TBI

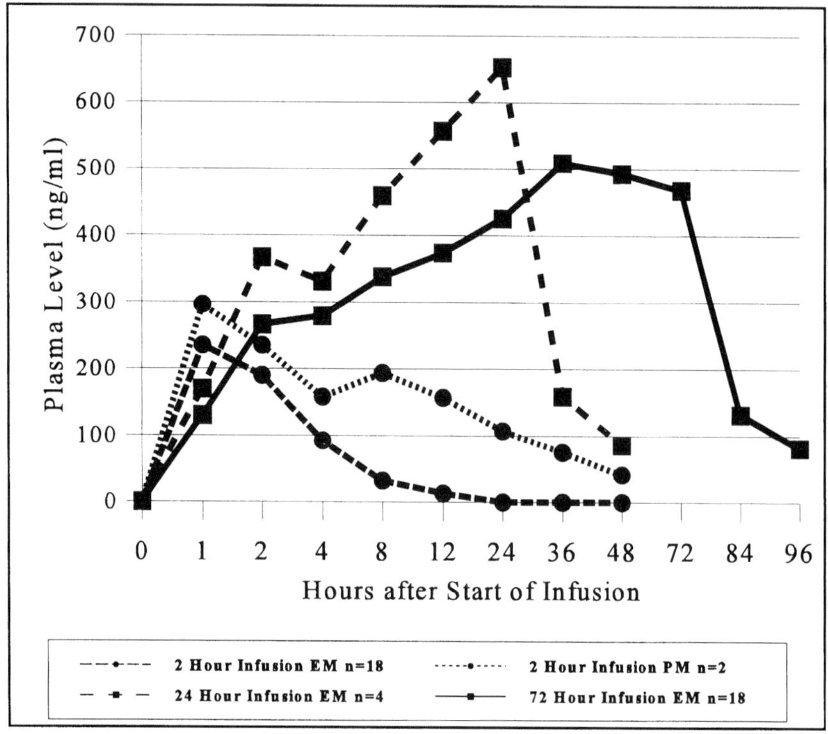

FIGURE 1. Pharmacokinetics of CP-101,606 in TBI patients.

subjects' injuries as revealed by CT scan was quite varied and included nearly every possible type such as cerebral contusions, subdural and epidural hematomas, intraventricular hemorrhage, and diffuse axonal injury. Cerebral contusions, however, were the most common finding, occurring in 21 of the 45 TBI cases.

The neurological status of all patients was characterized upon admission using the GCS. For the 45 TBI patients, this assessment categorized 26 (58%) as having suffered a moderate injury (GCS 9–12) and 19 (42%) a mild head injury (GCS 13–14). Subjects who met eligibility criteria were randomized in a double-blind fashion to receive CP-101,606 or placebo (4 drug:1 placebo). Drug/placebo was administered by i.v. infusion (0.75 mg/kg/hr) for 2 hours and then stopped or continued for 22 hours or 70 hours at a rate of 0.37 mg/kg/hr. Twenty-five subjects (22 TBI, 3 stroke) received the two-hour treatment, four TBI subjects received the 24-hour infusion, and 24 subjects (19 TBI, 5 stroke) were given the 72-hour infusion. Over the course of treatment and up to seven days after the start of infusion, blood pressure, heart rate, and body temperature were regularly monitored (data not shown). In addition, at 2 and 12 hours and then daily from the start of infusion until day seven or discharge, routine laboratory analyzes of blood and urine and ECGs were performed. The results of this monitoring showed that all the subjects tolerated their drug or pla-

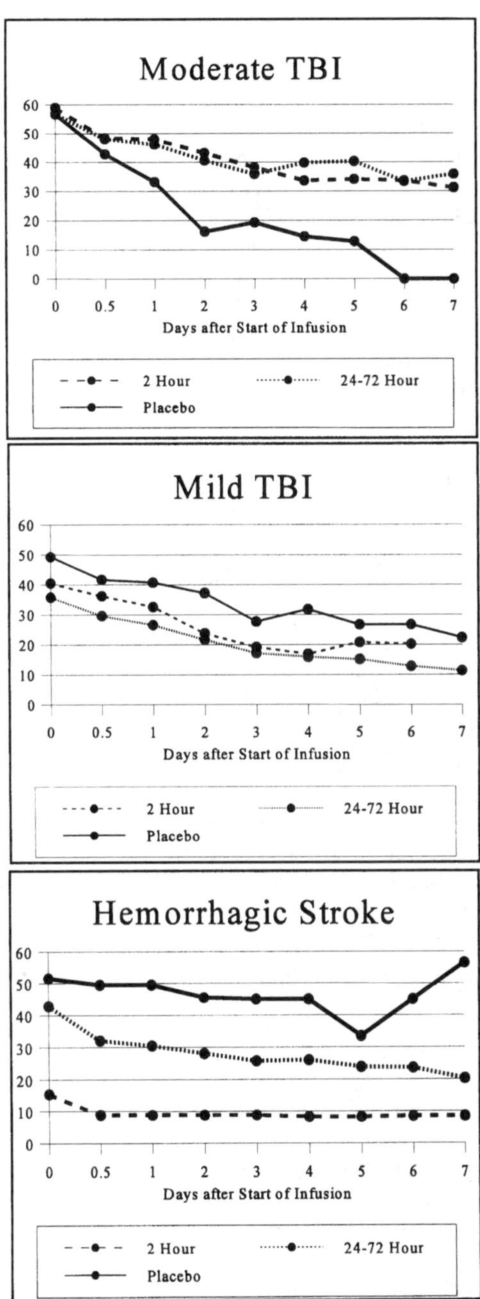

FIGURE 2. Neurobehavioral rating scale results.

cebo treatment and, irrespective of dose or type of head injury, there were no clinically significant cardiovascular or hematological abnormalities. No adverse events were attributed to study medication.

Plasma concentrations of CP-101,606 were determined from blood samples drawn at 0, 2, 4, 8, 12, 24, 36, 48, 72, 84, and 96 hours from the start of infusion. Mean plasma CP-101,606 concentrations were well above the predicted therapeutic concentration of 200 ng/ml within two hours of initiating treatment and were sustained as long as drug was infused (FIG. 1). For the 2-hour infusion, the mean plasma concentrations of CP-101,606 in both EMs ($n = 18$) and PMs ($n = 2$) were already above 200 ng/ml by the end of the first hour and were sustained over the next hour. For the EMs, the mean plasma concentration fell by 50% within two hours of stopping the infusion, while for PMs, plasma CP-101,606 concentrations were measurable up to 48 hours. For the four EM patients who received a 24-hour infusion, their mean plasma concentration of CP-101,606 peaked at the end of infusion at 653 ng/ml and then decreased rapidly by more than 80% after 24 hours. With a 72-hour infusion, the mean plasma concentration of drug appeared to plateau around 450 ng/ml at 24 hours into the infusion. For these patients, who were all EMs, mean plasma levels fell by 90% 24 hours after stopping the treatment.

The GCS score of patients was recorded at 1, 2, 4, 8, 12, 24, 36, 48, 72, 84, and 96 hours and then daily from the start of infusion until two consecutive scores of 15 were obtained. The GCS assessments of most patients indicated a rapid and steady improvement over the course of the infusion and afterward (data not shown). There were no apparent differences, however, in the speed of this improvement with regard to total dose of CP-101,606/placebo or type of head injury.

A Neurobehavioral Rating Scale, scored by a neuropsychologist, was used to detect personality changes and behavioral disturbances during and/or following infusion of CP-101,606 or placebo. This 10-item assessment was made at 0, 1, 2, 12, 24, 48, and 96 hours from the start of infusion and examined: attention, somatic concern, orientation, expression, conceptual disorganization, disinhibition, memory, agitation, motor retardation, and hallucinatory behavior. The patient's level of functioning was scored on a 4-point scale: not present (0), mild (1), moderate (2), severe (3). Therefore, the lower the score, the more normal a patient's behavior. Patients' scores from each assessment were totaled, and the averages for the various treatment groups are presented in FIGURE 2. All groups showed an improvement from baseline but did not significantly differ from each other with respect to type of head injury or if their treatment had been with CP-101,606 or placebo.

The Kurtzke Neurologic Status Evaluation was done to assess the functional neurological status of patients at 0, 12, 24 hours and then daily from the start of infusion for up to seven days. The results of this assessment indicated a pattern and rate of improvement comparable to that of the Neurobehavioral Scale. This evaluation indicated there were no significant differences in functional neurological status between types of head injury or whether or not the patients had been treated with CP-101,606 or placebo (data not shown).

At three months post-head injury, outcome was assessed using the GOAT, NIH Stroke Scale, and a battery of nine neuropsychological tests, which included the Wechsler Memory Scale-Revised Logical Memory I & II, Rey Osterreith Complex Figure, Grooved Pegboard, Trail Making Test A & B, Controlled Oral Word

Association, Symbol Digit Modalities Test, Rey Auditory Verbal Learning Test, Beck Depression Inventory, and Paced Auditory Serial Addition Test. While all of the participants could perform the tests, due to the relatively small numbers of patients in the different head injury groups and for each infusion rate, no statistical differences in outcome could be determined between treatment groups with these assessments. A much larger, double-blind, placebo-controlled trial will, therefore, be needed to show if treatment with CP-101,606 affects recovery from head injury as demonstrated by these neuropsychological tests.

Studies of CP-101,606 using animal models of neurotrauma and brain ischemia showed that a plasma level of 200 ng/ml was neuroprotective.[4–8] The present clinical trial demonstrates that in subjects who have suffered a mild or moderate TBI or hemorrhagic stroke, plasma levels of CP-101,606 could be sustained above 200 ng/ml for as long as 72 hours without any significant adverse physical, hematological, cardiovascular or neurobehavioral effects.

CONCLUSIONS

At all three doses tested in this double-blind placebo-controlled study, CP-101,606 was well-tolerated and there were no clinically significant cardiovascular or hematological abnormalities. Furthermore, no adverse events or behaviors were observed that could be considered related to or possibly related to CP-101,606. Mean plasma drug concentrations well above 200 ng/ml, the therapeutic concentration in animal models of brain injury, were attained within two hours of initiating treatment and were sustained as long as drug was infused. The results of this study suggest that unlike other NMDA receptor antagonists, CP-101,606 had no psychotropic effects and was well-tolerated in patients who had sustained either a mild or moderate TBI or an atraumatic hemorrhagic stroke.

REFERENCES

1. CHENARD, B.L., J. BORDNER, T.W. BUTLER, L.K. CHAMBERS, M.A. COLLINS, D.L. DECOSTA, M.F. DUCAT, M.L. DUMONT, C.B. FOX, E.E. MENA, F.S. MENNITI, J. NIELSEN, M.J. PAGNOZZI, K.E.G. RICHTER, R.T. RONAU, I.A. SHALABY, J.Z. STEMPLE & W.F. WHITE. 1995. (1*S*,2*S*)-1-(4-hydroxyphenyl)-2-(4-hydroxy-4-phenylpiperidino)-1-propanol: a potent new neuroprotectant which blocks *N*-methyl-D-aspartate responses. J. Med. Chem. **38:** 3138–3145.
2. BRIMECOMBE, J.C., M.J. GALLAGHER, D.R. LYNCH & E. AIZENMAN. 1998. An NR2B point mutation affecting haloperidol and CP-101,606 sensitivity of single recombinant *N*-methyl-D-aspartate receptors. J. Pharmacol. Exp. Ther. **286:** 627–634.
3. MENNITI, F.S., B.L. CHENARD, M. COLLINS, M. DUCAT, I. SHALABY & W.F. WHITE. 1997. CP-101,606, a potent neuroprotectant selective for forebrain neurons. Eur. J. Pharmacol. **331:** 117–126.
4. OKIYAMA, K., D.H. SMITH, W.F. WHITE & T.K. MCINTOSH. 1998. Effects of the NMDA antagonist CP-98,113 on regional cerebral edema and cerebrovascular, cognitive, and neurobehavioral function following experimental brain injury in the rat. Brain Res. **792:** 291–298.
5. OKIYAMA, K., D.H. SMITH, W.F. WHITE, K. RICHTER & T.K. MCINTOSH. 1997. Effects of the novel NMDA antagonists CP-98,113, CP-101,581 and CP-101,606 on cogni-

tive function and regional cerebral edema following experimental brain injury in the rat. J. Neurotrauma **14:** 211–222.

6. MENNITI, F.S., M.J. PAGNOZZI, P. BUTLER, B.L. CHENARD, S.S. JAW-TSAI & W.F. WHITE. 1998. CP-101,606, an NR2B subunit selective NMDA receptor antagonist, inhibits NMDA and injury induced c-fos expression and cortical spreading depression in rodents. Eur. J. Pharmacol. Submitted.

7. TSUCHIDA, E., M. RICE & R. BULLOCK. 1997. The neuroprotective effect of the forebrain-selective NMDA antagonist CP-101,606 upon focal ischemic damage caused by acute subdural hematoma in the rat. J. Neurotrauma **14:** 409–417.

8. DI, X., R. BULLOCK, J. WATSON, P. FATOUROS, B. CHENARD, F. WHITE & F. CORWIN. 1997. Effect of CP-101,606, a novel NR2B subunit antagonist of the N-methyl-D-aspartate receptor, on the volume of ischemic brain damage and cytotoxic brain edema after middle cerebral artery occlusion in the feline brain. Stroke **28:** 2244–2251.

9. MUIR, K.W. & K.R. LEES. 1995. Clinical experience with excitatory amino acid antagonist drugs. Stroke **26:** 503–513.

10. LEVIN, H.S., W.M. HIGH, C.A. MEYERS *et al.* 1987. Neurobehavioral outcome of minor head injury: a three center study. J. Neurosurg. **66:** 234-243.

11. KURTZKE, J.F. 1995. A new scale for evaluating disability in multiple sclerosis. Neurology **5:** 580-583.

An Open-Label Study of CP-101,606 in Subjects with a Severe Traumatic Head Injury or Spontaneous Intracerebral Hemorrhage

M. ROSS BULLOCK,[a] RANDALL E. MERCHANT,[a,c] CYNTHIA A. CARMACK,[a] EGON DOPPENBERG,[a] AJIT K. SHAH,[b] KEITH D. WILNER,[b] GRANT KO,[b] AND STEPHEN A. WILLIAMS[b]

[a]Virginia Commonwealth University, Medical College of Virginia, Richmond, Virginia 23298-0631, USA

[b]Central Research Division, Pfizer Inc., Groton, Connecticut 06340, USA

ABSTRACT: CP-101,606 is a postsynaptic antagonist of N-methyl-D-aspartate (NMDA) receptors bearing the NR2B subunit. When administered intravenously (i.v.), it decreases the effects of traumatic brain injury (TBI) and focal ischemia in animal models. Therapeutic plasma concentrations (200 ng/ml) in animals, have been well tolerated in healthy human volunteers. The purpose of the present dose escalation study was to assess the safety, tolerability, and pharmacokinetics of CP-101,606 in subjects who had suffered either an acute severe TBI (Glasgow Coma Scale 3–8) or spontaneous intracerebral hemorrhage. Thirty patients, 20 with a TBI and 10 with a stroke, were enrolled in the trial and began receiving an i.v. infusion of CP-101,606 for 2 hours, 24 hours, or 72 hours within 12 hours of brain injury. For the first two hours, the drug was given a rate of 0.75 mg/kg/hr and then stopped ($n = 17$) or continued for 22 ($n = 2$) or 70 hours ($n = 11$) at 0.37 mg/kg/hr. Plasma and cerebrospinal fluid (CSF) were collected at serial times during and after treatment. There were no consistent changes in blood pressure or pulse nor any clinically significant hematological or electrocardiogram (ECG) abnormalities attributable to CP-101,606. No adverse events or behavioral changes were considered to be related to the drug. Plasma concentrations of CP-101,606 over 200 ng/ml were rapidly achieved in the blood and CSF within two hours and were sustained there as long as the drug was infused. CSF concentrations were slightly higher than that in plasma by the end of infusion suggesting good penetration of CP-101,606 into the CSF. Outcome in the severe TBI patients, as measured by the Glasgow Outcome Score at six months, suggested that a two-hour infusion yielded a range of scores similar to contemporary patients with a severe TBI treated at our hospital while the outcomes of the patients treated with either a 24- or 72-hour infusion were better on average. Thus, these results indicate that CP-101,606 infused for up to 72 hours is well tolerated, penetrates the CSF and brain, and may improve outcome in the brain-injured patient.

[c]Corresponding author: Randall E. Merchant, Ph.D., Division of Neurosurgery, Virginia Commonwealth University, Box 980631 MCV Station, Richmond, VA 23298-0631. Phone, 804/828-9528; fax, 804/828-0374.

e-mail, rmerchant@hsc.vcu.edu

TABLE 1. *In vivo* activity of CP-101,606 in animal models of TBI and ischemia

Rodent models of TBI[2–4]
Decreases posttraumatic amnesia
Decreases posttraumatic neurological dysfunction
Decreases posttraumatic edema
Decreases posttraumatic elevation of ICP
Decreases posttraumatic c-fos induction
Decreases cortical spreading depression
Rodent model of subdural hematoma[5]
Decreases infarct volume
Rodent models of ischemic stroke
Improves neurological score
Increases survival
Cat model of ischemic stroke[6]
Decreases infarct volume
Decreases lactate accumulation

INTRODUCTION

CP-101,606 antagonizes glutamate at an allosteric regulatory site on the *N*-methyl-D-aspartate (NMDA) receptor. In rats, the drug readily crosses the blood-brain barrier and inhibits forebrain NMDA receptors.[1,2] CP-101,606 appears to act selectively on neurons with the NR2B receptor subtype, which are distributed mainly in the cortex and hippocampus, areas especially vulnerable to injury from trauma and ischemia. At plasma concentrations of 200 ng/ml or higher, CP-101,606 decreases the effects of traumatic brain injury (TBI) and focal ischemia in animal models (TABLE 1).[3–7] Phase I clinical trials in normal volunteers have shown that it is well tolerated at plasma concentrations two to three times the therapeutic level in animal models. The plasma half-life ranged from 3–6 hours for volunteers who were extensive metabolizers (EMs) of dextromethorphan and twice as long for poor metabolizers (PMs). No clinically significant laboratory test abnormalities were seen, but some adverse events were reported including facial numbness, nausea, headache, dizziness, fatigue, spacey feeling, amnesia, anxiety, and inflammation at the injection site. All adverse events cleared spontaneously and did not recur after discontinuation of infusion.

The principal objective of the present clinical trial was to assess the safety and tolerability of CP-101,606 when given for two hours at a dose of 0.75 mg/kg/hr and then for 22 or 70 more hours at a dose of 0.37 mg/kg/hr in subjects with either a severe traumatic brain injury or a spontaneous intracerebral hemorrhage. Secondarily, we measured the concentrations of CP-101,606 in the plasma and cerebrospinal fluid (CSF) at different times during and after the drug's intravenous (i.v.) infusion.

TABLE 2. Distribution of TBI subjects by injury, baseline GCS and dosing

Dosing	Stroke	TBI (GCS)						Total
		3	4	5	6	7	8	
2 Hour	8	0	2	0	1	4	2	17
24 Hour	0	0	0	0	1	0	1	2
72 Hour	2	1	4	0	3	1	0	11
Total	10	1	6	0	5	5	3	30

SUBJECTS

This study utilized 30 patients, 20 of whom had suffered a severe TBI (Glasgow Coma Scale (GCS) 3–8) and 10 of whom had an atraumatic hemorrhagic stroke (TABLE 2). There were 21 men and 9 women, and they ranged in age from 14 to 72 years. They all had a demonstrable brain abnormality on computerized tomography (CT) scan.

Upon admission, patients were stabilized, and their eligibility for the study was determined (TABLE 3). Information relevant to the study, including medical history, baseline labs, electrocardiogram (ECG), and neurological exams was then obtained. In addition, in order to establish whether a patient was either an EM or PM of dextromethorphan, a sample of whole blood was obtained for assessment to determine their cytochrome P450 2D6 status by genotyping. Within 12 hours of brain injury, treatment with the investigational drug was begun. The first series of patients ($n = 17$) had CP-101,606 administered by i.v. infusion at a dose of 0.75 mg/kg/hr for 2 hours. The next two series of patients received an i.v. infusion for a total of 24 ($n = 2$) or 72 ($n = 11$) hours. All these subjects received an initial loading infusion at 0.75 mg/kg/hr for 2 hours followed by either 22 or 70 hours at a rate of 0.37 mg/kg/hr.

Over the course of infusion and for up to seven days after the start of infusion, safety parameters including vitals and intracranial pressure (when available) were constantly monitored. In addition, laboratory tests of blood and urine, ECGs, and GCS examinations were performed at regular intervals. Plasma and CSF (when available) samples for CP-101,606 determination were obtained at 0 (predose), 1, 2, 4, 8, 12, 24, 36, 48, 72, 84, and 96 hours from the start of infusion. In one patient, microdialysis was used to determine the concentration of CP-101,606 in the extracellular fluid.[8]

RESULTS AND DISCUSSION

All patients had to have an acute abnormality on CT scan and begin receiving treatment with the investigational drug within 12 hours of injury. In all, 30 patients ranging in age from 14 to 72 years were enrolled and, of these, 20 had a severe TBI and 10 had a hemorrhagic stroke. For the 20 patients with a severe TBI, two-thirds were injured as a result of a motor vehicle accident, six were injured from a fall, and two had been assaulted. While all types of injury were seen, the most common ab-

TABLE 3. Enrollment criteria

Inclusion criteria

    Between the ages of 14 and 75 years, inclusive

    Enrolled within 12 hours of head injury or positive diagnosis of hemorrhage

    Positive admission CT scan

    Females of non-childbearing potential or have a negative urine pregnancy test

    No known life-threatening disease prior to head injury or hemorrhage

    Stable cardiovascular and respiratory function

    Legal representative present who can give Informed Consent

Exclusion criteria

    No motor response

    Both pupils fixed and dilated

    Severe illnesses that could affect assessment of the investigational drug

    Known major previous cerebral damage, e.g., major stroke, severe head trauma

    Dominant hemisphere intracerebral hematoma incompatible with survival

    Severe multiple trauma that could affect assessment of investigational drug

    Known exposure to an investigational drug within 30 days of injury

    Gross hematuria or anuria

    CT evidence of brainstem hemorrhage or ischemia

    CT evidence of massive anoxia

    Creatinine of >2 mg/dl

    Known diagnosis of epilepsy or history of convulsions

TABLE 4. Six month outcome as measured by the GOS

Infusion	Good	Moderate	Severe	Vegetative	Dead
2 Hour ($n = 9$)	22%	33%	11%	0	33%
24 Hour ($n = 2$)	50%	0	50%	0	0
72 Hour ($n = 9$)	78%	22%	0	0	0
Overall ($n = 20$)	50%	25%	10%	0	15%
Controls[a] ($n = 250$)	8%	12%	29%	8%	43%

[a]All patients with a severe TBI admitted to the MCVH from 1992–1997.

normalities indicated by CT scan were cerebral contusions, subdural hematoma, or subarachnoid hemorrhage.

Patients were treated with an i.v. infusion of CP-101,606 for 2 hours ($n = 17$), 24 hours ($n = 2$), or 72 hours ($n = 11$). For the first two hours, the drug was given at a rate of 0.75 mg/kg/hr and then stopped or continued for 22 or 70 hours at 0.37 mg/kg/hr. Before, during and after the infusion, safety parameters including vitals, GCS and intracranial pressure (when available) were constantly monitored. In addition, analyzes of blood, urine, and ECGs were performed at regular intervals. Results with brain injured patients were comparable to those of healthy subjects, that is, there were no consistent changes in cardiovascular function nor any clinically significant hematological or ECG abnormalities attributable to CP-101,606. There was also no adverse event or behavioral change considered to be related to the drug.

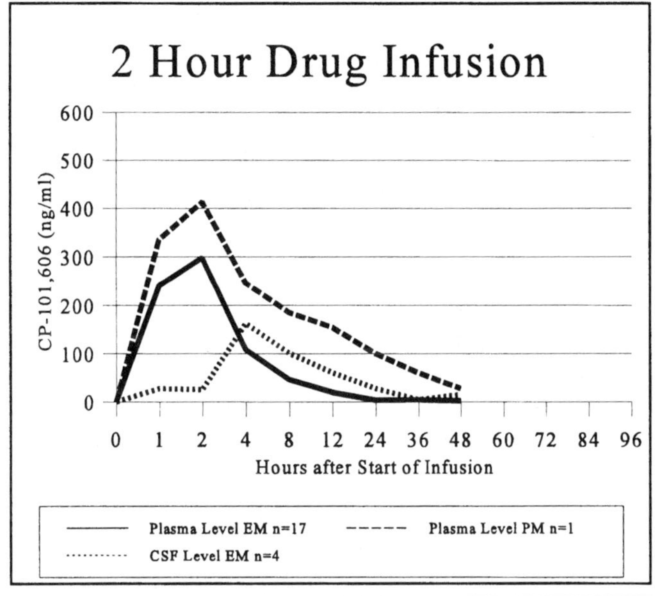

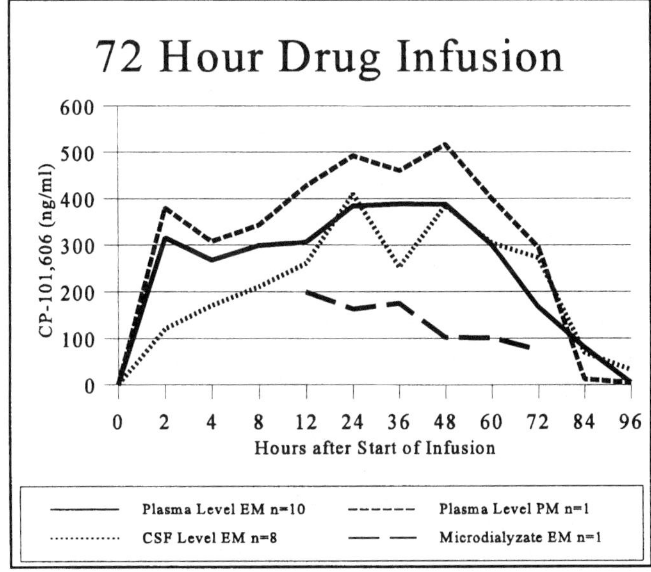

FIGURE 1. Pharmacokinetics in severe TBI patients.

Samples of plasma and when available, CSF, were taken at baseline and then at 1, 2, 4, 8, 12, 24, 36, 48, 72, 84, and 96 hours from the start of infusion for determination of CP-101,606 pharmacokinetics (FIG. 1). At the dose of 0.75 mg/kg/hr, plasma concentrations of CP-101,606 above 200 ng/ml, the therapeutic drug concentration in animal models, were achieved within an hour for both EM and PM patients. The plasma CP-101,606 concentrations in the 17 EM patients who received only the two-hour infusion fell below the 200 ng/ml level within two hours of stopping the infusion while, it took nearly six hours for the single PM. Three EM patients' CSF concentrations of drug were examined. CP-101,606 entered the CSF, but its concentration lagged behind that of the plasma, peaking at 162 ng/ml two hours after stopping the infusion. For the EM patients, CSF concentrations of CP-101,606 then remained higher than plasma concentrations until hour 36, when the drug could no longer be detected in either fluid.

Plasma drug concentrations for the 11 subjects in the 72-hour infusion group reached 200 ng/ml within an hour and were maintained above this concentration as long as the drug was infused (FIG. 1). The level in the one PM patient was approximately 20% higher than that of the 10 EMs. CSF was available from 8 of the EM subjects. As had been the case in the two-hour infusion group, the CP-101,606 concentration in the CSF lagged behind that of the plasma for the first four hours after the start of infusion. Thereafter, the CSF concentrations were higher than the plasma concentrations and were measurable up to 48 hours. Twelve hours after concluding the 72-hour infusion, plasma and CSF concentrations of CP-101,606 dropped by 75% and was nearly cleared from both after another 12 hours (i.e., at 96 hours post-initiation of treatment).

Microdialysis was performed on one patient in the 72-hour infusion group in order to detect the presence of the drug in the brain extracellular fluid[8] (FIG. 1). The first microdialysate sample taken at 12 hours after the start of infusion contained 200 ng CP-101,606 per ml. This level was maintained for up to 36 hours but then decreased to 102 ng/ml at the 48-hour time point after the start of infusion. It remained at approximately this concentration until the end of the infusion period of 72 hours. This is, to our knowledge, the first such use of clinical microdialysis to confirm adequate brain penetration by a neuroprotective drug.

At one, three, and six months post-brain injury, patients who had had a severe TBI were interviewed in order to determine their Glasgow Outcome Score (GOS). For the seven patients in the two-hour infusion group who survived to one month, one patient was good, three were moderate, and three were vegetative. At three months, one of the vegetative patients was rated moderate and one had died in the meantime. The status of the remaining patients was unchanged. For the two patients treated with a 24-hour infusion of CP-101,606, one was rated moderate and the other vegetative at one month post-injury, and both improved by one category by three months after injury. All nine of the patients treated for 72 hours survived to one month. At the time of this evaluation, six were rated moderate and three severe. After another two months, all six of the moderates and one of the severes were rated good. The other two remained severe.

The GOS of TBI patients at six months (TABLE 4) indicated that for the six survivors of the two-hour infusion group, two were good, three moderate, and one severe. The GOS of the two who had received the 24-hour treatment group was unchanged; i.e., one good and one severe. For the nine who were treated with CP-101,606 for 72 hours, seven were categorized as good and two moderate. These results suggested that a two-hour infusion of CP-101,606 yielded a range of GOS scores similar to historical controls who had received treatment for their severe TBI at the Medical College of Virginia Hospitals (MCVH) in the six years preceding this trial (TABLE 4). The outcomes of the patients treated with 72-hour infusions, however, appeared to be significantly better. Looking at our study population as a whole and disregarding the length of time CP-101,606 was infused, ten (50%) of our patients had a GOS of good, and five (25%) had a score of moderate. This compared quite favorably with our MCVH controls, who were 8% and 12%, respectively.

The purpose of the present study was to assess the safety, tolerability, and pharmacokinetics of CP-101,606 in subjects with either a severe TBI (GCS 3–8) or a spontaneous intracerebral hemorrhage. Our findings suggest that the doses infused in this study were well tolerated, and no adverse events occurred that could be attributed to the drug. Furthermore, for patients with a severe TBI, there was a strong trend for improved outcome. A large, multicenter, placebo-controlled clinical trial is presently underway to test for any beneficial effect CP-101,606 may have on limiting "excitotoxic" secondary brain injury and improving outcome in patients with a severe TBI.

CONCLUSIONS

The results of this dose escalation trial of CP-101,606 suggest that an i.v. infusion of 0.75 mg/kg/hr for 2 hours and continued for 22 or 70 hours at 0.37 mg/kg/hr is well tolerated by the brain-injured patient. Within an hour, all three doses tested achieved a plasma concentration that has been shown to be therapeutic in animal models of brain trauma and ischemia. The drug was also detected in the CSF of patients in concentrations comparable to that in the plasma. The outcomes of TBI patients measured at six months suggested that compared to our hospital's historical controls, there was a strong trend for improved outcome following treatment with CP-101,606.

REFERENCES

1. PAGNOZZI, M.J., L.K. CHAMBERS, F.S. MENNITI, B.L. CHENARD & W.F. WHITE. 1995. CP-101,606, a potent and selective antagonist of forebrain NMDA receptors, *in vivo* neuroprotective activity. Soc. Neurosci. Abstr. **21**(Suppl.): Part 1–3.
2. MENNITI, F.S., B.L. CHENARD, M. COLLINS, M. DUCAT, I. SHALABY & W.F. WHITE. 1997. CP-101,606, a potent neuroprotectant selective for forebrain neurons. Eur. J. Pharmacol. **331**: 117–126.
3. OKIYAMA, K., D.H. SMITH, W.F. WHITE & T.K. MCINTOSH. 1998. Effects of the NMDA antagonist CP-98,113 on regional cerebral edema and cerebrovascular, cognitive, and neurobehavioral function following experimental brain injury in the rat. Brain Res. **792**: 291–298.
4. OKIYAMA, K., D.H. SMITH, W.F. WHITE, K. RICHTER & T.K. MCINTOSH. 1997. Effects of the novel NMDA antagonists CP-98,113, CP-101,581 and CP-101,606 on cognitive function and regional cerebral edema following experimental brain injury in the rat. J. Neurotrauma **14**: 211–222.
5. MENNITI, F.S., M.J. PAGNOZZI, P. BUTLER, B.L. CHENARD, S.S. JAW-TSAI & W.F. WHITE. 1998. CP-101,606, an NR2B subunit selective NMDA receptor antagonist, inhibits NMDA and injury induced c-fos expression and cortical spreading depression in rodents. Eur. J. Pharmacol. Submitted.

6. TSUCHIDA, E., M. RICE & R. BULLOCK. 1997. The neuroprotective effect of the fore-brain-selective NMDA antagonist CP-101,606 upon focal ischemic damage caused by acute subdural hematoma in the rat. J. Neurotrauma **14:** 409–417.
7. DI, X., R. BULLOCK, J. WATSON, P. FATOUROS, B. CHENARD, F. WHITE & F. CORWIN. 1997. Effect of CP-101,606, a novel NR2B subunit antagonist of the *N*-methyl-D-aspartate receptor, on the volume of ischemic brain damage and cytotoxic brain edema after middle cerebral artery occlusion in the feline brain. Stroke **28:** 2244–2251.
8. BULLOCK, R., A. ZAUNER, J.J. WOODWARD, J. MYSEROS, S.C. CHOI, J.D. WARD, A. MARMAROU & H.F. YOUNG. 1998. Factors affecting excitatory amino acid release following severe human head injury. J. Neurosurg. **89:** 507–518.

Neuroprotective "Agents" in Surgery

Secret "Agent" Man, or Common "Agent" Machine?

RUSSELL J. ANDREWS[a]

NASA Ames Research Center, Moffett Field, California 94035
Division of Neurosurgery, Texas Tech University Health Sciences Center, El Paso,
Texas 79905

ABSTRACT: The search for clinically-effective neuroprotective agents has received enormous support in recent years—an estimated $200 million by pharmaceutical companies on clinical trials for traumatic brain injury alone. At the same time, the pathophysiology of brain injury has proved increasingly complex, rendering the likelihood of a single agent "magic bullet" even more remote.

On the other hand, great progress continues with technology that makes surgery less invasive and less risky. One example is the application of endovascular techniques to treat coronary artery stenosis, where both the invasiveness of sternotomy and the significant neurological complication rate (due to microemboli showering the cerebral vasculature) can be eliminated.

In this paper we review aspects of intraoperative neuroprotection both present and future. Explanations for the slow progress on pharmacologic neuroprotection during surgery are presented. Examples of technical advances that have had great impact on neuroprotection during surgery are given both from coronary artery stenosis surgery and from surgery for Parkinson's disease. To date, the progress in neuroprotection resulting from such technical advances is an order of magnitude greater than that resulting from pharmacologic agents used during surgery.

The progress over the last 20 years in guidance during surgery (CT and MRI image-guidance) and in surgical access (endoscopic and endovascular techniques) will soon be complemented by advances in our ability to evaluate biological tissue intraoperatively in real-time. As an example of such technology, the NASA Smart Probe project is considered.

In the long run (i.e., in 10 years or more), pharmacologic "agents" aimed at the complex pathophysiology of nervous system injury in man will be the key to true intraoperative neuroprotection. In the near term, however, it is more likely that mundane "agents" based on computers, microsensors, and microeffectors will be the major impetus to improved intraoperative neuroprotection.

INTRODUCTION

For many years, protection of the nervous system during operative surgery appeared something of a holy grail. … the pharmacological industry has of course been active [in pursuing protection of the nervous system]. Scarcely a year goes by without some new trial designed to demonstrate the efficacy of a particular pharmacological agent.

[a]Address for correspondence: Division of Neurosurgery, Texas Tech University Health Sciences Center, 4800 Alberta Avenue. El Paso, TX 79905. Phone, 915/545-6676; fax, 915/545-7584.
e-mail, nserja@ttuhsc.edu

One hopes that in the end this expensive effort will prove justified.

Lindsay Symon, CBE, TD, FRCS, FACS (Hon)
Professor of Neurological Surgery (Retired)
The National Hospital, Queen Square, London, UK
(Foreword to *Intraoperative Neuroprotection*[1])

In my contribution for the Third International Conference on Neuroprotective Agents two years ago, the historical development of protection of the nervous system during surgery was divided into three eras.[2] In the first era, from 1880 to 1960, contributions to neuroprotection came largely from the personal efforts of the early "giants" of neurosurgery, such as Harvey Cushing. In the second era, from 1960 to 1990, advances came largely from technology, such as the operating microscope and neuroimaging (e.g., computerized tomography (CT) and magnetic resonance imaging (MRI)). In the third era, beginning about 1990, progress in intraoperative neuroprotection appeared ready to come from our increasing understanding of the pathophysiology of injury to the nervous system, and our ability to devise pharmacologic interventions to block the events that lead to neuronal death following an injury such as ischemia.

This paper is in essence a revision—one might even call it a retraction—of the position put forth in the paper two years ago that "the realm of pharmacologic agents ... possesses the greatest potential for improvement in intraoperative neuroprotection in the near future."[2] For the reasons given below, I now believe that truly *significant* protection of the nervous sytem during surgery from pharmacologic interventions is unlikely to occur soon, as Lindsay Symon's quote at the beginning of this paper intimates. That is not to say that the "expensive effort" is unjustified, but rather that the payoff or benefit in terms of significantly improved intraoperative neuroprotection is likely to be quite far down the road (perhaps 10 years or more). The era of technology now appears healthier than ever with respect to protection of the nervous system during surgery. To paraphrase Mark Twain: "The report of the death of technology for neuroprotection is premature."

The reader deserves a brief explanation of the somewhat cryptic and punning title of this paper. Because of the increasing complexity of the pathophysiology of nervous system injury, we might consider "man" (i.e., nervous system injury) to be "secret" (i.e., enigmatic or elusive). On the other hand, advances in the "machine" (i.e., computers and technology) that continue to improve neuroprotection are for the most part quite "common" (i.e., basic and ubiquitous).

WHY HAS PHARMACOLOGIC NEUROPROTECTION BEEN SO ELUSIVE?

There are two major reasons why disappointing progress has been made in pharmacologic neuroprotection: (1) the pathophysiology of nervous system injury has proven to be increasingly complex; and (2) the pharmaceutical industry has chosen short-term politics over long-term efficacy in drug development and implementation for clinical use.

FIGURE 1 is one example of a flow chart for the "ischemic cascade" that occurs in the nervous system following a decrease in blood flow below that level necessary to sustain neuronal integrity. Other figures could be given that emphasize one or an-

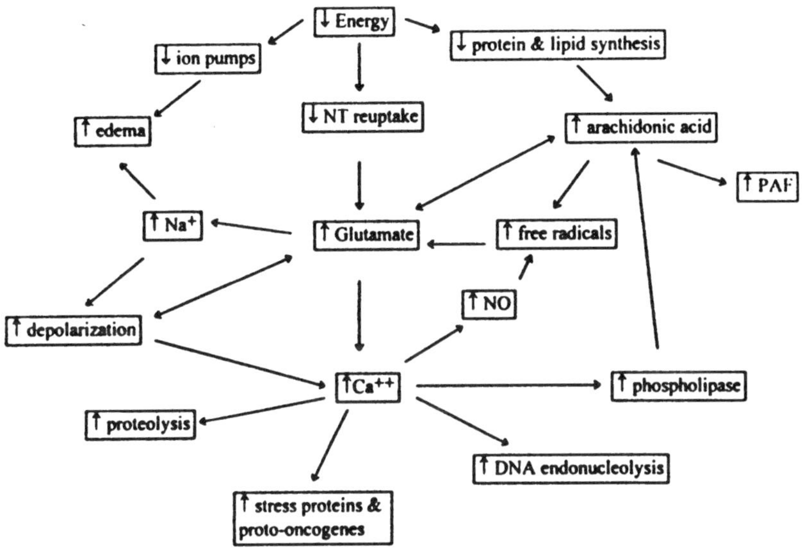

FIGURE 1. Schematic of some of the events in the "ischemic cascade" resulting from decreased cerebral blood flow. (From Pullan.[3] Reprinted by permission from Humana Press.)

other of the many pathophysiologic mechanisms that contribute to eventual neuronal death following ischemic injury. When one considers the proliferation of receptor types for calcium channel antagonism and excitatory amino acid antagonism, for example, the pharmacologic possibilities for therapeutic intervention—especially if multidrug "cocktails" are considered—become virtually endless.

Despite all the points at which pharmacologic intervention could be predicted to improve outcome—and the many encouraging reports in laboratory animals with a wide range of drugs[4]—only two agents appear to have stood the two tests of efficacy (i.e., randomized prospective trials in man) and time: (1) the calcium channel antagonist nimodipine for vasospasm-induced injury following subarachnoid hemorrhage; and (2) the corticosteroid methylprednisone for spinal cord injury. Interestingly, the most efficacious pharmacologic intervention for acute stroke presently is thrombolysis with tissue plasminogen activator (tPA).[5] Since the endpoint of tPA is reestablishing blood flow, rather than a pharmacologic effect at the cellular level, this intervention is more comparable to surgical thrombus removal than to pharmacologic neuroprotection.

The second reason for slow progress on pharmacologic neuroprotection, the politics of drug development for clinical use, is much simpler to perceive but may prove harder to do something about. During the early 1990s, pharmaceutical companies spent an estimated $200 million dollars on clinical trials for traumatic brain injury alone[6]—each company searching for that single agent ("magic bullet") that would pass statistical muster in a long-term outcome study. Unfortunately, agencies involved in these studies such as the Food and Drug Administration (FDA) and the

American Brain Injury Consortium (ABIC) have for the most part been limited to a regulatory role in the former instance (Is this trial safe?) or to an administrative role in the latter. Examples of pharmacologic agents undergoing large clinical trials include superoxide dismutase, tirilazad mesylate, cerestat and selfotel. The issues and some recommendations for improving the efficacy of such trials were offered in a paper presented at the Third International Conference on Neuroprotective Agents.[6]

However, it is likely that only combination drug therapy will have a truly significant impact on ischemic or traumatic brain injury.[7] For this, the pharmaceutical companies will need to act in concert rather than in competition to carry out multi-drug "cocktail" trials. It may also be necessary for "disinterested" (economically speaking) third parties such as the National Institutes of Health (NIH) to become involved, given that some pharmacologic agents likely to be of benefit in a drug "cocktail" do not possess financial incentive for a pharmaceutical company.[7] Examples of these "profitless" drugs include mannitol and tromethamine (THAM).[2]

Our current "Decade of the Brain" is doing a better job at defining the issues in neuroprotection than it is in solving them. The state-of-the-art in understanding the pathophysiology of brain injury still appears to be one of increasing complexity. No pharmacologic key or keys to reversing the "ischemic cascade" are on the immediate horizon. When combined with the political and economic difficulties in implementing a multifactorial approach to pharmacologic therapy for ischemic and traumatic brain injury, the near-term "return on investment" for pharmacologic neuroprotection is poor. In the long run, however, elucidating the pathophysiology of brain injury will be essential for mechanistic approaches to therapy. The secret "agent"—the complexity of man's response to brain injury—will hopefully be unraveled early in the 21st century.

AN EXAMPLE OF PROGRESS IN INTRAOPERATIVE NEUROPROTECTION

As noted in the section above, it is perhaps a prognostic indicator that the only drug for acute stroke therapy that has stood the test of clinical trials is not a neuroprotective agent at all in the true sense of metabolic protection at the cellular level, but rather a clot-lysing agent—tissue plasminogen activator (tPA)—which acts in essence like a mechanical thrombectomy. Another example of improvement in neuroprotection in cardiac surgery underscores the notion of technological advances providing improvement in intraoperative neurprotection.

It is well recognized that not only overt stroke but also persistent cognitive deficit are common sequelae of coronary artery bypass graft (CABG) surgery. Stroke complicates 5% or more of CABG operations,[8,9] and appears to be related to showering of emboli into the cerebral circulation according to transcranial doppler (TCD) studies during CABG surgery.[10] Persistent cognitive deficits that can be devastating for the patient, the patient's family, and the patient's employer are even more frequent—on the order of 20% of all CABG patients.[11,12] Techniques such as transesophageal echocardiography (TEE) have identified certain groups at high risk for stroke during CABG surgery, e.g., those patients with mobile plaque of the aortic arch (33% stroke rate in one study).[13] Cognitive deficits resulting from CABG surgery are likely re-

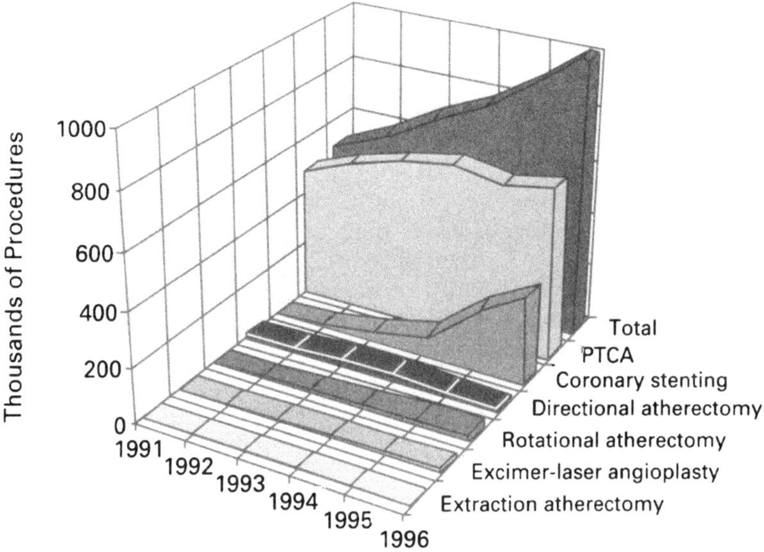

FIGURE 2. Growth in the number of interventional cardiovascular procedures worldwide from 1991 to 1996. (From Bittl.[14] Reprinted by permission from the *New England Journal of Medicine.*)

lated to cerebral microemboli; thus advances in CABG surgery that can reduce the number of microemboli may be expected to reduce the 20% complication rate.[13]

Interventional cardiovascular procedures have developed remarkably over the last decade as a substitute for open CABG operations (FIG. 2). The number performed worldwide doubled between 1991 and 1996, to nearly one million procedures per year.[14] Although balloon angioplasty procedures have plateaued since 1994, coronary artery stenting procedures continue to grow in number.[14] And although balloon angioplasty and stenting have significant risks of myocardial infarction or vessel stenosis/thrombosis (approximately 5% each), as well as need for CABG surgery (3–8%), the risk of stroke is much less than for CABG: 0.4–0.8% in some series, and 0% in others.[14–16] Cognitive deficits not accompanied by frank stroke following balloon angioplasty and/or stenting are rare (in contrast to CABG surgery), since they are not customarily noted. Presumably the decreased risk of stroke in interventional procedures for coronary artery stenosis—in comparison with CABG surgery—is due to the lack of microemboli showering into the cerebral circulation.

Balloon angioplasty and/or stenting has reduced the neurologic morbidity of coronary revascularization surgery perhaps tenfold—the stroke rate has gone from up to 5% to less than 0.5%. Thus a technological advance has improved neuroprotection during coronary revascularization much more than any pharmacologic agents given during CABG surgery.

A NEUROLOGIC DISORDER AND
INTRAOPERATIVE NEUROPROTECTION

Parkinson's disease (PD) is a nervous system movement disorder whose pathophysiology is reasonably well understood, and whose treatment has extensive roots in both pharmacologic and surgical interventions.[17–19] The pathological hallmark of PD is a loss of dopaminergic neurons in the substantia nigra compacta. Among the etiologies of PD are idiopathic, postencephalitic (encephalitis lethargica or von Economo's disease), and drug-induced. Drug-induced PD (DIPD) occurs following the use of dopamine receptor blocking agents, although the list of pharmacologic agents that can cause DIPD includes, in addition to dopamine receptor blockers, the false neurotransmitter methyldopa, antiemetics (e.g., chlorpromazine), anticonvulsants (e.g., valproic acid), cholinomimetics (e.g., bethanecol), sympatholytics (e.g., reserpine), and calcium channel blockers (e.g., flunarizine).[20] Although DIPD is relatively common among those taking one of the offending drugs, it fortunately resolves in most cases with stopping the drug.

Idiopathic PD unfortunately runs a relentlessly progressive course in most cases, with postencephalitic PD usually being less devastating. The severe disability of PD and other movement disorders has led to many surgical explorations in the search for relief from the uncontrollable movements. This began with resection of the precentral gyrus by Horsley in 1876, continued with caudate nucleus ablation by Myers in 1939, and was followed by stereotactic lesioning of the globus pallidus or thalamus by Cooper, Hassler, and others in the 1950s. Although cortical resection in particular was of questionable benefit (the movement disorder was replaced by a hyperreflexic and dyspraxic extremity), the localized stereotactic ablations in the globus pallidus and the thalamus were of considerably greater benefit with a significant reduction in morbidity.

The discovery that the dopamine precursor L-dopa, which readily crosses the blood-brain barrier, could ameliorate the dopamine deficit in PD resulted in a dramatic reduction in the number of surgical procedures for PD when L-dopa came into widespread clinical use in the late 1960s. A pharmacologic treatment (if not a cure) had been discovered that obviated the need for stereotactic surgery (or so it appeared in 1968!). For approximately 20 years after the late 1960s, only a few major academic medical centers routinely performed stereotactic procedures for PD and other movement disorders (Fig. 3).[21] L-dopa and other dopaminergic agents such as bromocriptine and pergolide, monoamine oxidase inhibitors such as deprenyl, and various anticholinergic agents all demonstrated varying degrees of success in treating PD.

These pharmacologic treatments for PD have several drawbacks, however. All the agents appear to be symptomatic rather than curative in their efficacy. Side effects—notably nausea, confusion, and hallucinations—are common to all as well. Their benefit is not universal, in that only 1/2–2/3 of patients experience significant benefit. Bradykinesia and rigidity usually respond better than tremor. Perhaps most importantly, within 2–5 years of beginning L-dopa therapy (usually combined with the peripheral decarboxylase inhibitor carbidopa) the majority of patients experience a gradual but progressive decrease in efficacy. This decrease takes the form of either a diurnal variation in, or recurrence of, the Parkinsonian dyskinesias and rigidity ("off" stage) alternating with periods of relative mobility ("on" stage). The failure of

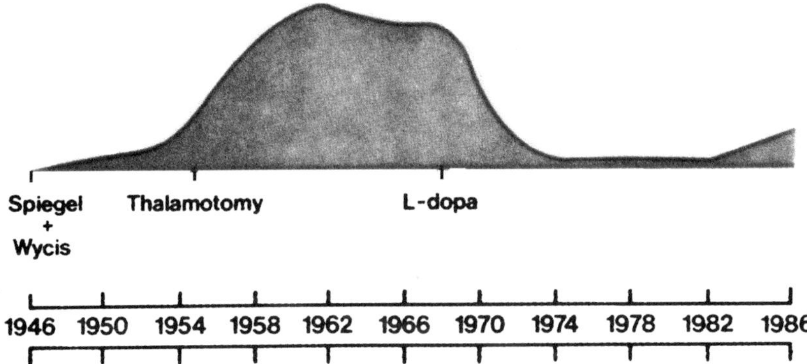

FIGURE 3. Relative frequency of stereotactic neurosurgical procedures from 1946 to 1986. (From Gildenberg.[21] Reprinted with permission from *Neurosurgery*.)

pharmacologic therapy to be an effective long-term treatment for PD, together with improvements in neuroimaging (CT and MRI) and electrophysiologic recording, have rekindled interest in the surgical treatment of PD and other movement disorders.

Stereotactic surgery for movement disorders such as PD and essential tremor has thus undergone a resurgence over the last 10 years. There has been a refinement or elaboration of the appropriate targets for ablation (including the subthalamic nucleus as well as the thalamus and globus pallidus). The trend toward minimally invasive surgery has led to the use of radiosurgery for lesion-making (Gamma Knife and linear accelerator techniques), with clinical results in PD comparable to precise radiofrequency ablation.[22]

A further refinement in surgical technique is chronic stimulation with a microelectrode implanted in the target of choice (e.g., the thalamus or globus pallidus), connected to a battery and microprocessor placed subcutaneously in the region of the clavicle.[23] As a result of extensive testing in Europe, safety and efficacy have been established. FDA approval was granted in 1997 to market a device in the US for deep brain stimulation of the thalamus. There is considerable conceptual appeal to stimulation rather than destruction of neural tissue. Deep brain stimulation may in fact be "safer" than L-dopa for PD in the long run, since it appears that the effect is truly reversible when the stimulation is turned off (i.e., irreversible dyskinesias are not seen).

An additional surgical technique for PD—tranplantation of autologous adrenal medullary or fetal nigral tissue, or genetically modified cells—has even greater appeal than deep brain stimulation. Such transplantation aims at "curing" the deficiency of dopamine in PD. Although the poor long-term outcome in PD treated with autologous adrenal medullary grafting (performed by various neurosurgical groups in the late 1980s) has tempered the initial enthusiasm for transplantation, circumspect studies involving the transplantation of fetal and genetically modified cells for PD and other movement disorders continue.[24]

In sum, PD is an example of a nervous system disorder where risky surgical treatments were replaced by what initially appeared to be a pharmacologic "cure," L-dopa. In time, however, the long-term side effects as well as the waning efficacy of the pharmacologic treatment came to be recognized. This, together with technical advances that are making the surgical treatments safer and more efficacious, has led to the common "agent"—the stereotactic surgical "machine"—being at least an alternative to, if not a replacement for, the pharmacologic treatment of PD.

HOW TO GET THERE, AND HOW TO KNOW WHEN WE HAVE ARRIVED

Surgical neuroprotection requires as little disturbance of neural tissue as possible. In the example of surgery for coronary artery occlusion discussed above, the endovascular route has permitted minimally invasive techniques (balloon angioplasty and stenting) to replace the sternum-splitting and vein-grafting that are the hallmark of CABG surgery. In the treatment of nervous system lesions, the endovascular route has also been taken to minimize morbidity and invasiveness. Examples include (1) embolization of arteriovenous malformations, (2) coil-induced thrombosis or stent exclusion of cerebral aneurysms, and (3) tPA for clot lysis in acute stroke (as discussed above).

Unfortunately, a lesion whose address is not on the cerebrovascular "roadmap" is not presently amenable to an endovascular approach. As catheters become increasingly delicate it will no doubt be possible to climb more and more distally up the cerebrovascular tree, but whether the majority of brain tumors will be within the interventional neuroradiologist/neurosurgeon's reach in the near future is questionable. Furthermore, regions of the brain involved in functional neurosurgery such as those ablated or stimulated in PD (e.g., thalamus or globus pallidus, as discussed above) are even less likely to be reached effectively by an endovascular approach.

Regarding "How to get there," for the near term at least (probably 5–10 years), we are thus left with the task of maximizing neuroprotection during neurosurgical procedures by minimizing trauma on direct (straight line) approach to the lesion or region in question. This drive to minimize trauma on access to deep regions of the brain has been a major impetus both for stereotactic techniques and for neuroendoscopy.

Both stereotaxy and neuroendoscopy, as currently practiced, have significant drawbacks. Stereotactic techniques that do not involve a craniotomy—i.e., where a needle is placed through a small hole in the skull—are minimally invasive but "blind," in that the neurosurgeon does not know what is occurring at the tip of the needle. Apart from miniature electrodes for recording brain electrical activity (e.g., in functional neurosurgery) and miniature ultrasound probes used to detect blood vessels or provide a grey-scale image of the brain immediately ahead of the needle, little has been done to provide the neurosurgeon with a "needle's eye" view of the brain.[25]

Neuroendoscopy has taken the approach of "minifying" the corridor through which the neurosurgeon operates in order to decrease tissue trauma. As the field of view narrows and visual aids such as miniature (1 mm diameter or less) fiber optic imaging become necessary, the view that the neurosurgeon receives is increasingly degraded. The loss both of depth perception and of image resolution with "minification" has led to such techniques as virtual reality head-mounted displays for enhancing the neurosurgeon's visual capabilities. Neuroendoscopy presumes that enhancements for the neurosurgeon's vision are preferable to sensors that detect and interpret deep tissues directly.

Because of the capabilities of miniature sensors used in industry, and the advancements in neural net learning, data fusion, and real-time computation (even on inexpensive desk- or lap-top PCs), we decided to pursue a somewhat different method for minimizing trauma to brain tissue on direct approach to deep lesions. Localization (Where is this region in relation to the rest of the brain?) and characterization (What kind of tissue is here?) are determined by the unique signature provided by summing the information gathered from a small number of microsensors (presently three). This is somewhat similar to sending a heavily instrumented unmanned space probe to a distant celestial body rather than a manned spacecraft. There is certainly a unique experience for the astronauts in going personally into outer space (and perhaps vicariously for those who remain earthbound), but one can hardly dispute that a manned spacecraft offers the possibility of gathering more information about the nature of some distant celestial body than the various instruments that can interpret and analyze that body. One might argue that the expense of making the spacecraft habitable for the astronauts could be better spent on additional analytical instrumentation, if the gathering of information about that distant celestial body is the primary goal of the mission.

Regarding "How to know when we have arrived," the NASA Smart Probe project is tasked with developing a device that will identify a unique "signature" for any location in the brain. In broader terms, the Smart Probe is a device for medical/surgical applications that can provide real-time biological tissue characterization. The classic example of a "signature" for tissue localization or characterization is the use of electrophysiologic recording. In the heart, the ECG is used to assess the status of the myocardium (Has there been an infarct? Is there ischemia? Is there hypokalemia?). In the brain, microelectrodes are used to identify the location of such areas as the nuclei of the thalamus and regions of the globus pallidus, as well as the location of abnormalities such as epileptic foci. The term "characterization" is preferred for the Smart Probe, since characterization can include both (1) localization, and (2) status identification (e.g., abnormalities such as ischemic changes, neurotransmitter imbalances, and degrees of malignancy).

The concept behind the Smart Probe is to use neural net learning and fuzzy logic to combine data gathered from sensors covering multiple modalities in order to uniquely characterize tissue in real-time. The sensors or techniques to be used include the following: microelectrodes (electrophysiology); optical reflectance or optical scattering (spectrometry using broad band light—roughly 300–1000 nm); color analysis of fiber optic neuroendoscopy output; optical fluorescence or absorbance for measuring pH, PCO_2, and PO_2; ion-sensitive microelectrodes; microstrain gauge for tissue stiffness and interstitial fluid pressure; laser Doppler blood flow; microultrasound; and microdialysis. For virtually all the above techniques, miniature sensors are available "off the shelf" that are 1 mm in diameter or less.

The initial purpose of the Smart Probe was to improve the safety and efficacy of stereotactic brain biopsy.[26] The two major goals are (1) to improve the diagnostic

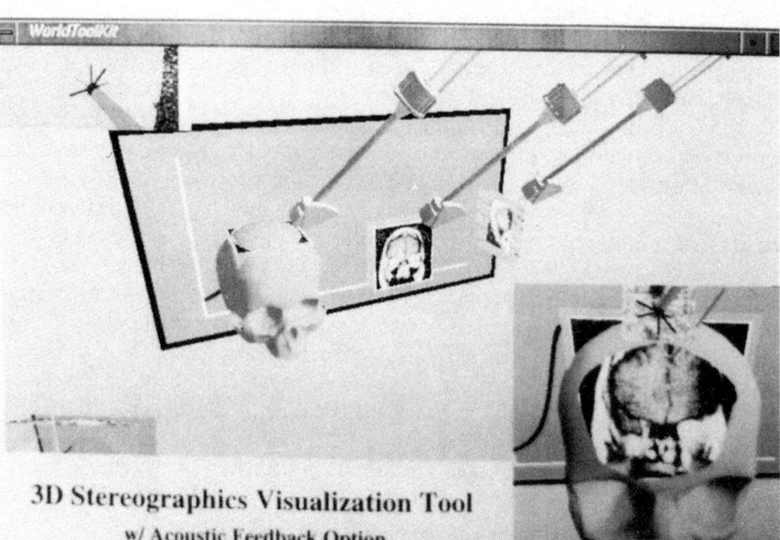

FIGURE 4. The NASA Smart Probe 3-D visualization of the Probe penetrating the brain in a stereotactic brain biopsy. Other panels provide real-time plots of data acquired from the three microsensors, as well as identification of the tissue at the tip of the Probe—based on the neural net software (normal brain, tumor of various types, edematous brain, etc.).

yield of tumor biopsy (since there is a 5% or higher rate of failure to obtain diagnostic tissue), and (2) to reduce the risk of hemorrhage (which can cause major morbidity or death in up to 5% of cases).[27–29] The Smart Probe can detect blood vessels before the probe/needle traverses them, and can determine whether the tissue about to be biopsied is indeed frank neoplasia, necrotic tissue, or surrounding brain.

In its present configuration (August, 1998) the Smart Probe is a 2.7-mm-diameter cannula that houses three sensors (each approximately 1 mm in diameter) in triangular configuration (FIG. 4). Neural net software (developed at the NASA Ames Research Center) running on a Windows NT-based PC analyzes the output from the three sensors in near real-time (< 0.1 second delay). The output is then compared with the data bank it has "learned" through prior experience (normal gray and white matter, blood vessels, and various types of tumors). The video display includes not only the result of the neural net analysis and the output of the individual sensors as desired, but also a 3-D representation of the probe penetrating the brain. The probe can be robotically advanced through the brain, and can be programmed to stop if certain conditions are fulfilled (e.g., the "signature" is that of a blood vessel to be avoided, or that of the globus pallidus internus (in surgery for Parkinson's disease)).

A GLIMPSE OF NEUROSURGERY IN THE 21ST CENTURY

Beyond the obvious applications of NASA's Smart Probe to areas such as cancer diagnosis, tissue identification during surgery, and cerebral monitoring (e.g., in head-injured patients), the technology can be used to provide the tactile feedback for "simulators" to train surgeons (much like flight simulators).

Perhaps even more important in the long run, however, is the development of multimodality effectors. Preliminary studies employ a microlaser that is guided by feedback from the multimodality sensors. One can easily imagine a robotic microlaser ablating a tumor deep within the brain. Tissue ablation would stop as soon as normal brain was encountered. Also within the realm of possibility in the near future is the use of "smart" effectors to place radiotherapy and/or chemotherapy seeds or pellets accurately within tumorous tissue, sparing injury to surrounding normal brain. Another exciting application is the precise placement of antibodies and other vectors of use in gene therapy—for conditions as diverse as Parkinson's disease and brain tumors.

From NASA's standpoint the ultimate goal of "smart" neurosurgery may be given in the following scenario:

Circa the year 2020, the space mission to Mars has begun: a two-year mission that involves nine months' travel time each way plus six months on the Martian surface. All astronauts undergo a premission high-resolution MRI head and body scan (including MR spectroscopy) and are fitted with a body-conforming space suit for EVA (extra vehicular activity). The space suit incorporates continuous multifunction medical monitoring (e.g., body temperature, electrocardiogram, blood gases, and blood pressure) and a helmet with an array of high-resolution ultrasound probes, electrodes, and near-infrared spectroscopy oximeter probes. The space suit and helmet permit correlation of the astronaut's medical status and brain function with premission studies. A compact robot, guided principally by preprogrammed routines (but also directly from the Houston Space Center if necessary for very specialized procedures) can place a probe anywhere in the brain or body with minimal morbidity. Thus an event such as a stroke or a head injury can not only be localized, but in many cases be treated definitively, during the space mission.

While exploring the Martian surface, one of the astronauts strikes his/her head and becomes unconscious. The ultrasound probes and the near-infrared oximeters soon indicate abnormalities consistent with blood clots both over the surface of the right hemisphere of the brain as well as within the right hemisphere. The astronaut is quickly taken into the space vehicle, where the robot injects a local anesthetic and drills a small hole in the skull over the region of blood clot. From there on, the multimodality sensor probe compares information obtained from the brain of the astronaut on the space mission with the data bank established over thousands of previous procedures by neural net learning—as well as with information obtained from the premission scans of that astronaut. First the abnormal regions are localized, and then identified, by their characteristics from a variety of sensory modalities. Then the blood clots are aspirated under robotic control with feedback from the multimodality sensor probe, and, if necessary, the bleeding is stopped with a coagulating laser (again under robotic control, with feedback to localize the bleeding and confirm that it is completely stopped). The diagnosis and treatment are performed by the robot under local anesthesia (i.e., the astronaut can be awake during the procedure).

The above scenario is speculative, but all the techniques described either are presently available or will be feasible for application to medicine shortly. Given the rapid progress in neurosurgery over the last 25 years, it is by no means unrealistic to expect such capabilities within the next 25 years.

CONCLUSION

The complexity of nervous system injury is only beginning to be understood. The hope of many researchers in the 1990s (not to mention several pharmaceutical companies) that a "magic bullet" might be on the immediate horizon appears premature. Much like the search for genetic answers to the riddle of cancer, the search to unravel the pathophysiology of neuronal cell injury and death is proving elusive. The human nervous system is slow to yield up its secrets, and our therapeutic agents to prevent or reverse nervous system injury are so far only marginally effective.

The computer, that ubiquitous agent in our lives as the 20th century concludes, bears an uncanny resemblance to the nervous system. From the elementary dichotomy of off or on, firing or silent, to the billions of "connections" common both to a computer and to the nervous system, it is perhaps the ultimate tribute to man's brain that it has been able to conceive and construct devices of such great but subtle computational power.[30] No doubt computer modeling and neural net learning will contribute to our understanding of the pathophysiology of nervous system injury.

In *1898*, few would have predicted that the 20th century would have man inhabiting space, but would have made precious little headway curing the "common" cold. In time we will unlock the "secret" of nervous system injury, but at the outset of the 21st century it is more likely that "common" devices (i.e., computers, microsensors, and microeffectors) will provide the greatest advances in intraoperative neuroprotection. Indeed, much as art can help reveal the inner workings of the psyche, the common inventions of the mind (e.g., computers and neural network heuristics) may provide—through modeling—insights into the pathophysiology of nervous system injury. Our "common" inventions may help us come closer to the ultimate goals of both prophylactic and therapeutic neuroprotective "agents."

REFERENCES

1. ANDREWS, R.J., Ed. 1996. Intraoperative Neuroprotection. Williams & Wilkins. Baltimore.
2. ANDREWS, R.J. 1997. Neuroprotection in surgery: development of a pharmacologic cocktail for intraoperative use. Ann. N.Y. Acad. Sci. **825:** 288–304.
3. PULLAN, L.M. Neuroprotective strategies for treatment of acute ischemic stroke. *In* Neurotherapeutics: Emerging Strategies. L. Pullan & J. Patel, Eds. 275–322. Humana. Totowa, NJ.
4. GROTTA, J. 1994. The current status of neuronal protective therapy: why have all the neuronal protective drugs worked in animals but none so far in stroke patients? Cerebrovasc. Dis. **4:** 115–120.
5. KASNER, S.E. & J.C. GROTTA. 1997. Emergency identification and treatment of acute ischemic stroke. Ann. Emerg. Med. **30:** 642–653.

6. DOPPENBERG, E.M.R., S.C. CHOI & R. BULLOCK. 1997. Clinical trials in traumatic brain injury: what can we learn from previous studies? Ann. N.Y. Acad. Sci. **825:** 305–323.
7. ADAMS, R.J., M. FISHER, A.J. FURLAN *et al.* 1995. Acute stroke trials in the United States: rethinking strategies for success. Stroke **26:** 2216–2218.
8. SHAW, P.J., D. BATES, N.E.F. CARTLIDGE *et al.* 1985. Early neurological complications of coronary artery bypass surgery. Br. J. Med. **291:** 1384–1387.
9. GOLD, J.P., M.E. CHARLSON, P. WILLIAMS-RUSSO *et al.* 1995. Improvement of outcomes after coronary artery bypass: a randomized trial comparing intraoperative high versus low mean arterial pressure. J. Thorac. Cardiovasc. Surg. **110:** 1302–1314.
10. BARBUT, D., Y.-W. LO, J.P. GOLD *et al.* 1997. Impact of embolization during coronary artery bypass grafting on outcome and length of stay. Ann. Thorac. Surg. **63:** 998–1002.
11. MURKIN, J.M., D.L. BAIRD, J.S. MARTZKE *et al.* 1996. Long-term neurological and neuropsychological outcome 3 years after coronary artery bypass surgery [abstract]. Anesth. Analg. **82:** S328.
12. HAMMON, J.W., D.A. STUMP, N.D. KON *et al.* 1997. Risk factors and solutions for the development of neurobehavioral changes after coronary artery bypass grafting. Ann. Thorac. Surg. **63:** 1613–1618.
13. BARBUT, D., Y.-W. LO, G.S. HARTMAN *et al.* 1997. Aortic atheroma is related to outcome but not numbers of emboli during coronary bypass. Ann. Thorac. Surg. **64:** 545–549.
14. BITTL, J.L. 1996. Advances in coronary angioplasty. N. Engl. J. Med. **335:** 1290–1302.
15. CHAUCHAN, A., E. VU, D.R. RICCI *et al.* 1998. Multiple coronary stenting in unstable angina: early and late clinical outcomes. Catheterization Cardiovasc. Diagn. **43:** 11–16.
16. LINDSAY, J., E.E. PINNOW & A.D. PICHARD. 1998. New devices enhance hospital results of coronary angioplasty. Catheterization Cardiovasc. Diagn. **43:** 1–6.
17. FRIEDMAN, A. & D.A. TURNER. 1996. Movement disorders. *In* The Practice of Neurosurgery. G.T. Tindall, P.R. Cooper & D.L. Barrow, Eds. 3225–3244. Williams & Wilkins. Baltimore.
18. SLUSHER, B.S., P.F. JACKSON & L.A. ARVANTIS. 1996. Parkinson's disease. *In* Neurotherapeutics: Emerging Strategies. L. Pullan & J. Patel, Eds. 343–388. Humana. Totowa, NJ.
19. GOETZ, C.G. 1998. Parkinson's disease. *In* Neurobase. S. Gilman, G.W. Goldstein & S.G. Waxman, Eds. CD-ROM. Arbor. San Diego.
20. DIEDERICH, N.J. & C.G. GOETZ. 1998. Drug-induced movement disorders. Neurol. Clin. North Am. **16:** 125–139.
21. GILDENBERG, P.L. 1987. Whatever happened to stereotactic surgery? Neurosurgery **20:** 983–987.
22. YOUNG, R.F., A. SHUMWAY-COOK, S.S. VERMEULEN *et al.* 1998. Gamma knife radiosurgery as a lesioning technique in movement disorder surgery. J. Neurosurg. **89:** 183–193.
23. BENABID, A.-L., P. POLLAK, D. HOFFMANN *et al.* 1998. Chronic stimulation for Parkinson's disease and other movement disorders. *In* Textbook of Stereotactic and Functional Neurosurgery. P.L. Gildenberg & R.R. Tasker, Eds. 1199–1212. McGraw-Hill. New York.
24. FELER, C.A. 1998. Adrenal medullary grafting in the treatment of Parkinsonism. *In* Textbook of Stereotactic and Functional Neurosurgery. P.L. Gildenberg & R.R. Tasker, Eds. 1213–1216. McGraw-Hill. New York.
25. GILSBACH, J., M. MOHADJER & F. MUNDINGER. 1987. A new safety device to prevent bleeding complications during stereotactic biopsy: the "stereotactic" Doppler sonography. Acta Neurochir. (Vienna) **89:** 77–79.

26. ANDREWS, R., R. MAH, A. GALVAGNI *et al.* 1997. Robotic multimodality stereotactic brain tissue identification: work in progress. Stereotactic Funct. Neurosurg. **68:** 72–79.
27. SOO, T.M., M. BERNSTEIN, J. PROVIAS *et al.* 1996. Failed stereotactic biopsy in a series of 518 cases. Stereotactic Funct. Neurosurg. **64:** 183–196.
28. KONDZIOLKA, D., A.D. FIRLIK & L.D. LUNSFORD. 1998. Complications of stereotactic brain surgery. Neurol. Clin. North Am. **16:** 35–54.
29. KULKARNI, A.V., A. GUHA & A. LOZANO. 1998. Incidence of silent hemorrhage and delayed deterioration after stereotactic brain biopsy. J. Neurosurg. **89:** 31–35.
30. RIEKE, F., D. WARLAND, R. DE RUYTER VAN STEVENICK *et al.* 1997. Spikes: Exploring the Neural Code. The MIT Press. Cambridge, MA.

Questions and Answers

QUESTIONS FOR DR. ANDREWS

From Dr. Maynard

Like you, I think that a pharmacologic cocktail may be the future. However, I think it is important to think of the treatment paradigm since irreversible damage due to stroke may involve (1) protecting the brain during ischemia, (2) determining whether the stroke is ischemic or hemorrhagic, and (3) protecting against reperfusion injury.

ANSWER: Your comment raises a number of important issues. I will only consider a couple of them. (1) Rapid determination of the type of stroke (ischemic or hemorrhagic) is crucial to the in-hospital management of stroke, and will depend on both (a) improvements in pre-hospital triage and (b) quicker diagnostic tests (e.g., CT, which currently takes a minute or less of actual scanning time to image the brain). However, it is likely that we can formulate a "cocktail" that might be safely given in the field by paramedics to patients suffering from either an ischemic or hemorrhagic stroke. (2) Protecting the brain against ongoing ischemic injury vs reperfusion injury will very likely involve two different drug "cocktails." Timing the initial onset of the stroke may prove to be quite important, i.e., drugs that may be helpful during the first couple of hours may prove to be contraindicated after, say, eight hours. The efficacy of steroids in the acute period following spinal cord injury (but not later) is an example.

From Dr. Schmued

Are clinicians presently combining dyes or tracers to help with the use of visual microprobes used in neurosurgery?

ANSWER: Perhaps the best example of dyes used to aid clinicians is the use of hematoporphryins in the treatment of certain types of cancer (photodynamic therapy). Fluorescent dyes have been used to aid in visualization. The beauty of spectroscopy for "optical biopsy" is the vast amount of information contained in the light analyzed (the visual and near infrared spectrum, e.g., 300–1000 nm). This information allows differentiation of tissues that could not be accomplished by the human eye, and—when combined with other modalities (e.g., tissue pressure, pH) such as is done by the NASA Smart Probe—provides a redundancy that is essential in the "hostile" operating room environment.

From Dr. Marchionni

This is a fascinating technology, but isn't the time lag between Mars and Earth a factor in implementing this technology to surgical intervention?

ANSWER: Exactly! The time lag precludes a "Houston-operated" robot. It will be essential that the "astrosurgeon" robot have both sensors and effectors—and that the two be interconnected (with feedback, in both directions)—i.e., "brainlike." The astrosurgeon, like the human surgeon, will need to be taught all the basic diagnostic and therapeutic information, and, again like the (talented) human surgeon, will eventually have the ability to make "intelligent" decisions when faced with novel situations. That does not mean that Earth-bound humans cannot have some input into the astrosurgeon, but the astrosurgeon will need to be largely self-sufficient. For an eye-opening account of the possibilities for robots, I suggest the book *March of the Machines* by Kevin Warwick, Director of Cybernetics at the University of Reading, UK (Century, 1997).

QUESTIONS FOR DR. NISHIO

From Dr. Obrenovitch

Have you considered that this phenomenon may be linked to induction of hibernation rather than equivalent to stress-induced preconditioning?

ANSWER: The underlying mechanisms of hypothermia-induced tolerance remain to be established. It is possible that this phenomenon shares features with hibernation and/or stress-induced preconditioning. It is important to note that the time course of hypothermia-induced tolerance is shorter than tolerance induced by some other preconditioning stimuli. Consequently, it is also possible that hypothermia-induced tolerance shares only a subset of the mechanisms induced by other conditioning stimuli.

From Dr. Manev

Does hypothermia induce heat shock proteins, and would the preconditioning by increasing temperature also induce neuroprotection?

ANSWER: We have no direct evidence on this point in our studies. Hypothermia has previously been shown to induce Hsp72 mRNA; however, the mechanism of heat shock factor activation by hypothermia may differ from that typically observed in response to heat shock (see Cullen & Sarge. 1997. J. Biol. Chem.).

From Dr. Narahashi

Your *in vivo* hypothermic preconditioning experiments are quite interesting. Will it be possible to reproduce the effects *in vitro*? For example, one could use cultured neurons to improve hypothermic preconditioning. Such *in vitro* experiments will be useful to dissect out the factors responsible for the effects.

ANSWER: We are currently examining this issue in co-cultured hippocampal neurons and glia. Preliminary evidence suggests that *in vitro* hypothermic conditioning may limit excitotoxic injury in these cells. We agree that a model system of this type will be extremely valuable to identify and characterize mechanisms underlying tolerance.

From Dr. Maynard

Have you looked at later time points following ischemia to show if hypothermia preconditioning protects against delayed neuronal death such as in apoptosis?

ANSWER: We have no evidence regarding the effect of hypothermic preconditioning on apoptotic injury, but this is a very important topic for investigation.

From Dr. Bowyer

Is the transient cold stress you subjected the animals to affecting adrenal function and cortisol levels, and could it be that such an effect is producing the neuroprotection you are seeing?

ANSWER: Our current results cannot rule out this possibility. However, our preliminary results in cell culture (see response to T. Narahashi) suggest that a direct effect on cells in the brain parenchyma occurs.

From Dr. Marini

Why use two doses of anisomycin?

ANSWER: Hypothermia-induced tolerance appears to develop over 6 or more hours after preconditioning. We sought to block protein synthesis during this key period (i.e., during, and for 6–8 hours after, preconditioning). Because the peak inhibitory effects of anisomycin on protein synthesis decay over a few hours, we administered a second injection of anisomycin to sustain the inhibition.

From Dr Marini

Hasn't it been shown that Hsp70 mRNA increases in hyperthermia but CA1 neurons still die?

ANSWER: The role of all potential underlying mechanisms for tolerance, including the induction of heat shock protein, remains to be fully established. There is strong evidence demonstrating the induction of heat shock protein in response to various types of conditioning stimuli; however, the time course of this induction does not always correlate perfectly with the tolerance phenomenon.

From Dr. Lin

During cardiac surgery, a bypass circulation is provided by a machine. After recovery from surgery, patients develop neurologic deficits. Whether hypothermia is an effective neuroprotection requires more investigation.

ANSWER: We agree.

From Dr. Abbracchio

I have a question on hypothermia-induced preconditioning. Do you have any idea on the nature of the intracellular targets responsible for hypothermia-induced increased tolerance? In particular, have you looked at the possible involvement of the cytoskeleton? I am asking this because we have raised the hypothesis that adenosine may be involved in ischemic preconditioning of the brain, and we have demonstrated that the *in vitro* exposure of mammalian astrocytes to selected adenosine agonists results in a reinforcement of the actin cytoskeleton and protection against spontaneous apoptosis.

ANSWER: We are at the early stages of evaluating a variety of potential intracellular mechanisms involved in hypothermia preconditioning. The possible roles of adenosine and cytoskeletal changes are interesting, but we have no direct data on these points.

QUESTIONS FOR DR. YOUDIM

From Dr. Marini

I believe that apomorphine may play a greater role (i.e., neuroprotectant) than by just reducing the dose of L-dopa.

ANSWER: The European studies of Lees *et al.* in London and of Powve in Innsbruck have shown that L-dopa dosage can be reduced in apomorphine-treated patients. This is also seen with other dopamine agonists such as bromocritine and pergolid. However, apomorphine may be even more effective, since unlike other dopamine agonist it is an agonist of both D_1 and D_2 dopamine receptors. It is possible that aopmorphine may have a neuroprotective activity because of its iron chelating and radical scavenging actions. We are now investigating this problem in Parkinsonian subjects treated with apomorphine with PET.

From Dr. Maynard

Have you looked to see if apomorphine improves Parkinson's disease-like symptoms? I think it is important to show neuroprotection at the cellular level, but it may also be useful to show functional benefit.

ANSWER: This has been shown in the last few years by numerous studies. There is no question that apomorphine is probably the most potent antiParkinson drug available. However, its pharmacokinetic and delivery has a drawback because of its short half-life and rapid oxidation.

From Dr. Sobotka

What effects do dietary iron imbalances (dietary iron deficiency and iron excess) have on incidence or progression of neurodegenerative diseases? On toxicity of neurotoxicants such as MPTP? On treatment with neuroprotectants?

ANSWER: This is an important question. As you may know we were the first group that actually studied the role of iron in brain function, and we have been doing work since 1973. I will first deal with iron deficiency. Rats made nutritionally iron deficient have cognitive impairment similar to what has been reported in infants and children with iron deficiency. Brain iron can be reduced by nutritional means in animals. This affects the dopamine by downregulating dopaminergic activity. We have published numerous papers on this. However, iron cannot be increased in brain, because once the blood-brain barrier is formed, serum iron has no access to the brain. All the iron that is in the brain is conserved and remains there for life. But in Parkinson's disease and Alzheimer's disease there is a highly significant increase of iron at the site of neurodegeneration. In fact, all neurodegenerative diseases show this. The question that has intrigued us for years is: Where is iron coming from? We have no answer to this, and we know that it is accumulated in the neurons and microglia. Indeed, one of the most fascinating and puzzling aspects of neurodegenration with 6-OHDA and MPTP is that both these neurotoxins also induce increases in iron at the site of neurodegeneration, and, indeed, we were the first to show that the iron chelator desferal (desferrioxamine) is neuroprotective against these neurotoxins. Finally, as I showed in my presentation of the new studies that we have done, namely, rats made nutritionally iron deficient are protected against MPTP, 6-OHDA and kainate neurotoxicity—supporting the importance of iron to the process of neuronal cell death. In fact, several studies from our own laboratory and those of others have shown that these neurotoxins have the ability to release iron from ferritin. This may be the reason why iron chelators are neuroprotective.

From Dr. Sobotka

Assuming inflammatory reactions may be involved in the cascade of events underlying neurodegenerative diseases, do antiinflammatory drugs affect the onset or progression of neurodegenerative disease?

ANSWER: We have some evidence that iron may be the endogenous activator of NFκB, the transcription factor that is responsible for gene transcription activation of inflammatory cytokine TNFα, IL-1β, and IL-6, which are increased in Parkinson's disease and Alzheimer's disease as well as in rats treated with 6-OHDA. Thus antiinflammatory drugs could be an important therapy. It is most interesting that aspirin has been shown to be neuroptoective against glutamate and MPTP toxicity.

From Dr. Sobotka

Have antibiotics been shown to affect onset of neurodegenerative diseases?

ANSWER: No. But you never know. The anti-Parkinson action of amantadine, an antiviral drug, was discovered by an observant clinician who was treating a viral infection of a Parkinsonian subject, who reported to him that his Parkinsonian syndrome was better. We now know that anti-Parkinson action of amatadine may be due to its antiglutaminergic action.

From Dr. Hall

Is there any evidence for a role of peroxynitrite-induced neurotoxicity in Parkinson's disease?

ANSWER: This is an open question, and no clear-cut evidence is available. The fact that glutamate has been implicated in neurodgeneration indirectly may involve nitric oxide. Indeed our *in vitro* studies has shown that nitric oxide is a potent releaser of iron, and in cell culture studies glutamate and nitric oxide toxicity can be prevented again with the iron chelartor.

From Dr. Jonas

How do you prevent vomiting in patients receiving apomorphine?

ANSWER: By giving a peripheral dopamine antagonist such as domperidone.

From Dr. Trembly

What might be the role of antiinflammatory agents such as indomethacin in changes surrounding Alzheimer's plaques, as well as in other neurodegenerative disorders?

ANSWER: The simple answer would be either prevention or protection against oxidative stress factors or prevention to progression of apoptosis, which has received so much publicity recently. One thing that is certain is that in Parkinson's disease and Alzheimer's disease there is proliferation of (reactive) microglia around the dying as well as dead neurons.

Brain Adenosine Receptors as Targets for Therapeutic Intervention in Neurodegenerative Diseases

MARIA P. ABBRACCHIO[a] AND FLAMINIO CATTABENI

Institute of Pharmacological Sciences, Milan, Italy

ABSTRACT: Adenosine acts as a neurotransmitter in the brain through the activation of four specific G-protein-coupled receptors (the A_1, A_{2A}, A_{2B}, and A_3 receptors). The A_1 receptor has long been known to mediate neuroprotection, mostly by blockade of Ca^{2+} influx, which results in inhibition of glutamate release and reduction of its excitatory effects at a postsynaptic level. However, the development of selective A_1 receptor agonists as antiischemic agents has been hampered by their major cardiovascular side effects. More recently, apparently deleterious effects have been reported following the activation of other adenosine receptor subtypes, namely, the A_{2A} and the A_3 receptors. In particular, selective A_{2A} receptor antagonists have been demonstrated to markedly reduce cell death associated with brain ischemia in the rat, suggesting that the cerebral A_{2A} receptor may indeed contribute to the development of ischemic damage. The beneficial effects evoked by A_{2A} antagonists may be due to blockade of presynaptic A_{2A} receptors (which are stimulatory on glutamate release) and/or to inhibition of A_{2A} receptor-mediated activation of microglial cells. Even more puzzling data have been reported for the A_3 receptor subtype, which can indeed mediate both cell protection and cell death, simply depending upon the degree of receptor activation and/or specific pathophysiological conditions. In particular, a mild subthreshold activation of this receptor has been associated with a reinforcement of the cytoskeleton and reduction of spontaneous apoptosis, which may play a role in "ischemic preconditioning" of the brain, according to which a short ischemic period may protect the brain from a subsequent, sustained ischemic insult that would be lethal. In contrast, a robust and prolonged activation of the A_3 receptor has been shown to trigger cell death by either necrosis or apoptosis. Such apparently opposing actions may be reconciled by hypothesizing that adenosine-mediated cell killing during ischemia may be aimed at isolating the most damaged areas to favor those parts of the brain that still retain a chance for functional recovery. In fact, both A_3 receptor-mediated cell death and A_{2A} receptor-mediated actions may be viewed as an attempt to selectively kill irreversibly damaged cells in the "core" ischemic area, in order to save space and energy for the surrounding live cells in the "penumbra" area. Hence, the pharmacological modulation of the A_{2A} and A_3 receptors via selective ligands may represent a novel strategy in the therapeutic approach to pathologies characterized by acute or chronic neurodegenerative events.

[a]To whom correspondence and reprint requests should be addressed at the Institute of Pharmacological Sciences, University of Milan, Via Balzaretti 9, 20133 Milan, Italy. Phone, +39-02-20488316; fax, +39-02-29404961.

e-mail, abbracch@mailserver.unimi.it

INTRODUCTION

The role of adenosine in neurotransmission is relatively well established.[1] Either adenosine per se or its precursor adenosine triphosphate (ATP) is colocalized with a variety of excitatory "classic" neurotransmitters in both central and peripheral presynaptic vesicles. Purines are released upon depolarization of presynaptic terminals during physiological neurotransmission, and modulate nerve cell activity via both pre- and postsynaptic specific receptors. Uptake sites for adenosine and four distinct G-protein-coupled receptors (the A_1, A_{2A}, A_{2B}, and A_3 receptors)[2,3] have been identified on both neurons and glial cells.[4] These receptors have been linked to both inhibition (A_1 and A_3 receptors) and activation (A_{2A} and A_{2B} receptors) of adenylyl cyclase activity, stimulation of phosphoinositide metabolism (A_1 and A_3 receptors), as well as modulation of K^+ and Ca^{2+} conductances (A_1 receptors, see also below). The potent depressant, anticonvulsant and sedative properties of adenosine have been known for years, and adenosine has indeed been proposed to represent the brain endogenous "natural" anticonvulsant agent.[5] A protective role for adenosine in epilepsy and against trauma- and ischemia-associated brain injury has also been proposed; such neuroprotective activities have been hypothesized to be mainly mediated by the adenosine A_1 receptor[4,5] (see also below) and have so far been interpreted in terms of a short-term functional antagonism of the neurotoxicity produced by excitatory amino acids (e.g., glutamate, see also below). However, the concept that adenosine may also function as a direct regulator of cell viability via mechanisms other than activation of the A_1 adenosine receptor subtype (i.e., by activating fully independent intracellular pathways modulatory on cell survival) has recently been explored. Both cell protection and cell death have been reported, depending upon activation of distinct receptor subtypes and specific pathophysiological conditions.[6] The aim of the present review is to summarize the currently available data on modulation of cell survival by adenosine, with particular emphasis on recent data supporting a role for the A_{2A} and A_3 receptors in specific pathophysiological conditions.

MODULATION OF BRAIN CELL VIABILITY BY ADENOSINE: ROLE OF DIFFERENT RECEPTOR SUBTYPES

Role of the Adenosine A_1 Receptor

As mentioned above, most of the depressant, sedative and anticonvulsant effects of adenosine are mediated by the activation of pre- and postsynaptic A_1 receptors. Adenosine has a potent feed-back inhibitory effect on excitatory neurotransmission, which is due both to presynaptic inhibition of neurotransmitter release and to blockade of postsynaptic excitatory action potentials. Both these effects are mediated by the A_1 receptor, which is linked to modulation of K^+ and Ca^{2+} conductances and inhibition of adenylyl cyclase activity via Gi/Go proteins.[7] In brain, A_1 receptor-mediated inhibition of Ca^{2+} influx through voltage-gated channels seems to play a particularly important role, since, by limiting the availability of Ca^{2+}, it contributes to reducing the presynaptic release of excitatory transmitters as well as to counteracting their excitatory effects at the postsynaptic level.[7] These two mechanisms have been implicated as major determinants in adenosine-mediated antiglutamatergic and protective activities, during both physiological transmission as well as cerebral ischemia and brain trauma.[5]

Based on the above evidence, there have been several attempts during the years to develop selective A_1 receptor agonists that may prove useful as antiischemic and antiepileptic agents.[8] However, the development of such agents as novel therapeutic entities has been hampered by their marked side effects, namely, sedative, hypothermic and cardiovascular effects (e.g., dose-dependent bradycardia and hypotension). Thus, systemically-administered A_1 agonists elicit profound sedation and hypotension at doses that have relatively weak anticonvulsant and neuroprotective effects, which would make them therapeutically useless.[5] The separation of the desirable effects of A_1 agonists from the unwanted action has always been a problem, although some advancement has recently been reported in this respect, through the design and synthesis of novel A_1 receptor agonists characterized by selectivity towards brain receptors and hence by little or no effect on cardiovascular parameters or body temperature (ibidem). Another problem that may arise from the therapeutic use of A_1 agonists, especially in the case of chronic dosing (i.e., epilepsy), is agonist-induced receptor desensitization, which may progressively reduce the efficacy of the treatment upon repeated drug administration.[9,10] Hence, the future success of the agonist approach to ischemia and epilepsy may depend upon the availability of either A_1 partial agonists (which may reduce the extent of desensitization) or the identification of brain-specific A_1 receptor subtypes that can lead to more selective pharmacological manipulation.[5] An alternative approach to potentiating the neuroprotective actions mediated by the A_1 receptor resides in the development of Regulators of Endogenous Adenosine Levels (REAL agents).[11] These agents do not act at receptor level, but influence adenosine transport, metabolism and/or release.[11] In particular, inhibitors of adenosine deaminase and adenosine kinase, the two enzymes responsible for the transformation of adenosine to inosine and AMP, respectively, have been suggested to be potentially useful in augmenting cerebral adenosine levels during trauma and ischemia. Three desirable therapeutic objectives may be achieved by these agents. First, levels of endogenous adenosine might be selectively elevated by such agents only where and when adenosine is being produced. Secondly, due to its extremely short half-life, adenosine-induced actions may be limited to the area(s) where adenosine is being made. Thirdly, side effects for REAL agents are expected to be less than those of metabolically stable, longer-acting adenosine receptor agonists.

Role of the Adenosine A_{2A} Receptor

A_{2A} adenosine receptors were originally shown to be abundant in discrete brain areas such as c. striatum, and have hence been implicated in regulation of motor functions via a specific interaction with the dopaminergic system.[12,13] More recently, the presence of A_{2A} receptors, although to a lower expression level, has also been confirmed in hippocampus and cortex, where these receptors have been linked to augmentation of neurotransmission release.[13] In the past, A_{2A} receptors have also been implicated in adenosine-mediated neuroprotection following trauma and ischemia.[4] However, their protective role has mainly been attributed to nonneuronal receptors, i.e., those located on the arterial wall and on platelets and neutrophils.

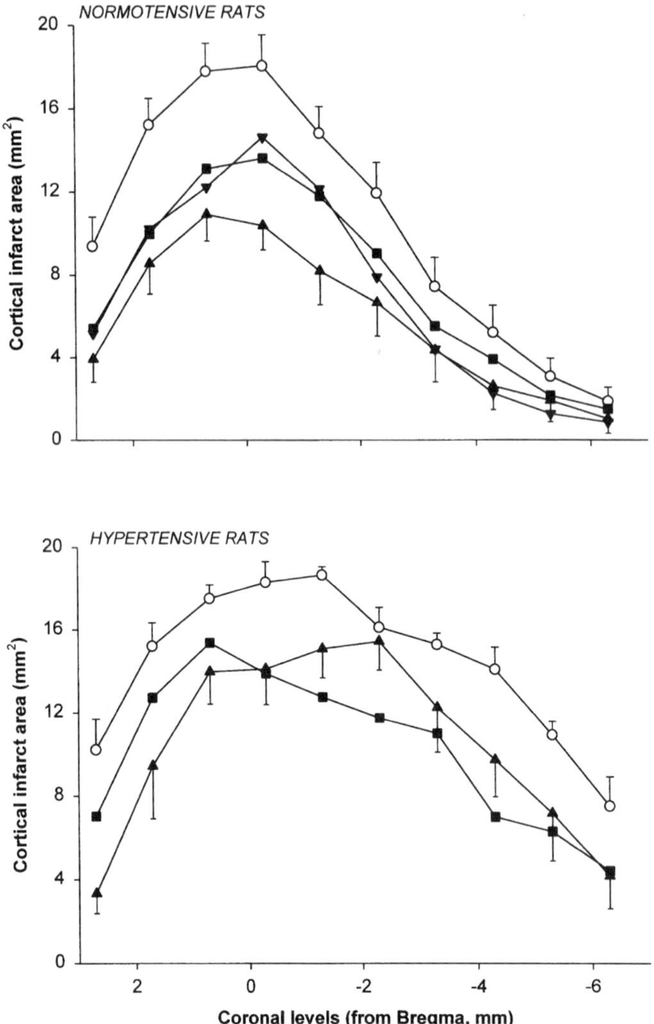

FIGURE 1. Effects of the A_{2A} adenosine receptor antagonist SCH 58261, 0.01 mg/kg, i.p. (■) or i.v. (▼), on brain infarct area in normotensive or hypertensive rats. The NMDA receptor antagonist, MK 801, 3 mg/kg, i.p. (▲), was used as refererence drug. Vehicle (○) or drugs were given 10 min after left middle cerebral artery occlusion. Data (mean ± SE) represent the areas of infarct in ten coronal sections for drug-treated groups vs controls in the left cerebral hemisphere. Both compounds significantly reduced infarct area as compared with controls (ANOVA, $p < 0.95$). (From Monopoli *et al.*[21] Reprinted by permission from *NeuroReport*.)

Hence, stimulation of these receptors by increasing adenosine concentrations during ischemia would synergize with the neuroprotective events mediated by the neuronal

A_1 receptor via increased blood flow, inhibition of platelet activation and thrombi formation, and reduced activation of neutrophils, which would eventually result in a reduction of damaging radical formation.

More recently, a role for neuronal A_{2A} receptors in the modulation of ischemic brain damage has also emerged. In an opposite fashion with respect to A_1 inhibitory receptors, activation of presynaptic A_{2A} receptors enhances the release of excitatory amino acids.[14,15] An enhancement of A_{2A} receptor-induced glutamate release seems to occur during ischemia, likely as a result of an imbalance between inhibitory A_1 and stimulatory A_{2A} receptors,[9,14] which may contribute to glutamate-dependent damage. Accordingly, blockade of these receptors reduces neuronal damage in various animal models.[13] Early evidence in this respect came from studies employing the nonselective A_{2A} receptor antagonists CGS 15943 (5-amino-9-chloro-2-(2-furyl)-1,2,4-triazolo[1.5-c]quinazoline) and CP 66,713 (4-amino-1-phenyl[1,24]triazolo[4,3-a]quinoxaline), which were proved to effectively reduce cerebral ischemic damage in the gerbil.[16,17] More recently, these data have received further confirmation by employing two more selective blockers, such as ZM 241385 (4-92-[7-amino-2-(2-furyl)[1,2,4]triazolo[2,3-a][1,3,5]triazin-5-yl-amino]ethyl-phenol) which reduced neuronal injury in the rat model of kainate-induced hippocampal damage,[18] and SCH 58261 (5-amino-7-(β-phenylethyl)-2-(8-furyl)pyrazolo[4,3-e]-1,2,4-triazolo[1,5-c]pyrimidine, which indeed represents the first really selective A_{2A} receptor antagonist.[19,20] With respect to CGS 15943, which shows only a 7-fold selectivity for A_{2A} receptors with respect to A_1 receptors (ibidem), SCH 58261 is 50- or 500-fold selective for A_{2A} versus the rat and human A_1 receptor, respectively; moreover, it does not interact with either A_{2B} or A_3 receptors. SCH 58261 (0.01 mg/Kg either i.p. or i.v.) administration to rats 10 min after occlusion of the left middle cerebral artery markedly reduced cortical infarct volume as measured 24 hr later (FIG. 1).[21] A similar effect was observed when SCH 58261 was administered to hypertensive rats (also shown in FIG. 1). Such *in vivo* neuroprotective properties of SCH 58261 indicate that, despite the above-mentioned data demonstrating benefical antiischemic effects mediated by "peripheral" A_{2A} receptors in blood vessels, platelets and neutrophils, blockade of neuronal A_{2A} receptors is a potentially useful target for the reduction of brain injury. Additional mechanisms that may contribute to the *in vivo* SCH 58261 protective effects may involve the microglial cells. Under pathological conditions, these cells start to proliferate and adopt a number of immune functions, including upregulation of cyclooxygenase-2 (COX-2) and production of inflammatory mediators such as prostaglandin E_2, cytokines and interleukins.[13] Activation of microglial A_{2A} receptors has been shown to stimulate the proliferation of these cells and to upregulate COX-2 expression, hence resulting in inflammation and production of prostaglandins.[22] Induction of COX-2 may contribute to both ischemia-associated neurotoxicity and neurodegeneration in aging-associated chronic neurodegenerative diseases, such as Alzheimer's and Parkinson's disease.[23] Therefore, blockade of A_{2A} receptors may also be protective by preventing the stimulatory actions of adenosine on resting microglial cells.

Role of the Adenosine A_3 Receptor

Within the four adenosine receptor subtypes, the recently discovered A_3 receptor is the most intriguing one. Similar to the A_1 receptor, its activation is coupled to both inhibition of adenylyl cyclase activity and stimulation of phospholipase C (see Introduction); however, at variance with the A_1 receptor subtype, which shows a very discrete brain regional distribution, the cerebral distribution of the A_3 receptor is very widely diffused. A_3 receptors can be detected in virtually all brain areas, although to a much lower density with respect to the other receptor subtypes. Moreover, differently from the A_1 and A_{2A} receptors, which are activated by nanomolar concentrations of adenosine, the A_3 receptor subtype responds to micromolar concentrations.[24] This has raised the hypothesis that at physiological interstitial adenosine concentrations (approx. 20–300 nM) this receptor may be functionally dormant, and may instead be activated under specific pathophysiological conditions characterized by elevation of local adenosine concentrations. One of such conditions is brain trauma and ischemia, when brain levels of adenosine are massively increased, as a consequence of augmented presynaptic release of transmitters (see Introduction), rapid intraischemic breakdown of ATP, and degradation of nucleic acids of dead cells (see also below). It may well be that in brain this receptor is recruited only under emergency conditions.

Initial evidence for the involvement of adenosine A_3 receptors in modulation of brain cell survival came from *in vivo* studies.[25] Administration of the selective A_3 receptor agonist IB-MECA (N^6-(3-iodobenzyl)-adenosine-5′-N-methyl-uronamide) to ischemic gerbils resulted in either reduction or enhancement of brain damage depending upon the protocol of agonist administration. A single acute IB-MECA administration immediately before the induction of global ischemia markedly worsened both animal survival and the extent of neuronal damage in the hippocampus with respect to control animals; in contrast, a one-week pretreatment of animals with IB-MECA before the induction of ischemia resulted in marked protection, as shown by both significantly increased rate of animal survival and reduced histopathological damage in the hippocampus.[25] On this basis, it was suggested that the adenosine A_3 receptor may contribute to brain damage during trauma and ischemia, and hence a subchronic treatment of animals with a selective A_3 receptor agonist prior to ischemia would reduce the contribution of this receptor to neuronal death via the induction of agonist-induced desensitization.[25] Subsequent *in vitro* studies have confirmed that the adenosine A_3 receptor is indeed involved in modulation of the survival of a variety of different cell types, including lymphoid cells,[26–27] eosinophils,[28] cardiomyocytes,[29] and, more relevant to this review, cerebellar granule cells[30] and astroglial cells.[31,32] When used in the higher micromolar range, the selective adenosine A_3 receptor agonist IB-MECA induced necrosis of cerebellar granule cells in a concentration-dependent fashion. Incubation of cultures with comparable concentrations of agonists of A_1, A_{2A}, and A_{2B} receptors (i.e., cyclopentyl-adenosine, 5′-N-ethylcarboxamidoadenosine, NECA, and 2-[4-[(2-carboxyethyl)-phenyl]ethylamino]-5′-N-ethylcarboxamidoadenosine, CGS 21680) had no effect on neuronal survival, suggesting a specific role for the A_3 receptor. Furthermore, a subcytotoxic (1 micromolar) concentration of the Cl-derivative of IB-MECA (Cl-IB-MECA) significantly augmented the receptor-mediated neurotoxicity of 50 micromolar glutamate.[30] In the Sei *et al.* study,[30] neuronal cell death induced by Cl-IB-MECA appeared to be related to inhibition of cyclic AMP production (see also Introduction), and not related to protein kinase C activation through modulation of phosphoinositide metabolism. Adding the stable and cell-permeating analog of cy-

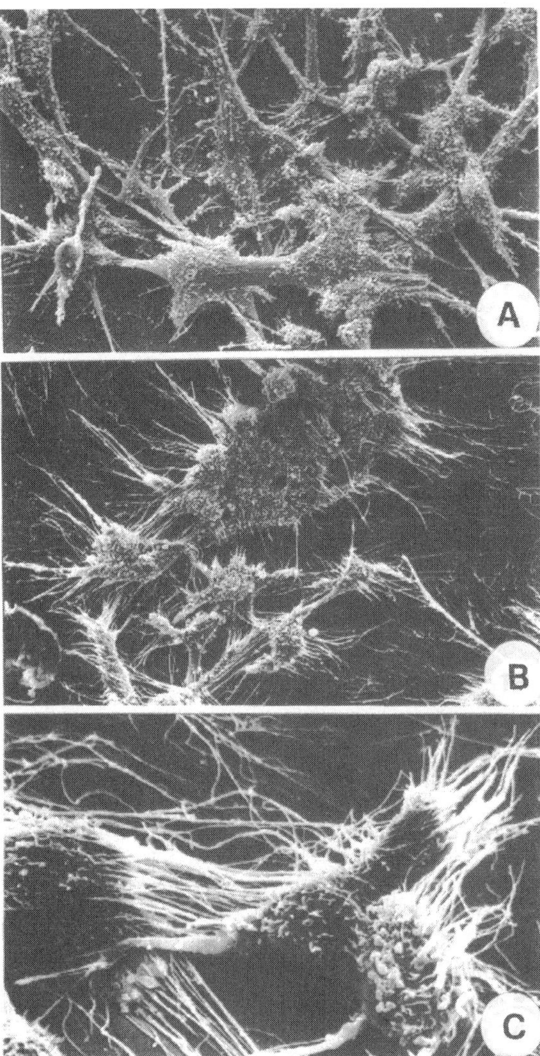

FIGURE 2. Scanning electron micrographs of human astrocytoma ADF control cells (**A**) and ADF cells treated with 100 nanomolar Cl-IB-MECA for 72 hr (**B,C**). Control cells show a typical bipolar shape with a relatively low number of cell protrusions (A). Exposure to the selective A_3 receptor agonist Cl-IB-MECA induced marked morphological changes represented by a dramatic increase of both the number and length of astrocytic processes (B,C). (Original magnification: A,B 1000×; C 3300×). (From Abbracchio et al.[31] Reprinted by permission from *Biochemical and Biophysical Research Communications*.)

clic AMP (cAMP), dibutyryl-cAMP, to the culture to activate cyclic AMP-dependent protein kinases indeed attenuated Cl-IB-MECA-induced neurotoxicity.[30] Besides confirming the role of this receptor subtype in regulation of cell survival, these results also highlight the possibility of a functional relationship with the glutamatergic system. Hence, it could be hypothesized that activation of the adenosine A_3 receptor such as believed to occur during ischemia may contribute to augmenting glutamate-mediated neuronal death (see also below). The existence of a synergism between the A_3 receptor and the glutamatergic system is also supported by recent electrophysiological findings showing that A_1 receptor-mediated inhibition of glutamate release is markedly attenuated by activation of the A_3 receptor,[33] hence resulting in a potentiation of glutamate-evoked effects (see also below).

The role of the A_3 receptor in cells of astroglial cells, a cell type crucially involved in brain response to trauma and ischemia, has been studied in detail.[31,32] A 48–72-hr exposure of both rat primary astrocytes and human astrocytoma ADF cells to the selective A_3 receptor agonists IB-MECA and Cl-IB-MECA resulted in a biphasic regulation of cell survival, with "trophic" protective effects at nanomolar concentrations[31,32] and cell death at high micromolar concentrations.[32] The exact role of the A_3 receptor in the latter effect is still under study, since this effect could not be reversed by several selective A_3 antagonists.[32] It could well be that an atypical A_3 receptor characterized by insensitivity to the currently available antagonists is involved in A_3 agonist-induced cell death. A clearcut role for the A_3 receptor was instead demonstrated for the trophic effect induced by nanomolar A_3 agonists on these same cells. Such effect consisted in an increase of cellular protrusions (FIG. 2), likely due to a reinforcement of the actin cytoskeleton, with the appearance of F-actin-positive stress fibers in agonist-treated cells with respect to control cells.[31] The morphological changes induced by A_3 receptor agonists in these cells did have a functional counterpart, since they were associated with a reduction of the degree of spontaneous apoptotic cell death, as evaluated with the fluorescent nuclear dye Hoechst 33258 in cells detached in the culture medium.[32] A specific role for the adenosine receptor was also confirmed by the fact that the selective A_3 receptor antagonist MRS1191 could completely prevent the antiapoptotic effects evoked by A_3 agonists.[32] To shed some light on the mechanisms responsible for A_3 agonist-induced cytoprotection, we have recently focussed our attention on proteins belonging to the bcl-2 family. This family has been shown to encompass both antiapoptotic proteins such as Bcl-2 and Bcl-XL, as well as proapoptotic proteins such as bak, bad or bax.[34] Immunocytochemical studies have shown that ADF cells do not express Bcl-2 but do express significant amounts of Bcl-XL, which in these cells can be detected as a specific doublet of proteins of 31 and 37 kDa.[31] Although exposure of cells to A_3 agonists was found not to alter the total amount of immunodetectable protein with respect to control untreated cells,[31] marked changes of its intracellular distribution were detected. In fact, whereas in control cells, Bcl-XL was mainly located to the cytoplasm, in agonist-exposed cultures immunoreactivity was detected as bright spots specifically located in cellular protrusions.[31,32] Such a highly specific location may suggest association with cytoskeleton elements. This effect was antagonized by the selective A_3 antagonist MRS1191 (FIG. 3), confirming that it is indeed mediated by activation of the adenosine A_3 receptor. These results raise the hypothesis that the A_3 receptor may modulate cell adhesion (and ultimately cell viability) by influencing the intracellular distribution of the Bcl-XL protein and by promoting its association with the cytoskeleton. To support a link between expression of Bcl-XL, cell

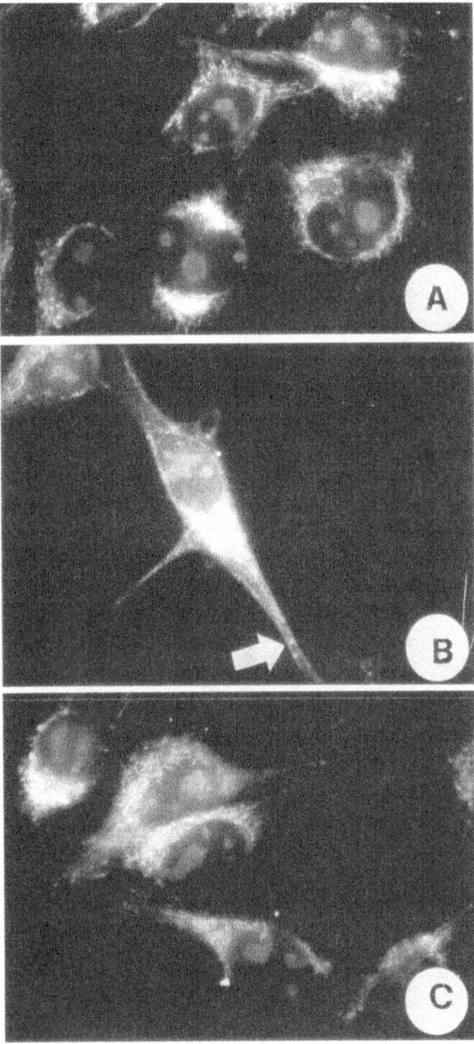

FIGURE 3. Modulation of the intracellular distribution of Bcl-XL by A_3 agonists in human astrocytoma ADF cells. In the majority of control cells (**A**), immunoreactivity is located to the cytoplasm. After exposure of cultures to 100 nanomolar Cl-IB-MECA for 48 hr, immunoreactivity to the anti-Bcl-XL antibody is also found as very bright spots that are particularly abundant in cell protrusions (see *arrow* in (**B**)). Similar data were obtained after a 48-hr treatment with 100 nanomolar IB-MECA (data not shown). The concomitant exposure of cultures to 10 nM MRS1191 counteracted agonist-induced accumulation of Bcl-XL in cellular protrusions (**C**). Cultures exposed to MRS1191 alone showed no differences with respect to control cultures (data not shown). Note that all micrographs were taken at the same high magnification (1800×) in order to compare the biological effect and to better point out intracellular labeling. (From Abbracchio *et al.*[32] Reprinted by permission from *Drug Development Research*.)

adhesion and cell survival, in this same experimental model, spontaneously detached cells in culture supernatants were all Bcl-XL-negative, suggesting that turning off of the Bcl-XL gene may represent a key signal in directing cells towards detachment and apoptosis.[31] Moreover, these data are consistent with the recent demonstration that Bcl-2 promotes growth and regeneration of retinal axons[35] and support the existence of a close relationship between the cytoskeleton, adhesion processes and Bcl-2-like proteins. It may be hypothesized that, at least in part, the protective effects of these proteins are mediated by a target effect on the cytoskeleton, and hence by modifications of cell-substrate interactions that eventually influence cell survival and death.

The dual effects induced by A_3 agonists on cells of the astroglial lineage are consistent with what has been reported on cardiac myocytes. In chick ventricular cardiomyocytes, exposure to nanomolar concentrations of A_3 agonists prior to the induction of ischemia markedly protected against injury.[36] In these cells, protection could be achieved also by exposure to selective A_1 receptor agonists: however, protection associated to A_3 receptor activation was significantly higher. Prior exposure of myocytes to a brief ischemic period also protected them against injury induced by a subsequent exposure to prolonged ischemia (a phenomenon known as "ischemic preconditioning"), suggesting that adenosine, which is released in large amounts during myocardial ischemia, may protect the myocardium via the activation of the A_3 adenosine receptor.[36] Such an hypothesis was further supported by data showing that the A_3 receptor selective antagonist MRS1191 inhibited A_3 agonist-induced protection. Moreover, transfection of atrial cells (which lack native A_3 receptors and exhibit a shorter duration of cardioprotection) with cDNA encoding the human adenosine A_3 receptor caused a sustained A_3-agonist-mediated cardioprotection.[36] While nanomolar concentrations of selective agonists for either A_1 or A_3 receptors protected cardiac myocytes, micromolar concentrations of A_3 selective agonists induced cell death in cardiomyocytes.[29] This cell death occurred exclusively through an apoptotic rather than a necrotic mechanism.

Globally these data suggest a remarkable similarity between the cardiac and the brain A_3 receptor in modulation of cell survival. A subthreshold activation of this receptor subtype by low (nanomolar) agonist concentrations is associated with cytoprotection in both cell types; it may be hypothesized that a phenomenon similar to the well-known ischemic preconditioning of the heart may also exist in brain, and that activation of the cerebral adenosine A_3 receptor during a brief ischemic period (or in the "penumbra" area, see also below) activates a series of protective mechanisms (e.g., cytoskeletal reinforcement), resulting in cytoprotection and reduced sensitivity to subsequent insults. In this respect, a brief ischemic period obtained by carotid occlusion has been demonstrated to protect the brain against a subsequent, stronger ischemic insult that would be lethal.[37] Conversely, a robust activation of this receptor by elevated adenosine concentrations may contribute to cell death and to the elimination of irreversibly damaged cells (see also below).

An hypothesis that may reconcile the opposite effects evoked by the A_3 receptor on cell survival and give them a pathophysiological significance has recently been raised by von Lubitz.[38] This hypothesis is based on the existence of a gradient of adenosine concentrations within the infarct area following an ischemic insult to the brain. It may be hypothesized that, in the ischemic "core," extracellular concentrations of adenosine are raised to the level sufficient for sustained stimulation of A_3 receptors. Once activated, the latter attenuates the inhibitory control that is normally exerted on glutamate release by the A_1 receptor,[33] resulting in further release of the neurotransmitter and hence in a potentiation of excitotoxicity. Besides this interaction at a presynaptic level, the A_3 receptor would work in concert with glutamate in enhancing the deleterious effects mediated by the postsynaptic N-methyl-D-aspartate (NMDA) receptor,[30] leading to massive neuronal killing. The process is compounded by killing of astroglial cells,[32] which would interrupt astrocytic glutamate uptake, and hence further increase glutamate-induced excitotoxicity. In contrast, in the "penumbra" area, cells are damaged but are still alive, and adenosine concentrations would be progressively reduced depending upon distance from the ischemic "core." Under these conditions, a subthreshold stimulation of the A_3 adenosine receptor by much lower adenosine concentrations would be favored, leading to the activation of protective trophic mechanisms aimed at favoring the survival and recovery of neurons. A_3 receptor-mediated activation of astrocytes in the "penumbra" area, with elongation of astrocytic processes and differentiation to a more specialized phenotype,[31] would contribute both to the formation of the gliotic scar (and hence to isolating the most severely damaged tissue from the surrounding recovering cells), and to the recovery of damaged neurons via a potentiation of the astrocytic support to these cells.

According to this hypothesis, all these actions are aimed at killing irreversibly damaged cells in the "core" area (in order to reroute energy resources to the surrounding live cells) and at favoring rescue of suffering neurons in the "penumbra" area by a potentiation of the astrocytic support to neurons. Such an hypothesis is also consistent with the concept that in some cases induction of cell death in the ischemic brain may be beneficial.[39]

CONCLUSIONS

The evidence summarized above supports the hypothesis that adenosine may play a key role in the modulation of ischemic brain damage. Apparently opposite effects seem to be mediated by selected adenosine receptor subtypes (namely, cytoprotection by the A_1 and cell death by the A_3 receptor), which would obscure the dogma that adenosine is a neuroprotective agent. However, despite such differential roles, it is tempting to suggest that all adenosine actions, at least those mediated by the A_1 and A_3 receptors, are indeed aimed at limiting brain damage and favoring functional recovery. If seen in the context of survival as the ultimate goal, the apparently deleterious effects evoked by the A_3 receptor can also be interpreted as an attempt to isolate the most damaged areas and support the recovery of those parts of the brain still retaining a chance for functional recovery. Also some of the actions evoked by the A_{2A} receptor during ischemia (e.g., potentiation of glutamate release and activation of microglial cells) may be viewed in terms of selective killing of most damaged cells and remodeling of brain circuitries in the postischemic period.

On this basis, it may be speculated that a reduction of the detrimental effects evoked by the A_{2A} and A_3 receptors via selective antagonists would reduce brain damage, an hypothesis that is already partially supported by experimental data.[21,25]

Moreover, the antagonist approach would have significant advantages with respect to the use of A_1 agonist to improve adenosine neuroprotection, due to the wide array of side effects associated with agonist administration and with the induction of receptor desensitization.

ACKNOWLEDGMENTS

The authors are grateful to Dr. Ennio Ongini (Schering-Plough Research Institute, Milan, Italy) and to Dr. Dag von Lubitz (Department of Emergency Medicine, University of Michigan, Ann Arbour, MI, USA) for useful discussion and critical reading. MPA is the recipient of contract grants from the Consiglio Nazionale delle Ricerche (96.03340.CT04 and 98.01047.CT04).

REFERENCES

1. RUDOLPHI, K.A. & P. SCHUBERT. 1996. Purinergic interventions in traumatic and ischemic injury. *In* Novel Therapies for CNS Injuries. Rationales and Results. P.L. Peterson & J.W. Phillis, Eds.: 327–346. CRC Press. Boca Raton, FL.
2. FREDHOLM, B.B., M.P. ABBRACCHIO, G. BURNSTOCK, J.W. DALY, T.K. HARDEN, K.A. JACOBSON, P. LEFF & M. WILLIAMS. 1994. Nomenclature and classification of purinoceptors. Pharmacol. Rev. **46:** 143–156.
3. FREDHOLM, B.B., M.P. ABBRACCHIO, G. BURNSTOCK, G.R. DUBYAK, T.K. HARDEN, K.A. JACOBSON, U. SCHWABE & M. WILLIAMS. 1997. Towards a revised nomenclature for P1 and P2 receptors. Trends Pharmacol. Sci. **18:** 79–82.
4. SCHUBERT, P., T. OGATA, C. MARCHINI, S. FERRONI & K. RUDOLPHI. 1997. Protective mechanisms of adenosine in neurons and glial cells. Ann. N.Y. Acad. Sci. **825:** 1–10.
5. KNUTSEN, L.J.S. & T.F. MURRAY. 1997. Adenosine and ATP in epilepsy. *In* Purinergic Approaches in Experimental Therapeutics. K.A. Jacobson & M.F. Jarvis, Eds.: 423–447. Wiley Liss. New York.
6. JACOBSON, K.A., C. HOFFMANN, F. CATTABENI & M.P. ABBRACCHIO. 1999. Adenosine-induced cell death: evidence for receptor-mediated signalling. Apoptosis **4:** 197–211.
7. FREDHOLM, B.B., G. ARSLAN, B. KULL, E. KONTNY & P. SVENNINGSSON. 1996. Adenosine (P1) receptor signalling. Drug Dev. Res. **39:** 262–268.
8. SPEDDING, M. & M. WILLIAMS. 1996. Developments in purine and pyrimidine receptor-based therapeutics. Drug Dev. Res. **39:** 436–441.
9. ABBRACCHIO, M.P., G. FOGLIATTO, A.M. PAOLETTI, G.E. ROVATI & F. CATTABENI. 1992. Prolonged *in vitro* exposure of rat brain slices to adenosine analogues: selective desensitization of A_1 but not A_2 adenosine receptors. Eur. J. Pharmacol. (Mol. Pharmacol.) **227:** 317–324.
10. ADAMI, M., R. BERTORELLI, N. FERRI, M.C. FODDI & E. ONGINI. 1996. Effects of repeated administration of selective adenosine A_1 and A_{2A} receptor agonists on pentylentetrazole-induced convulsions in the rat. Eur. J. Pharmacol. **294:** 383–389.
11. GEIGER, J.D., F.E. PARKINSON & E.A. KOWALUK. 1997. Regulation of endogenous adenosine levels as therapeutic agents. *In* Purinergic Approaches in Experimental Therapeutics. K.A. Jacobson & M.F. Jarvis, Eds.: 55–84. Wiley Liss. New York.
12. ONGINI, E., S. DIONISOTTI, M. MORELLI, S. FERRÉ, P. SVENNINGSSON, K. FUXE & B.B. FREDHOLM. 1996. Neuropharmacology of the adenosine A_{2A} receptor. Drug Dev. Res. **39:** 450–460.
13. ONGINI, E. & P. SCHUBERT. 1998. Neuroprotection induced by stimulating A_1 or blocking A_{2A} adenosine receptors: an apparent paradox. Drug Dev. Res. **45:** 387–393.

14. O'REGAN, M.H., R.E. SIMPSON, L.M. PERKINS & J.W. PHILLIS. 1992. The selective A_2 adenosine receptor agonist CGS 21680 enhances excitatory amino acid release from the ischaemic rat cerebral cortex. Neurosci. Lett. **138:** 169–172.

15. POPOLI, P., P. BETTO, R. REGGIO & G. RICCIARELLO. 1995. Adenosine A_{2A} receptor stimulation enhances striatal extracellular glutamate levels in rats. Eur. J. Pharmacol. **287:** 215–217.

16. GAO, Y. & J.W. PHILLIS. 1994. CGS 15943, an adenosine A_2 receptor antagonist, reduces cerebral ischemia injury in the Mongolian gerbil. Life Sci. **55:** PL61–PL65.

17. PHILLIS, J.W. 1995. The effects of selective A_1 and A_2 adenosine receptor antagonists on cerebral ischaemic injury in the gerbil. Brain Res. **705:** 79–84.

18. JONES, P.A., R.A. SMITH & T.W. STONE. 1998. Protection against kainate-induced excitotoxicity by adenosine A_{2A} receptor agonists and antagonists. Neuroscience **85:** 229–237.

19. JACOBSON, K.A. & F. SUZUKI. 1996. Recent developments in selective agonists acting at purine and pyrimidine receptors. Drug Dev. Res. **39:** 289–300.

20. ONGINI, E. 1997. SCH 58261: a selective A_{2A} adenosine receptor antagonist. Drug Dev. Res. **42:** 63–70.

21. MONOPOLI, A., G. LOZZA, A. FORLANI, A. MATTAVELLI & E. ONGINI. 1998. Blockade of adenosine A_{2A} receptors by SCH 58261 results in neuroprotective effects in cerebral ischaemia in rats. NeuroReport **9:** 3955–3959.

22. FIEBICH, B.L., K. BIBER, K. LIEB, D. VAN CALKER, M. BERGER, J. BAUER & P.J. GEBICKE-HAERTER. 1996. Cyclo-oxygenase-2 expression in rat microglia is induced by adenosine A_{2A} receptors. Glia **18:** 152–160.

23. TOCCO, G., J. FREIRE-MOAR, S.S. SCHREIBER, S.H. SAKHI, P.S. AISEN & G.M. PASINETTI. 1997. Maturational regulation and regional induction of cyclooxygenase-2 in rat brain: implications for Alzheimer's disease. Exp. Neurol. **144:** 339–349.

24. JACOBSON, K.A. 1998. Adenosine A_3 receptors: novel ligands and paradoxical effects. Trends Pharmacol. Sci. **19:** 184–191.

25. VON LUBITZ, D.K.J.E., R.C.-S. LIN, P. POPIK, M.F. CARTER & K.A. JACOBSON. 1994. Adenosine A_3 receptor stimulation and cerebral ischemia. Eur. J. Pharmacol. **263:** 59–67.

26. KOHNO, Y., Y. SEI, M. KOSHIBA, H.O. KIM & K.A. JACOBSON. 1996. Induction of apoptosis in HL-60 human promyelocytic leukemia cells by selective adenosine A_3 receptor agonists. Biochem. Biophys. Res. Commun. **219:** 904–910.

27. BARBIERI, D., M.P. ABBRACCHIO, S. SALVIOLI, D. MONTI, A. COSSARIZZA, S. CERUTI, R. BRAMBILLA, F. CATTABENI & K.A. JACOBSON. 1998. Apoptosis by 2-chloro-2′-deoxy-adenosine and 2-chloro-adenosine in human peripheral blood mononuclear cells. Neurochem. Int. **32:** 493–504.

28. KOHNO, Y., X.-D. JI, S.D. MAWHORTER, B. BOCHNER, Y. SEI, M. KOSHIBA & K.A. JACOBSON. 1996. Activation of adenosine A_3 receptor on human eosinophils raises intracellular Ca^{2+} and induces apoptosis. Drug Dev. Res. **37:** 182.

29. SHNEYVAIS, V., H. NAWRATH, K.A. JACOBSON & A. SHAINBERG. 1998. Induction of apoptosis in cardiac myocytes by an A_3 adenosine receptor agonist. Exp. Cell Res. **243:** 383–397.

30. SEI, Y., D.K.J.E. VON LUBITZ, M.P. ABBRACCHIO, X.-D. JI & K.A. JACOBSON. 1997. Adenosine A_3 receptor agonist-induced neurotoxicity in rat cerebellar granule neurons. Drug Dev. Res. **40:** 267–273.

31. ABBRACCHIO, M.P., G. RAINALDI, A.M. GIAMMARIOLI, S. CERUTI, R. BRAMBILLA, F. CATTABENI, D. BARBIERI, C. FRANCESCHI, K.A. JACOBSON & W. MALORNI. 1997. The A_3 adenosine receptor mediates cell spreading, reorganization of actin cyto-

skeleton and distribution of Bcl-XL. Studies in human astroglioma cells. Biochem. Biophys. Res. Commun. **241:** 297–304.

32. ABBRACCHIO, M.P., S. CERUTI, R. BRAMBILLA, D. BARBIERI, A. CAMURRI, C. FRANCE-SCHI, A.M. GIAMMARIOLI, K.A. JACOBSON, F. CATTABENI & W. MALORNI. 1998. Adenosine A_3 receptors and viability of astrocytes. Drug Dev. Res. **45:** 379–386.

33. DUNWIDDIE, T.V., L. DIAO, H.O. KIM, J.-L. JIANG & K.A. JACOBSON. 1997. Activation of hippocampal adenosine A_3 receptors produces a heterologous desensitization of A_1 receptor mediated responses in rat hippocampus. J. Neurosci. **17:** 607–614.

34. BROWN, R. 1997. The bcl-2 family of proteins. Br. Med. Bull. **53:** 451–465.

35. CHEN, D.F., G.E. SCHNEIDER, J.-C. MARTINOU & S. TONEGAWA. 1997. Bcl-2 promotes regeneration of severed axons in mammalian CNS. Nature **385:** 434–439.

36. LIANG, B.T. & K.A. JACOBSON. 1998. A physiological role of the adenosine A_3 receptor: sustained cardioprotection. Proc. Natl. Acad. Sci. USA **95:** 6995–6999.

37. KITAGAWA, K., M. MATSUMOTO, M. TAGAYA, R. HATA, H. UEDA, M. NIINOBE, N. HANDA, R. FUKUNAGA, K. KIMURA, K. MIKOSHIBA & T. KAMADA. 1990. "Ischemic tolerance" phenomenon found in the brain. Brain Res. **528:** 21–24.

38. VON LUBITZ, D.K.J.E. 1999. Stimulation of adenosine A_3 receptors in cerebral ischemia: neuronal death, recovery, or both? This volume.

39. NEARY, J.T., M.P. RATHBONE, F. CATTABENI, M.P. ABBRACCHIO & G. BURNSTOCK. 1996. Trophic actions of extracellular nucleotides and nucleosides on glial and neuronal cells. Trends Neurosci. **19:** 13–18.

Stimulation of Adenosine A_3 Receptors in Cerebral Ischemia

Neuronal Death, Recovery, or Both?

DAG K.J.E. von LUBITZ,[a,c] WEN YE,[a] JENNIFER McCLELLAN,[a] AND RICK C.-S. LIN[b]

[a]*Emergency Medicine Research Laboratories, Department of Emergency Medicine, University of Michigan Health System, Ann Arbor, Michigan 48109-0303, USA*

[b]*Department of Anatomy, University of Mississippi Medical Center, Jackson, Mississippi 39216-4505, USA*

ABSTRACT: The role of the adenosine A_3 receptor continues to baffle, and, despite an increasing number of studies, the currently available data add to, rather than alleviate, the existing confusion. The reported effects of adenosine A_3 receptor stimulation appear to depend on the pattern of drug administration (acute vs. chronic), dose, and type of the target tissue. Thus, while acute exposure to A_3 receptor agonists protects against myocardial ischemia, it is severely damaging when these agents are given shortly prior to cerebral ischemia. Mast cells degranulate when their A_3 receptors are stimulated. Degranulation of neutrophils is, on the other hand, impaired. While reduced production of reactive nitrogen species has been reported following activation of A_3 receptors in collagen-induced arthritis, the process appears to be enhanced in cerebral ischemia. Indeed, immunocytochemical studies indicate that both pre- and postischemic treatment with A_3 receptor antagonist dramatically reduces nitric oxide synthase in the affected hippocampus. Even more surprisingly, low doses of A_3 receptor agonists seem to enhance astrocyte proliferation, while high doses induce their apoptosis. This review concentrates on the studies of cerebral A_3 receptors and, based on the available evidence, discusses the possibility of adenosine A_3 receptor serving as an integral element of the endogenous cerebral neuroprotective complex consisting of adenosine and its receptors.

THE NATURE OF THE ADENOSINE A_3 RECEPTOR

In the very beginning of the present decade, the family of adenosine receptors (A_1, A_{2A}, and A_{2B}) increased by the addition of another distinct type—the A_3 receptor. Cloning of the cDNA from the rat testis library revealed approximately 40% identity with A_1 and A_{2A} types.[1] Further cloning studies[2–4] revealed intriguing differences in the degree of homologies among different species, indicating a possibility that A_3 receptors may, in fact, exist as a range of subtypes.[5]

[c]Corresponding author: Dr. Dag K.J.E. von Lubitz, Emergency Medicine Research Laboratories, Department of Emergency Medicine, University of Michigan Health System, TC/B1354/0303, 1500 E. Medical Center Drive, Ann Arbor, MI 48109-0303. Phone, 734/936-6020; fax, 734/936-9414.

e-mail, dvlubitz@umich.edu

The A_3 receptor is a G-protein-coupled entity and, like all other known receptors of this type, consists of a long polypeptide chain with seven α-helices residing within the cellular membrane ending in an extracellular N- and an intracellular C-terminus.[6] The region between the central and the extracellular region of V–VII helices appears to constitute the active site of the receptor.[6] Signal transduction at the A_3 receptor is mediated by G_i/G_o proteins,[7,8] and the receptor appears to regulate their expression. The latter process is, however, somewhat heterogenous, and the responses of different subunits to the receptor's prolonged exposure to an agonist differ.[7] Long-lasting stimulation of A_3 receptors *in vitro* also results in their functional desensitization[9] and a noticeable reduction of high-affinity binding sites.[7] A detailed discussion can be found in the reviews by Palmer and Stiles[8] and Olah and Stiles.[10] In the context of the present paper, the finding that A_3 receptors desensitize rapidly may provide at least partial explanation for rather striking outcome differences observed following acute or chronic exposure to A_3 receptor agonists *in vivo* (see below).

Adenyl cyclase and phospholipase C serve as the second messenger systems of the A_3 receptor. Its stimulation results in depression of cyclic adenosine-5',3'-monophosphate (cAMP) synthesis[2,3] or activation of phospholipase C[11] and subsequent stimulation of inositol-1,4,5-triphosphate synthesis.[12] Although it is unlikely that both second messengers are triggered into action at the same time, there are presently no studies analyzing these processes in detail. However, recent observations on the dependence of astrocytic response on the concentration of the stimulating A_3 agonist[13] (see below) indicate the possibility that the intensity and/or duration of receptor activation may have a possibly preferential impact on the selection of the second messenger system.

Probably the most striking aspect of A_3 receptor pharmacology is its very low affinity for adenosine. Although more recent studies reduced the original estimates of K_i from 30 μM[2] to 1 μM,[5] the value is still approximately two orders of the magnitude higher than that characterizing either A_1 or A_2 receptors (10 and 30 nM, respectively). The low affinity of A_3 receptors for adenosine poses one of many difficulties in envisaging the biological role of the receptor since, under the normal conditions, the extracellular concentration of adenosine in the brain does not exceed 300 nM (for review, see Ref. 14). However, none of the currently available methods of measuring adenosine concentration in the normal brain offers any indication of its value in the "operational" areas of neurons, i.e., perisynaptic space. Hence, intense synaptic activity, even under the normal conditions, may elevate local adenosine concentration to the level that is sufficient for A_3 receptor activation. Recent physiological studies of Dunwiddie *et al.*[15] indicate such a possibility. While interspecies differences in the affinity of A_3 receptors for antagonists are also striking, it is more likely that they mirror differences of receptor structure rather than function as such.[16] Much less pronounced, the variability in agonist affinity has been demonstrated as well.[16]

The progress in understanding of the 3-dimensional structure of A_3 receptors that derived from introduction of new techniques[17] is paralleled by a continuously increasing availability of selective A_3 receptor agonists and antagonists.[18–20] Regrettably, the development of these agents is not matched by the corresponding effort to synthesize equally selective radio-labeled ligands. Hence, our knowledge of A_3 receptor distribution is comparatively meagre, although considerable variation both in its distribution and density among several nonhuman mammalian species has been reported.[5,16] The exact cellular location of A_3 receptors is still unknown as much in the brain as elsewhere.

THE ACTIONS OF ADENOSINE A_3 RECEPTOR

Nonneural Tissues

Most of the hitherto known effects elicited by the stimulation of A_3 receptors have been reviewed in the volume of *The Annals of the New York Academy of Sciences* devoted to the preceding Conference on Neuroprotective Agents held at Lake Como, Italy in 1996.[14] Since that time, experimental work concentrated predominantly (and unsurprisingly in view of the clinical uses of adenosine) on cardiovascular involvement of A_3 receptors shown to participate in hypotensive and vasoconstrictive responses,[21–24] and in cardioprotection both in myocytes[25–27] and in perfused rabbit hearts.[28] While there are indications that A_3 receptors may also be involved in ischemic preconditioning (IP) of the heart, the exact nature of their contribution to the phenomenon appears to need further clarification. Thus, while showing that the agonists of both A_1 and A_3 receptors mimic cardiac IP, Hill *et al.*[29] also indicated that A_1 rather than A_3 receptors are the principal source of the adenosine-mediated component of preconditioning. Other authors[30] concluded, however, that both receptors seem to play a role, while others described a complex interaction of adenosine A_1/A_3 and bradykinin B_2 receptors.[31]

Several recent studies focused their attention on the antiinflammatory effect of adenosine A_3 receptor agonists, e.g., prevention of neutrophil degranulation,[24] attenuation of inflammatory mediator,[33] and chemo- and cytokine release.[33–35] Moreover, since stimulation of A_3 receptors markedly decreases eosinophil chemotaxis,[35,36] it has been suggested that A_3 receptor agonists may be potentially useful in treatment of the pulmonary (asthma) and rheumatoid disorders.[32,33]

Nervous System

Astrocytes and hippocampal neurons have been the primary target of *in vitro* studies of the effects elicited by A_3 receptors. Fleming and Mogul[37] showed that exposure to the nonselective A_3 receptor agonist N^6-2-(4-aminophenyl)ethyl-adenosine (APNEA) potentiated high threshold Ca^{2+} current. The potentiating effect was sustained in the presence of A_1 and A_2 receptor antagonists and of protein kinase C (PKC) peptide inhibitor. The inhibitor of protein kinase A, on the other hand, blocked the potentiation. Since activation of A_3 receptors also results in the depression of adenylyl cyclase,[2,3] the authors concluded that PKA is negatively coupled to the Ca^{2+} current. The latter finding may have a significance in explaining at least some of the consequences following preischemic exposure of A_3 to selective agonists (see below; also the review of Domanska-Janik[38] on the importance of various protein kinases in the generation of ischemic damage). Of similar importance are the studies of Dunwiddie *et al.*[15] showing that stimulation of A_3 receptors with a selective agonist 2-chloro-N^6-(iodobenzyl)-adenosine-5′-N-methyluronamide (Cl-IB-MECA) antagonizes adenosine A_1 receptor-mediated inhibition of excitatory neurotransmission. Similar functional disinhibition results from A_3 receptor inhibitory influence on the function of presynaptic group III metabotropic glutamate receptors (metGluRs)[39] that are responsible for the reduction of glutamatergic neurotransmission at a wide variety of synapses.[40]

A series of papers by Abbracchio *et al.*[13,41] and Yao *et al.*[42] indicated that the response of astrocytes to A_3 receptor stimulation is clearly dependent on its intensity, confirming theoretical arguments of von Lubitz *et al.*[43] based on their studies of acute and chronic administration of A_3 receptor agonists. Thus, Abbracchio *et al.*[13,41] reported that exposure of human astrocytoma ADF cells to nanomolar concentration of the selective A_3 receptor agonist Cl-IB-MECA results in increased ramification of astrocytes accompanied by reorganization of cytoskeleton, accompanied by Bcl-XL protein expression within the newly appeared astrocyte protrusions. Higher (micromolar) concentrations of the drug resulted in apoptosis.[41] Similar, concentration-dependent results were also obtained in the studies of human leukemia (HL-6) and lymphoma (U-937) cells.[42] Finally, a very high concentration of Cl-IB-MECA (>10 μM) is required to induce necrosis of cerebellar granule cells in culture.[44] However, when the cells were exposed to 1 μM Cl-IB-MECA in the presence of nontoxic glutamate concentration (50 μM), the necrosis was very rapid and virtually complete. Glutamate alone had no effect.

The data on the effect of adenosine A_3 receptor stimulation obtained in isolated cell systems may explain, at least in part, the outcome of *in vivo* acute exposure to A_3 agonist IB-MECA prior to global and focal cerebral ischemia[43] (see also this conference). Significant delay in the normalization of the postischemic cortical blood flow was the most immediate sign of the effect of the drug. Postischemic mortality

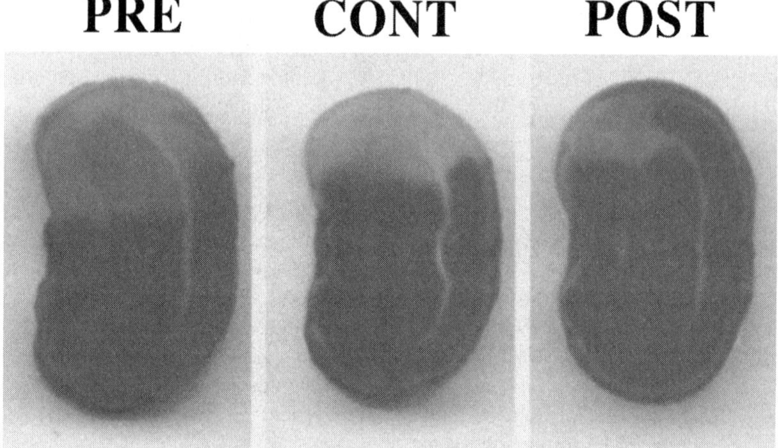

FIGURE 1. Acute administration of IB-MECA (100 μg/kg) 20 min prior to (PRE) or 20 min after (POST) initiation of permanent middle cerebral artery occlusion (MCAO) in mice. Following removal, brain slices were stained with the 2,3,5-triphenyltetrazolium chloride monohydrate (TTC) method. Preischemic administration results in a larger infarct (approximately 40% increase compared to control animals (CONT), $p > 0.01$, $n = 15$/group). Compared to saline injected controls, administration of the drug after initiation of MCAO shrunk the infarcted volume by approximately 20% ($p > 0.05$, $n = 15$/group).

was substantially elevated, especially during the initial 3 days of postischemic recovery, while neuronal damage (cortex, hippocampus, striatum) was intensified in the surviving drug-treated animals at 7 days postischemia.[14,43] These results are similar to those obtained in the model of permanent middle cerebral artery occlusion in mice, where the initial mortality among IB-MECA-treated (100 µg/kg) mice increased by almost 30% (von Lubitz *et al.*, this conference, and in preparation). Increase in the infarct size was also very significant ($p > 0.01$, FIG. 1). Moreover, acute preischemic treatment with IB-MECA elevated the presence of nitric oxide synthase (NOS) and accelerated deterioration of cytoskeletal protein MAP-2 as shown using quantitative and semiquantitative immunocytochemical methods.[14,45] Chronic treatment with daily IB-MECA doses as low as 5 µg/kg (daily for 60 days) had, on the other hand, a diametrically opposite effect, i.e., improved postischemic blood flow, reduced mortality, and a significantly better neuropathological and neurological (e.g., improved postischemic memory and learning ability[14]) outcome. Finally, immunocytochemical expression of NOS was fully suppressed, and there was an excellent preservation of MAP 2, accompanied by a striking increase in the density of glial fibrillary acidic protein (GFAP, i.e., activated) astrocytes.[45] Importantly, acute preischemic treatment with the selective adenosine A$_3$ receptor MRS 1191 reproduced the effects of chronic exposure to IB-MECA, indicating that the observed phenomena were indeed A$_3$ receptor-induced (Ref. 46, and in preparation).

It is unclear what mechanism is directly responsible for the *in vivo* effects of A$_3$ receptor activation. As indicated in the preceding section, stimulation of A$_3$ receptors elicits a broad range of effects. Some of these, e.g., degranulation of mast cells and vasoconstriction (which may be the mechanism behind retarded normalization of the postischemic blood flow), attenuation of the inhibitory effects of A$_1$ and IIImetGLU receptors on glutamatergic neurotransmission, activation of NOS, or liberation of intracellular Ca^{2+} stores and facilitation of extracellular Ca^{2+} influx[47] are highly damaging in the context of cerebral ischemia and the subsequent recovery. Others, such as depression of eosinophil chemotaxis, reduction of neutrophil recruitment, or inhibition of tumor necrosis factor-α (TNF-α) and macrophage inflammatory protein (MIP)1-α release are quite beneficial, since studies have shown that reduction of inflammatory phenomena results in improvement of postischemic outcome in the brain.[48–50] Astrocyte activation appears to be equally recovery-enhancing.[51,52] One is thus presented with a complex mix of A$_3$ receptor-induced effects, some of which clearly promote, while others retard, the demise of ischemia-injured neurons, and make the interpretation of A$_3$ receptor involvement in brain pathology a seemingly hopeless task. Yet, the studies that have emerged recently offer a number of alluring clues which, taken together, indicate that adenosine A$_3$ receptor may be a very important constituent of a very efficient endogenous system defending brain against injury.

ADENOSINE A$_3$ RECEPTOR AND BRAIN INJURY: A SPECULATION ON FACTS

All known, and often contradictory, aspects of adenosine A$_3$ receptor-mediated actions notwithstanding, two facts are strikingly prominent: their very wide interspe-

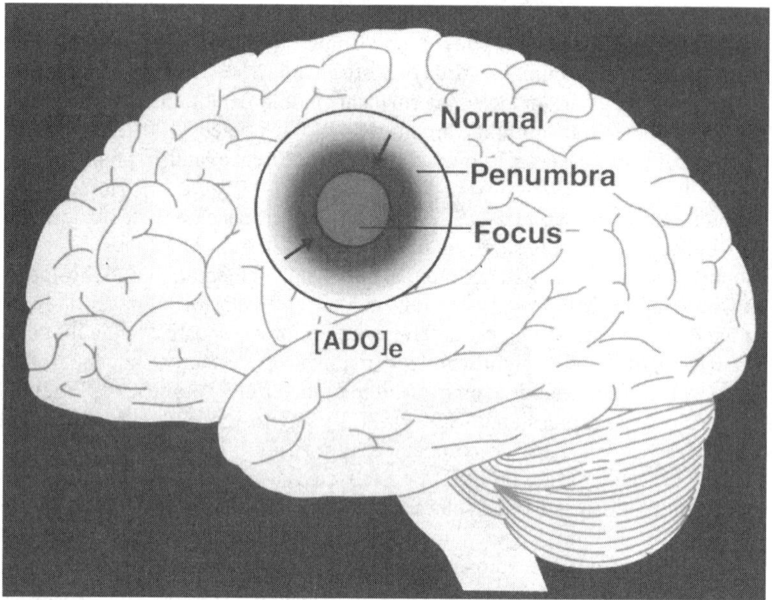

FIGURE 2. Schematic representation of the ischemic focus and the penumbra zone. It is very likely that the concentration of interstitial adenosine released during ischemia ($[ADO]_e$) increases progressively in the direction of the ischemic focus, attaining its highest value within the focus itself.

cies distribution,[16] and their very low affinity for adenosine.[5] In the evolutionary sense, its retention across the spectrum of several species, and its development into a functionally identical entity of a significantly varying molecular structure indicate that A_3 receptor must have an important survival value. On the other hand, the very low affinity of A_3 receptor for its endogenous agonist, adenosine, and a very low extracellular concentration of the latter under normal conditions,[53] also indicate that the receptor is, most likely, dormant under most but the most extreme conditions. Conditions such as encountered during ischemia, traumatic brain injury, or seizures, where the brain is exposed to extreme metabolic stress, where the bulk of adenosine released into the extracellular space originates from a furious pace of adenosine triphosphate (ATP) catabolism,[54] and where its extracellular level rapidly reaches and exceeds the threshold necessary for stimulation of A_3 receptors.[55–57] But, even before that level is reached, enough adenosine is already present to activate the neuroprotective A_1 receptors strategically located in the perisynaptic regions of neurons (see Ref. 58 for the most recent review). An important aspect of this process is the fact that enhancement of adenosine release is not a global, indiscriminate process but rather a localized "adenosine pulse" that is both event and site specific event.[59] While it has not been demonstrated due to the substantial technical difficulties in measurement of its interstitial concentration,[60] it may be expected that the level of adenosine released into the extracellular space diminishes with the distance from the center of the metabolic disturbance (FIG. 2). Thus, in focal ischemia, the territory of the intensely hypoxic/ischemic tissue enveloping the immediate proximity of the occluded vessel will be rapidly surrounded by a zone of elevated extracellular adenosine in which the concentration of the latter is high enough to sustain continuous stimulation of A_1 receptors. Since the main effects induced by such stimulation manifest as the reduction of glutamate release, depression of N-methyl-D-aspartate (NMDA) receptor hyperstimulation, lowered influx of Ca^{2+}, etc., the net result shows as diminished electrical activity, reduced metabolic pace, and hypothermia (for reviews, see Refs. 58 and 60–62). Consequently, the progression of the infarct enlargement may be slowed down and, in cases of very mild ischemia, arrested entirely. There is, indeed, indirect evidence for such a possibility. Thus, studies of Matsumoto *et al.*[63] have shown that depression of the local cerebral blood flow (CBF_L) to 25 ml/100 g/min (i.e., above the level of bona-fide ischemia) is sufficient to raise adenosine 5–15-fold above its resting concentration, i.e., enough to activate A_1 receptors. Extracellular concentration of glutamate, on the other hand, begins to increase when CBF_L decreases to 20 ml/100g/min. Since activation of A_1 receptors results in hyperpolarization of the presynaptic terminals and attenuation of glutamate release, the latter process will be operational at CBF_L values that are depressed below normal but are still above the level necessary to induce neuronal damage.[64] There are thus good reasons to believe that adenosine A_1 receptors may be an important element sustaining the existence of the "penumbra zone,"[64] i.e., metabolically depressed but still viable volume of cerebral tissue surrounding the infarct core. Eventually, since the stimulation of A_1 receptors effectively increases the threshold of critical NMDA receptor input frequencies (i.e., depresses receptor excitability[65]), and since activity-dependent release of adenosine is, in turn, directly related to the intensity of NMDA and AMPA receptor stimulation,[66–68] the local extracellular concentration of adenosine will decrease due to the attenuation of glutamate receptor excitability, and due to the rapid metabolic removal of extracellular adenosine. In consequence, and providing the original insult is mild (e.g., occlusion of a minor arteriole), the tissue within the penumbra zone will regain its normal (or almost normal) function. Anti-inflammatory actions elicited by stimulation of A_{2A} receptors (reviewed in Ref. 69) will unquestionably assist in this process. Thus, but for the existence of A_3 receptors, the endogenous mechanism aimed at the reduction of neuronal injury would be an ideal example of interaction among several receptor systems whose joint task is to maintain functional integrity of the brain. However, many hitherto described effects elicited by the stimulation of A_3 receptors appear to contradict that goal entirely.

As discussed above, activation of A_3 receptors results in the desensitization of A_1 receptor-mediated inhibition of excitatory synaptic transmission.[15] With the inhibitory effect of A_3 receptors on IIImetGluR, whose stimulation modulates glutamate signaling,[39] the net effect induced by the A_3 receptors may be the enhancement of glutamate release, invigoration of ischemic NMDA receptor activity, and actual amplification of the subsequent neurotoxic phenomena. Since enhanced activity of NMDA/AMPA receptors increases concentration of interstitial adenosine, the process of "egotropic inhibition" sustained by the interaction of A_1 and NMDA receptors transforms rapidly into a self-fueling "egotropic excitation," in which the continuously increasing production of adenosine caused by intraischemic catabolismm of ATP activates A_3 receptors. A_3 receptors interact, in turn, with A_1 and IIImetGluRs and decrease their inhibitory impact on glutamate release. The constant presence of the latter sustains activation of NMDA and non-NMDA receptors contributing to further release of adenosine, etc. The intensity of neurodestructive processes initiated by the initial intraischemic "glutamate burst" increases rapidly and sustains propagation of the neuronal destruction. Stimulation of A_3 receptors with micromolar concentration of their agonists results in apoptotic death of astrocytes.[13,41] While it is unknown whether A_3 receptors participate directly in the ischemia-evoked failure of glutamate uptake,[70] it is plausible that the process of A_3 receptor-induced apoptosis may be the source of such failure, contributing even further to the continuous presence of extracellular glutamate. The fairly rapid process of ischemia-induced apoptosis of astrocytes[52,71] is, most likely, hastened by A_3 receptor-mediated induction of NOS,[14,45] since nitric oxide pathway has been implicated in both glial and neuronal apoptosis.[72–74] Thus, activation of adenosine A_3 receptors by maximal intraischemic concentration of extracellular adenosine appears to trigger a massive destruction of cellular components within the entire volume of the tissue exposed to the most severe ischemia. This intensely "suicidal" role of A_3 receptors has been confirmed by the studies of global and focal ischemia, where preischemic administration of the selective A_3 receptor IB-MECA vastly amplified the subsequent brain damage[43] (see FIG. 1). While such paradoxical function of a receptor may have a remote evolutionary value in the context of removing from the population its members handicapped by the intense brain damage incurred, for example, during a mating fight, there are other, and unquestionably more efficient, mechanisms to achieve this goal. More importantly, from the point of *individual survival*, the "killer" role of cerebral A_3 receptor offers no biological advantage at all, especially that in the other tissues (e.g., heart, see Refs. 29, 30) stimulation of A_3 receptors is clearly protective. Very recent studies of von Lubitz *et al.* (this conference, and in preparation), in which administration of A_3 receptor agonist (IB-MECA) shortly after induction of permanent middle cerebral artery in mice resulted in a highly significant reduction of the infarct size (FIG. 1), may offer some indications on the likely function of A_3 receptors in the context of brain injury.

As indicated, it is very likely that the concentration of interstitial adenosine decreases with the distance from the ischemic core (FIG. 2). Hence, within the core itself, adenosine will reach a micromolar level adequate to fully stimulate A_3 receptors, and resulting in the full range of their destructive effects (FIG. 3). Further away, where the concentration decreases to high nanomolar values, more "benign" effects of A_3 receptors will predominate, i.e., activation and proliferation of astrocytes[13,41] (see also Ref. 52), antiinflammatory effects.[24,32–34] Combining their effects with the inhibitory and antiinflammatory effects mediated by A_1 and A_2 receptors, respectively, the A_3 receptors will enhance the chances of survival of the tissue within the volume that, most likely, constitutes the center of the penumbra zone. Finally, at the periphery of the penumbra, the concentration of adenosine will be, most likely, high enough to sustain prolonged activity of A_1 and A_2 but not A_3 receptors, resulting in "prophylactic" effects, i.e., reduction of the intensity of glutamatergic neurotransmission (and hence metabolism) by A_1 and vasodilation by A_{2A} to assure adequate blood supply to the outer rim of penumbra. Viewed in such light, adenosine A_3 receptor becomes an "*in situ* surgeon" rather than a "killer:" metabolic and physical excision of the ischemic core is afforded by the isolation of the affected volume from further blood supply through areteriolar vasoconstriction,[21]

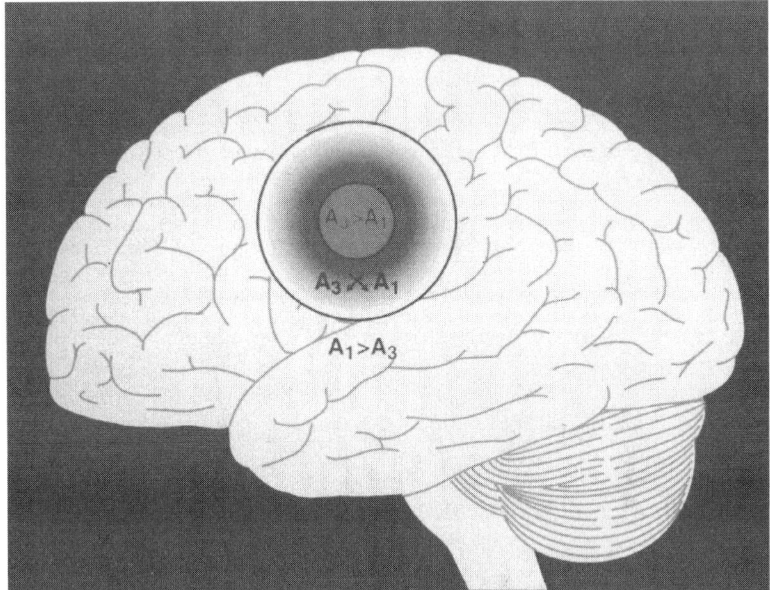

FIGURE 3. Schematic representation of the possible interactions between adenosine receptors and their effects during stroke/brain injury. In the focal volume, the actions of A$_3$ receptors predominate, resulting in enhanced excitotoxic phenomena and diminished astrocytic efficacy. Within the penumbra, there is a gradual transition from A$_3$ receptor-mediated effects (close to the focus) to weak A$_3$ receptor stimulation accompanied by the intense stimulation of A$_1$ receptors induced by endogenously released adenosine. As a result, at the periphery of the penumbra, one may expect enhanced A$_1$ receptor-mediated inhibition of glutamate release, and lowered intensity of stimulation accompanied by astrocyte activation resulting from activation of A$_3$ receptors. In the unaffected volume of the brain, A$_1$ receptor-mediated effects predominate. See text for further discussion.

and through A$_3$ receptor-mediated intensification of tissue damage (astrocytes and neurons). Activation of astrocytes within the inner rim of the penumbra promotes rapid scar development,[52] while, at the same time, enhancing neuronal protection through neurotrophin synthesis, potassium buffering, and neurotransmitter uptake[50] within the rest of penumbra volume. Hence, the damage may be contained more easily, and the continuing survival with less than debilitating neurological deficit becomes more likely. Thus, the adenosine A$_3$ receptor becomes an indispensable component of the "graded injury response complex," and finds a place in Newby's[75] concept of adenosine as a "retaliatory metabolite" that is as important as that of the other two adenosine types—A$_1$ and A$_2$,

Much of the preceding discussion is speculative, and the evidence is missing, although the emerging data point compellingly in the direction outlined above. The overriding question of the A$_3$ receptor biological role is still awaiting a plausible answer. Likely, there may be several roles, their nature depending on the studied tissue, and the context of function within the continuum of functions. But, indisputably, the A$_3$ receptor is more than just a variation on the "adenosine theme."

REFERENCES

1. MYERHOF, W.R., R. MÜLLER-BRECHLIN & D. RICHTER. 1991. Molecular cloning of a novel putative G protein-coupled receptor expressed during rat spermiogenesis. FEBS Lett. **284:** 155–160.

2. ZHOU, Q.Y., C.Y. LI, M.E. OLAH, R.A. JOHNSON, G.L. STILES & O. CIVELL. 1992. Molecular cloning and characterization of an adenosine receptor: the A_3 adenosine receptor. Proc. Natl. Acad. Sci. USA **89:** 7432–7436.

3. LINDEN, J., E. TAYLOR, A.S. ROBEVA, A.L. TUCKER, J.H. STEHLE, S.A. REEVES, J.S. FINK & S.M. REPPERT. 1993. Molecular cloning and functional expression of a sheep A_3 adenosine receptor with widespread tissue distribution. Mol. Pharmacol. **44:** 524–532.

4. SALVATORE, C.A., M.A. JACOBSON, H.E. TAYLOR, J. LINDEN & R.G. JOHNSON. 1993. Molecular cloning and characterization of the human A_3 adenosine receptor. Proc. Natl. Acad. Sci. USA **90:** 10365–10369.

5. JACOBSON, K.A., H.O. KIM, S.M. SIDIQQI, M.E. OLAH, G. STILES & D.K.J.E. VON LUBITZ. 1995. Adenosine A_3 receptors: design of selective ligands and therapeutic prospects. Drugs Future **20:** 689–699.

6. VAN RHEE A.M. & K.A. JACOBSON. 1996. Molecular architecture of G-protein coupled receptor. Drug. Dev. Res. **37:** 1–38.

7. PALMER, T.M., T.W. GETTYS & G.L. STILES. 1995. Differential interaction with and regulation of multiple G proteins by the rat adenosine A_3 receptor. J. Biol. Chem. **28:** 16895–16902.

8. PALMER, T.M. & G.L. STILES. 1997. Structure-function analysis of inhibitory adenosine receptor regulation. Neuropharamacology **36:** 1141–1147.

9. PALMER, T.M., J.L. BENVIC & G.L. STILES. 1996. Molecular basis for subtype-specific desensitization of inhibitory adenosine receptors: analysis of chimeric A_1-A_3 receptor. J. Biol. Chem. **270:** 29607–29613.

10. OLAH, M.E. & G.L. STILES. 1995. Adenosine receptor subtypes: characterization and therapeutic regulation. Annu. Rev. Pharmacol. Toxicol. **35:** 581–606.

11. ABBRACCHIO, M.P., R. BRAMBILA, S. CERUTI, H.O. KIM, D.K.J.E. VON LUBITZ & K.A. JACOBSON. 1995. G-protein-dependent activation of phospholipase C by adenosine A_3 receptors in rat brain. Mol. Pharmacol. **48:** 1038–1045.

12. RAMKUMAR, V., G.L. STILES, M.A. BEAVEN & H. ALI. 1993. The A_3 AR is the unique adenosine receptor which facilitates release of allergic mediators in mast cells. J. Biol. Chem. **268:** 16887–16890.

13. ABBRACCHIO, M.P., S. CERUTI, R. BRAMBILA, C. FRANCESCHI, W. MALORNI, K.A. JACOBSON, D.K.J.E. VON LUBITZ & F. CATTABENI. 1997. Modulation of apoptosis by adenosine in the central nervous system: a possible role for the A_3 receptor. Ann. N.Y. Acad. Sci. **825:** 11–22.

14. VON LUBITZ, D.K.J.E. 1997. Adenosine A_3 receptor and brain: a culprit, a hero, or merely yet another receptor? Ann. N.Y. Acad. Sci. **825:** 49–67.

15. DUNWIDDIE, T.V., L. DIAO, H.O. KIM, J.-L. JIANG & K.A. JACOBSON. 1997. Activation of hippocampal adenosine A_3 receptors produces a desensitization of A_1 receptor-mediated responses in rat hippocampus. J. Neurosci. **17:** 807–814.

16. JI, X.-D., D.K.J.E. VON LUBITZ, M.E. OLAH, G.L. STILES & K.A. JACOBSON. 1994. Species differences in ligand affinity at central A_3 adenosine receptors. Drug Dev. Res. **33:** 51–59.

17. MORO, S., A.H. LI & K.A. JACOBSON. 1998. Molecular modeling studies of human A_3 adenosine antagonists: structural homology and receptor dockling. J. Chem. Inf. Comput. Sci. **38:** 1239–1248.

18. BARALDI, P.G., B. CACCIANI, M.J. PINEDA DE LAS INFANTAS, R. ROMAGNOLI, G. SPALLUTO, R. VOLPINI, S. COSTANZI, S. VITTORI, G. CRISTALLI, N. MELMAN, K.S. PARK, X.-D. JI & K.A. JACOBSON. 1998. Synthesis and biological activity of a new series of N^6-arylcarbamoyl,2-(Ar)alkynyl-N^6-arylcarbamoyl, and N^6-carboxamido deri-

vation of adenosine-5′-*N*-ethyluronamide as A_1 and A_3 adenosine receptor agonists. J. Med. Chem. **41:** 3174–3185.

19. VAN MIJLWIJK-KOEZEN, J.E., H. TIMMERMAN, R. LINK, H. VAN DER GOOT & A.P. IJZERMAN. 1998. A novel class of adenosine A_3 receptor ligands. 1. 3-(2-Pyridinyl)isoquinoline derivatives. J. Med. Chem. **41:** 3987–3993.

20. VAN MIJLWIJK-KOEZEN, J.E., H. TIMMERMAN, R. LINK, H. VAN DER GOOT & A.P. IJZERMAN. 1998. A novel class of adenosine A_3 receptor ligands. 2. Structure affinity profile of a series of isoquinoline and quinazoline compounds. J. Med. Chem. **41:** 3994–4000.

21. SHEPHERD, R.K., J. LINDEN & B.R. DULING. 1996. Adenosine-induced vasoconstriction *in vivo*. Role of the mast cell and A_3 adenosine receptor. Circ. Res. **78:** 627–634.

22. ZHAO, Z., C.E. FRANCIS & K. RAVID. 1997. An A_3-subtype adenosine receptor is highly expressed in rat vascular smooth muscel cells: its role in attenuating adenosine-induced increases in cAMP. Microvasc. Res. **54:** 243–252.

23. VAN SCHAICK, E.A., K.A. JACOBSON, H.O. KIM, A.P. IJZERMAN & M. DANHOF. 1996. Hemodynamic effects and histamine release elicited by the selective adenosine A_3 receptor agonist 2-Cl-IB-MECA in conscious rats. Eur. J. Pharmacol. **308:** 311–314.

24. BOUMA, M.G., T.M. JEUNHOMME, D.L. BOYLE, M.A. DENTENER, N.N. VOITENOK, F.A. VAN DEN WILDENBERG & W.A. BUURMAN. 1997. Adenosine inhibits neutrophil degranulation in activated human whole blood: involvement of A_2 and A_3 receptors. J. Immunol. **11:** 5400–5008.

25. STAMBAUGH, K., K.A. JACOBSON, J.-L. JIANG & B.T. LIANG. 1997. A novel cardioprotective function of adenosine A_1 and A_3 receptors during prolonged simulated ischemia. J. Physiol. **273** (Heart Circ. Physiol. **42**): H501–505.

26. DOUGHERTY, C., J. BARUCHA, P.R. SCHFIELD, K.A. JACOBSON & B.T. LIANG. 1998. Cardiac myocytes rendered ischemia resistant by expressing the human adenosine A_1 or A_3 receptor. FASEB J. **12:** 1785–1792.

27. LIANG, B.T & K.A. JACOBSON. 1998. A physiological role of the adenosine A_3 receptor: sustained cardioprotection. Proc. Natl. Acad. Sci. USA **95:** 6995–6999.

28. TRACEY, W.R., W. MAGES., H. MASAMUNE, S.P. KENNEDY, D.R. KNIGHT, R.A. BUCHHOLZ & R.J. HILL. 1997. Selective adenosine A_3 receptor stimulation reduces ischemic myocardial injury in the rabbit heart. Cardiovasc. Res. (Netherl.) **33:** 410–415.

29. HILL, R.J., J.J. OLEYNEK, W. MAGEE, D.R. KNIGHT & W.R. TRACEY. 1998. Relative importance of adenosine A_1 and A_3 receptors in mediating physiological or pharmacological protection from ischemic myocardial injury in the rabbit heart. J. Mol. Cell. Cardiol. **30:** 579–585.

30. LIU, G.S., S.C. RICHARDS, R.A. OLSSON, K. MULLANE, R.S. WALSH & J.M. DOWNEY. 1994. Evidence that the adenosine A_3 receptor may mediate the protection afforded by preconditioning in the isolated rabbit heart. Cardiovasc. Res. **28:** 1057–1061.

31. GIANELLA, E., H.C. MOCHMANN & R. LEVI. 1997. Ischemic preconditioning prevents the impairment of hypoxic coronary vasodilation caused by ischemia/reperfusion: role of adenosine A_1/A_3 receptors and bradykinin B_2 receptor activation. Circ. Res. **81:** 415–422.

32. SZABO, C., G.S. SCOTT, L. VIRAG, G. EGNACZYK, A.L. SALZMAN, T.P. HANLEY & G. HASKO. 1998. Suppression of macrophage inflammatory protein (MIP)-1α production and collagen-induced arthritis by adenosine receptor agonists. Br. J. Pharmacol. **125:** 379–387.

33. MCWHINNEY, C.D., M.W. DUDLEY, T.L. BOWLIN, N.P. PEET, L. SCHOOK, M. BRADSHAW, D.R. DE M. BORCHERDING & C.K. EDWARDS. 1996. Activation of adenosine

A_3 receptors on macrophages inhibits tumor necrosis factor-alpha. Eur. J. Pharmacol. **310**(2–3): 209–216.

34. BOWLIN, T.L., D.R. BORCHERDING, C.K. EDWARDS III & C.D. MCWHINNEY. 1997. Adenosine A_3 receptor agonists inhibit murine macrophage tumor necrosis factor-α production *in vitro* and *in vivo*. Cell. Mol. Biol. **43:** 345–349.

35. KNIGHT, D., X. ZHENG, C. ROCCHINI, M. JACOBSON, T. BAI & B. WALKER. 1997. Adenosine A_3 receptor stimulation inhibits migration of human eosinophils. J. Leukocyte Biol. **62:** 465–468.

36. WALKER, B.A., M.A. JACOBSON, D.A. KNIGHT, C.A. SALVATORE, T. WEIR, D. ZHOU & T.R. BAI. 1997. Adenosine A_3 receptor expression and function in eosinophils. Am. J. Respir. Cell Mol. Biol. **16:** 531–537.

37. FLEMING, K.M. & D.J. MOGUL. 1997. Adenosine A_3 receptors potentiate hippocampal calcium by a PKA-dependent/PKC-independent pathway. Neuropharmacology **36:** 353–362.

38. DOMANSKA-JANIK, K. 1996. Protein serine/threonine kinases (PKA, PKC, and CaMKII) involved in ischemic brain pathology. Acta Neurobiol. Exp. **2:** 579–585.

39. MACEK, T.A., H. SCHAFFHAUSER & J. CONN. 1998. Protein kinase C and A_3 adenosine receptor activation inhibit presynaptic metabotropic glutamate receptor (mGluR) function and uncouple mGluRs from GTP-binding proteins. J. Neurosci. **18:** 6136–6146.

40. GLAUM, S.R. & R.J. MILLER. 1994. Acute regulation of synaptic transmission by metabotropic glutamate receptors. *In* The Metabotropic Glutamate Receptors. P.J. Conn & J. Patel, Eds.: 147–172. Humana Press. Tatawa, NJ.

41. ABBRACCHIO, M.P., G. RAINALDI, A.M. GIAMMARIOLI, S. CERUTI, R. BRAMBILA, F. CATABENI, D. BARBIERI, C. FRANCESCHI, K.A. JACOBSON & W. MALORNI. 1997. The A_3 adenosine receptor mediates cell spreading, reorganization of actin cytoskeleton, and distribution of Bcl-x_2: studies in human astroglioma cells. Biochem. Biophys. Res. Commun. **241**(2): 297–304.

42. YAO, Y., Y. SEI, M.P. ABBRACCHIO, J.L. JIANG, Y.C. KIM & K.A. JACOBSON. 1997. Adenosine A_3 receptor agonists protect HL-60 and U-937 cells from apoptosis induced by A_3 antagonists. Biochem. Biophys. Res. Commun. **232:** 317–322.

43. VON LUBITZ, D.K.J.E., R.C.-S. LIN, P. POPIK, M.F. CARTER & K.A. JACOBSON. 1994. Adenosine A_3 receptor stimulation and cerebral ischemia. Eur. J. Pharmacol. **263:** 59–67.

44. SEI, Y., D.K.J.E. VON LUBITZ, M.P. ABBRACCHIO, X.-D. JI & K.A. JACOBSON. 1997. Adenosine A_3 receptor agonist-induced neurotoxicity in rat cerebellar granule neurons. Drug Dev. Res. **40:** 267–273.

45. VON LUBITZ, D.K.J.E., R.C.-S. LIN, M. BOYD, N. BISCHOFBERGER & K.A. JACOBSON. 1999. Chronic administration of adenosine A_3 receptor agonist and cerebral ischemia: neuronal and glial effects. Eur. J. Pharmacol. In press.

46. VON LUBITZ, D.K.J.E., R.C.-S. LIN & K.A. JACOBSON. 1997. Adenosine A_3 receptor antagonists and protection against cerebral ischemia [abstract 745.16]. Soc. Neurosci. Abstr. **23/2:** 1924.

47. KOHNO, Y., X. JI, S.D. MAWHORTER, M. KOSHIBA & K.A. JACOBSON. 1996. Activation of A_3 adenosine receptors on human eosinophils elevates intracellular calcium. Blood **88:** 3569–3574.

48. YAMASAKI, Y., Y. ITOYAMA & K. KOGURE. 1996. Involvement of cytokine production in pathogenesis of transient cerebral ischemic damage. Keio J. Med. **3:** 225–229.

49. HALLENBECK, J.M. 1996. Significance of the inflammatory response in brain ischemia. Acta Neurochir. Suppl. **66:** 27–31.

50. STOLL, G., S. JANDER & M. SCHROETER. 1998. Inflammation and glial responses in ischemic brain lesions. Prog. Neurobiol. **56:** 149–171.

51. LOUW, D.F., T. MASADA & G.R. SUTHERLAND. 1998. Ischemic neuronal injury is ameliorated by astrocyte activation. Can. J. Neurol. Sci. **25:** 102–107.

52. PETITO, C.K., J.P. OLARTE, B. ROBERTA, T.S. NOWAK, JR & W.A. PULSINELLI. 1998. Selective glial vulnerability following transient global ischemia in rat brain. J. Neurobiol. Exp. Neurol. **57:** 231–238.

53. BALLARIN, M., B.B. FREDHOLM, S. AMBROSI & N. MAHY. 1991. Extracellular levels of adenosine and its metabolites in the striatum of awake rats: inhibition of uptake and metabolism. Acta Physiol. Scand. **142:** 97–103.

54. WHITTINGHAM, T.S. 1990. Aspects of brain energy metabolism and cerebral ischemia. *In* Cerebral Ischemia and Resuscitation. A. Schurr & B.M. Rigor, Eds.: 101–121. CRC Press. Boca Raton, FL.

55. HAGBERG, H., P. ANDERSSON, J. LACAREWICZ, I. JACOBSON, S. BUTCHER & M. SANDBERG. 1987. Extracellular adenosine, inosine, hypoxanthine, and xanthine in relation to tissue nucleotides and purines in rat striatum during transient ischemia. J. Neurochem. **49:** 227–231.

56. PHILLIS, J.W. 1990. Adenosine, inosine, and oxypurines in cerebral ischemia. *In* Cerebral Ischemia and Resuscitation. A. Schurr & B.M. Rigor, Eds.: 189–204. CRC Press. Boca Raton, FL.

57. BELL, M.J., P.M. KOCHANEK, J.A. CARCILLO, Z. MI, J.K. SCHIDING, S.R. WISNIEWSKI, R.S.B. CLARK, C.E. DIXON, D.W. MARION & E. JACKSON. 1998. Interstitial adenosine, inosine, and hypoxanthine are increased after experimental traumatic brain injury in the rat. J. Neurotrauma **15**(3): 163–170.

58. VON LUBITZ, D.K.J.E. 1999. Adenosine and cerebral ischemia: therapeutic future or death of a brave concept? Eur. J. Pharmacol. In press.

59. VON LUBITZ, D.K.J.E. & P.J. MARANGOS. 1990. Self-defense of the brain: adenosinergic strategies in neurodegeneration. *In* Emerging Strategies in Neurodegeneration. P.J. Marangos & H. Lal, Eds.: 151–186. Birkhauser. Boston.

60. FREDHOLM, B.B. 1997. Adenosine and neuroprotection. Int. Rev. Neurobiol. **40:** 259–280.

61. RUDOLPHI, K.A., P. SCHUBERT, F.E. PARKINSON & B.B. FREDHOLM. 1992. Adenosine and brain ischemia. Cerebrovasc. Brain Metab. Rev. **4:** 346–369.

62. VON LUBITZ, D.K.J.E. 1997. Acute treatment of cerebral ischemia and stroke: put out more flags. *In* Purinergic Approaches in Experimental Therapeutics. K.A. Jacobson & M.F. Jarvis, Eds.: 449–470. Wiley-Liss. New York.

63. MATSUMOTO, K., R. GRAF, G. ROSNER, N. SHIMADA & W.D. HEUISS. 1992. Flow thresholds for extracellular purine catabolite elevation in cat brain ischemia. Brain Res. **579:** 309–314.

64. ASTRUP, J., B.K. SIESJÖ & L. SYMON. 1981. Thresholds in cerebral ischemia: the ischemic penumbra. Stroke **12:** 723–725.

65. SCHUBERT, P. & R. MAGER. 1990. The critical input frequency for NMDA-mediated Ca^{2+} frequency depends on endogenous adenosine. Int. J. Purine Pyrimidine Res. **2:** 11–16.

66. HOEHN, K. & T.D. WHITE. 1990. *N*-Methyl-D-aspartate, kainate, and quisqualate release endogenous adenosine from rat cortical slices. J. Neurochem. **54**.

67. HOEHN, K. & T.D. WHITE. 1990. Role of excitatory amino acids receptors in K$^+$ and glutamate-evoked release of endogenous adenosine from rat cortical slices. J. Neurochem. **54:** 256–265.

68. DELANEY, S.M. & J.D. GEIGER. 1998. Levels of endogenous adenosine in rat striatum II: regulation of basal and *N*-methyl-D-aspartate-induced levels by inhibitors of adenosine transport and metabolism. J. Exp. Pharmacol. Ther. **285:** 568–572.

69. CRONSTEIN, B. 1997. Adenosine regulation of neutrophil function and inhibition of inflammation via adenosine receptors. *In* Purinergic Approaches in Experimental

Therapeutics. K.A. Jacobson & M.F. Jarvis, Eds.: 285–299. Wiley-Liss. New York.

70. SWANSON, R.A., K. FARELL & R.P. SIMON. 1995. Acidosis causes failure of astrocyte glutamate uptake during hypoxia. J. Cereb. Blood Flow Metab. **3:** 417–424.

71. CONTI, A.C., R. RAGHUPATHI, J.Q. TROJANOWSKI & T.K. MCINTOSH. 1998. Experimental brain injury induces regionally distinct apoptosis during acute and delayed posttraumatic period. J. Neurosci. **18:** 5663–5672.

72. HU, J. & D.J. VAN ELDIK. 1996. S100-ß induces apoptotic cell death in cultured astrocytes via a nitric oxide-dependent pathway. Biochem. Biophys. Acta **131:** 239–245.

73. BONFOCO, E., M. LEIST, B. ZHIVOTOVSKY, S. ORRENIUS, S.A. LIPTON & P. NICOTERA. 1996. Cytoskeletal breakdown and apoptosis elicited by NO donors in cerebellar grunule cells require NMDA receptor activation. J. Neurochem. **67:** 2484–2493.

74. NOMURA, Y., T. UEHARA & M. NAKAZAWA. 1996. Neuronal apoptosis by glial NO: involvement of inhibition af glyceraldehyde 3-phosphate. Hum. Cell **9:** 205–214.

75. NEWBY, A.C. 1984. Adenosine and the concept of "retaliatory metabolites." Trends Pharmacol. Sci. **9:** 42–48.

Excitotoxicity, Oxidative Stress, and the Neuroprotective Potential of Melatonin

S.D. SKAPER,[a] M. FLOREANI, M. CECCON, L. FACCI,[a] AND P. GIUSTI[b]

Department of Pharmacology, University of Padua, Padua 35131, Italy

ABSTRACT: The brain consumes large quantities of oxygen relative to its contribution to total body mass. This, together with its paucity of oxidative defense mechanisms, places this organ at risk for damage mediated by reactive oxygen species. The pineal secretory product melatonin possesses broad-spectrum free radical scavenging and antioxidant activities, and prevents kainic acid-induced neuronal lesions, glutathione depletion, and reactive oxygen species-mediated apoptotic nerve cell death. Melatonin's action is thought to involve electron donation to directly detoxify free radicals such as the highly toxic hydroxyl radical, which is a probable end-product of the reaction between NO• and peroxynitrite. Moreover, melatonin limits NO•-induced lipid peroxidation, inhibits cerebellar NO• synthase, scavenges peroxynitrite, and alters the activities of enzymes that improve the total antioxidative defense capacity of the organism. Melatonin function as a free radical scavenger and antioxidant is likely facilitated by the ease with which it crosses morphophysiological barriers, e.g., the blood-brain barrier, and enters cells and subcellular compartments. Pinealectomy, which eliminates the nighttime rise in circulating and tissue melatonin levels, worsens both reactive oxygen species-mediated tissue damage and brain damage after focal cerebral ischemia and excitotoxic seizures. That melatonin protects against hippocampal neurodegeneration linked to excitatory synaptic transmission is fully consistent with the last study. Conceivably, the decreased melatonin secretion that is documented to accompany the aging process may be exaggerated in populations with dementia.

INTRODUCTION

The selective vulnerability of neuronal systems is a remarkable characteristic of age-related degenerative disorders of the brain, including Alzheimer's disease, Parkinson's disease, Huntington's disease, and amyotrophic lateral sclerosis. Considerable evidence now points to excessive stimulation of glutamate-gated ion channels in provoking neuronal degeneration in animal models of these disorders as well as in stroke, epilepsy, and head trauma.[36] However, one must reconcile the rapid kinetics of glutamate-linked ion channel activity with the gradual process of neuronal loss in age-associated neurodegenerative disorders.

[a]Present address: Neuroscience Research Department, SmithKline Beecham Pharmaceuticals, New Frontiers Science Park, Third Avenue, Harlow, Essex CM19 5AW, United Kingdom.

[b]Corresponding author: Prof. Pietro Giusti, Department of Pharmacology, University of Padua, Largo Meneghetti, 2, 35131 Padua, Italy. Phone, +39 049-827-5103; fax, +39 049-827-5093.

e-mail, giusti@ux1.unipd.it

Independent investigations have focused on the role of oxidative stress as the proximate cause of a number of these degenerative disorders. Oxidative stress refers to the cytotoxic consequences of oxygen radicals—which are generated as by-products of normal and aberrant metabolic processes that utilize molecular oxygen. This hypothesis is attractive in that it can account for cumulative damage associated with the delayed onset and progressive nature of these conditions.[23,59] Emerging evidence indicates that activation of glutamate-gated cation channels may be an important source of oxidative stress and that these two mechanisms may act in a sequential as well as reinforcing manner, leading to selective neuronal degeneration. Comprehending the relationship between oxidative stress and glutamatergic neurotransmission may lead to the development of pharmacologic interventions that disrupt this chain of pathological events without compromising excitatory neurotransmission.

Melatonin, the principal secretory product of the pineal gland, was recently found to possess free radical scavenging and antioxidant properties. Melatonin likely works via electron donation to directly detoxify free radicals. In *in vitro* and *in vivo* experiments, melatonin has been found to protect cells, tissues and organs against oxidative damage induced by a variety of free radical-generating agents and processes, including cyanide poisoning, glutathione depletion, ischemia-reperfusion, kainic acid-induced excitotoxicity, and 1-methyl-4-phenyl-1,2,3,6-tetrahydropyridine (MPTP).[19,22,54] Melatonin as an antioxidant is not only effective in protecting nuclear DNA, membrane lipids and possibly cytosolic proteins from oxidative damage, but is also reported to alter the activities of enzymes that improve the total antioxidative defense capacity of the organism.[2,4,19,53] Most studies have used pharmacological concentrations of melatonin to protect against free radical damage, although physiological levels of the indole have been shown to be beneficial against oxidative stress.[44,48] Whether the quantities of melatonin produced are sufficient to influence significantly the overall antioxidative defense capacity of the organism remains unknown. Given the low toxicity of the molecule, however, melatonin and/or melatonin derivatives may be considered putative neuroprotectants useful for the treatment of brain pathologies that involve excitotoxicity or where oxidative damage may contribute to neuropathogenesis.[11,15,43] This article will briefly review the experimental findings supporting the above proposal.

OXIDATIVE STRESS

Oxidation reactions are essential biological reactions necessary for formation of high-energy compounds used to fuel cellular metabolic processes. Oxidation and reduction reactions involve the transfer of electrons and can generate by-products known as free radicals. The fact that oxygen is ubiquitous in aerobic organisms has led to the concept of the oxygen paradox; namely, the fact that this life-supporting molecule is also a precursor to the formation of harmful reactive oxygen species (ROS). The term "oxidative stress" was first coined by Sies[58] to account for the imbalance between ROS and the antioxidant opposing forces. ROS may be oxygen-centered radicals possessing unpaired electrons, such as superoxide anion and hydroxyl radical, or covalent molecules such as hydrogen peroxide.[23] ROS can react with and damage virtually any biological molecule, including DNA, essential proteins, and membrane lipids.[25,66]

A series of naturally occurring antioxidant defense mechanisms normally prevent or limit ROS production and tissue damage. (1) Oxidative phosphorylation primarily takes place within mitochondria where reactive oxidant species are tightly bound and can be safely reduced to water. (2) Superoxide radical is dismutated by superoxide dismutase to H_2O_2, which can then be cleared by either catalase or glutathione peroxidase (GPx). (3) Chain-breaking antioxidants or free-radical scavengers such as α-tocopherol and ascorbic acid can react directly with ROS. The oxidative damage potential and the antioxidant defense capacity are in a dynamic equilibrium at all times.

Brain cells may be at particular risk to oxidant stress. The brain consumes approximately 20% of total body oxygen, yet it comprises less than 2% of total body weight. Polyunsaturated fatty acids are a major constituent of neural cell membranes and substrates for free radicals and the chain reaction of lipid peroxidation. The brain derives its energy almost exclusively from oxidative metabolism of the mitochondrial respiratory chain. Mitochondria are found in neuronal cell bodies but are also distributed throughout neuritic processes, where ATPases maintain ion gradients across the neuronal membrane. The genes encoding the components of the mitochondrial respiratory chain are located on both nuclear and mitochondrial DNA. The latter has a mutation rate that is 10 times greater than that of nuclear DNA and has less effective repair mechanisms.[31] Consistent with the proximity of mitochondrial DNA to a major source of cellular oxidants, there is a striking 15-fold increase in oxidized nucleotides in brain mitochondrial DNA.[31] Against this backdrop, the brain is relatively deficient in protective mechanisms compared to other tissues, such as liver. It contains almost no catalase and reduced quantities of GPx, reduced glutathione (GSH), and vitamin E.[41] Moreover, the central nervous system (CNS) has limited capacity for regeneration.

GLUTATHIONE HOMEOSTASIS, OXIDATIVE DAMAGE, AND KAINIC ACID NEUROTOXICITY

Glutathione functions as a major antioxidant in tissue defense against oxidative stress, including the brain. Intracellular levels of GSH are maintained by glutathione reductase (GRx), a dimeric cytosolic enzyme that uses the reduced form of nicotinamide adenine dinucleotide phosphate (NADPH) as a cofactor to catalyze the reduction of oxidized glutathione (GSSG).[32] GSH participates nonenzymatically and enzymatically (GSH *S*-transferases) in supporting cellular redox balance and in protecting against oxidative damage by ROS.[33] Most GSH is localized to the cytoplasm, although approximately 10% of total cellular GSH is compartmentalized within mitochondria.[50] Because mitochondria also contain GPx, GRx and NADPH, a complete system for detoxifying hydroperoxides is contained within these organelles. The mitochondrial pool of GSH is also likely to be involved in maintaining intramitochondrial protein thiols in the reduced state. The latter are essential for a number of functions of these organelles, including selective membrane permeability and Ca^{2+} homeostasis. Thus, excessive production of H_2O_2 within mitochondria may lead to depletion of mitochondrial GSH, oxidation of protein thiols, and impairment of mitochondrial function.

Mitochondrial GSH originates from the cytosol.[29] Therefore, any decrease in cellular levels of GSH is likely to reflect mitochondrial function via loss of mitochondrial GSH. That inborn errors of the GSH biosynthetic machinery produce neurological abnormalities attests to the importance of GSH in normal brain function.[14] Inhibition of GSH synthesis leads to a pronounced decrease of GSH in cerebral cortices and to a striking enlargement and degeneration of mitochondria and loss of citrate synthase activity (a mitochondrial matrix marker enzyme) in brains of newborn rats.[26] If loss of GSH may cause mitochondrial damage, it is also conceivable that impaired mitochondrial function can lead to a decrease in cytosolic GSH. GSH synthesis requires adenosine triphosphate (ATP), and thus a deficiency of energy supplies by mitochondria is likely to affect cellular turnover of GSH.

Kainic acid (KA) is a potent CNS excitotoxin producing acute and subacute epileptoform activity that can last for hours to days, ultimately resulting in widespread irreversible neuropathological changes involving not only nerve cells, but also glia, myelin sheaths, and blood vessels.[61] KA binds to and activates a subtype of ionotropic glutamate receptor.[42] Besides inducing brain lesions directly, KA can provoke the release of potentially neurotoxic amounts of glutamate.[15] Convincing evidence for a role of ROS in non-N-methyl-D-aspartate (non-NMDA) receptor-mediated neurotoxicity is mounting. Lipid peroxidation and protein oxidation have been detected in brain concurrent with KA-induced neurotoxicity.[9,62] Furthermore, the neurotoxic effects of intracerebrally administered KA or quisqualic acid, an α-amino-3-hydroxy-5-methyl-4-isoxazole-4-propionate (AMPA) receptor agonist, were blocked by the centrally acting antioxidant idebenone, which did not affect NMDA receptor-mediated neurotoxicity.[38] Results *in vitro* have demonstrated that KA-induced lipid peroxidation and neurodegeneration were attenuated with antioxidants.[49] Xanthine oxidase has been implicated as a source of ROS, because allopurinol, a xanthine oxidase inhibitor, as well as the combination of superoxide dismutase and catalase protected against KA toxicity in mouse cerebellar granule neurons in culture.[17]

A single intraperitoneal injection of KA was sufficient to trigger a time-dependent decrease in forebrain GSH (maximal reduction at 48 hours).[19] KA also markedly lowered GSH levels in amygdala and hippocampus (FIG. 1), but not in the corpus striatum, which is resistant to KA injury and relatively poor in KA receptors.[19] The mechanism whereby KA causes intracellular GSH content to fall is not fully understood. Oxygen radicals have been reported to inactivate GRx[24] and GPx;[47] KA-triggered ROS formation[8,17,49,62] could thus disrupt the GSH redox cycle at the enzyme level. Indeed, reductions in GRx and GPx activities were observed in the forebrains of KA-treated rats at 48 hours, but not over the first several hours.[19] Cellular damage induced by KA was maximal at the former time.[21,22] The timing of the observed KA-induced decrease in GSH indicates that the latter may represent an index of cellular damage prior to death. Although GSH content was already significantly reduced in the forebrain, hippocampus and amygdala by 2.5 hours after KA administration (FIG. 1), no tissue injury was evident at this time.[19] The GSH/(GSH + GSSG) ratio was also altered in the same brain areas at 2.5 hours in KA-treated rats, further indicative of an oxidative imbalance.[19] The neuronal nature of the precocious influence of KA on glutathione status was strengthened by showing that cytotoxic concentrations of KA provoked, in cultured rat cerebellar granule neurons

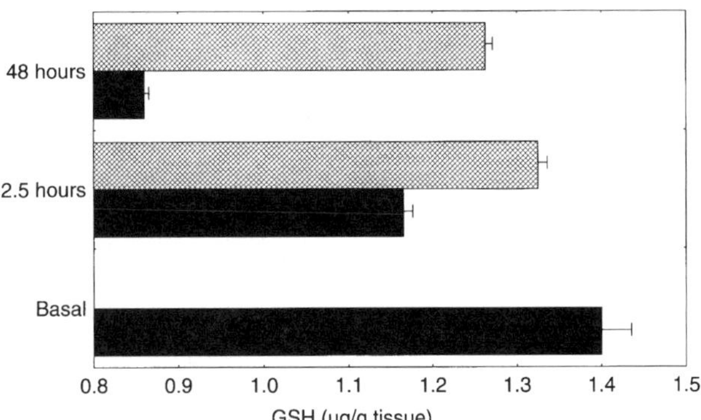

FIGURE 1. Melatonin limits KA-induced GSH loss in adult rat hippocampus. Animals were treated with KA (10 mg/kg, i.p.) alone, or with melatonin (2.5 mg/kg, i.p., 20 min before, immediately after, and 1 and 2 hr after KA). Rats were sacrificed 2.5 hr and 48 hr following KA administration, and GSH content measured. Basal refers to the control group. Values are mean ± SD. Melatonin + KA treatment (*hatched columns*) differed significantly (p <0.001) from KA alone (*filled columns*).

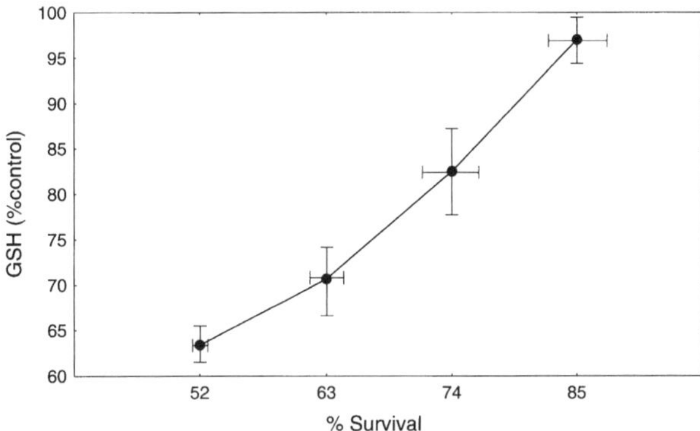

FIGURE 2. Kainic acid causes a coordinated decrease in cerebellar granule neuron survival and GSH content. Granule neurons at 14 days *in vitro* were exposed to KA (50, 100, 250, and 500 μM) for 30 min (22°C) in Locke's solution. After this time, cells were either processed immediately for GSH measurement, or returned to their original conditioned culture medium for a further 24 hr prior to assessment of viability. Values are means ± SD.

but not astrocytes, a clear fall in GSH within 30 minutes of excitotoxin challenge;[19] no changes in granule neuron integrity could be detected in the first 2 hours after KA removal. In fact, a good correlation can be shown between KA-induced loss of neuron vitality and fall in GSH level (FIG. 2). Interestingly, while both rat cerebellar granule neurons[40] and astrocytes[37] express functional KA receptors, only the former display KA receptor-mediated injury.[20,49]

PHARMACOLOGICAL ACTIONS OF MELATONIN
IN OXYGEN RADICAL NEUROTOXICITY

The effects of the pineal gland and melatonin were initially defined in terms of the endocrine physiology, particularly in relation to the neuroendocrine-reproductive axis.[51] In recent years, it has become apparent that melatonin's actions go well beyond those a hormonal modulator. In 1993, Tan and co-workers[64] reported on the ability of melatonin to quench hydroxyl radicals. Subsequently, melatonin was described as also capable of scavenging another toxic oxygen-related radical, the peroxyl radical.[45] The peroxyl radical is produced during the peroxidation of lipids and is sufficiently reactive that it propagates the chain reaction thereby leading to extensive destruction of fatty acids. Free radicals can destroy virtually any molecule that they encounter. Oxidative destruction, however, is most often assessed in terms of the damage done to macromolecules, i.e., carbohydrates, lipids, proteins, and DNA. To date the ability of melatonin to protect against oxidative modification of lipids, proteins and DNA has been described in a number of studies (see Refs. 53, 54 for reviews).

In primary cortical neuron cultures, free radical scavengers such as the vitamin E analog trolox protect from excitotoxicity triggered by agonists for non-NMDA glutamate receptors, but not from the toxicity of NMDA.[13] On the basis of the reported free radical scavenging properties of melatonin, the indole was subsequently examined for its antiexcitotoxic efficacy. When mature cerebellar granule neurons were exposed to glutamate, KA, and NMDA, cotreatment with melatonin (500 µM) protected the cells completely from the toxicity of KA (up to 1 mM) and shifted the LC_{50} for glutamate from 50 to 100 µM; no protection was afforded against NMDA toxicity.[20] Melatonin did not appear to exert any direct inhibitory action on KA-sensitive glutamate receptors.[20] Moreover, melatonin prevented KA-induced neuronal death as well as behavioral and biochemical disturbances,[22] and reduced mortality.[21] Importantly, melatonin partially prevented all decreases in GSH of KA-treated rats (FIG. 1).[19] Moreover, melatonin counteracted the changes in GSH induced by KA in cultured cerebellar granule neurons. These neuroprotective effects of melatonin may result from a sparing of GRx and GPx, which decreased in KA-treated but not in KA/melatonin-treated animals.[19] Melatonin is known to cause rapid and sustained increases in GSH-dependent enzyme activities in the rat brain[4] as well as mRNA levels for superoxide dismutases.[2] The pineal hormone has also been demonstrated to stimulate the activity of glucose-6-phosphate dehydrogenase in both liver and brain.[46] The importance of this lies in the fact that this enzyme resupplies the cell with reduced nicotinamide dinucleotide phosphate, which is required for regenerating GSH from GSSG via GRx. Melatonin, by neutralizing the extremely reactive hydroxyl radical[30,53,64] (which cannot be detoxified enzymatically like the superoxide anion radical and hydrogen peroxide) could spare crucial antioxidant enzymes, thereby maintaining GSH levels. The precocious nature of the KA-triggered alterations in GSH content both in individual brain areas and in cultured neurons makes it unlikely that the observed melatonin effects at these times resulted from a reduction in cell death. Recovery of glutathione balance (GSH levels and GSH/GSH + GSSG) ratio) at longer (48 hours) times *in vivo* might be attributable, in part, to cytoprotection afforded by melatonin.

Melatonin has been shown to prevent neuronal apoptosis triggered by ROS[10] and brain injury caused by singlet oxygen,[27] and to be effective in reducing KA[34] and hydrogen peroxide[56] -induced lipid peroxidation in homogenates of various brain regions. Extraneuronally, melatonin protects also against oxidative damage.[35,57] Collectively, these data suggest that the neuroprotective effect of melatonin involves the antioxidant activity of this hormone.

Seizures alter many chemical and biophysical processes in the CNS, and there are several reports indicating that ROS may play a role in seizure phenomena. The generation of superoxide anion in brain may increase during seizure activity,[3] and superoxide dismutase administration affords some protection against kindling-induced seizures.[39] Brief electroconvulsive shock is sufficient to cause elevated rates of ROS formation in rat cerebral cortex.[7] A reciprocal relation between seizures and ROS appears to exist, since free radicals induced in the brain by hyperbaric oxygen can precede, and may provoke, convulsions.[65] Using an *in vitro* primary cell culture model in which hippocampal pyramidal neurons undergo a gradual and delayed degeneration induced by enhanced network activity, Skaper *et al.*[60] showed that both melatonin and inhibitors of NO• synthase were neuroprotective. A role for ROS in the injury process was strengthened by the finding that, while neurons cocultured with astroglia were more resistant to killing, agents capable of lowering intracellular GSH negated this protection.[60] Consistent with this last study is the observation that pinealectomy, which eliminates the nighttime rise in circulating and tissue melatonin levels, worsens both ROS-mediated tissue damage and brain damage after focal cerebral ischemia and excitotoxic seizures.[28] In mice treated intracerebroventricularly with L-cysteine, melatonin reduced the seizure activity as well as the rise in neutral lipid peroxidation.[67] In addition, melatonin administration protected CA1 hippocampal neurons after transient forebrain ischemia in rats.[12] The cytoprotective action of melatonin against synaptic transmission-linked neurodegeneration could be attributed to its ability to limit NO•-induced lipid peroxidation,[18] and inhibit NO• synthase at or near physiological concentrations.[6,48] The pineal hormone may also scavenge peroxynitrite,[16] the end-product of the reaction between NO• and superoxide anion. The fact that the kinetics of neuroprotection afforded by delayed melatonin addition closely mirrored those for NO• synthase inhibitors lends support to this premise.[60]

Two major neurodegenerative conditions, Parkinson's disease and Alzheimer's disease, are theorized to involve ROS during the course of their development. There are partial experimental models for these conditions that allow tests of treatments that may ameliorate them. The drug MPTP and its metabolite 1-methyl-4-phenylpyridium ion (MPP^+) produce behavioral signs and neurochemical changes similar to those observed in humans with Parkinson's disease.[63] Recently, Acuña-Castroviejo and co-workers[1] used MPTP to induce oxidative changes in the brain of mice, and showed that treatment with melatonin (10 mg/kg) completely reversed the rises in lipid peroxidation products. MPTP-treated mice displayed a significant decrease in striatal tyrosine hydroxylase-immunoreactive nerve terminals, an effect that was also prevented by melatonin. Finally, the severity of morphological damage to cells in the nigrostriatal system, hippocampus, cerebellum, and sensorimotor cortex was reduced after melatonin administration compared to that in MPTP-only-treated mice.[1] The finding that amyloid β peptide (Aβ) has neurotoxic properties and that

TABLE 1. Models demonstrating melatonin cytoprotection

Paradigm	Reference
Kainic acid neurotoxicity	Giusti *et al.* (1995, 1996)
	Melchiorri *et al.* (1995)
	Floreani *et al.* (1997)
Brain ischemia	Cho *et al.* (1997)
Synaptic activity-induced neurodegeneration	Skaper *et al.* (1998)
L-Cysteine induced seizures	Yamamoto and Tang (1996)
Singlet oxygen-induced neurotoxicity	Cagnoli *et al.* (1995)
MPTP-induced lesions	Acuña-Castroviejo *et al.* (1997
Amyloid β-peptide neurotoxicity	Pappolla *et al.* (1997)
Ischemia-reperfusion (liver)	Sewerynek *et al.* (1996)
Paraquat toxicity	Melchiorri *et al.* (1996)
Carrageenan-induced inflammation	Cuzzocrea *et al.* (1997)
NO· –induced peroxidation	Escames *et al.* (1997)
Antioxidant enzyme expression	Antolin *et al.* (1996)

such effects are, in part, mediated by ROS[5] provides an avenue to explore melatonin protective actions. In neuroblastoma cells cultured in the presence of toxic amounts of Aβ, melatonin (10 μM) prevented cell death, the accumulation of lipid peroxidation products, and the large increases in intracellular calcium induced by Aβ.[44] The diverse models that have to date been used to show melatonin protection against cell injury are summarized in TABLE 1.

CONCLUDING REMARKS

The generation of ROS and the resultant lipid peroxidation are a crucial component in the pathogenesis of ischemic brain injury and of nerve cell loss after status epilepticus. Oxidative stress may also participate in the pathology of certain neuro-degenerative disorders. The pineal hormone melatonin exerts a protective action against oxidative stress-induced neuronal apoptosis, brain ischemia, and neuronal degeneration caused by network activity or neurotoxins that selectively mimic neu-rodegenerative disease. Moreover, melatonin-deficient rats exhibit increased brain damage after stroke or excitotoxic seizures. KA-induced neurotoxicity is linked with an imbalance of neuronal GSH, and melatonin administration is capable of restoring tissue GSH homeostasis. Treatment with GSH may also protect against KA-dependent neuropathological changes in rat brain,[55] suggesting the value of pharmacological strategies directed toward the regulation of endogenous melatonin levels. Melatonin has the capability of entering cells because of its high lipophilicity and it readily crosses all morphophysiological barriers. Entering the brain is particularly important, since this organ is highly susceptible to oxidative damage, coupled with its relatively weak antioxidative defense system.

The bulk of the studies published to date have used pharmacological levels of me-latonin to achieve protection against ROS. Certainly a major question is whether the quantity of melatonin produced by the pineal gland, and by other organs, is sufficient to significantly resist oxidative attack. This may be important especially in advanced age, where endogenous melatonin production is often severely attenuated.[52] Even if only pharmacologically relevant, however, the findings are significant in view of the ease with which melatonin is absorbed and its apparently low toxicity. Melatonin or related derivatives may thus be considered as potential neuroprotective molecules for the treatment of neuropathological conditions where oxidative damage may contribute to pathogenesis.

ACKNOWLEDGMENTS

This work was partially supported by Ricerca Sanitaria Finalizzata-Anno 1997, Regione Veneto and MURST Anno 1998-prot. 9805089988_007.

REFERENCES

1. ACUÑA-CASTROVIEJO, D., A. COTO-MONTES, M.G. MONTI, G.G. ORTIZ & R.J. REITER. 1997. Melatonin is protective against MPTP-induced striatal and hippocampal lesions. Life Sci. **60:** PL23–PL29.
2. ANTOLIN, I., C. RODRIGUEZ, R.M. SAINZ, J.C. MAYO, H. URIA, M.L. KOTLER, M.J. RODRIGUEZ-COLUNGA, D. TOLIVIA & A. MENENDEZ-PELAEZ. 1996. Neurohormone melatonin prevents cell damage: effect on gene expression for antioxidant enzymes. FASEB J. **10:** 882–890.
3. ARMSTEAD, W.M., R. MIRRO, C.W. LEFFLER & D.W. BUSYA. 1989. Cerebral superoxide anion generation during seizures in newborn pigs. J. Cereb. Blood Flow Metab. **9:** 175–179.
4. BARLOW-WALDEN, L.R., R.J. REITER, M. ABE, M.I. PABLOS, A. MENENDEZ-PELAEZ, L.-D. CHEN & B. POEGGELER. 1995. Melatonin stimulates brain glutathione peroxidase activity. Neurochem. Int. **26:** 497–502.
5. BEHL, C., J.B. DAVIS, R. LESLIE & D. SCHUBERT. 1994. Hydrogen peroxide mediates amyloid protein toxicity. Cell **77:** 817–827.
6. BETTAHI, I., D. POZO, C. OSUNA, R.J. REITER, D. ACUÑA-CASTROVIEJO & J.M. GUERRERO. 1996. Melatonin reduces nitric oxide synthase activity in rat hypothalamus. J. Pineal Res. **20:** 205–210.
7. BONDY S.C. & C.P. LEBEL. 1993. The relationship between excitotoxicity and oxidative stress in the central nervous system. Free Radical Biol. Med. **14:** 633–642.
8. BONDY, S.C. & D.K. LEE. 1993. Oxidative stress induced by glutamate receptor agonists. Brain Res. **610:** 229–233.
9. BRUCE, A.J. & M. BAUDRY. 1995. Oxygen free radicals in rat limbic structures after kainate-induced seizures. Free Radical Biol. Med. **18:** 993–1002.
10. CAGNOLI, C.M., C. ATABAY, E. KHARLAMOV & H. MANEV. 1995. Melatonin protects neurons from singlet oxygen-induced apoptosis. J. Pineal Res. **18:** 222–226.
11. CHAN, P.H. 1996. Role of oxidants in ischemic brain damage. Stroke **27:** 1124–1129.
12. CHO, S., T.H. JOH, H.H. BAIK, C. DIBINIS & B.T VOLPE. 1997. Melatonin administration protects CA1 hippocampal neurons after transient forebrain ischemia in rats. Brain Res. **755:** 335–338.
13. CHOW, H.S., J.J. LYNCH III, K. ROSE & D.W. CHOI. 1994. Trolox attenuates cortical neuronal injury induced by iron, ultraviolet light, glucose deprivation, or AMPA. Brain Res. **639:** 102–108.
14. COOPER, A.J.L. & A. MEISTER. 1993. Glutathione in the brain: disorders of glutathione metabolism. *In* The Molecular and Genetic Basis of Neurological Disease.

R. Rosenberg, S. Prusiner, S. Di Mauro, R. Barchi & L. Kunkel, Eds.: 209–238. Butterworths. Stoneham, Massachusetts.

15. COYLE, J.T. & P. PUTTFARCKEN. 1993. Oxidative stress, glutamate, and neurodegenerative disorders. Science **262:** 689–695.

16. CUZZOCREA, S., B. ZINGARELLI, E. GILAD, P. HAKE, A.L. SALZMAN & C. SZABO. 1997. Protective effect of melatonin in carrageenan-induced models of local inflammation: relationship to its inhibitory effect on nitric oxide production and its peroxynitrite scavenging activity. J. Pineal Res. **23:** 106–116.

17. DYKENS, J.A., A. STERN & E. TRENKNER. 1988. Mechanism of kainate toxicity to cerebellar neurons *in vitro* is analogous to reperfusion tissue injury. J. Neurochem. **49:** 1222–1228.

18. ESCAMES, G., J.M. GUERRERO, R.J. REITER, J.J. GARCIA, A. MUNOZ-HOYOS, G.G. ORTIZ & C.S. OH. 1997. Melatonin and vitamin E limit nitric oxide-induced lipid peroxidation in rat brain homogenates. Neurosci. Lett. **230:** 147–150.

19. FLOREANI, M., S.D. SKAPER, L. FACCI, M. LIPARTITI & P. GIUSTI. 1997. Melatonin maintains glutathione homeostasis in kainic acid-exposed rat brain tissues. FASEB J. **11:** 1309–1315.

20. GIUSTI, P., M. GUSELLA, M. LIPARTITI, D. MILANI, W. ZHU, S. VICINI & H. MANEV. 1995. Melatonin protects primary cultures of cerebellar granule neurons from kainate but not from N-methyl-D-aspartate excitotoxicity. Exp. Neurol. **131:** 39–46.

21. GIUSTI, P., D. FRANCESCHINI, M. PETRONE, H. MANEV & M. FLOREANI. 1996. *In vivo* and *in vitro* protection against kainate-induced excitotoxicity by melatonin. J. Pineal Res. **20:** 226–231.

22. GIUSTI, P., M. LIPARTITI, D. FRANCESCHINI, N. SCHIAVO, M FLOREANI & H. MANEV. 1996. Neuroprotection by melatonin from kainate-induced excitotoxicity in rats. FASEB J. **10:** 891–896.

23. HALLIWELL, B. & J.M.C. GUTTERRIDGE. 1989. Free Radicals in Biology and Medicine. 2nd edit. Clarendon Press. Oxford.

24. HUANG, J. & M.A. PHILBERT. 1996. Cellular responses of cultured cerebellar astrocytes to ethacrynic acid-induced perturbation of subcellular glutathione homeostasis. Brain Res. **711:** 184–192.

25. IMLAY, J.A. & S. LINN. 1988. DNA damage and oxygen radical toxicity. Science **240:** 1302–1309.

26. JAIN, A., J. MÅRTENSSON, E. STOLE *et al.* 1991. Glutathione deficiency leads to mitochondrial damage in brain. Proc. Natl. Acad. Sci. USA **88:** 1913–1917.

27. MANEV, H., C.M. CAGNOLI, A. KHARLAMOV, C. ATABAY & E. KHARLAMOV. 1995. *In vitro* and *in vivo* neuroprotection with melatonin against toxicity of singlet oxygen. Soc. Neurosci. Abstr. **21:** 1518.

28. MANEV, H., T. UZ, A. KHARLAMOV & J.-Y. JOO. 1996. Increased brain damage after stroke or excitotoxic seizures in melatonin-deficient rats. FASEB J. **10:** 1546–1551.

29. MÅRTENSSON, J., J.C.K. LAI & A. MEISTER. 1990. High-affinity transport of glutathione is part of a multicomponent system essential for mitochondrial function. Proc. Natl. Acad. Sci. USA **87:** 7185–7189.

30. MATUSZAK, Z, K. RESZKA & C.F. CHIGNELL. 1997. Reaction of melatonin and related indoles with hydroxyl radicals: EPR and spin trapping investigations. Free Radical Biol. Med. **23:** 367–372.

31. MECOCCI, P., U. MACGARVEY & M.F. BEAL. 1994. Oxidative damage to mitochondrial DNA is increased in Alzheimer's disease. Ann. Neurol. **36:** 747–751.

32. MEISTER, A. 1995. Strategies for increasing cellular glutathione. *In* Biothiols in Health and Disease. L. Packer & E. Cardenas, Eds.: 165–188. Marcel Dekker. New York.

33. MEISTER, A. & M.E. ANDERSON. 1983. Glutathione. Annu. Rev. Biochem. **52:** 711–760.

34. MELCHIORRI, D., R.J. REITER, E. SEWERYNEK, L.D. CHEN & G. NISTICÒ. 1995. Melatonin reduces kainate-induced lipid peroxidation in homogenates of different brain regions. FASEB J. **9:** 1205–1210.

35. MELCHIORRI, D., R.J. REITER, E. SEWERYNEK, M. HARA, L.D. CHEN & G. NISTICÒ. 1996. Paraquat toxicity and oxidative damage: reduction by melatonin. Biochem. Pharmacol. **51:** 1095–1099.

36. MELDRUM, B. 1993. Amino acids as dietary excitotoxins: a contribution to understanding neurodegenerative disorders. Brain Res. Rev. **18:** 293–314.

37. MILANI, D., L. FACCI, D. GUIDOLIN, A. LEON & S.D. SKAPER. 1989. Activation of polyphosphoinositide metabolism as a signal-transducing system coupled to excitatory amino acid receptors in astroglial cells. Glia **2:** 161–169.

38. MIYAMOTO, M. & J.T. COYLE. 1990. Idebenone attenuates neuronal degeneration induced by intrastriatal injection of excitotoxins. Exp. Neurol. **108:** 38–45.

39. MORI, N., J.A. WADA, M. WATANABE & H. KUMASHIRO. 1991. Increased activity of superoxide dismutase in kindled brain and suppression of kindled seizure following intra-amygdaloid injection of superoxide dismutase in rats. Brain Res. **557:** 313–315.

40. NICOLETTI, F., J.T. WROBLEWSKI, A. NOVELLI, H. ALHO, A. GUIDOTTI & E. COSTA. 1986. The activation of inositol phospholipid metabolism as a signal-transducing system for excitatory amino acids in primary cultures of cerebellar granule cells. J. Neurosci. **6:** 1905–1911.

41. OLANOW, C.W. 1992. An introduction to the free radical hypothesis in Parkinson's disease. Ann. Neurol. **32:** S2–S9.

42. OLNEY, J.W., V. RHEE & O.L. HO. 1974. Kainic acid: a powerful toxic analogue of glutamate. Brain Res. **77:** 507–512.

43. PACE, G.W. & C.D. LEAF. 1995. The role of oxidative stress in HIV disease. Free Radical Biol. Med. **19:** 523–528.

44. PAPPOLLA, M.A., M. SOS, R.A. OMAR, R.J. BICK, D.L.M. HICKSON-BICK, R.J. REITER, S. EFTHIMIOPOULOS & N.K. ROBAKIS. 1997. Melatonin prevents death of neuroblastoma cells exposed to the Alzheimer amyloid peptide. J. Neurosci. **17:** 1683–1690.

45. PIERI, C., M. MARRA, F. MORONI, R. RECCHIONI & F. MARCHESELLI. 1994. Melatonin: a peroxyl radical scavenger more effective than vitamin E. Life Sci. **55:** PL271–PL276.

46. PIERREFICHE, G. & H. LABORIT. 1995. Oxygen free radicals, melatonin, and aging. Exp. Gerontol. **30:** 213–227.

47. PIGEOLET, E. & J. REMACLE. 1991. Susceptibility of glutathione peroxidase to proteolysis after oxidative alterations by peroxides and hydroxyl radicals. Free Radical Biol. Med. **11:** 191–195.

48. POZO, D., R.J. REITER, J.R. CALVO & J.M. GUERRERO. 1994. Physiological concentrations of melatonin inhibit nitric oxide synthase in rat cerebellum. Life Sci. **55:** PL455–PL460.

49. PUTTFARCKEN, P.S., R.L. GETZ & J.T. COYLE. 1993. Kainic acid-induced lipid peroxidation: protection with butylated hydroxytoluene and U78517F in primary cultures of cerebellar granule cells. Brain Res. **624:** 223–232.

50. REED, D.J. 1990. Glutathione: toxicological implications. Annu. Rev. Pharmacol. Toxicol. **30:** 603–631.

51. REITER, R.J. 1980. The pineal and its hormones in the control of reproduction in mammals. Endocr. Rev. **1:** 109–131.

52. REITER, R.J. 1992. The aging pineal gland and its physiological consequences. BioEssays **14:** 169–175.

53. REITER, R.J. 1995. Oxidative processes and antioxidative defense mechanisms in the aging brain. FASEB J. **9:** 526–533.
54. REITER, R., L. TANG, J.J. GARCIA & A. MUÑOZ-HOYOS. 1997. Pharmacological actions of melatonin in oxygen radical pathophysiology. Life Sci. **60:** 2255–2271.
55. SAIJA, A., P. PRINCI, A. PISANI, M. LANZA, M. SCALESE, E. ARAMNEJAD, E. CESARANI & G. COSTA. 1997. Protective effect of glutathione on kainic acid-induced neuro-pathological changes in rat brain. Gen. Pharmacol. **25:** 97–102.
56. SEWERYNEK, E., D. MELCHIORRI, G.G. ORTIZ, B. POEGGELER & R.J. REITER. 1995. Melatonin reduces H_2O_2-induced lipid peroxidation in homogenates of different brain regions. **19:** 51–56.
57. SEWERYNEK, E., R.J. REITER, D. MELCHIORRI, G.G. ORTIZ & A. LEWINSKI. 1996. Oxidative damage in the liver induced by ischemia-reperfusion: protection by melatonin. Hepatogastroenterology **43:** 898–905.
58. SIES, H. 1985. Oxidative stress: introductory remarks. *In* Oxidative Stress. H. Sies, Ed.: 1–5. Academic Press. London.
59. SIESJO, B.K. 1989. Free radicals and brain damage. Cerebrovasc. Brain Metab. Rev. **1:** 165–211.
60. SKAPER, S.D., B. ANCONA, L. FACCI, D. FRANCESCHINI & P. GIUSTI. 1998. Melatonin prevents the delayed death of hippocampal neurons induced by enhanced excitatory neurotransmission and the nitridergic pathway. FASEB J. **12:** 725–731.
61. SPERK, G. 1994. Kainic acid seizures in the rat. Prog. Neurobiol. **42:** 1–32.
62. SUN, A.Y., Y. CHENG, Q. BU & F. OLDFIELD. 1992. The biochemical mechanisms of the excitotoxicity of kainic acid. Free radical formation. Mol. Chem. Neuropathol. **17:** 51–63.
63. SUNDSTROM, E., I. SUNDSTROM, T. TSUTSUMI, L. OLSON & G. JONSSON. 1987. Studies on the effect of 1-methyl-4-phenyl-1,2,3,6-tetrahydropyridine (MPTP) on central catecholamine neurons in C57BL/6 mice. Comparison with three other strains of mice. Brain Res. **405:** 26–38.
64. TAN, D.-F., L.-D. CHEN, B. POEGGLER, L.C. MANCHESTER & R.J. REITER. 1993. Melatonin: a potent, endogenous hydroxyl radical scavenger. Endocr. J. **1:** 57–60.
65. TORBATI, D., D.F. CHUCH, J.M. KELLER & W.A. PRYOR. 1992. Free radical generation in the brain precedes hyperbaric oxygen-induced convulsions. Free Radical Biol. Med. **13:** 101–114.
66. WOLFF, S.P., A. GARNER & R.T. DEAN. 1986. Free radicals, lipids and protein degradation. Trends Biol. Sci. **11:** 27–31.
67. YAMAMOTO, H. & H. TANG. 1996. Melatonin attenuates L-cysteine-induced seizures and lipid peroxidation in the brain of mice. J. Pineal Res. **21:** 108–113.

Neuroprotective Role of Melatonin in Methamphetamine- and 1-Methyl-4-phenyl-1,2,3,6-tetrahydropyridine-induced Dopaminergic Neurotoxicity

SYED F. ALI,[a,c] JULIO L. MARTIN,[b] M. DEAN BLACK,[b] AND YOSSEF ITZHAK[b]

[a]*Neurochemistry Laboratory, Division of Neurotoxicology, National Center for Toxicological Research/FDA, Jefferson, Arkansas, USA*

[b]*Department of Biochemistry and Molecular Biology, University of Miami School of Medicine, Miami, Florida, USA*

Methamphetamine (METH)- and 1-methyl-4-phenyl-1,2,3,6-tetrahydropyridine (MPTP)-induced dopaminergic neurotoxicity is thought to be associated with the formation of free radicals. Since evidence suggests that melatonin may act as a free radical scavenger and antioxidant, the present study was undertaken to investigate the effect of melatonin on METH- and MPTP-induced neurotoxicity. In addition, the effect of melatonin on METH-induced locomotor sensitization was investigated.

The administration of METH (5 mg/kg × 3) or MPTP (20 mg/kg × 3) to Swiss Webster mice resulted in 45–57% depletion in the content of striatal dopamine and its metabolites, 3,4-dihydroxyphenylacetic acid and homovanillic acid, and 57–59% depletion in dopamine transporter binding sites. The administration of melatonin (10 mg/kg) before each of the three injections of the neurotoxic agents (on day 1), and thereafter for 2 additional days, afforded a full protection against METH-induced depletion of dopamine and its metabolites and dopamine transporter binding sites. In addition, melatonin significantly diminished METH-induced hyperthermia.

However, the treatment with melatonin had no significant effect on MPTP-induced depletion of the dopaminergic markers tested. In the set of behavioral experiments, we found that the administration of 1 mg/kg METH to Swiss Webster mice for 5 days resulted in marked locomotor sensitization to a subsequent challenge injection of METH, as well as context-dependent sensitization (conditioning). The pretreatment with melatonin (10 mg/kg) prevented neither the sensitized response to METH nor the development of conditioned locomotion.

Results of the present study suggest that melatonin has a differential effect on the dopaminergic neurotoxicity produced by METH and MPTP. Since it is postulated the METH-induced hyperthermia is related to its neurotoxic effect, while regulation of body temperature is unrelated to MPTP-induced neurotoxicity or METH-induced locomotor sensitization, the protective effect of melatonin observed in the present study may be due primarily to diminishing METH-induced hyperthermia.

[c]Corresponding author: Syed F. Ali, Ph.D., Neurochemistry Laboratory, Division of Neurotoxicology, National Center for Toxicological Research/FDA, Jefferson, AR 72079-9502. Phone, 870/543-7203; fax, 870/543-7745.

e-mail, sali@nctr.fda.gov

Neuroprotective and Cognitive Enhancing Effects of Novel Small Peptides

A.I. FADEN,[a] G. FOX, L. FAN, S. KNOBLACH, G.L. ARALDI,
AND A.P. KOZIKOWSKI

*Georgetown Institute for Cognitive and Computational Sciences,
Washington, DC 20007, USA*

Treatment with thyrotropin-releasing hormone (TRH) or certain TRH analogs improves neurological recovery in experimental neurotrauma models. Beneficial effects have proved superior to other major neuroprotective classes, and mechanisms appear to be multifactorial. However, TRH (analogs) have other physiological actions—autonomic, endocrine, analeptic—that may be suboptimal for the treatment of traumatic brain injury (TBI) or for chronic administration.

We have developed a series of tripeptides partially related to TRH, with substitutions at both the N-terminus and imidazole ring, as well as dipeptide derivatives. These compounds show considerable neuroprotective activity with little or none of the other classical physiological effects of TRH. Administration of the tripeptides 53a or 57a, or the diketopiperazine 35b as a single i.v. bolus injection 30 min after injury, significantly improved motor recovery at 1 and 2 weeks after lateral fluid percussion induced TBI in rats. Similar post injury treatment with 53a or 35b in mice subjected to controlled cortical impact (CCI) TBI significantly improved both motor recovery and cognitive performance up to 1 month following trauma. Treatment with 35b beginning 1 month after CCI in mice, administered as a single bolus injection prior to each training trial, significantly improved both spatial learning and memory. None of the compounds had effects on release, whereas 53a had a significantly smaller effect than the well studied TRH analog YM14673. All three compounds significantly reduced neuronal death following mechanical trauma to rat neuronal/glial cultures. Preliminary *in vitro* and *in vivo* studies suggest that these compounds modify a number of proposed secondary injury factors.

[a]Corresponding author: Alan Faden, M.D., Georgetown Institute for Cognitive and Computational Sciences, 3970 Reservoir Road, NW NRB, EP-04, Washington, DC 20007. Phone, 202/687-0492; fax, 202/687-0617.
e-mail, fadena@giccs.georgetown.edu

Estrogens: Neuroprotective or Neurotoxic?

ANDREW C. SCALLET[a]

*Division of Neurotoxicology, National Center for Toxicological Research/FDA,
Jefferson, Arkansas, USA*

ABSTRACT: **The present paper reviews the major modes of action of estrogen on the molecular, cellular, tissue, and neurobehavioral levels of mammalian physiology, with an emphasis on the brain as an estrogen target tissue. We draw a distinction between receptor- and nonreceptor-mediated actions, as well as delineate the range of different signal transduction pathways that might be available within a given tissue to mediate estrogenic effects. We consider species differences relevant to understanding the predictability of effects in humans from data obtained in rats or monkeys. Finally, we emphasize the importance of developmental stage in determining whether estrogenic effects are beneficial or harmful; "neuroprotective" or "neurotoxic."**

INTRODUCTION

Types of Action of Estrogen

Understanding the actions of estrogens on brain tissue first requires a general introduction to estradiol's actions on receptors, cells, and tissues. Two estrogen receptor (ER) genes termed alpha and beta, encoding structurally related proteins, but found on different chromosomes, are expressed differentially in many tissues, including uterus, ovary, liver, mammary glands, and brain.[1,2] The actions of estradiol and related compounds are pleiotropic, depending on the presence or absence of ER-alpha and ER-beta, their relative abundance, the presence in the tissue of other phosphorylation-regulated proteins, and the particular mix of active genes containing estrogen response elements (EREs) in the cell.

Some estrogenic effects are "completely" receptor mediated; that is, they require liganding of the estrogen to its receptor, then the formation of dimers with other receptor molecules, and finally binding to EREs in the nuclear DNA. The liganded EREs may then activate the expression of any genes they reside in, as well as perhaps a related response cascade involving other genes.

Still other estrogenic effects may be "partially" receptor mediated; requiring receptor binding of the lipophilic estrogen in order for it to transit the phospholipid membrane into the cytoplasm. Thereupon, the bound estrogen-ER complex may enhance a cytoplasmic enzyme activity such as mitogen-activated protein kinase,[3] with no requirement for first binding to an ERE. The activated tyrosine kinase activity may then also phosphorylate a variety of other proteins, including the estrogen receptor proteins themselves, which must have a phosphotyrosine at position 537 (ER-alpha) or 443 (ER-beta) in order to form dimers capable of successfully binding to the ERE.

[a]Address for correspondence: Andrew C. Scallet, Ph.D., Division of Neurotoxicology, NCTR/FDA, 3900 NCTR Drive, Jefferson, AR 72079-9502. Phone, 870/543-7203; fax, 870/543-7745.
 e-mail, ascallet@nctr.fda.gov

Other effects of estrogens may be mediated completely independently of the ER. For example, steroids may locate and orient themselves within the plasma membrane solely based on their hydrophobic and lipophilic character, in the absence of any binding proteins. Once in place, they may effect membrane properties such as fluidity, the probability of channel-opening events, or the activity of membrane-bound insulin or neurotrophin receptors.[4] Thus there are at least three different modes of action of estrogenic compounds (receptor-mediated promotion of ERE-initiated gene transcription, receptor-mediated regulation of tyrosine phosphorylation of proteins, and membrane effects not mediated by the known ER alpha and beta receptors) that should be considered in evaluating the potential for neurotoxicity or neuroprotection of estrogenic compounds.

Sites of Action of Estrogen

In brain, as in other tissues, any one or more of a subset of the cellular/molecular effects described above may be operative. It is useful to consider the location of ER-alpha and ER-beta receptors in brain, since at least some neuroprotective or neurotoxic actions mediated in whole or in part by estrogenic compounds might best be detected in tissues containing significant numbers of receptors. The distribution of ER-alpha expression in the rat brain is primarily limited to ventral midline structures, many of which are related to neuroendocrine and reproductive functions. For this reason, a single immunostained sagittal section just lateral to the midline can reveal nearly all of the main concentrations of ER-alphas: the bed nucleus of the stria terminalis (BNST), the medial preoptic area of the hypothalamus (MPO), the ventromedial nucleus of the hypothalamus (VMH), the arcuate nucleus of the hypothalamus (AH), the septohypothalamic nucleus, and the septum and the central grey of the midbrain[5] (FIG. 1). Slightly more lateral lies the ER-containing medial amygdala, which must be evaluated in a separate section. Distribution of ER-beta neurons largely overlaps the distribution of ER-alpha, but includes additionally groups of cells in the paraventricular nucleus of the hypothalamus and the hippocampus.[6] Neither type of receptor has been reported to be expressed in the caudate nucleus, where dopaminergic terminals normally mediate the control of movements. The hypothalami of male and female *castrated* rodents generally contain comparable amounts and distributions of ERs, as evaluated either by neurochemistry[7,8] or by immunohistochemistry.[9] However, either the estrogen formed in the male (when circulating testosterone in the intact adult male is aromatized to estrogen) or the estrogen surge in cycling females can downregulate ER expression in the VMH and MPO. The result may be the *appearance* of diffferent ER concentrations between females and males, although actually there may be a similar number and distribution of ER-positive cells in both sexes. For this reason, the endocrine state of the animal has to be considered in interpreting the number and/or distribution of ERs in experimental studies.

NEUROTOXICITY OF ESTROGENS

The various neuroanatomical groupings of ERs each contain different types of neurons, with different connections to other brain regions, differing densities of other receptors, different resting potentials, P450-aromatase activity, calcium handling,

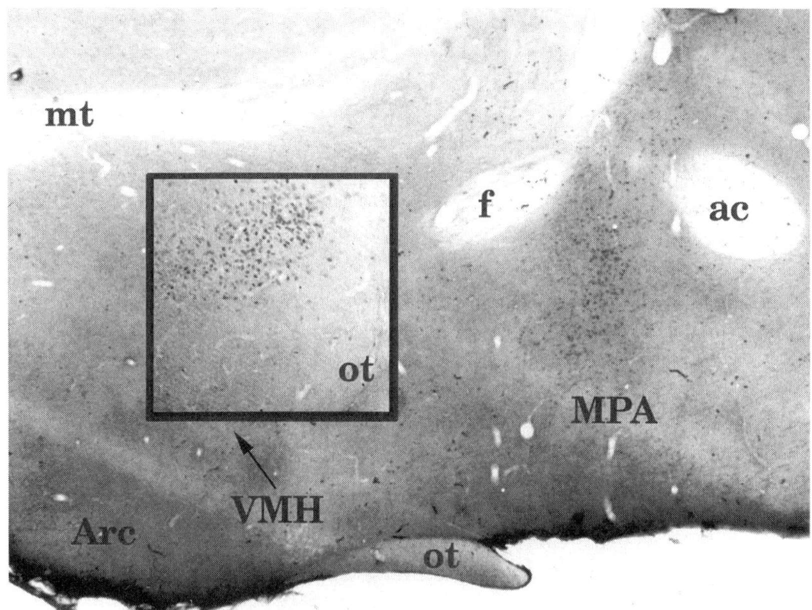

FIGURE 1. A sagital section of the entire hypothalamus (10×) of an ovariectomized female, immunohistochemically stained with the Abbott H-222 monoclonal antibody,[5] illustrates the location of the alpha-estrogen receptors (ERs). The largest concentration of ER-containing neurons is in the anterior hypothalamus (to the *right* of the micrograph). The medial preoptic area (MPA) and the bed nucleus of the stria terminalis, which is located between the fornix (f) and the anterior commissure (ac), contain most of the immunopositive nuclei in the hypothalamus. In the medial and posterior portions of the hypothalamus (to the *left* of the micrograph), both the ventromedial nucleus (VMH, shown enlarged 20× as an *inset*) and the arcuate nucleus (Arc) contain a smaller, but still considerable number of ER immunopositive nuclei. *Abbreviations*: ot, optic tract; mt, mammilothalamic tract.

resistance to oxidative stress, etc. Therefore, it is unlikely that each brain region would be affected identically by estrogenic compounds. As a practical matter, the existing literature describing the neurotoxicity of estradiol or testosterone (which can be converted to estradiol by aromatase) can identify those brain areas most likely to be susceptible to other estrogenic compounds. An examination of the literature suggests that there are two major types of *irreversible* syndromes resulting from neurotoxic exposure to estrogens. Both of these involve estrogen receptor-rich subregions of the hypothalamus, but they are completely different otherwise.

Necrotic

One of the two syndromes occurs with adult exposure to estradiol valerate[10,11] and results in direct neuronal death, as indexed by loss of beta-endorphin neurons[12] in the arcuate nucleus of the hypothalamaus, one of the brain's circumventricular organs. The estrogenic lesions are quite comparable to those produced by monosodium glutamate.[13–16] Such lesions have well-documented neurohistological, neurochemical, neuroendocrine, reproductive and neurobehavioral effects (reviewed by Scallet, 1999). This syndrome may be diagnosed by documenting one or more of the following: necrotic arcuate neurons shortly after exposure: persistent immunohistochemical or neurochemical loss of hypothalamic beta-endorphin or growth hormone-releasing hormone, hyperinsulinemia, low circulating levels of growth hormone, hyperalgesia and supersensitivity to opiate analgesia, and increased latency to male mounting, decreased frequency of female lordosis reflex, and decreased fertility.

Organizational (Apoptotic): Atypical Sexual Differentiation of the SDN/MPO

The other irreversible syndrome requires exposure during a perinatal critical period. It results in alterations of the typical pattern of development of ER-containing neurons of the sexually dimorphic nucleus of the medial-preoptic area of the hypothalamus (SDN/POA), and also results in a distinctive pattern of neurobehavioral alterations.[17] It is thought that the typical adult female hypothalamus develops according to an orchestrated removal of neurons by programmed cell death (apoptosis).[18] The typical male pattern is maintained whenever this process of programmed cell death is blocked or suspended throughout the critical period. In the latter case, the hypothalamic neuronal ERs remain liganded with estrogen produced by enzymatic aromatization *in situ* of the male's circulating testosterone. These liganded ERs then may directly promote activation by phosphorylation of the receptors for nerve growth factors (NGFs), the "trk-A" family of tyrosine kinase receptors. Alternately, after forming dimers and binding to nuclear EREs, the liganded ER dimers may cause EREs to promote the synthesis of NGF and/or its trk-A receptors. The end result of either or both processes would presumably be the suspension of apoptosis in the neuronal target cells. This estrogen-induced suspension of apoptosis could occur either in developing or adult animals.[19–21] We will discuss below the implications for "neuroprotection" vs "neurotoxicity" of estrogenic compounds, which depends not only on their mode of action, but also on the developmental stage of the subject.

Genetic females may become "masculinized" by exposure to testosterone, excessive levels of estrogen, or moderate amounts of any estrogenic compounds that fail to bind to the protective alpha-fetoproteins normally found in the perinatal circulation, since any of these conditions may mediate the suspension of the typical pattern of apoptotic remodeling in the female. Genetic males may become "feminized" if insufficient testosterone is available to be aromatized to estrogen, or if anti-estrogenic compounds are present; in this case the typical hormonal blockade of apoptosis in the male can be bypassed. Masculinization of genetic female rats may be suggested by documenting a perinatal reduction in apoptosis, an increased size of the SDN/POA and/or a decreased frequency of the female lordosis reflex. Feminization of genetic male rats may be observed as an increase in perinatal apoptosis, a decrease in the size of the SDN/POA and/or an increased latency to show a mounting reflex, and a capability of showing a lordosis reflex after appropriate hormonal priming.

The rat medial preoptic area is anatomically interconnected to spinal, uterine and cervical regions in such a way as to be able to respond to and/or influence reproductive behaviors.[22–24] The capability of expressing either lordosis or mounting reflexes depends ultimately on the sexually differentiated portions of the spinal cord that mediate the appropriate neuromuscular fixed action patterns.[25] However, this spinal sexual differentiation, unlike in hypothalamus, is mediated by androgen receptors (ARs), not ERs. For this reason, deviations from the sex-typical pattern of reproductive behaviors may occur following hypothalamic alterations, spinal cord alterations, or both. In addition to ARs and ERs themselves, there are a number of hypothalamic and spinal cord neuropeptides with sexually dimorphic expression. Therefore, it should be possible to develop neurochemical tests for "organizational" estrogenic and androgenic neurotoxicity, although such tests are not yet available.

NEUROPROTECTIVE ACTIONS OF ESTROGENS

Another interesting feature of the "organizational/apoptotic" effects of estrogens is their protective action in post-menopausal females. For example, following menopause, the rate of endothelial cell turnover in coronary vessels increases greatly. The elimination of damaged cells from the vessel walls proceeds by apoptosis, and 17-beta-estradiol inhibits this process in cultured endothelial cells,[26] as well as stimulates the tyrosine phosphorylation of focal adhesion kinase. In other tissues, such as MCF-7 human breast carcinoma cells, estradiol has been observed to *decrease* tyrosine phosphorylation of focal adhesion kinase.[27] In brain, the post-menopausal neuronal loss in aging females may also be apoptotic.[28] An important group of cells lost in the brains of aging patients, especially those with Alzheimer's disease symptoms, are the cholinergic neurons of the nucleus basalis of Meynert,[29] which are located very close to the ER-immunopositive neurons of the BNST. This neuronal loss in ovariectomized, aging rat brain can be suspended or reversed by estrogen replacement therapy, which also has been reported to normalize cognitive losses in aging human females.[30] Estrogenic action to slow or prevent post-menopausal apoptosis of cholinergic neurons is best viewed as a highly beneficial effect; it is important to evaluate it appropriately so that it will become possible to perform a "risk & benefit" analysis of various estrogens that may have differential activity profiles for neuroprotection, neurotoxicity, and carcinogenesis. Such evaluations may be especially important in light of the fact that mixtures of up to 10 or so different estrogenic compounds, both natural and synthetic, are either currently being used or are being proposed for use as replacement hormonal therapy in post-menopausal women.

ACTIVATIONAL EFFECTS OF ESTROGENS

Of course, some actions of estrogen on brain tissue that *are* reversible ("activational" effects, either neuroprotective or neurotoxic) may also occur. Some of these are feedback actions of steroids onto their receptors in pituitary, hypothalamus, hippocampus, etc. at doses within a range that does not result in necrotic damage, or that occur outside the critical period and dose requirements for the occurrence of organizational neurotoxicity or post-menopausal rescue from apoptosis. For example, a protocol for hormone-induced birth control would fall in this category, because the negative feedback actions of the estrogens are used to disrupt the normal neuroendocrine control of ovulation. If fertility is desireable, this could be considered a "neurotoxic" effect, because any adverse action of a chemical compound, even its expected pharmacological action, may be considered neurotoxic whether or not it is permanent or involves any structural changes. Similarly, "activational" effects of hormones may condition the hypothalamus to produce sexual receptivity, such as by artificially "priming" an ovariectomized female rat with estradiol followed by progesterone. "Activational" effects from unknown estrogenic compounds could be expressed as either persistent estrus or persistent lack of sexual receptivity that is reversible upon suspending the exposure. Estrogens may also confer some clearly neuroprotective, albeit reversible, benefits from its "activational" effects. For example, short-term treatments with estrogens might be expected to reduce or prevent the occurrence of neuronal death by apoptosis that otherwise occurs in the penumbral areas of damage around the central core of necrotic neurons produced by a stroke.

Still other "activational" estrogenic actions on brain may be completely nonreceptor mediated; these must also be considered, although they may produce completely different signs and symptoms due to the larger number of possible separate brain regions involved. Since all neurons have phospholipid membranes and fluidity responses, a broad range of activational effects of estrogens could occur, even in brain regions lacking ER-alpha or ER-beta. Although membrane-bound "receptors" for transducing the effects of steroid residency into channel opening/membrane permeabilty have been proposed,[31] their structure/activity requirements and even their existence have not been well described or accepted. A promising system in which to study such potential effects of estrogens *in vivo* is microdialysis of the caudate (corpus striatum). Our own data, measuring both total (Meredith *et al.*, unpublished observations) and extracellular (Ferguson *et al.*, unpublished observations) levels of dopamine and its metabolites suggest increased dopaminergic turnover following treatment with estrogenic compounds. Consistent with these observations, although the caudate lacks specific estrogen receptor expression (alpha or beta), several dopamine-mediated behaviors have been reported to be initiated upon direct infusion of 17-beta estradiol to the striatum.[32] The local infusion of estradiol or related estrogenic compounds should release dopamine, which should then produce increased movement of its target neuromuscular junctions (on the opposite side of the body), which may become measureable as rotation toward the side of the cannula implant, suggesting a way to screen for purely nonclassical–receptor-mediated, nongenomic actions of novel estrogenic compounds. Although a purely nonreceptor-mediated activational effect could be identified this way, further testing would be required to understand how dopamine in the rest of the brain is affected, and what the functional consequences of such a nonreceptor-mediated activational effect would be in the case of whole-animal exposure.

NEUROACTIVITY TEST BATTERY FOR ESTROGENIC COMPOUNDS

The preceding considerations suggest that a battery of evaluations might be used together in order to address several aims: to identify whether a particular estrogenic compound may be neuroprotective or neurotoxic, to categorize its activity as necrotic, organizational/apoptotic, or activational, and to apply appropriate biomarkers and measurement strategies in order to estimate the benefits and risks associated with exposure to a given tissue at a given age.

TABLE 1. Neurotoxic and neuroprotective effects of estrogenic compounds

		Males			Females		
		Perinatal	Adult	Aged	Perinatal	Adult	Aged
Neuroanat	Apoptosis	SDN Over-masculine (enlarged)	OK	Cort/Hipp Dendrites spared?	SDN Masculinized (enlarged)	OK	Cort/Hipp Dendrites spared?
	Necrosis	?	Arcuate N. lesioned ?	?	?	Arcuate N. lesioned ?	
	Activation	N/E	N/E	N/E	N/E	N/E	N/E
Neurochem	Apoptosis	NGF up	NGF up	NGF up ACh OK?	NGF up	NGF up	NGF up ACh OK
	Necrosis	BE loss?	BE loss?	BE loss?	BE loss?	BE loss?	BE loss?
	Activation	DA up	DA up	DA up	DA up	DA up	DA up
Neurobehav	Apoptosis	Excessive mounts/ aggress.?	OK	Cognitive sparing?	IRREV. reduced lordosis	OK	Cognitive sparing?
	Necrosis	?	IRREV. delayed mounting	?	?	IRREV. delayed lordosis	?
	Activation	?	Turns toward inj. side	?	?	Turns toward inj. side	?
Neuroendoc	Apoptosis	OK	OK	OK	No E-induced LH surge	OK	Normal decline
	Necrosis	?	Blocks GH, LH release?	?	?	Blocks GH, LH release.	?
	Activation	?	Inhibits LHRH/LH ?		?	Induces LHRH/LH ?	

A sample of a scheme for evaluating estrogenic compounds is listed in TABLE 1. The anticipated effects of the estrogen (characterized by necrotic, organizational/apoptotic, or activational effects as its predominant mode of action) in producing toxic or protective outcomes are predicted as a function of tissue type, sex and developmental stage of exposure. The reversible activational effects of estrogens on reproductive or sexually dimorphic behaviors are also shown.

COMPARISONS TO HUMANS

Ultimately, we wish to extrapolate our estrogenic compound evaluations from the experimental animal model to the human exposure situation. Since certain cases are more readily extended than others, we will consider each of the major estrogen neuroactivities to try to anticipate what difficulties will be encountered.

Necrotic

It has been somewhat controversial whether or not the primate arcuate nucleus shows a similar sensitivity to chemical damage as the rat's arcuate nucleus, which has been shown to be highly sensitive to neuronal necrosis from estrogen valerate[10,12] or monosodium glutamate (MSG) treatment.[13,16] However, MSG-induced lesions have been described in the neonatal rhesus monkey,[33,34] and their location has been identified as the infundibular nucleus. To our knowledge, no studies of the capability of estrogenic compounds to damage the arcuate nucleus of a primate have been conducted. No data as to the effects of any such chemical lesions in primates on neurochemistry, immunohistochemistry, or reproductive behavior have been reported. However, arcuate/infundibular nucleus damage produced in an adult rhesus monkey using stereotaxically implanted electrodes resulted in a complete cessation of LH secretion from the pituitary to plasma.[35] This result suggests that chemically-induced arcuate nucleus damage in *primates* might be inferred from a large decrease of circulating luteinizing hormone (LH) as measured noninvasively in a plasma sample. MSG-treated *rats* with arcuate nucleus lesions experience only a modest reduction in circulating LH, which is probably not sufficiently distinctive from controls to infer the presence of hypothalamic damage (Scallet, 1999, in press).

Organizational/Apoptotic

In monkeys, prenatal hormonal treatments have produced animals exhibiting at least some aspects of the play, sexual behavior, and neuroendocrine characteristics normally associated with the opposite sex.[36,37] However, although a sexually dimorphic SDN/POA has been identified in human primates,[38] we have seen no similar report of dimorphic neuroanatomy of the monkey hypothalamus. Thus, there are also no controlled studies of hormonal effects on sexually differentiated parts of the hypothalamus in any primate. Some research using human postmortem tissues has claimed a decrease in size of the SDN/POA and/or other sexually dimorphic hypothalamic regions such as the suprachiasmatic nucleus (SCN) and the bed nucleus of the stria terminalis (BNST), in male homosexuals;[39] while other studies have disagreed.[40,41] However, human studies have inherent limitations in terms of controls for medications, illnesses, postmortem effects, etc., and they represent correlational rather than experimental research designs.

Although our approach to determine estrogenic organizational neurotoxicity in rats cannot be readily extended to primates, it may be possible to do so if we develop a better understanding of which nuclei in the primate are functionally homologous to those in the rat, and whether they respond similarly to organizational neurotoxicity of an estrogenic neurotoxicant. We may then have a better approach to predicting neurotoxicity in humans from an appropriate endpoint in the primate, and more security about predictions from rodent models.

Activational

Adult ovariectomy of the female rhesus macaque prevents her initiation of sexual behavior and copulation. This effect can be reversed by restoring estradiol, and the female will initiate sexual behavior directed toward even disinterested males during the nonbreeding season.[42] Lesions of the anteromedial hypothalamus, including the MPO and BNST, but not the VMH, reduce proceptivity behaviors in female marmosets.[43] In the female macaque monkey, electrical stimulation of the VMH or the MPO results in her taking a proceptive "presenting" posture, where her hindquarters were directed toward a nearby male in order to solicit a mount.[44,45] In humans, there is some evidence of activational effects of estrogen on women's sexual behavior. It has been reported that at the time of ovulation, women are more likely to engage in autosexual activity and more likely to initiate sex with their partners than at other times of the menstrual cycle.[46] Androgens also are reported to have activational effects on human female sexual behavior. Frequency of intercourse in well-established heterosexual relationships is correlated to the woman's peak testosterone level and women with high testosterone are more likely to report sexual gratification.[46]

Adult castration of male rhesus monkeys completely eliminates their mounting behavior, but normal mounting behavior is restored upon testosterone replacement therapy. Lesions of the medial preoptic area in male rhesus monkeys or marmosets, like castration, have also been reported to eliminate mounting behavior.[47,48] Electrical stimulation of the MPO, on the other hand, elicits mounting behavior and extends its duration in rhesus macaques.[49]

In human males, sexual behavior is greatly reduced by adult castration; they lose ejaculatory and erectile capability over a period of time. Most of these effects are reversible by testosterone replacement.[46] The hypothalamic sites of action controlling sexual activity or hormonal effects in male and female humans are unknown.

REFERENCES

1. KUIPER, G.G., P.J. SHUGHRUE, I. MERCHENTHALER & J.A. GUSTAFSSON. 1998. The estrogen receptor beta subtype: a novel mediator of estrogen action in neuroendocrine systems. Front. Neuroendocrinol. **19:** 253–286.
2. SIMONIAN, S.X. & A.E. HERBISON. 1997. Differential expression of estrogen receptor alpha and beta immunoreactivity by oxytocin neurons of rat paraventricular nucleus. J. Neuroendocrinol. **9:** 803–806.
3. SINGER, C.A., X.A. FIGUEROA-MASOT, R.H. BATCHELOR & D.M. DORSA. 1999. The mitogen-activated protein kinase pathway mediates estrogen neuroprotection after glutamate toxicity in primary cortical neurons. J. Neurosci. **19:** 2455–2463.

4. Wu, C., S. Butz, Y. Ying & R.G. Anderson. 1997. Tyrosine kinase receptors concentrated in caveolae-like domains from neuronal plasma membrane. J. Biol. Chem. **272:** 3554–3559.

5. Henry, W.W., Jr., K.L. Medlock, D.M. Sheehan & A.C. Scallet. 1991. Detection of estrogen receptor (ER) in the rat brain using rat anti-ER monoclonal IgG with the unlabeled antibody method. Histochemistry **96:** 157–162.

6. Laflamme, N., R.E. Nappi, G. Drolet, C. Labrie & S. Rivest. 1998. Expression and neuropeptidergic characterization of estrogen receptors (ERalpha and ERbeta) throughout the rat brain: anatomical evidence of distinct roles of each subtype. J. Neurobiol. **36:** 357–378.

7. Cidlowski, J.A. & T.G. Muldoon. 1976. Sex-related differences in the regulation of cytoplasmic estrogen receptor levels in responsive tissues of the rat. Endocrinology **98:** 833–841.

8. Brown, T.J., N.J. MacLusky, M. Shanabrough & F. Naftolin. 1990. Comparison of age- and sex-related changes in cell nuclear estrogen-binding capacity and progestin receptor induction in the rat brain. Endocrinology **126:** 2965–2972.

9. Yokosuka, M., H. Okamura & S. Hayashi. 1997. Postnatal development and sex difference in neurons containing estrogen receptor-alpha immunoreactivity in the preoptic brain, the diencephalon, and the amygdala in the rat. J. Comp. Neurol. **389:** 81–93.

10. Desjardins, G.C., J.R. Brawer & A. Beaudet. 1993. Estradiol is selectively neurotoxic to hypothalamic beta-endorphin neurons. Endocrinology **132:** 86–93.

11. Brawer, J.R., A. Beaudet, G.C. Desjardins & H.M. Schipper. 1993. Pathologic effect of estradiol on the hypothalamus. Biol. Reprod. **49:** 647–652.

12. Desjardins, G.C., A. Beaudet, M.J. Meaney & J.R. Brawer. 1995. Estrogen-induced hypothalamic beta-endorphin neuron loss: a possible model of hypothalamic aging. Exp. Gerontol. **30:** 253–267.

13. Olney, J.W. 1969. Brain lesions, obesity, and other disturbances in mice treated with monosodium glutamate. Science **164:** 719–721.

14. Scallet, A.C. & J.W. Olney. 1986. Components of hypothalamic obesity: bipiperidyl-mustard lesions add hyperphagia to monosodium glutamate-induced hyperinsulinemia. Brain Res. **374:** 380–384.

15. Caputo, F.A., S.F. Ali, G.L. Wolff & A.C. Scallet. 1996. Neonatal MSG reduces hypothalamic DA, beta-endorphin, and delays weight gain in genetically obese (A viable yellow/alpha) mice. Pharmacol. Biochem. Behav. **53:** 425–432.

16. Desjardins, G.C., J.R. Brawer & A. Beaudet. 1992. Monosodium glutamate-induced reductions in hypothalamic beta-endorphin content result in mu-opioid receptor upregulation in the medial preoptic area. Neuroendocrinology **56:** 378–384.

17. Davis, E.C., J.E. Shryne & R.A. Gorski. 1995. A revised critical period for the sexual differentiation of the sexually dimorphic nucleus of the preoptic area in the rat. Neuroendocrinology **62:** 579–585.

18. Davis, E.C., P. Popper & R.A. Gorski. 1996. The role of apoptosis in sexual differentiation of the rat sexually dimorphic nucleus of the preoptic area. Brain Res. **734:** 10–18.

19. Toran-Allerand, C.D. 1996. Mechanisms of estrogen action during neural development: mediation by interactions with the neurotrophins and their receptors? J. Steroid Biochem. Mol. Biol. **56:** 169–178.

20. Toran-Allerand, C.D. 1996. The estrogen/neurotrophin connection during neural development: is co-localization of estrogen receptors with the neurotrophins and their receptors biologically relevant? Dev. Neurosci. **18:** 36–48.

21. Gibbs, R.B. 1998. Levels of trkA and BDNF mRNA, but not NGF mRNA, fluctuate across the estrous cycle and increase in response to acute hormone replacement. Brain Res. **787:** 259–268.

22. Papka, R.E., S. Williams, K.E. Miller, T. Copelin & P. Puri. 1998. CNS location of uterine-related neurons revealed by trans-synaptic tracing with pseudorabies

virus and their relation to estrogen receptor-immunoreactive neurons. Neuroscience **84:** 935–952.

23. VAN DER HORST, V.G. & G. HOLSTEGE. 1998. Sensory and motor components of reproductive behavior: pathways and plasticity. Behav. Brain Res. **92:** 157–167.

24. KOW, L.M. & D.W. PFAFF. 1998. Mapping of neural and signal transduction pathways for lordosis in the search for estrogen actions on the central nervous system. Behav. Brain Res. **92:** 169–180.

25. MATSUMOTO, A. 1997. Hormonally induced neuronal plasticity in the adult motoneurons. Brain Res. Bull. **44:** 539–547.

26. ALVAREZ, R.J. *et al.* 1997. 17Beta-estradiol inhibits apoptosis of endothelial cells. Biochem. Biophys. Res. Commun. **237:** 372–381.

27. BARTHOLOMEW, P.J., J.M. VINCI & J.A. DEPASQUALE. 1998. Decreased tyrosine phosphorylation of focal adhesion kinase after estradiol treatment of MCF-7 human breast carcinoma cells. J. Steroid Biochem. Mol. Biol. **67:** 241–249.

28. GIBBS, R.B. & P. AGGARWAL. 1998. Estrogen and basal forebrain cholinergic neurons: implications for brain aging and Alzheimer's disease-related cognitive decline. Horm. Behav. **34:** 98–111.

29. GIBBS, R.B. 1998. Impairment of basal forebrain cholinergic neurons associated with aging and long-term loss of ovarian function. Exp. Neurol. **151:** 289–302.

30. GIBBS, R.B., A.M. BURKE & D.A. JOHNSON. 1998. Estrogen replacement attenuates effects of scopolamine and lorazepam on memory acquisition and retention. Horm. Behav. **34:** 112–125.

31. NEMERE, I. & M.C. FARACH-CARSON. 1998. Membrane receptors for steroid hormones: a case for specific cell surface binding sites for vitamin D metabolites and estrogens. Biochem. Biophys. Res. Commun. **248:** 443–449.

32. VAN HARTESVELDT, C. & J.N. JOYCE. 1986. Effects of estrogen on the basal ganglia. Neurosci. Biobehav. Rev. **10:** 1–14.

33. OLNEY, J.W. & L.G. SHARPE. 1969. Brain lesions in an infant rhesus monkey treated with monsodium glutamate. Science **166:** 386–388.

34. OLNEY, J.W., L.G. SHARPE & R.D. FEIGIN. 1972. Glutamate-induced brain damage in infant primates. J. Neuropathol. Exp. Neurol. **31:** 464–488.

35. PLANT, T.M. *et al.* 1978. The arcuate nucleus and the control of gonadotropin and prolactin secretion in the female rhesus monkey (Macaca mulatta). Endocrinology **102:** 52–62.

36. GOY, R.W., F.B. BERCOVITCH & M.C. MCBRAIR. 1988. Behavioral masculinization is independent of genital masculinization in prenatally androgenized female rhesus macaques. Horm. Behav. **22:** 552–571.

37. RESKO, J.A. & C.E. ROSELLI. 1997. Prenatal hormones organize sex differences of the neuroendocrine reproductive system: observations on guinea pigs and nonhuman primates. Cell. Mol. Neurobiol. **17:** 627–648.

38. SWAAB, D.F. & E. FLIERS. 1985. A sexually dimorphic nucleus in the human brain. Science **228:** 1112–1115.

39. LEVAY, S. 1991. A difference in hypothalamic structure between heterosexual and homosexual men [see comments]. Science **253:** 1034–1037.

40. SWAAB, D.F., L.J. GOOREN & M.A. HOFMAN. 1992. Gender and sexual orientation in relation to hypothalamic structures. [Review]. Horm. Res. **38**(Suppl. 2): 51–61.

41. SWAAB, D.F., L.J. GOOREN & M.A. HOFMAN. 1995. Brain research, gender and sexual orientation. [Review]. J. Homosex. **28:** 283–301.

42. ZEHR, J.L., D. MAESTRIPIERI & K. WALLEN. 1998. Estradiol increases female sexual initiation independent of male responsiveness in rhesus monkeys. Horm. Behav. **33:** 95–103.

43. KENDRICK, K.M. & A.F. DIXSON. 1986. Anteromedial hypothalamic lesions block

proceptivity but not receptivity in the female common marmoset (Callithrix jacchus). Brain Res. **375:** 221–229.

44. KOYAMA, Y., I. FUJITA, S. AOU & Y. OOMURA. 1988. Proceptive presenting elicited by electrical stimulation of the female monkey hypothalamus. Brain Res. **446:** 199–203.

45. OOMURA, Y., S. AOU, Y. KOYAMA, I. FUJITA & H. YOSHIMATSU. 1988. Central control of sexual behavior. Brain Res. Bull. **20:** 863–870.

46. MONEY, J. & A.A. EHRHARDT. 1975. Man & Woman, Boy and Girl.: 1–311. Johns Hopkins University Press. Baltimore, MD.

47. SLIMP, J.C., B.L. HART & R.W. GOY. 1978. Heterosexual, autosexual and social behavior of adult male rhesus monkeys with medial preoptic-anterior hypothalamic lesions. Brain Res. **142:** 105–122.

48. LLOYD, S.A. & A.F. DIXSON. 1988. Effects of hypothalamic lesions upon the sexual and social behaviour of the male common marmoset (Callithrix jacchus). Brain Res. **463:** 317–329.

49. PERACHIO, A.A., L.D. MARR & M. ALEXANDER. 1979. Sexual behavior in male rhesus monkeys elicited by electrical stimulation of preoptic and hypothalamic areas. Brain Res. **177:** 127–144.

Role of Glycemia in Acute Spinal Cord Injury

Data from a Rat Experimental Model and Clinical Experience

FRANCESCO SALA,[a,c] GAETANO MENNA,[b] ALBINO BRICOLO,[a]
AND WISE YOUNG[b]

[a]*Department of Neurological and Visual Sciences, Section of Neurosurgery,
Verona University, Verona, Italy*

[b]*Neuroscience Center, Spinal Cord Injury Project, Rutgers State University,
Brunswick, New Jersey, USA*

ABSTRACT: While experimental and clinical evidence indicates that in brain injury blood glucose increases with injury severity and hyperglycemia worsens neurological outcome, the role of blood glucose in secondary mechanisms of neuronal damage after acute spinal cord injury has not yet been investigated. Data from spinal cord ischemia models suggests a deleterious effect of hyperglycemia, likely due to enhanced lactic acidosis, which is primarily dependent on the amount of glucose available to be metabolized. The purpose of this study is to summarize preliminary experimental and clinical observations on the role of blood glucose in acute spinal cord injury.

Between 1995 and 1996 we used the New York University (NYU) rat spinal cord injury model to test the following hypotheses: 1) Blood glucose levels increase with injury severity. 2) Fasting protects from hyperglycemia and prevents secondary damage to the spinal cord. 3) Postinjury-induced hyperglycemia (dextrose 5% 2 gm/Kg) enhances spinal lesion volume.

From a clinical perspective, we reviewed blood glucose records of 47 patients admitted to the Department of Neurosrgery in Verona, between 1991 and 1995, within 24 hours of acute spinal cord injury in order to determine: a) the incidence of hyperglycemia (>140 mg/dl); b) the correlation between blood glucose and injury severity; and c) the role of methylprednisolone in affecting blood glucose.

Results indicate that in a graded spinal cord injury model: 1) Early after injury, more severe contusions support significantly higher blood glucose levels. 2) Fasting overnight does not directly affect spinal cord lesion volume but influences blood gases, and we observed that a slightly systemic acidosis plays a minor neuroprotective role. Fasting also ensures more consistent normoglycemic baseline blood glucose values. 3) Postinjury-induced moderate hyperglycemia (160–190 mg/dl) does not significantly affect spinal cord injury.

In the clinical study, we observed that during the first 24 hours after spinal cord injury: a) Glycemia ranges between 90 and 243 mg/dl (mean value 143 mg/dl), and close to 50% of the patients present blood glucose values higher than normal. b) Methylprednisolone administration is not associated to significantly higher blood glucose levels. c) There is a trend for larger glucose rises with more severe injury.

[c]Corresponding author: Francesco Sala, M.D., Department of Neurological and Visual Sciences, Section of Neurosurgery, Ospedale Civile Maggiore Piazzale Stefani 1, 37100 Verona, Italy. Phone, 011-39-045-8072695; fax, 011-39-045-916790.
e-mail, Francescosala@yahoo.com

INTRODUCTION

Several studies have suggested a deleterious effect of hyperglycemia and lactoacidosis in brain ischemia. In ischemic conditions the production of lactic acidosis mainly depends on the amount of glucose available to be metabolized through the anaerobic glycolisis. Hyperglycemia enhances the production of lactic acid inducing a decrease in intracellular pH. This phenomenon, together with cellular energy failure, exacerbates cellular damage through a cascade of secondary mechanisms, which include: loss of selective membrane permeability and calcium homeostasis, abnormalities in protein synthesis and enzymatic activities, and derangements in neurotransmitters release-reuptake and free-radical reactions.[1–27] Experimental data[28–35] suggest that similar mechanisms may account for the deleterious role played by hyperglycemia during spinal cord ischemic injury.

Observations in head injured patients documented that in traumatic brain injury admission hyperglycemia is a frequent component of the stress response to head injury, a significant indicator of injury severity and a predictor of outcome.[36–40] Conversely, time course and consequences of posttraumatic hyperglycemia are unknown in traumatic spinal cord injury (SCI).

If SCI raises blood glucose and hyperglycemia is deleterious, glucose may play an important role in traumatic SCI models as well as clinical management of SCI. From an experimental perspective, if glucose affects SCI, pre- and postinjury nutritional management of animals must be carefully standardized and glucose rigorously monitored. In clinical practice, a detrimental effect of hyperglycemia would refrain from glucose-containing solution administration to spinal cord-injured patients and would suggest correcting the nutrition of these patients with substrates other than glucose.

We systematically investigated the role of blood glucose (BG) in a standardized graded rat spinal cord injury model in order to test the following hypotheses: 1) BG levels increase with injury severity (Experiment 1). 2) Fasting protects from hyperglycemia and prevents spinal cord damage (Experiment 2). 3) Postinjury-induced hyperglycemia enhances spinal lesion volume (Experiment 3). From a clinical perspective, we reviewed blood glucose records of patients admitted to the Department of Neurosurgery in Verona, between 1991 and 1995, within 24 hours of acute SCI in order to: a) determine the incidence of hyperglycemia (>140 mg/dl) and its correlation with injury severity; and b) rule out the possibility that high doses of glucocorticoids, currently administered in the first 24 hours after SCI, may significantly affect blood glucose values (Clinical Study).

EXPERIMENTAL

In this section we briefly describe the procedures that were common to all three experimental studies.

Animals were anesthetized with intraperitoneal pentobarbital. During surgery rectal temperatures were maintained at $37 \pm 1°C$ with a heating pad. The surgical sites were shaved and both the tail artery and the femoral vein were catheterized. Blood gases and glucose were tested several times before and after injury. The determination of glucose in whole blood (Chemstrip bG Test Strips and Accu-Chek III Blood Glucose Monitor) was based on a modification of the colorimetric glucose oxidase/peroxidase reaction that showed a 0.99 correlation coefficient compared to the hexokinase method. Initial blood drops collected from the catheter were discarded to ensure that the blood came from the body and not from the catheter. Blood gases were measured in the arterial blood samples using a CIBA/CORNING 238 pH Blood Gas Analyzer.

Injury to the spinal cord was obtained using the New York University (NYU) impactor. In this model, described in detail elsewhere,[41–43] SCI is achieved by dropping a rod from a height of 12.5 up to 50 mm onto the thoracic spinal cord exposed by a laminectomy at T-9. Digital optical potentiometers are then used to monitor rod and vertebral movements during the impact and allow precise measurements of the extent and time course of spinal cord compression. A computer program calculates impact velocities from the rod trajectory during the 2-ms period before impact. The program also subtracts vertebral column and cord movements to obtain the maximum compression depth (Cd) and time (Ct) of cord compression. The ratio Cd:Ct reflects the mean compression rate (Cr) which linearly predicts 24-hour lesion volumes in contused spinal cords.[41–43]

Blood pressure was continuously recorded from 5 minutes before until 5 minutes after injury. After injury, the surgical wound was immediately sutured, and the animals remained on a heating pad until they woke up. Then they were maintained at room temperature (approximately 22°C).

At 24 hours, under pentobarbital anesthesia, animals were sacrificed. Urine, whole blood, urine and blood hematocrit, plasma and the spinal cord were collected for the analysis of the lesion volume. This was obtained by the ratio of intracellular/extracellular tissue volume calculated from the values of total tissue Na and K in a 9-mm length of cord centered on the injury site and measured by atomic absorption spectroscopy.[42,43]

Statistical Analysis

The program StatView 4.02 (Abacus Concepts, Berkeley, CA) was used to generate summary statistics, including data counts, mean values, standard errors of the mean, and graphs of pre- and postinjury data. Variances given in the text, tables, and figures represent standard errors of the mean unless otherwise specified. Regression plots were generated with StatView 4.02. To assess differences between treatment-injury groups, we applied analysis of variance (ANOVA), using SuperANOVA 1.1 (Abacus Concepts, Berkeley, CA). Because cord compression rate (Cr) correlates linearly with lesion volumes, we used analysis of covariance (ANCOVA) with Cr as a covariate to assess the effects of treatments on lesion volumes.

Details of each experiment and results are provided in the following paragraphs.

Experiment 1

Objective

To determine if blood glucose increases after SCI and if this increase is related to injury severity.

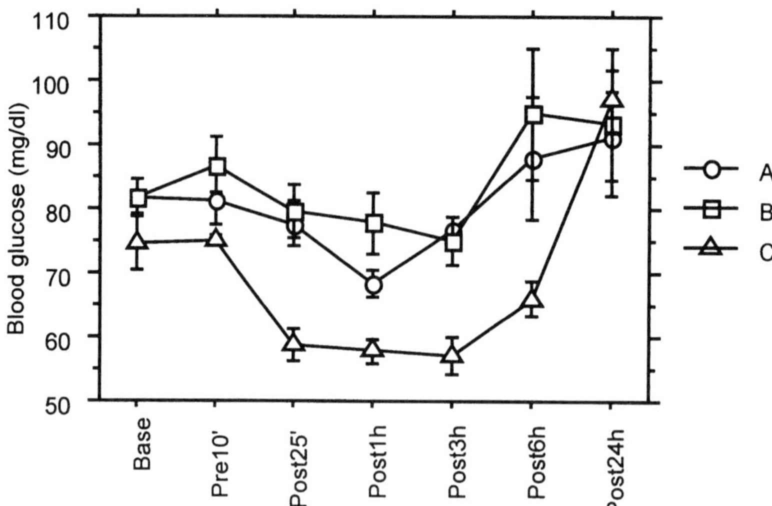

FIGURE 1. Time course of blood glucose pre- and postinjury in group A (mild injury), (severe injury), and C (control laminectomy).

Materials and Methods

Eighteen adult female rats were fasted overnight and split into three groups (6 rats each) according to injury severity. Group A was subjected to a mild injury (12.5-mm drop), and group B to a severe injury (50-mm drop); control group C underwent only laminectomy but no SCI.

Blood glucose was tested before surgery, 10 minutes before injury and 25 minutes and 1, 3, 6, and 24 hours after injury. Lesion volume determination at 24 hours was obtained as described above.

Results

Due to technical problems, such as catheter obstruction or saline in the blood sample, 15 out of 126 samples (12%) were excluded. Measured blood glucose levels

TABLE 1. ANOVA comparing blood glucose values at different time pre- and postinjury, among group A (mild injury), B (severe injury), and C (control laminectomy)

Dependent Variable	Cases (n)	F-Value	p-Value
Gl/base (mg/dl)	18	1.420	0.2621
Gl/pre 10′ (mg/dl)	16	0.075	0.7871
Gl/post 25′ (mg/dl)	16	11.150	**0.0005**
Gl/post 1 h (mg/dl)	15	9.939	**0.0010**
Gl/post 3 h (mg/dl)	17	7.788	**0.0043**
Gl/post 6 h (mg/dl)	14	2.716	0.0931
Gl/post 24 h (mg/dl)	15	0.180	0.8364

NOTE: Significant values ($p < 0.05$) are *bold*.

TABLE 2. Scheffe's post-hoc test for mean blood glucose values in the first 3 hours postinjury

Dependent Variable	Group A 12.5 mm	Group B 50.0 mm	Group C Laminectomy	Scheffe's Test
Gl/post 25′ (mg/dl)	75.8 ± 3.4	79.3 ± 2.2	58.8 ± 3.0	A and B > C
Gl/post 1 h (mg/dl)	66.4 ± 2.7	75.3 ± 2.5	57.8 ± 2.2	B > C
Gl/post 3 h (mg/dl)	74.3 ± 2.5	76.2 ± 3.9	57.0 ± 4.4	A and B > C

ranged between 50 and 141 mg/dl, with a mean value of 77 mg/dl. FIGURE 1 describes the time course of blood glucose in the 3 groups. A tendency toward normo-slightly hypoglycemic blood glucose values was present up to the third hour postinjury; then, glycemia gradually recovered to normal values. ANOVA showed significantly different blood glucose values in the 3 groups during the first 3 hours after injury (TABLE 1). Scheffe's posthoc test revealed higher glycemia in the injured groups A and/or B compared to the control group at 25 minutes and 1 and 3 hours after injury (TABLE 2).

Lesion volumes at 24 hours reflected the amount of tissue damage, confirming a very significant effect of drop height (*p*-value <0.0001) (FIG. 2). However, this difference was not significant when the analysis was corrected for injury severity (Cr). Linear regression revealed a positive correlation between lesion volume and blood glucose levels in the first hour after injury, confirming that rats subjected to a more severe injury had higher glucose levels.

Conclusions

Spinal cord injury unexpectadely did not result in a hyperglycemic response. In a normo- slightly hypoglycemic range, however, more severe SCI supported significantly higher blood glucose values up to 3 hours postinjury.

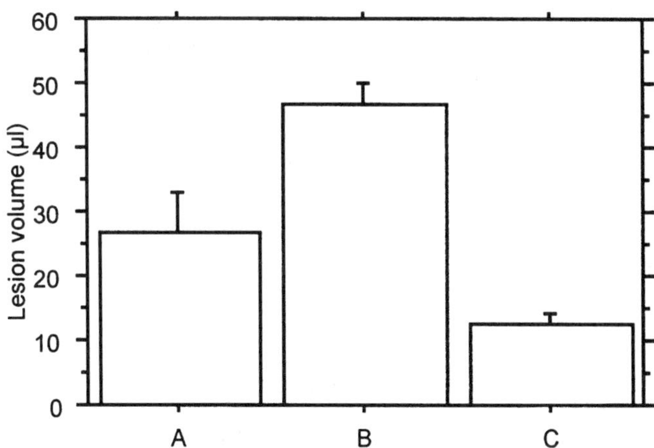

FIGURE 2. Lesion volumes at 24 hours in group A (mild injury), B (severe injury), and C (control laminectomy). *p* <0.0001.

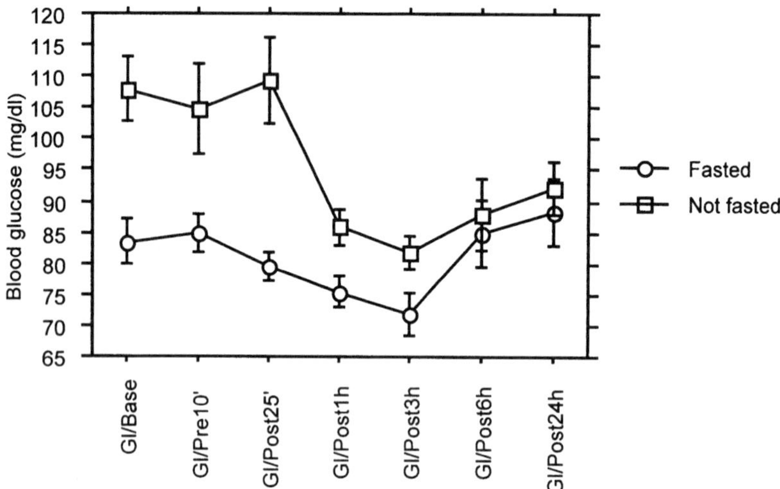

FIGURE 3. Time course of blood glucose in fasted and not fasted rats.

Experiment 2

Objective

To demonstrate that fasting protects from hyperglycemia and prevent spinal cord damage.

Materials and Methods

Twenty-four adult females, 12 of them fasted overnight, were subjected to severe SCI (50-mm drop). Blood glucose was tested before surgery, 10 minutes before injury and 25 minutes and 1, 3, 6, and 24 hours after injury. Blood gases (PaO_2, $PaCO_2$, HCO_3_-, pH) were tested 10 minutes before and 25 minutes after injury. After injury half the rats (6 fasted and 6 not fasted) were allowed free access to food and water,

TABLE 3. ANOVA comparing blood glucose values at different time pre- and postinjury between fasted and not fasted animals

Dependent variable	Fasted	Cases (n)	Not Fasted	Cases (n)	p-Value
Gl/base (mg/dl)	83.4 ± 3.5	12	107.1 ± 5.1	11	**0.0007**
Gl/pre 10′ (mg/dl)	84.1 ± 2.9	12	104.7 ± 7.3	12	**0.0208**
Gl/post 25′ (mg/dl)	79.3 ± 2.2	11	109.3 ± 7.0	12	**0.0008**
Gl/post 1 h (mg/dl)	75.3 ± 2.5	11	85.8 ± 2.9	13	**0.0149**
Gl/post 3 h (mg/dl)	71.8 ± 3.5	8	81.6 ± 2.6	12	**0.0354***
Gl/post 6 h (mg/dl)	84.9 ± 5.3	11	88.0 ± 5.7	10	0.7031*
Gl/post 24 h (mg/dl)	90.1 ± 4.9	12	90.4 ± 4.5	12	0.5724*

NOTE: Significant values ($p < 0.05$) are *bold*. The *asterisk* (*) indicates p-values corrected for the postinjury supplementation (per os or intravenous) with a 2 factor ANOVA.

and half received a minimum intravenous dextrose support (0.1 gm/24 h) starting at 1 hour postinjury.

Results

FIGURE 3 illustrates the time course of blood glucose in fasted and not fasted rats. TABLE 3 summarizes comparisons of blood glucose values at different times before and after injury. Fasted animals presented more consistent baseline (83.4 mg/dl ± 3.5 SEM vs 107.1 mg/dl ± 5.1 SEM) and preinjury (84.1 mg/dl ± 2.9 SEM vs 104.7 ± 7.3 SEM) blood glucose values when compared to not fasted rats. ANOVA showed that fasting significantly reduced blood glucose levels up to 3 hours after injury, regardless of the early postinjury intravenous or per os supplementation. However, lesion volume was not significantly different in fasted and not fasted animals (FIG. 4). Similarly, blood glucose values, either before or after injury, never correlated with lesion volume (TABLE 4).

Beside blood glucose values, $PaCO_2$ and HCO_{3^-} were also significantly lower in fasted rats before and after injury (TABLE 5).

Preinjury pH as well as pre- and postinjury bicarbonates, $PaCO_2$ and PaO_2 did not correlate with lesion volume. Conversely, we observed a significant correlation between postinjury pH and lesion volume, even when the analysis was corrected for Cr (TABLE 6): lower pH was associated to smaller lesion volume (FIG. 5).

Conclusions

Fasting overnight did not directly affect lesion volume but significantly influenced blood gases; this is noteworthy because of a minor neuroprotective role of mild acidosis. Fasting ensured more consistent baseline blood glucose values.

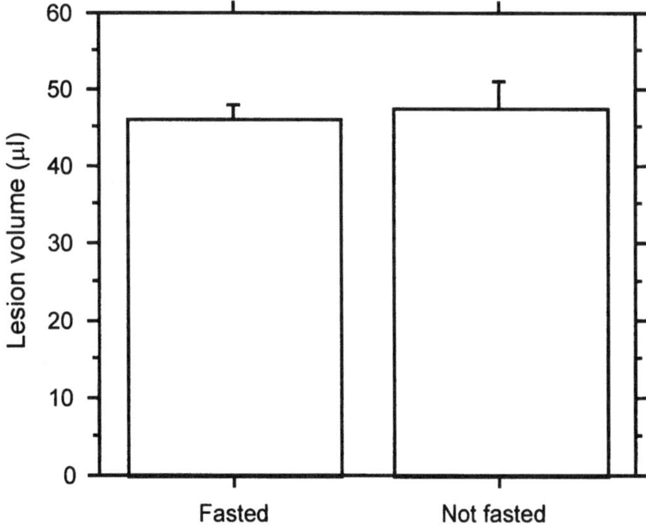

FIGURE 4. Lesion volumes at 24 hours in fasted and not fasted rats. *p* >0.05.

TABLE 4. Multiple regression of pre- and postinjury blood glucose vs lesion volume, adjusted for Cr

Independent variable	Cases (n)	F-Value	p-Value
Gl/base	21	0.485	0.4950
Gl/pre 10′	22	1.739	0.4006
Gl/post 25′	21	0.017	0.8986
Gl/post 1 h	21	0.100	0.7556
Gl/post 3 h	19	0.093	0.7641
Gl/post 6 h	20	0.239	0.6311
Gl/post 24 h	23	0.296	0.5925

NOTE: Lesion volume is the dependent variable.

TABLE 5. ANOVA comparing blood gases at different times pre- and postinjury between fasted and not fasted animals

Dependent Variable	Fasted	Cases (n)	Not Fasted	Cases (n)	p-Value
Pre PaO_2	80.1 ± 1.6	12	77.9 ± 2.8	13	0.5084
Post PaO_2	72.9 ± 2.3	11	71.1 ± 1.8	13	0.5530
Pre $PaCO_2$	41.0 ± 1.3	12	46.1 ± 1.0	13	**0.0030**
Post $PaCO_2$	42.5 ± 1.3	11	49.0 ± 1.1	13	**0.0012**
Pre pH	7.36 ± 0.01	12	7.35 ± 0.005	13	0.4635
Post pH	7.32 ± 0.009	11	7.33 ± 0.09	13	0.2752
Pre HCO_3	23.2 ± 0.5	12	24.6 ± 0.3	13	**0.0498**
Post HCO_3	21.2 ± 0.4	11	24.1 ± 0.5	13	**0.0007**

NOTE: Significant values ($p < 0.05$) are *bold*.

TABLE 6. Multiple regression of pre- and postinjury PaO_2, $PaCO_2$, pH, and HCO_3 vs lesion volume, adjusted for Cr

Independent variable	Cases (n)	F-Value	p-Value
Pre PaO_2	23	2.081	0.1646
Post PaO_2	22	2.097	0.1639
Pre $PaCO_2$	23	0.038	0.8480
Post $PaCO_2$	22	0.199	0.6603
Pre HCO_3	23	1.711	0.2057
Post HCO_3	22	2.548	0.1270
Pre pH	23	1.275	0.2721
Post pH	22	6.469	**0.0198**

NOTE: Lesion volume is the dependent variable. Significant values ($p < 0.05$) are *bold*.

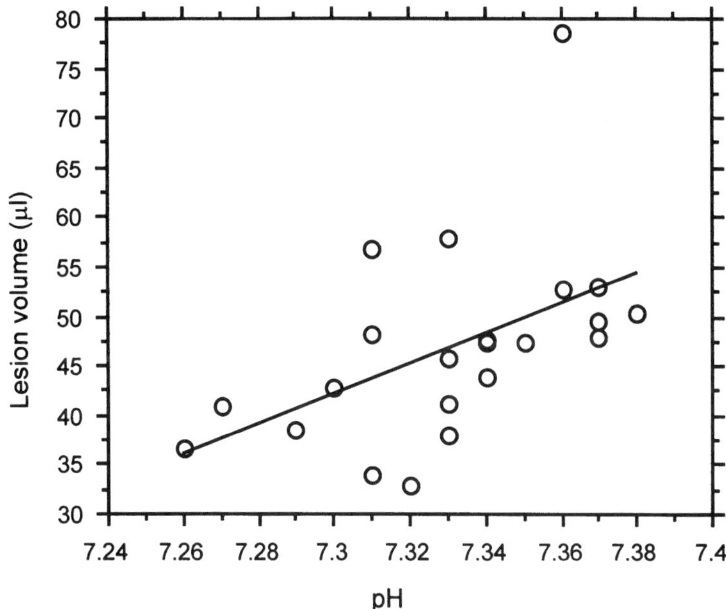

FIGURE 5. Linear regression between postinjury pH and lesion volume. $p < 0.05$.

Experiment 3

Objective

To determine the role of hyperglycemia induced early (5 minutes) and late (45 minutes) after spinal cord injury.

Materials and Methods

Eighteen adult fasted rats (9 males and 9 females) received moderate SCI (25-mm drop height) and were then split into 3 groups by postinjury treatment: Dextrose 5% 2 gm/Kg was injected intraperitoneally respectively 5 minutes after SCI in group E (early) and 45 minutes after injury in group D (delayed). Control group C received the same volume of saline 5 minutes postinjury. Blood glucose levels were tested 10 minutes before injury. Additional blood glucose samples were collected immediately before and then 10, 25, and 55 minutes after dextrose/saline administration.

Results

FIGURE 6 describes mean blood glucose levels in the 3 groups. In groups D and E, dextrose administration accounted for a moderate hyperglycemic response, which lasted almost 45 minutes. Mean plasma glucose values in groups D and E ranged from 161 to 186 mg/dl in the first 30 minutes after dextrose administration (absolute value range 138–214 mg/dl).

Because of the different timing in dextrose administration, group E presented significantly ($p < 0.005$) higher blood glucose levels than control group C between 15

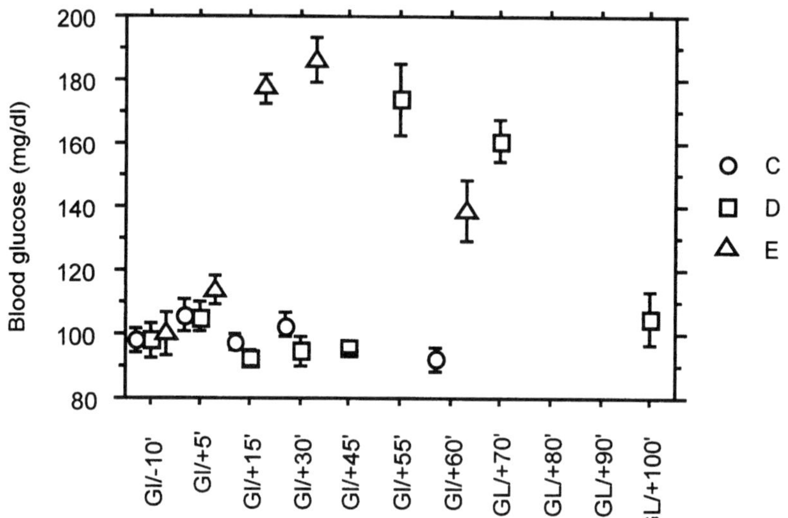

FIGURE 6. Blood glucose levels pre- and postinjury in group E (early glucose over-load), D (delayed glucose overload), and C (control saline).

TABLE 7. Scheffe's post-hoc test for blood glucose values recorded postinjury

Time after-injury	Group C	Group D	Group E	p-Value	Scheffe's test
5 minutes	105.6 ± 4.9	105.1 ± 4.5	113.6 ± 4.9	0.3981	—
15 minutes	97.5 ± 2.8*	92.3 ± 2.6	177.3 ± 4.4	**0.0001**	E > D and C
30 minutes	102.6 ± 3.7**	94.6 ± 4.3	186.1 ± 6.9	**0.0001**	E > D and C
55 minutes	—	174 ± 11*	—	**0.0001**	D > C
60 minutes	92.3 ± 3.7***	—	138.5 ± 9.7	**0.0013**	E > C
70 minutes	—	160.8 ± 6.6**	—	**0.0001**	D > C
100 minutes	—	105.0 ± 8.5***	—	0.5276	—

NOTE: Significant values (p <0.05) are *bold*. Blood glucose values in group D after dextrose administration (*, **, ***) , were compared to the corresponding values in group C during the first hour after saline administration (**).

and 60 minutes after SCI. In group D this difference was observed between 55 and 70 minutes after injury (TABLE 7).

Despite of hyperglycemic values obtained in groups D and E, mean lesion volume in these 2 groups was not significantly higher than that of the control group (FIG. 7).

Conclusions

Moderate postinjury hyperglycemia induced within 1 hour after SCI does not affect lesion volume.

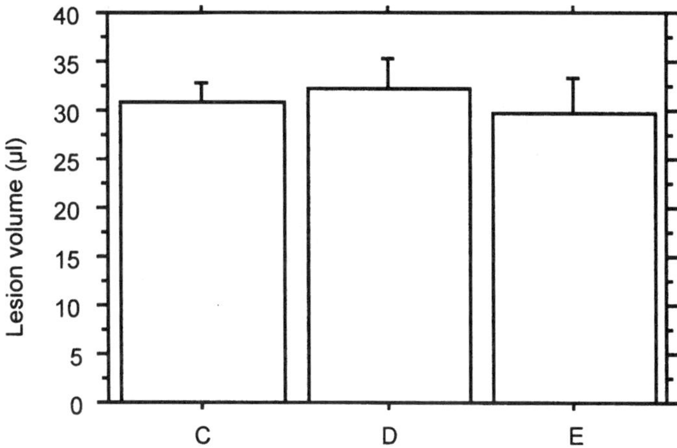

FIGURE 7. Lesion volume in group E (early glucose overload), D (delayed glucose overload), and C (control saline). *p* >0.05.

CLINICAL

Clinical Study

Objective

To detect the incidence of hyperglycemia, and to assess the effects of injury severity and glucocorticoids (methylprednisolone, MP) on blood glucose levels in the first 24 hours after SCI.

Materials and Methods

Between 1991 and 1995, over 200 patients were admitted to the Department of Neurosurgery in Verona for traumatic spinal cord injury. Exclusion criteria for this study were: documented history of diabetes; brain injury or other associated major injuries (abdominal or chest trauma, bone fractures, burns); administration of glucose-containing solutions before admission; lack of blood glucose data during the first 24 hours after injury.

According to these criteria, 47 patients were selected and split into groups according to injury severity and the timing of MP administration (30 mg/Kg intravenously (i.v.) over 15 minutes; 5.4 mg/Kg/h i.v. over 23 hours), before (MPb) or after (MPa) testing glucose levels. Patients who were tested for glucose within 60 minutes of MP administration were included in group MPa. Group MPa also included 9 patients who, according to the NASCIS 2 protocol,[44] did not receive MP at all because they were admitted to our department later than 8 hours after injury. Injury severity (complete or incomplete neurologic deficit) was assessed according to the American Spinal Injury Association scoring system (ASIA 92).

For statistical analyses, we considered the earliest recorded blood glucose value, whether at our department or in other hospitals. Blood glucose values were assessed

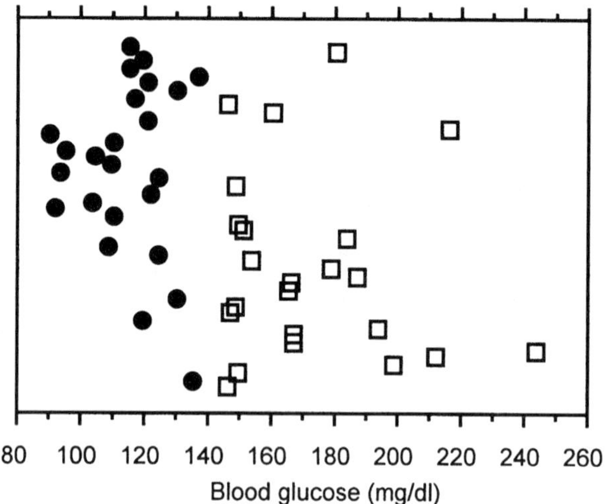

FIGURE 8. Distribution of blood glucose levels in the first 24 hours after spinal cord injury. Hyperglycemia (blood glucose >140 mg/dl; *empty squares*) was observed in 23 out of 47 patients.

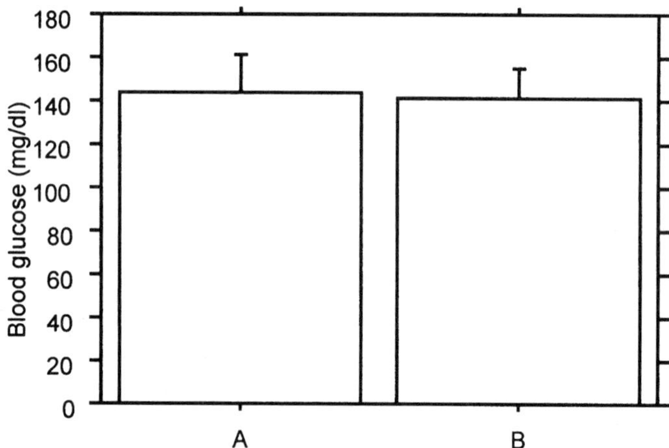

FIGURE 9. Blood glucose levels in patients who received methylprednisolone **(A)** after (MPa) and **(B)** before (MPb) testing blood glucose. *p* >0.05.

by the hexokinase method, and values >140 mg/dl were considered hyperglycemic. Because blood glucose was recorded at different times within the 24 hours postinjury, we performed a regression analysis, which excluded a relationship between blood glucose values and the time interval between injury and glucotest.

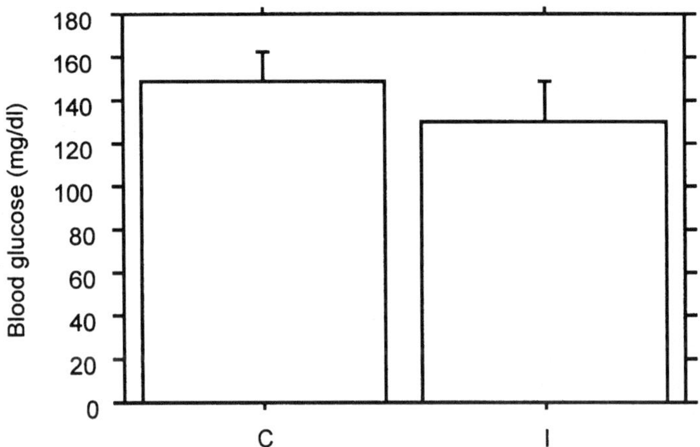

FIGURE 10. Blood glucose levels in patients with complete (C) and incomplete (I) spinal cord injury. There is a trend to larger glucose rises with more severe injury ($p = 0.077$).

Results

Mean time between injury and admission to the hospital was 4 hours and 28 minutes. Blood glucose was tested at a mean time of 6 hours and 36 minutes after injury, but this time ranged from as early as 30 minutes up to 22 hours after trauma.

Mean blood glucose in the 47 patients was 143 mg/dl (range 90–243). Hyperglycemia (blood glucose >140 mg/dl) was present in 23 patients (49%) with a mean value of 174 mg/dl (FIG. 8). Mean blood glucose values did not significantly differ in patients who received MP before (mean 141 mg/dl) or after (mean 144 mg/dl) the glucotest (FIG. 9), while there was a trend to larger glucose rises with more severe injury: 149 mg/dl in plegic patients versus 130 mg/dl in those with incomplete SCI ($p = 0.077$) (FIG. 10).

Conclusions

In this study, almost 50% of patients presented blood glucose values higher than normal in the first 24 hours after SCI. The hyperglycemic response slightly correlated to injury severity, while the administration of glucocorticoids did not significantly affect glycemia.

DISCUSSION

In this series of experimental and clinical observations we attempted to clarify the relationships between spinal cord injury and glycemia. The rationale for these studies comes from previous observations that documented the detrimental role of hyperglycemia in models of central nervous system ischemia.

In 1976 Myers and Yamaguchi observed that hyperglycemia worsened neurological recovery after cardiac arrest.[5] Since then, a large amount of data supported that hyperglycemia may be harmful during brain ischemia, because it enhances lactic acidosis. The accumulation of lactic acid aggravates falls in brain pH and exacerbates tissue damage due to disregulation of calcium homeostasis, energy failure and promotion of free radical reactions in injured cells.[6,7,9–27,45–49]

On the basis of these data, in the past 10 years clinicians have refrained from the administration of glucose-cointaining solutions to patients at risk for brain ischemia.[23,48,50,51] A similar attitude has been adopted in the treatment on brain-injured patients. Severe head injury, in fact, is associated with a sympathoadrenal response,[52–54] which includes hyperglycemia. Clinical studies have shown that hyperglycemia after head injury is an indicator of injury severity and a significant predictor of outcome.[36,37,40] Although a causal relationship between blood glucose and traumatic brain injury has not been unquestionably established yet,[38,39] different sources of calories have been proposed for brain-injured patients.[55]

Little attention has been paid, so far, to the role of glucose in spinal cord rather than brain injury. Studies that have investigated the role of hyperglycemia in spinal cord ischemia models suggest that secondary mechanisms of neuronal damage, similar to those involved in brain ischemia, may be implicated.[28,33,46] These studies, based on the aortic occlusion model, invariably showed that the neurological outcome after spinal cord ischemia was significantly worsened by hyperglycemia induced before or at the time of aortic occlusion. The point of demarcation for bad or good outcome were blood glucose values ranging between 180 to 290 mg/dl. The possibility that hyperglycemia and lactic acidosis directly affect the spinal cord damage was then supported by further data. First, Robertson and LeMay demonstrated a neuroprotective role of insuline and dichloroacetate.[32,35] Second, Lundy observed that the osmotic effects alone could not account for the exacerbation of ischemic injury.[28] Thus, evidence that metabolic changes were responsible for secondary mechanisms of spinal cord injury was accumulating. Vink *et al.* observed that spinal cord injury resulting in severe spastic paraparesis was accompanied by progressive, delayed depletion of intracellular ATP reserves, accumulation of lactic acid with profound tissue acidosis and compromised bioenergetic status.[56]

The results from our preliminary studies add some information to this background and are discussed in the following sections.

Experiment 1

From an experimental perspective we first tested the hypothesis that spinal cord inury induces an hyperglycemic response, likely secondary to the sympathoadrenal response to injury. After SCI, in fact, there is a prompt activation of both the adrenal medulla and the sympathetic nervous system, as well as the parasympathetic and the hypothalamic-hypophyseal-adrenal systems.[57–66] This response results in rises of blood pressure, heart rate and blood glucose.[57,59] Unexpectedly, in Experiment 1 blood glucose levels never exceed normoglycemic levels, and many of the rats were rather moderately hypoglycemic. At least two different explanations can be taken into account. First, rats were fasted overnight. Rats have high metabolic rates, and fasting may have caused relative hypoglycemia before injury, increasing the amount of glucose release required to reach hyperglycemic levels. Furthermore, fasting depletes liver and glycogen stores, so that a blunted injury-induced glucose response is not surprising. A second consideration is that if the hyperglycemic response occurred within 25 minutes after injury, we may not have sampled blood early enough to document the peak of this response. In experimental brain injury, however, the sympathoadrenal response clearly lasts longer than 25 minutes[54] and, from a clinical perspective, hyperglycemia has been recorded as late as on admission time after head injury.[36–38]

Despite the fact that we did not observe a real hyperglycemic response, glucose values were related to injury severity up to three hours after SCI: more severe contusions maintained blood glucose in a higher range. This suggests that, although blunted because of the fasting treatment, SCI was followed by a relative increase in blood glucose. We did not study catecholamine concentrations in the blood; nevertheless it is highly probable that this metabolic response is secondary to the sympathoadrenal response, as extensively demonstrated by others.[65,67–70]

Finally, because both lesion volume and glucose response correlated with injury severity, this experiment did not clarify whether or not blood glucose levels directly affect spinal cord damage.

Experiment 2

In experimental SCI, all the methodologic and physiological variables introduced during a relatively narrow time window before and after injury may affect the outcome. The possibility that fasting affects spinal cord lesion volume, which is the main outcome measurement in several SCI studies, must be investigated. If glucose affects tissue damage in SCI, the common practice of fasting animals overnight might deserve to be carefully standardized.

Beside blood glucose, other variables of interest are the blood gases. We previously reported that variations in blood gases within clinically normal ranges do not influence 24-hour lesion volume. In the same experiment, however, we observed a significant neuroprotective effect of a mild systemic acidosisis after mild and moderate, but not severe SCI.[42]

Results from Experiment 2 suggest that fasting significantly reduced glycemia up to 3 hours after injury and accounts for more consistent preinjury blood glucose levels. These data support findings from Experiment 1 and suggest that fasting overnight provides more uniform glycemia baseline conditions. With regard to postinjury supplementation, we obtained similar blood glucose values whether the animals were fed per os or received just a minimum intravenous caloric support. In our experience this second strategy appears to be less practical and not more advantageous than to allow free access to food and water.

A remarkable finding in this experiment was the lack of correlation between spinal cord lesion volume and both blood glucose levels and fasting treatment. This strongly suggest that pre- and postinjury nutritional management is not directly related to the lesion volume, as long as it does not shift blood glucose levels from a normo-slightly hypoglycemic range. These data are indirectly confirmed by the fact that in spinal cord ischemia models detrimental blood glucose levels were higher than those observed in our study;[28,29,33] this also explains why our results cannot rule out a deleterious effect of severe hyperglycemia. Conversely, the administration of insulin, and the subsequent decrease in glycemia down to levels similar to those that we observed, not only prevented from aggravating spinal cord damage, but even resulted in neuroprotection when compared to not pretreated control animals.[30,34]

In our Experiment 2, we also observed a relationship between fasting and blood gases. Either before or after injury, $PaCO_2$ and bicarbonates were significantly higher in not fasted rats. We expected all the animals to undergo a respiratory depression due to anesthesia. However, in hypoxic conditions, not fasted animals were also subjected to a higher risk for metabolic lactoacidosis, because of a larger availability of glycolitic substrate; they where somehow forced to compensate for a mixed respiratory and metabolic acidosis, in order to maintain a stable pH.

The role of fasting in influencing blood gases and, in general, the acid-base equilibrium, is noteworthy since we also observed a slight neuroprotective role of postinjury extracellular pH. Higher lesion volumes were associated to higher postinjury pHs. These data confirmed what we previously observed in mild and moderate SCI[42] and suggest that secondary mechanisms of SCI may be relevant after severe SCI as well. The role of acidosis in central nervous system ischemia is largely debated and will not be discussed here in detail. However, it is of interest to observe that previous dogma on the deleterious effect of acidosis, especially lactic acidosis, in brain and spinal cord ischemia has been at least partially revised in the light of new experimental evidence. Many data support the idea that a decrease in intracellular pH exacerbates cellular damage through a cascade of secondary mechanisms of injury.[14,16,20,22,26,35,56,71–76] Despite the known effects of extreme values of acidosis, however, other evidence supports the hypothesis that a mild acidosis may have a modulatory rather than a deleterious effect during spinal cord injury. Extracellular acidosis, for example, may improve spinal cord oxygenation by reducing the affinity of hemoglobin to oxygen through the Bohr effect. Recent studies, furthermore, revealed a role of pH in modulating the glutamate N-methyl-D-aspartate (NMDA) receptor activity.[77–80] A lowering of extracellular pH decreases NMDA receptor-gated currents, slowing the influx of calcium; this ultimately ameliorates neuronal damage by partially blunting the cascade of cellular excito-toxicity mechanisms.[1,2,81]

Experiment 3

In most of the studies that have investigated the role of blood glucose in the aorta occlusion model, hyperglycemia was induced before or during the ischemic event. From a clinical perspective, however, it would be of greater interest to know the effect of hyperglycemia in the first few hours after spinal cord ischemia. In fact, while we cannot affect preinjury blood glucose levels, we are directly involved in the medical care of these patients from the very early times after the accident. These first few hours are now known to be critical, because represent the time-window when secondary mechanisms of spinal cord injury take place and the therapeutical intervention may be effective.

Hemmila *et al.*[82] investigated the role of hyperglycemia induced immediately after or 30 minutes after an 8-minute aorta occlusion period. They gave treatment groups dextrose 5% 2 gm/Kg and the control group saline. The neurologic deficit score was determined at 1, 4, 18, and 24 hours after ischemia. They observed elevated baseline blood glucose values, around 170 mg/dl, which rose to 230 mg/dl in the control group and 390 mg/dl in the treatment groups, 1 hour after dextrose or saline administration. Treatment groups had significantly higher glycemia up to 4 hours after dextrose administration, but the neurologic deficit score was significantly worse only at 24 hours and only in the group that received dextrose immediately after aortic occlusion release.

Experiment 3 was designed to confirm these data in spinal cord traumatic more than ischemic injury, but we did not detect any significant effect of dextrose administration on lesion volume. We advance two explanations for this discrepancy. First, the rats in our study were fasted overnight, and baseline glucose values were much lower than those observed by Hemmila (100 vs 170 mg/dl). This may have prevented the rats from incurring a truly severe hyperglycemia, and the values we obtained (around 160–190 mg/dl) may have been too moderate to exacerbate spinal cord damage. A second possibility is that hyperglycemia may have a different role in ischemic and traumatic SCI, and different mechanisms may be involved. In recent studies, in fact, it has been hypothesized that blood glucose concentration may not be a significant factor affecting outcome in traumatic brain injury unless complicated by secondary ischemia.[24,83,84] This is a fascinating theory, which deserves further investigation with regard to SCI.

Clinical Study

The lack of clinical information on blood glucose levels in the acute phase after SCI prompted us to review the data of patients admitted to our hospital within 24 hours after traumatic SCI in order to detect the incidence of hyperglycemia and its correlation with injury severity. In addition, the conclusion of the third National Acute Spinal Cord Injury Study suggests us prolonging the administration of high doses of MP up to 48 hours after injury in patients where the MP protocol started more than 3 hours after injury.[85] These high doses of glucocorticoids may enhance the hyperglycemic response to injury. We therefore attempted to detect correlations between glycemia and administration of MP in patients treated according to the NASCIS 2 protocol.[44]

This clinical study unfortunately suffers from the major drawbacks of retrospective studies. A major limitation is that, although within the 24-hour time-window, blood glucose testing as well as MP administration were done at different times in different patients. Nevertheless, conclusions from this study provide first preliminary data on the relationship between glucose and spinal cord injury in humans.

Our results revealed a significant incidence (49%) of high blood glucose levels in spinal cord-injured patients, which we interpreted as the sympathoadrenal response to injury. It is of interest that the range of hyperglycemic values observed in this clinical study (90–243, mean 143 mg/dl) was definitely lower than the severe hyperglycemia induced in experimental models of spinal cord ischemia. This suggests that from an experimental perspective it is probably not necessary to work in a severe hyperglycemic range, since this is rarely the case in clinical practice.

The trend to higher glucose levels in more severely injured patients would confirm observations in head injury patients,[36,37,40] and it is likely the consequence of a greater catecholamine release.

Administration of methylprednisolone (30 mg/Kg i.v. over 15 minutes; 5.4 mg/Kg/h i.v. over 23 hours) did not significantly enhance this response, but we cannot exclude different results when MP administration is prolonged for 48 hours.

CONCLUSIONS

We presented our preliminary data on the relationships between SCI and blood glucose in experimental and clinical conditions. Similarly to what has been described in brain inury, SCI induces a hyperglycemic response that is likely the result of the stress response to injury. We suggest that blood glucose does not significantly affect damage to the spinal cord when it is maintained in a normo- slightly hypoglycemic range. Even moderate hyperglycemia induced early after injury does not further impair spinal cord lesion volume. We confirmed a minor neuroprotective effect of mild acidosis. Only future studies will clarify the effect of severe hyperglycemia and the possibility that glucose plays a different role in ischemic and traumatic central nervous system injury.

From a clinical perspective, we observed that one out of two patients presents hyperglycemia in the acute phase after SCI. However, we need to prospectively clarify the time course of the hyperglycemic response to SCI, its correlation with the administration of glucocorticoids, and the effects of glucose on the outcome after SCI.

While waiting for these results, we recommend monitoring blood glucose in experimental and clinical SCI in order to maintain normoglycemia.

ACKNOWLEDGMENTS

We would like to thank Bor Tom Ng and Hock Ng for their excellent technical assistance, Jing Hui Wu for her help in performing statistical analyses, and Prof. Antonio Cevese for reviewing the manuscript and providing invaluable suggestions.

REFERENCES

1. KRISTIAN, T. & B.K. SIESJO. 1996. Calcium-related damage in ischemia. Life Sci. **59:** 357–367.
2. KRISTIAN, T. & B.K. SIESJO. 1998. Calcium in ischemic cell death. Stroke **29:** 705–718.
3. TYMIANSKI, M. & C.H. TATOR. 1996. Normal and abnormal calcium homeostasis in neurons: a basis for the pathophysiology of traumatic and ischemic central nervous system injury. Neurosurgery **38:** 1176–1195.
4. WACHTLER, J., C. MAYER, F. RUCKER & P. GRAFE. 1996. Glucose availability alters ischaemia-induced changes in intracellular pH and calcium of isolated rat spinal roots. Brain Res. **725:** 30–36.
5. MYERS, R.E. & S. YAMAGUCHI. 1976. Effects of serum glucose concentration on brain response to circulation arrest. J. Neuropathol. Exp. Neurol. **35:** 301.
6. GINSBERG, M.D., F.A. WELSH & W.W. BUDD. 1980. Deleterious effect of glucose pretreatment on recovery from diffuse cerebral ischemia in the cat. I. Local cerebral blood flow and glucose utilization. Stroke **11:** 347–354.
7. WELSH, F.A., M.D. GINSBERG, W. RIEDER & W.W. BUDD. 1980. Deleterious effect of glucose pretreatment on recovery from diffuse cerebral ischemia in the cat. II. Regional metabolite levels. Stroke **11:** 355–363.
8. REHNCRONA, S., I. ROSEN & B.K. SIESJO. 1980. Excessive cellular acidosis: an important mechanism of neuronal damage in the brain? Acta Physiol. Scand. **110:** 435–437.
9. PULSINELLI, W.A., S. WALDMAN, D. RAWLINSON & F. PLUM. 1982. Moderate hyperglycemia augments ischemic brain damage: a neuropathologic study in the rat. Neurology **32:** 1239–1246.
10. PULSINELLI, W.A., D.E. LEVY, B. SIGSBEE, P. SCHERER & F. PLUM. 1983. Increased

damage after ischemic stroke in patients with hyperglycemia with or without established diabetes mellitus. Am. J. Med. **74:** 540–544.

11. SIEMKOWICZ, E. 1985. The effect of glucose upon restitution after transient cerebral ischemia: a summary. Acta Neurol. Scand. **71:** 417–427.

12. MARSH, W.R., R.E. ANDERSON & T.M. SUNDT, JR. 1986. Effect of hyperglycemia on brain pH levels in areas of focal incomplete cerebral ischemia in monkeys. J. Neurosurg. **65:** 693–696.

13. DUCKROW, R.B., D.C. BEARD & R.W. BRENNAN. 1987. Regional cerebral blood flow decreases during chronic and acute hyperglycemia. Stroke **18:** 52–58.

14. DE SALLES, A.A., J.P. MUIZELAAR & H.F. YOUNG. 1987. Hyperglycemia, cerebrospinal fluid lactic acidosis, and cerebral blood flow in severely head-injured patients. Neurosurgery **21:** 45–50.

15. COMBS, D.J., R.J. DEMPSEY, M. MALEY, D. DONALDSON & C. SMITH. 1990. Relationship between plasma glucose, brain lactate, and intracellular pH during cerebral ischemia in gerbils. Stroke **21:** 936–942.

16. KRAIG, R.P. & M. CHESLER. 1990. Astrocytic acidosis in hyperglycemic and complete ischemia. J. Cereb. Blood Flow Metab. **10:** 104–114.

17. ROBERTSON, C.S., J.C. GOODMAN, R.K. NARAYAN, C.F. CONTANT & R.G. GROSSMAN. 1991. The effect of glucose administration on carbohydrate metabolism after head injury. J. Neurosurg. **74:** 43–50.

18. MARIE, C. & J. BRALET. 1991. Blood glucose level and morphological brain damage following cerebral ischemia. Cerebrovasc. Brain Metab. Rev. **3:** 29–38.

19. TOMLINSON, F.H., R.E. ANDERSON & F.B. MEYER. 1993. Effect of arterial blood pressure and serum glucose on brain intracellular pH, cerebral and cortical blood flow during status epilepticus in the white New Zealand rabbit. Epilepsy Res. **14:** 123–137.

20. STAUB, F., B. MACKERT, O. KEMPSKI, J. PETERS & A. BAETHMANN. 1993. Swelling and death of neuronal cells by lactic acid. J. Neurol. Sci. **119:** 79–84.

21. DIETRICH, W.D., O. ALONSO & R. BUSTO. 1993. Moderate hyperglycemia worsens acute blood-brain barrier injury after forebrain ischemia in rats. Stroke **24:** 111–116.

22. SAPPEY MARINIER, D., L. CHILEUITT, M.W. WEINER, A.I. FADEN & P.R. WEINSTEIN. 1995. Hypoglycemia prevents increase in lactic acidosis during reperfusion after temporary cerebral ischemia in rats. NMR Biomed. **8:** 171–178.

23. SHAPIRA, Y., A.A. ARTRU, N. QASSAM, N. NAVOT & U. VALD. 1995. Brain edema and neurological status with rapid infusion of 0.9% saline or 5% dextrose after head trauma. J. Neurosurg. Anesthesiol. **7:** 17–25.

24. CHERIAN, L., J.C. GOODMAN & C.S. ROBERTSON. 1997. Hyperglycemia increases brain injury caused by secondary ischemia after cortical impact injury in rats. Crit. Care Med. **25:** 1378–1383.

25. KAWAI, N., R.F. KEEP & A.L. BETZ. 1997. Effects of hyperglycemia on cerebral blood flow and edema formation after carotid artery occlusion in Fischer 344 rats. Acta Neurochir. Suppl. **70:** 34–36.

26. LI, P.A. & B.K. SIESJO. 1997. Role of hyperglycaemia-related acidosis in ischaemic brain damage. Acta Physiol. Scand. **161:** 567–580.

27. SIESJO, B.K., K. KATSURA, P. MELLERGARD, A. EKHOLM, J. LUNDGREN & M.L. SMITH. 1993. Acidosis-related brain damage. Prog. Brain Res. **96:** 23–48.

28. LUNDY, E.F., T.D. BALL, M.A. MANDELL, G.B. ZELENOCK & L.G. D'ALECY. 1987. Dextrose administration increases sensory/motor impairment and paraplegia after infrarenal aortic occlusion in the rabbit. Surgery **102:** 737–742.

29. LEMAY, D.R., S. NEAL, S. NEAL, G.B. ZELENOCK & L.G. D'ALECY. 1987. Paraplegia in the rat induced by aortic cross-clamping: model characterization and glucose exacerbation of neurologic deficit. J. Vasc. Surg. **6:** 383–390.

30. LEMAY, D.R., A.C. LU, G.B. ZELENOCK & L.G. D'ALECY. 1988. Insulin administration protects from paraplegia in the rat aortic occlusion model. J. Surg. Res. **44:** 352–358.

31. LEMAY, D.R., G.B. ZELENOCK & L.G. D'ALECY. 1989. The role of glucose uptake and metabolism in hyperglycemic exacerbation of neurological deficit in the paraplegic rat. J. Neurosurg. **71:** 594–600.

32. LEMAY, D.R., G.B. ZELENOCK & L.G. D'ALECY. 1990. Neurological protection by dichloroacetate depending on the severity of injury in the paraplegic rat. J. Neurosurg. **73:** 118–122.

33. DRUMMOND, J.C. & S.S. MOORE. 1989. The influence of dextrose administration on neurologic outcome after temporary spinal cord ischemia in the rabbit. Anesthesiology **70:** 64–70.

34. ROBERTSON, C.S. & R.G. GROSSMAN. 1987. Protection against spinal cord ischemia with insulin-induced hypoglycemia. J. Neurosurg. **67:** 739–744.

35. ROBERTSON, C.S., J.C. GOODMAN, R.G. GROSSMAN & A. PRIESSMAN. 1990. Reduction in spinal cord postischemic lactic acidosis and functional improvement with dichloroacetate. J. Neurotrauma **7:** 1–12.

36. YOUNG, B., L. OTT, R. DEMPSEY, D. HAACK & P. TIBBS. 1989. Relationship between admission hyperglycemia and neurologic outcome of severely brain-injured patients. Ann. Surg. **210:** 466–72; discussion 472–473.

37. LAM, A.M., H.R. WINN, B.F. CULLEN & N. SUNDLING. 1991. Hyperglycemia and neurological outcome in patients with head injury. J. Neurosurg. **75:** 545–551.

38. MARGULIES, D.R., J.R. HIATT, D. VINSON, JR. & M.M. SHABOT. 1994. Relationship of hyperglycemia and severity of illness to neurologic outcome in head injury patients. Am. Surg. **60:** 387–390.

39. MICHAUD, L.J., F.P. RIVARA, W.T. LONGSTRETH & M.S. GRADY. 1991. Elevated initial blood glucose levels and poor outcome following severe brain injuries in children. J. Trauma **31:** 1356–1362.

40. YANG, S.Y., S. ZHANG & M.L. WANG. 1995. Clinical significance of admission hyperglycemia and factors related to it in patients with acute severe head injury. Surg. Neurol. **44:** 373–377.

41. GRUNER, J.A. 1992. A monitored contusion model of spinal cord injury in the rat. J. Neurotrauma **9:** 123–128.

42. HUANG, P.P. & W. YOUNG. 1994. The effects of arterial blood gas values on lesion volumes in a graded rat spinal cord contusion model. J. Neurotrauma **11:** 547–562.

43. CONSTANTINI, S. & W. YOUNG. 1994. The effects of methylprednisolone and the ganglioside GM1 on acute spinal cord injury in rats. J. Neurosurg. **80:** 97–111.

44. BRACKEN, M.B., M.J. SHEPARD, W.F. COLLINS, T.R. HOLFORD, D.S. BASKIN *et al.* 1992. Methylprednisolone or naloxone treatment after acute spinal cord injury: 1-year follow-up data. Results of the second National Acute Spinal Cord Injury Study. J. Neurosurg. **76:** 23–31.

45. MYERS, R.E. 1976. Anoxic brain pathology and blood glucose. Neurology **26:** 345.

46. LEMAY, D.R., L. GEHUA, G.B. ZELENOCK & L.G. D'ALECY. 1988. Insulin administration protects neurologic function in cerebral ischemia in rats. Stroke **19:** 1411–1419.

47. WIDMER, H., H. ABIKO, A.I. FADEN, T.L. JAMES & P.R. WEINSTEIN. 1992. Effects of hyperglycemia on the time course of changes in energy metabolism and pH during global cerebral ischemia and reperfusion in rats: correlation of 1H and 31P NMR spectroscopy with fatty acid and excitatory amino acid levels. J. Cereb. Blood Flow Metab. **12:** 456–468.

48. WASS, C.T. & W.L. LANIER. 1996. Glucose modulation of ischemic brain injury: review and clinical recommandations. Mayo Clin. Proc. **71:** 801–812.

49. SIESJO, B.K. & P. SIESJO. 1996. Mechanisms of secondary brain injury. Eur. J. Anaesthesiol. **13:** 247–268.

50. BROWNING, R.G., D.W. OLSON, H.A. STUEVEN & J.R. MATEER. 1990. 50% dextrose: antidote or toxin? Ann. Emerg. Med. **19:** 683–687.
51. FELDMAN, Z., S. ZACHARI, E. REICHENTHAL, A.A. ARTRU & Y. SHAPIRA. 1995. Brain edema and neurological status wuth rapid infusion of lactated Ringer's or 5% dextrose solution following head trauma. J. Neurosurg. **83:** 1060–1066.
52. BECKMAN, D.L. & S.G. IAMS. 1979. Circulating catecholamines in cats before and after lethal head injury. Proc. Soc. Exp. Biol. Med. **160:** 200–202.
53. CLIFTON, G.L., M.G. ZIEGLER & R.G. GROSSMAN. 1981. Circulating catecholamines and sympathetic activity after head injury. Neurosurgery **8:** 10–14.
54. ROSNER, M.J., H.H. NEWSOME & D.P. BECKER. 1984. Mechanical brain injury: the sympathoadrenal response. J. Neurosurg. **61:** 76–86.
55. CHERIAN, L., K. PEEK, C.S. ROBERTSON, J.C. GOODMAN & R.G. GROSSMAN. 1994. Calorie sources and recovery from central nervous system ischemia. Crit. Care Med. **22:** 1841–1850.
56. VINK, R., L.J. NOBLE, S.M. KNOBLACH, M.R. BENDALL & A.I. FADEN. 1989. Metabolic changes in rabbit spinal cord after trauma: magnetic resonance spectroscopy studies. Ann. Neurol. **25:** 26–31.
57. RAWE, S.E. & P.L. PEROT, JR. 1979. Pressor response resulting from experimental contusion injury to the spinal cord. J. Neurosurg. **50:** 58–63.
58. TIBBS, P.A., B. YOUNG, M.G. ZIEGLER & R.G. MCALLISTER, JR. 1979. Studies of experimental cervical spinal cord transection. Part II: Plasma norepinephrine levels after acute cervical spinal cord transection. J. Neurosurg. **50:** 629–632.
59. TIBBS, P.A., B. YOUNG, R.G. MCALLISTER, W.H. BROOKS & L. TACKETT. 1978. Studies of experimental cervical spinal cord transection. Part I: Hemodynamic changes after acute cervical spinal cord transection. J. Neurosurg. **49:** 558–562.
60. MUELHEIMS, G.H., K.E. WALTER & L. BILLY. 1969. Catecholamine release after spinal cord section. Proc. Soc. Exp. Biol. Med. **130:** 574–576.
61. NAFTCHI, N.E., M. DEMENY, V. DE CRESCITO, J.J. TOMASULA, E.S. FLAMM & J.B. CAMPBELL. 1974. Biogenic amine concentrations in traumatized spinal cords of cats. Effect of drug therapy. J. Neurosurg. **40:** 52–57.
62. OSTERHOLM, J.L. & G.J. MATHEWS. 1972. Altered norepinephrine metabolism following experimental spinal cord injury. 1. Relationship to hemorrhagic necrosis and post-wounding neurological deficits. J. Neurosurg. **36:** 386–394.
63. OSTERHOLM, J.L. 1974. The pathophysiological response to spinal cord injury. The current status of related research. J. Neurosurg. **40:** 5–33.
64. OSTERHOLM, J.L. & G.J. MATHEWS. 1972. Altered norepinephrine metabolism, following experimental spinal cord injury. 2. Protection against traumatic spinal cord hemorrhagic necrosis by norepinephrine synthesis blockade with alpha methyl tyrosine. J. Neurosurg. **36:** 395–401.
65. SCHOULTZ, T.W. & D.C. DE LUCA. 1974. Alterations in spinal cord norepinephrine levels following experimentally produced trauma in normal and adrenalectomized cats. Life Sci. **15:** 1485–1495.
66. SCHOULTZ, T.W., D.C. DE LUCA & D.L. REDING. 1976. Norepinephrine levels in traumatized spinal cord of catecholamine-depleted cats. Brain Res. **109:** 367–374.
67. RIZZA, R., M. HAYMOND, P. CRYER & J. GERICH. 1979. Differential effects of epinephrine on glucose production and disposal in man. Am. J. Physiol. **237:** 356–362.
68. RIZZA, R.A., P.E. CRYER, M.W. HAYMOND & J.E. GERICH. 1980. Adrenergic mechanisms for the effects of epinephrine on glucose production and clearance in man. J. Clin. Invest. **65:** 682–689.
69. KING, L.R., H.C. KNOWLES, JR., R.L. MCLAURIN & H.P. LEWIS. 1971. Glucose tolerance and plasma insulin in cranial trauma. Ann. Surg. **173:** 337–343.
70. FRAYN, K.N., R.A. LITTLE, P.F. MAYCOCK & H.B. STONER. 1985. The relationship of plasma catecholamines to acute metabolic and hormonal responses to injury in

man. Circ. Shock **16:** 229–240.

71. GOLDMAN, S.A., W.A. PULSINELLI, W.Y. CLARKE, R.P. KRAIG & F. PLUM. 1989. The effects of extracellular acidosis on neurons and glia *in vitro*. J. Cereb. Blood Flow Metab. **9:** 471–477.

72. REHNCRONA, S., H.N. HAUGE & B.K. SIESJO. 1989. Enhancement of iron-catalyzed free radical formation by acidosis in brain homogenates: differences in effect by lactic acid and CO_2. J. Cereb. Blood Flow Metab. **9:** 65–70.

73. NAGAI, Y., S. NARUSE & M.W. WEINER. 1993. Effect of hypoglycemia on changes of brain lactic acid and intracellular pH produced by ischemia. NMR Biomed. **6:** 1–6.

74. FAROOQUE, M., L. HILLERED, A. HOLTZ & Y. OLSSON. 1996. Effects of methyprednisolone on extracellular lactic acidosis and amino acids after severe compression injury of rat spinal cord. J. Neurochem. **66:** 1125–1130.

75. FOLBERGROVA, J., P.A. LI, H. UCHINO, M.L. SMITH & B.K. SIESJO. 1997. Changes in the bioenergetic state of rat hippocampus during 2.5 min of ischemia, and prevention of cell damage by cyclosporin A in hyperglycemic subjects. Exp. Brain Res. **114:** 44–50.

76. FAROOQUE, M., Y. OLSSON & L. HILLERED. 1997. Pretreatment with alpha-phenyl-*N*-tert-butyl-nitrone (PBN) improves energy metabolism after spinal cord injury in rats. J. Neurotrauma **14:** 469–476.

77. MUKHIN, A.G., S.A. IVANOVA, J.W. ALLEN & A.I. FADEN. 1998. Mechanical injury to neuronal/glial cultures in microplates: role of NMDA receptors and pH in secondary neuronal cell death. J. Neurosci. Res. **51:** 748–758.

78. CHEN, Y.H., M.L. WU & W.M. FU. 1998. Regulation of presynaptic NMDA responses by external and intracellular pH changes at developing neuromuscular synapses. J. Neurosci. **18:** 2982–2990.

79. GOTTFRIED, J.A. & M. CHESLER. 1994. Endogenous H^+ modulation of NMDA receptor-mediated EPSCs revealed by carbonic anhydrase inhibition in rat hippocampus. J. Physiol. **478:** 373–378.

80. SAYBASILI, H. 1998. The protective role of mild acidic pH shifts on synaptic NMDA current in hippocampal slices. Brain Res. **786:** 128–132.

81. IMAIZUMI, T., J.D. KOCSIS & S.G. WAXMAN. 1997. Anoxic injury in the rat spinal cord: pharmacological evidence for multiple steps in $Ca(^{2+})$-dependent injury of the dorsal columns. J. Neurotrauma **14:** 299–311.

82. HEMMILA, M.R., G.B. ZELENOCK & L.G. D'ALECY. 1993. Postischemic hyperglycemia worsens neurologic outcome after spinal cord ischemia. J. Vasc. Surg. **17:** 661–668.

83. CHERIAN, L., H.J. HANNAY, G. VAGNER, J.C. GOODMAN, C.F. CONTANT & C.S. ROBERTSON. 1998. Hyperglycemia increases neurological damage and behavioral deficits from post-traumatic secondary ischemic insults. J. Neurotrauma **15:** 307–321.

84. VINK, R., E.M. GOLDING, J.P. WILLIAMS & T.K. MCINTOSH. 1997. Blood glucose concentration does not affect outcome in brain trauma: A 31P MRS study. J. Cereb. Blood Flow Metab. **17:** 50–53.

85. BRACKEN, M.B., M.J. SHEPARD, T.R. HOLFORD, L. LEO-SUMMERS, E.F. ALDRICH, M. FAZL, M.G. FEHLINGS, D.L. HERR, P.W. HITCHON, L.F. MARSHALL, R.P. NOCKELS, V. PASCALE, P.L. PEROT, J. PIEPMEIER, V.K.H. SONNTAG, F. WAGNER, J.E. WILBERGER, H.R. WINN & W. YOUNG. 1997. Methylprednisolone or tirilazad mesylate administration after acute spinal cord injury: 1-year follow-up. Results of the third National Acute Spinal Cord Injury randomized controlled trial. J. Neurosurg. **89:** 699–706.

N-Acetylserotonin, Melatonin and Their Derivatives Improve Cognition and Protect against β-Amyloid-Induced Neurotoxicity

S. BACHURIN, G. OXENKRUG,[a] N. LERMONTOVA, A. AFANASIEV,
B. BEZNOSKO, G. VANKIN, E. SHEVTZOVA, T. MUKHINA, AND T. SERKOVA

Institute of Physiologically Active Compounds, Russian Academy of Sciences, Chernogolovka 142432, Russia

Pineal Research Laboratory, Department of Psychiatry, St. Elizabeth's Medical Center/ Tufts University, Boston, Massachusetts, USA

ABSTRACT: After a single injection of cholinergic neurotoxin ethylcholine aziridinium (AF64A, 3 nmol intracerebroventricularly (i.c.v.)), rats failed to perform the tasks in the active avoidance (learning and retention paradigms) and water maze tests. *N*-Acetylserotonin (NAS), melatonin and their newly synthesized derivatives, CA-15 and CA-18, (0.3–3.0 mg/kg daily for 12–14 days) reversed the effect of AF64A in a dose-dependent manner with CA-18 being the most active. Melatonin and NAS caused sedation absent in CA-18-treated rats. The studied compounds (25–500 μM for 72 hr) protected against β-amyloid peptide (βAP) fragment 25–35-induced neurotoxicity in cerebellar granule cell culture. Our results suggest that neuroprotecting properties of these compounds might mediate their cognition-enhancing effects. The results obtained warrant the further search for the novel types of safe neuroprotectors among the synthetic NAS/melatonin derivatives.

INTRODUCTION

It is known that dysfunction of circadian rhythms in Alzheimer's disease (AD) can be compensated by exogenous melatonin.[1] It was also suggested that the positive effect of chronic prophylactic administration of melatonin as gerontoprotector is based on its antioxidative properties.[2] Numerous studies indicate that melatonin as free radical scavenger displays pronounced neuroprotective effects against neurotoxic action of the excitatory amino acids (excitotoxicity) and toxic effect of beta-amyloid peptide (βAP)—one of the specific hallmarks of AD.[3] Recently neuroprotective activity was revealed for the melatonin precusor *N*-acetylserotonin (NAS).[4] Since neurodegenerative processes in AD are associated with the decreased cognitive functions, it was reasonable to study the effect of melatonin, NAS and their newly synthesized derivatives on cognitive functions in animal models of AD-type neurodegeneration.

[a]Corresponding author: Prof. G. F. Oxenkrug, M.D., Ph.D., Pineal Research Laboratory, Department of Psychiatry, St. Elizabeth's Medical Center, QN-3P, 736 Cambridge St., Boston, MA, 02135. Phone, 617/789-2925; fax, 617/789-2066.
e-mail, Oxenkrug@SEMC.ORG

In the present study both *in vivo* and *in vitro* models were used. The *in vivo* study involved the neurotoxin-induced animal model of AD, based on observation that intracerebroventricular (i.c.v.) administration of ethylcholine aziridinium ion (AF64A) produced chronic cholinergic hypofunction and learning and memory impairment in rat analogous to that observed in AD.[5] Currently this model is also used for screening of the compounds for their potential cognition-enhancing properties.[6,7] At the cellular level (*in vitro*) the adequate model of AD-type degeneration is believed to be the neuronal cell culture degeneration induced by βAP fragment 25–35.[8] In the present study we examined cognition-enhancing and neuroprotective properties of melatonin, NAS and their newly synthesized derivatives CA-15 and CA-18 in the above-mentioned animal and cell models of AD-type neurodegeneration.

MATERIALS AND METHODS

Chemicals

NAS and melatonin derivatives CA-15 and CA-18 were identified by H1-nuclear magnetic resonance (NMR) and elemental analysis. βAP fragment 25–35 was purchased from Bachem; AF64 was purchased from RBI. All other reagents were purchased from Sigma. Melatonin, NAS and CA-15 and CA-18 were preliminarily dissolved in dimethyl sulfoxide (DMSO) and diluted by water each day prior to use.

Animals

Male Wistar rats (12–16 weeks old, 280–450 g) were used in behavioral experiments. Rats were kept at 12 hr light:12 hr dark schedule (lights on/off at 4:00/16:00 hr) with free access to water and food.

Rats were anesthetized with ether and placed into a stereotaxic frame before the surgery. Freshly prepared from AF64 solutions of AF64A (3 nmol/3 ml) or vehicle (cerebrospinal fluid, CSF) were injected into each of lateral cerebral ventricles. After surgery, rats were given a recovery period (12 days) before being tested in behavioral experiment. Melatonin, NAS and their derivatives were administrated orally (in starch solutions) once a day around the time of circadian light-off during the whole recovery period.

Behavioral Studies

Active Avoidance Test

Training was conducted in a two-chamber shuttle box according to the procedure described earlier.[7] The conditioned stimulus was a 5-sec light followed by the unconditioned stimulus, a 1-mA shock, which was delivered to the grid in the lit chamber. The rat avoided the shock by crossing through to the other (dark) chamber. The avoidance during the conditioned stimulus was considered as a correct response. Training procedure consisted of 35 trials (learning test). Fifteen further trials were given 24 hr later (retention test).

TABLE 1. The influence of melatonin, NAS, and its *o*-benzil homologs on active avoidance performance of the AF64A-treated rats

No.	Compounds	Daily Dose mg/kg	Number of Rats	Correct Responses, %	
				Learning Test	Retention Test
1	Control (i.c.v. CSF)	solvent	33	79.3 ± 5.4*	76.3 ± 6.3*
2	AF64A alone	solvent	31	37.4 ± 9.8	43.8 ± 8.1
3	Melatonin	3	9	75.4 ± 7.0**	72.2 ± 5.8*
	Melatonin	0.3	11	79.0 ± 6.0*	83.0 ± 3.2*
4	NAS	1	10	65.4 ± 8.8*	56.0 ± 9.2
5	CA-15	3	9	61.4 ± 7.4	68.0 ± 8.4**
6	CA-18	1	10	50.0 ± 8.8	48.1 ± 9.8
	CA-18	0.3	11	84.0 ± 5.4*	82.7 ± 5.0*

NOTE: Rats were treated i.c.v. AF64A (3 nmol/3µl) or CSF (control groups) and were given a recovery period (12–14 days) before being tested in the behavioral experiment. The experimental rats were orally given the studied compounds during the recovery period. Shuttle-box avoidance performance: *Learning test.* Following 20 acquisition trials, rats were given 3 blocks of 5 trials. *Retention test.* Two blocks of 5 trials were given 24 hr after the learning trial. Data are presented as the mean ± SEM percentage of correct responses summarized over each block and were analyzed by a statistical test (ANOVA); *p <0.001, **p <0.05 vs the AF64A-treated group.

Statistical Treatment

Each experimental group, i.e., control, AF64A-treated groups and groups for each concentration of the tested compounds, contained 9–11 rats. Data of the number of correct responses from the last 15 trials of the first 35 trials (learning test) or first 15 trials of the retention test were collected for each rat. The mean ± SEM of correct responses was calculated for total number of rats in groups. Data were analyzed as the mean ± SEM in percentage of the maximum possible number of correct responses (= 100%) by anaylsis of variance (ANOVA) followed by post hoc comparisons.

Morris Water Maze Test

The test was started 2 days after the last injection of tested compounds and was performed daily for the period from 3 to 9 days. Round swimming pool (1.8 m diameter and 0.45 m high) with 22°C water was placed in the center of the room. The platform was located 1 cm below the surface of the water. Starting points for the swims were at the cardinal compass points (N, S, E, W), which were selected in a semirandom fashion for each rat on each trial.

Statistical Treatment

Each experimental group, i.e., control, AF64A-treated groups and groups for each concentration of the tested compounds, contained 9–11 rats. Results were estimated as time required for a rat having fallen into the water pool to reach the platform (a sum of 2 trials from a different position every day). Data were analyzed as the mean ± SEM (ANOVA followed by post hoc comparisons).

Neuronal Cell Culture

Cerebellar granule cells (CGC) were prepared from the postnatal rats (7–8 days old) by the following procedure based on the generally accepted methods.[9] The pieces of cerebellum were digested with 0.25 mg/ml trypsin for 25 min at 37°C and incubated for 5 min in 0.1% soybean trypsin inhibitor. After washing, cells were dissociated by triturating. Following 2 centrifugation-resuspension steps, the cells were plated at a density of 2.5–5 × 10 cells per ml on polylysine-coated 24-well plates (Corning) and maintained at 37°C in a humidified incubator with 5% CO_2/ 95% room air. The medium was composed of Eagle's minimum essential medium and fetal calf serum (10%) supplemented with 20 mM potassium chloride, 10 mM glucose, 2 mM glutamine, and 50 µg/ml gentamycin sulfate. Cytosine arabinoside (10 µM) was added 24–48 hr later to prevent the replication of nonneuronal cells.

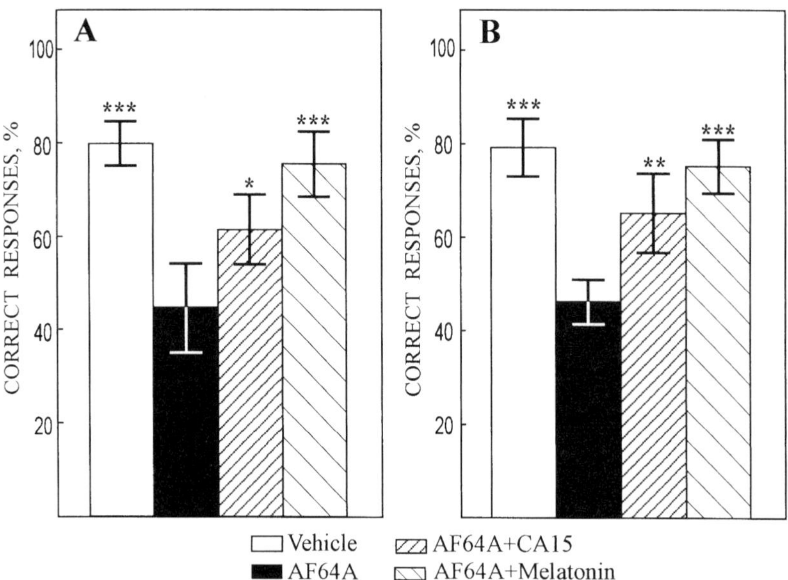

FIGURE 1. Cognition-enhancing effect of melatonin and CA15. Shuttle-box avoidance performance of vehicle-treated rats ($n = 11$), AF64A-treated rats and AF64A-treated rats receiving melatonin or CA-15 (3 mg/kg, once daily, 12–14 days, orally; $n = 10$), where n is the number of rats in each group. **(A)** Learning test. Following 20 acquisition trials, rats were given 3 blocks of 5 trials. **(B)** Retention test. Two blocks of 5 trials were given 24 hr after the learning trial. Data are presented as mean ± SEM percentage of correct responses summarized over each block; **p <0.05, ***p <0.001 vs AF64A-treated group, where p is the significance level; *not significant (post hoc ANOVA).

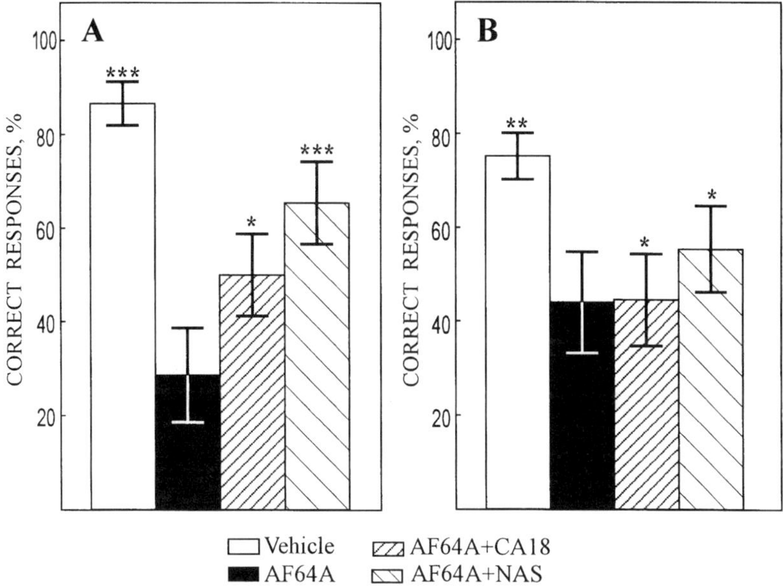

FIGURE 2. Cognition-enhancing effect of CA18 and NAS. Shuttle-box avoidance performance of vehicle-treated rats ($n = 11$), AF64A-treated rats and AF64A-treated rats receiving NAS or CA-18 (1 mg/kg, once daily, 12–14 days, orally; $n = 10$), where n is the number of rats in each group. **(A)** Learning test. Following 20 acquisition trials, rats were given 3 blocks of 5 trials. **(B)** Retention test. Two blocks of 5 trials were given 24 hr after learning trial. Data are presented as mean $\pm$ SEM percentage of correct responses summarized over each block; $**p < 0.05$, $***p < 0.001$ vs AF64A-treated group, where p is the significance level; *not significant (post hoc ANOVA).

Toxic Assays

The neurotoxic and neuroprotective effects of NAS, melatonin and their derivatives were tested in mature cultures at 7–8 days *in vitro* (7–8 DIV) after changing of medium to a fresh medium without serum with Supplement N1 (Sigma). The βAP 25–35 (Bachem) was dissolved by sonication in sterilized distilled water at a concentration of 1 mM. Solutions of all reagents were added to the wells with cultures at 25 μM, and the effect was observed during the next days by microscopy.

Quantitative Assessment

Neuronal viability was evaluated by morphometric cell counting using the presence of neurites and smooth, round cell bodies as criteria of survival. The cells were examined under the phase-contrast microscope Axiovert 25C with videocamera and Software miroMedia PCTV VideoCap program for image scanning and photography. Cell survival was quantified by counting the number of viable neurons in premarked microscope fields prior to, and 4 days after the exposure. The difference in numbers of living neurons before and after 4 days of treatment was determined.

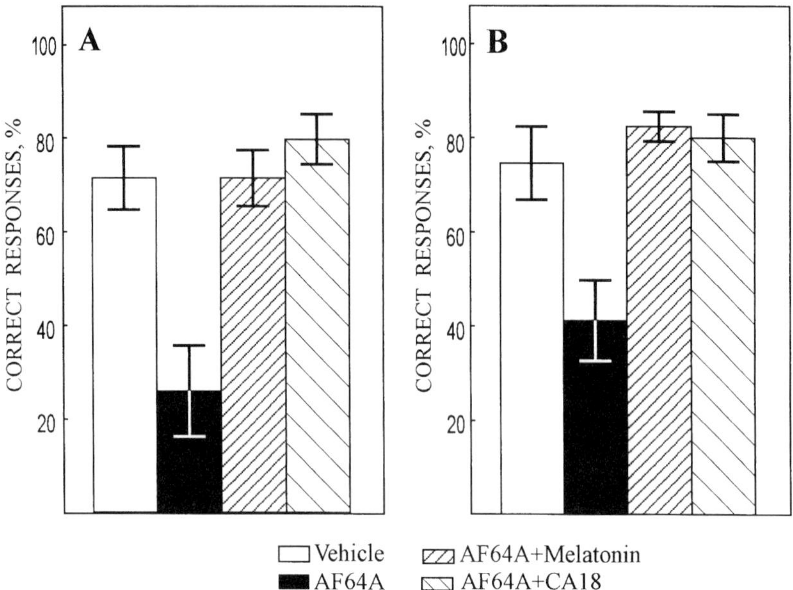

FIGURE 3. Cognition-enhancing effect of melatonin and CA18. Shuttle-box avoidance performance of vehicle-treated rats ($n = 11$), AF64A-treated rats ($n = 10$) and AF64A-treated rats receiving melatonin or CA-18 (0.3 mg/kg, once daily, 12–14 days, orally; $n = 11$), where n is the number of rats in each group. **(A)** Learning test. Following 20 acquisition trials, rats were given 3 blocks of 5 trials. **(B)** Retention test. Two blocks of 5 trials were given 24 hr after learning trial. Data are presented as the mean ± SEM percentage of correct responses summarized over each block; $p < 0.001$, where p is the significance level. The values of p illustrate that there was a significant difference in avoidance performance vs AF64A-treated group (post hoc ANOVA).

Statistical Analysis

For each experiment, we used 4–6 separate wells of a 24-well multiwell plate for control (with 0.05% DMSO) and for each concentration of compound or composition of compound with βAP. Each well equaled one observation (average of 25 cells per microscope field). Experiments are repeated 2–3 times ($n = 12–18$). For graphical presentation, average data from representative experiments were expressed as a percentage of survival cells in comparison with control ± SEM and analyzed by ANOVA and Student t-test.

RESULTS

Active Avoidance Test

AF64A (3 nmol/3 µl i.c.v.) dramatically decreased rats performance in learning and retention paradigms of the active avoidance test (FIGS. 1–3, TABLE 1).

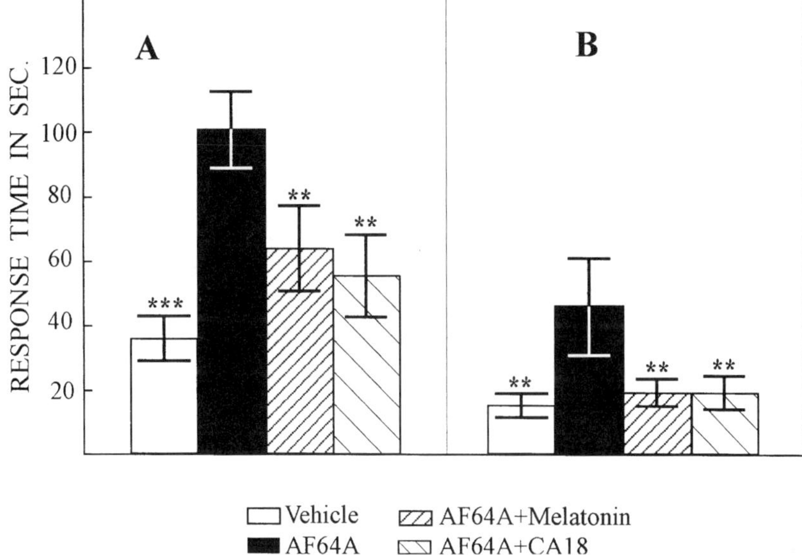

FIGURE 4. Average swim latency made by rats, when trained **(A)** 1 and **(B)** 5 days to find a platform in the Morris water maze test. Performance of vehicle-treated rats ($n = 11$), AF64A-treated rats ($n = 10$) and AF64A-treated rats receiving melatonin or CA-18 (0.3 mg/kg, once daily, 12–14 days, orally; $n = 11$) was started 3 days after the last injection of compound and was performed daily during the period from the 3rd to the 7th day (n is the number of rats in each group). Results were estimated as time required for rat having fallen into the water pool to reach a platform; **p <0.05, ***p <0.001 vs the AF64A-treated group, where p is the significance level (post hoc ANOVA).

NAS (1 mg/kg per os (p.o.) daily) improved the performance of AF64A-treated rats in learning (FIG. 2A) but not in retention (FIG. 2B) paradigms of the active avoidance test.

The effect of melatonin was studied in 2 doses: 0.3 and 3 mg/kg (p.o. daily). The lower dose of melatonin (0.3 mg/kg) completely restored rats performance in the learning (FIG. 3A) and retention (FIG. 3B) paradigms of the active avoidance test. The cognitive-enhancing effect of the higher dose of melatonin (3 mg/kg) was significant but somewhat less pronounced than the effect of the lower dose (0.3 mg/kg) (FIG. 1A and B).

CA-15 (3 mg/kg p.o. daily) improved the performance of AF64A-treated rats in retention paradigm of the active avoidance test (FIG. 1B). CA-15 demonstrated a strong tendency (although not reaching the level of statistical significancy) towards improvement of the learning ability of the AE64A-treated rats (FIG. 1A).

The effect of CA-18 was studied in 2 doses: 0.3 and 1 mg/kg (p.o. daily). The lower dose of CA-18 (0.3 mg/kg) completely restored rats' performance in the learning (FIG. 3A) and retention (FIG. 3B) paradigms of the active avoidance test. The higher dose of CA-18 (1 mg/kg) demonstrated a strong tendency (although not

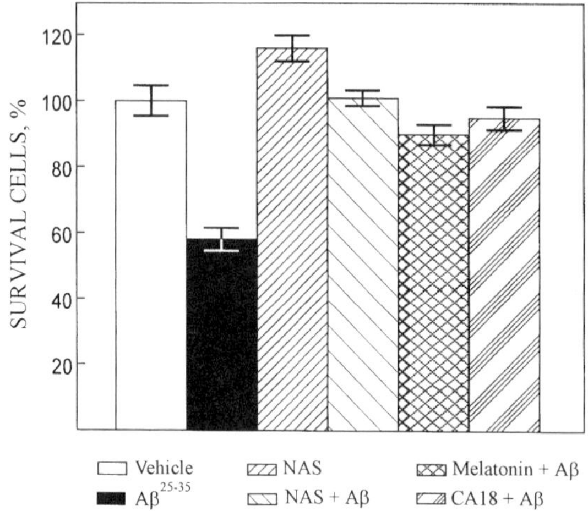

FIGURE 5. Protective effect of *N*-acetylserotonin (NAS), melatonin and CA-15 against the toxicity of βAP 25–35 in mature cultures of cerebellar granule cells. Cultures 8 DIV were treated with vehicle, 25 mM βAP, 25 mM βAP and 25 mM NAS, or 25 mM melatonin, or 25 mM CA-15 for 4 days. The difference in numbers of living neurons before and after 4 days of treatment were determined. The amount of viable neurons is expressed as mean (%) above viable in preliminary photography of the same place. Experiments were repeated 2–3 times (n = 12–18). For graphical presentation, average data from representative experiments are converted to percentages of control group's viability. Results are expressed as a percentage of survival cells to compare with control ± SEM and were analyzed by a statistical test (ANOVA).

reaching the level of statistical significance) towards the improvement of the learning (FIG. 2A) but not in the retention (FIG. 2B) ability of the AF64A-treated rats.

Although we did not plan to perform the special evaluation of the general locomotor activity, we did notice the unspecified sedative effect in rats treated with melatonin (3 mg/kg) starting from the third to fourth day of treatment and in rats treated with NAS (1 mg/kg) starting from the sixth day of treatment.

Melatonin (0.3 mg/kg) and CA-18 (0.3 and 1 mg/kg) did not induce sedation in rats.

Morris Water Maze Test

AF64A significantly increased the response time in comparison to rats treated with the vehicle (CSF) (FIG. 4A and B). Melatonin and CA-18 (0.3 mg/kg daily) decreased the response time of AF64A-treated rats. Only the results observed on day 1 (FIG. 4A) and day 5 (FIG. 4B) are presented.

Neuronal Cell Culture

Earlier it was shown that exposure of mature cultures of CGC against the fragment of βAP reduced the cell viability in a dose-dependent manner (IC_{50} = 25 μM).

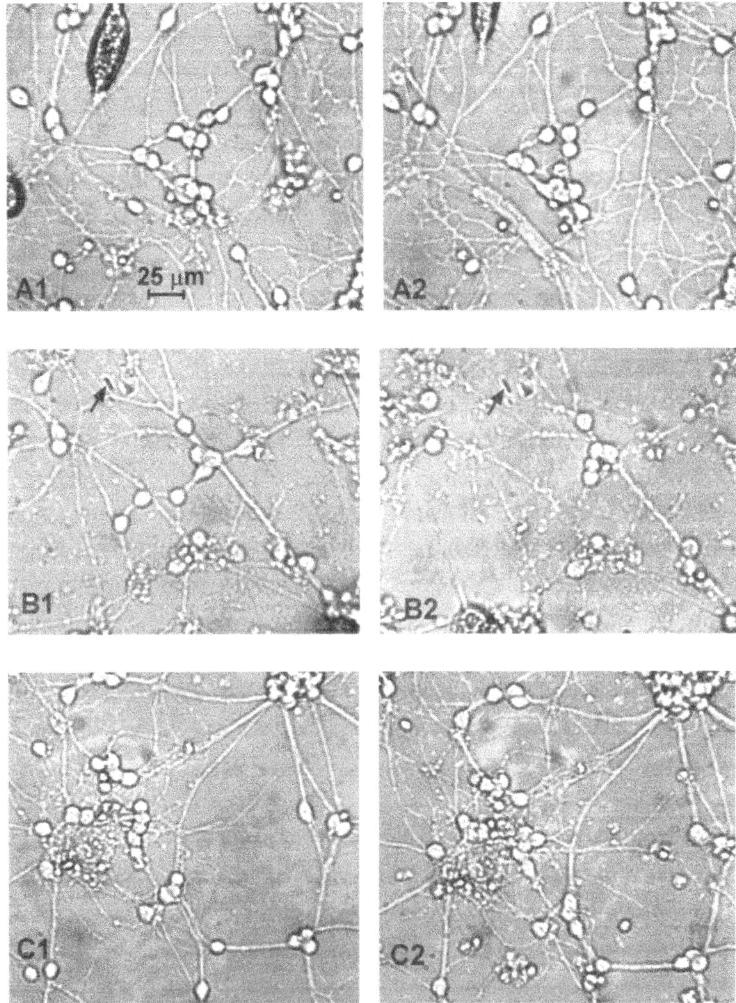

FIGURE 6. Protective effect of *N*-acetylserotonin (NAS) against the toxicity of βAP 25–35 in mature cultures of cerebellar granule cells. Cultures 8 DIV were treated with vehicle **(A1)**, 25 mM βA **(B1)** or 25 mM βA and 25 mM NAS **(C1)** for 4 days, at which time photographs of the same part of the microscope fields were taken **(A2)**, **(B2)** and **(C2)**, respectively. Living cultures, "darkfield" method (*arrowhead* shows the mark on a plate).

Morphological changes (shrinkage of the body and fragmentation of neurites) were observed only when cells were exposed to βAP for 3 days or longer.[10] In the present study we used βAP in concentration of 25 μM to evaluate the ability of the compounds to protect neurons against β-amyloid (βA) neurotoxicity. Incubation of cultures only with NAS or melatonin in the concentration range 25–200 μM increased the amount of living CGCs by 16–28% or 3–10% of control, respectively. The viability of neurons exposed to 25 μM βAP was 58 ± 7% (mean ± SEM) of control, while coincubation of cultures with 25 μM NAS and 25 mM βAP resulted in an increase of viable neurons up to 101 ± 5% of control (FIGS. 5 and 6) in the same conditions. Melatonin and CA-18 at 25 μM protected neurons against 25 μM βAP (90% and 93%, respectively) as well. Melatonin was less effective in preventing βA toxicity compared to NAS (FIG. 5).

DISCUSSION

The obtained results indicate that chronic administration of NAS, melatonin, and their newly synthesized derivatives, CA-15 and CA-18, improve cognitive performance of AF64A-treated rats in active avoidance and in water-maze tests. What is more, these compounds exerted the neuroprotective effect against the βA (25–35)-induced neurotoxicity in the cerebellar granule cell culture. It is known that the neurotoxic action of AF64A related, in part, to oxidative stress, and its indexes are persisting up to 4 months.[11] In this vein, one might suggest that antioxidative properties of melatonin, NAS and, possibly, their derivatives, CA-15 and CA-18, are responsible for their neuroprotective effects. Recent studies indicate that the antioxidant ability of melatonin is inferior in comparison to NAS,[24] and, at least in one model, melatonin exerted a prooxidant effect, while NAS exerted strong antioxidant action.[12] Traditionally, NAS was considered only as the precursor of melatonin in the process of melatonin biosynthesis from serotonin. Very few researchers pointed out the effects of NAS independent from melatonin, i.e., its memory facilitating,[13] hypothermic,[14] analgesic,[15] antihypertensive,[16–18] antidepressant[19] and antioxidative action.[20] NAS, therefore, might be considered not only as melatonin precursor but as endogenous indolamine with its own biological properties. Since about 30% of melatonin is demethylated back into NAS,[21] the antioxidant effect of supraphysiological concentrations of melatonin[22] might be ascribed to NAS formed from melatonin. It is noteworthy that the very first indication of the NAS involvement in the cognitive processes came from the observation that scotophobin A, the memory neuropeptide, increased dark avoidance behavior in goldfish via inhibition of NAS methylation into melatonin.[13]

Under the *in vivo* conditions rapid methylation of NAS into melatonin[23] might limit the effect of NAS. Therefore, the availability of NAS derivatives that would not undergo the *in vivo* transformation into melatonin might be of therapeutic advantage. Our preliminary experiments indicated that systemic administration of CA-15 and CA-18 did not change the rat pineal levels of NAS and melatonin (Oxenkrug & Requintina, unpublished data). Although all studied compounds attenuated the AF64A-induced cognitive impairment, there were noticeable differences between the effects of NAS, melatonin, and their derivatives (TABLE 1). NAS was apparently the weakest among the studied compounds in the active avoidance test, while it was the strongest in the attenuating of βA-induced neurotoxicity. Since NAS is rapidly converted into melatonin in rats,[23] the effect of NAS in our *in vivo* experiments could not be attributed only to NAS but rather to the mixture of NAS and melatonin.

The occurrence of the sedative effect in rats treated with NAS and melatonin, and somewhat delayed appearance of sedation in NAS- than in melatonin-treated rats suggest that melatonin but not NAS is responsible for the sedative action. The absence of the sedative effect in rats treated with CA-18 might be of therapeutic advantage of the synthetic NAS/melatonin derivatives.

We have found that CA-15 and CA-18 in addition to their positive effect on cognition exerted antihypertensive and antidepressant-like effects.[24] The antidepressant-like activity (decreasing the duration of immobility in the mouse tail suspension test) was more pronounced in CA-18- than in CA-15-treated rats. The combination of cognition-enhancing and antidepressant effect in the one and the same compound might be of additional therapeutic advantage.

The results of our studies warrant the further search of the novel types of safe neuroprotectors among the synthetic NAS/melatonin derivatives.

ACKNOWLEDGMENTS

This work was supported by the Russian Foundation for Basic Research (Grant No. 96-04-50318) and the International Science and Technology Center (Project No. 312-96).

REFERENCES

1. WITTING, W., I. KWA, P. EIKELENBOOM, M. MIRMIRAM & D. SWAAB. 1990. Alterations in the circadian rest-activity rhythm in aging and Alzheimer's disease. Biol. Psychiatry **27:** 563–572.
2. REITER, R.J., M.I. PABLOS, T.T. AGAPITO & J.M. GUERRERO. 1996. Melatonin in the context of the free radical theory of aging. Ann. N.Y. Acad. Sci. **786:** 362–378.
3. PAPOLLA, M.A., M. SOS, R.A. OMAR, D. BICK, L.M. HICKSONBICK, R.J. REITER, S. EPTHIMIOPOULUS & N.K. ROBAKIS. 1997. Melatonin prevents death of neuroblastoma cells exposed to the Alzheimer amyloid peptide. J. Neurosci. **17:** 1683–1690.
4. LONGONI, B., W.A. PRYOR & P. MARCHIAFAVA. 1997. Inhibition of lipid peroxidation by *N*-acetylserotonin and its role in retinal physiology. Biochem. Biophys. Res. Commun. **233:** 778–780.
5. FISHER, A. & I. HANIN. 1986. Potential animal models for senile dementia of Alzheimer's type with emphasis on AF64A-induced cholinotoxicity. Annu. Rev. Pharmacol. Toxicol. **26:** 161–181.
6. WALSH, T. & K. OPELLO. 1994. The use of AF64A to model Alzheimer disease. *In* Toxin-Induced Models of Neurological Disorders. M.I. Woodruff & A.J. Nonneman, Eds.: 259–279. Plenum Press. New York, London.
7. LERMONTOVA, N.N., N.V. LUKOYANOV, T.P. SERKOVA, E.A. LYKOYANOVA & S.O. BACHURIN. 1998. Effects of tacrine on memory deficits in rats treated with cholinergic neurotoxin AF64A. Mol. Chem. Neuropathol. **33:** 51–61.
8. GOZES, I., A. BARDEA, A. RESHEF, R. ZAMOSTIANO, S. ZHUKOVSKY, S. RUBINRAUT, M. FRIDKIN & D. BRENNEMAN. 1996. Neuroprotective strategy for Alzheimer disease: intranasal administration of a fatty neuropeptide. Proc. Natl. Acad. Sci. USA **93:** 427–432.
9. GALLO, V., A. KINGSBURY, R. BALAZS & O.S. JORGENSEN. 1987. The role of depolarisation in the survival and differentiation of cerebellar granule cells in culture. J. Neurosci. **7:** 2203–2213.
10. BACHURIN, S., N. LERMONTOVA, E. SHEVTZOVA, T. SERKOVA & E. KIREEVA. 1998. Prevention of β-amyloid-induced neurotoxicity by tacrine and dimebon. J. Neurochem. **71**(Suppl. 1): S68.

11. GULYAEVA, N.V., N.A. LAZAREVA & N.L. LIBE. 1996. Oxidative stress in the brain following intraventricular administration of ethylholine aziridinium (AF64A). Brain Res. **726:** 174–180.

12. BARSACCHI, R., C. KUSMIC, E. DAMIANI, P. CARLONI, L. GRECI & L. DONATO. 1998. Vitamin E consumption induced by oxidative stress in red blood cells is enhanced by melatonin and reduced by N-acetylserotonin. Free Radical Biol. Med. **24:** 1187–1192.

13. SATAKE, N. & B.E. MORTON. 1979. Scotophobin A causes dark avoidance in goldfish by elevating pineal N-acetylserotonin. Pharmacol. Biochem. Behav. **10:** 449–436.

14. MORTON, D.J. 1987. Both hydroxy- and methoxyindoles modify basal temperature in the rat. J. Pineal Res. **4:** 1–5.

15. PSARAKIS, S., G. BROWN & L.J. GROTA. 1988. Analgesia induced by N-acetyl-serotonin in the central nervous system. Life Sci. **42:** 1109–1116.

16. OXENKRUG, G.F. 1998. N-Acetylserotonin and the hypotensive effect of MAO-A inhibition (mini-review). Vopr. Med. Khim. **43:** 522–526 (Russian).

17. OXENKRUG, G.F. 1999. Antidepressive and antihypertensive effects of MAO-A inhibition: role of N-acetylserotonin. A review. J. Neurobiol. **7:** 213–224.

18. OXENKRUG, G.F. & P.J. REQUINTINA. 1999. Hypotensive effect of N-acetylserotonin in spontaneously hypertensive rats. Biol. Psychiatry. In press.

19. PRAKHIE, I.V. & G.F. OXENKRUG. 1998. The effect of nifedipine, Ca^{++} antagonist, on activity of MAO inhibitors, N-acetylserotonin and melatonin in the mouse tail suspension test. Int. J. Neuropsychopharmacol. **1:** 35–40.

20. LEZOUALC'H, F., M. SPARAPANI & C. BEHL. 1998. N-Acetyl-serotonin (normelatonin) and melatonin protect neurons against oxidative challenges and suppress the activity of the transcription factor NF-κB. J. Pineal Res. **24:** 168–178.

21. LEONE, R.M. & R.E. SILMAN. 1984. Melatonin can be differentially metabolized in the rat to produce N-acetyl-serotonin in addition to 6-hydroxy-melatonin. Endocrinology **114:** 1825–1832.

22. DUELL, P.B,. D.L. WHEATON, A. SHULTZ & H. NGUYEN. 1998. Inhibition of LDL oxidation by melatonin requires supraphysiologic concentrations. Clin. Chem. **44:** 1931–1936.

23. OXENKRUG, G.F. & P.J. REQUINTINA. 1994. Stimulation of rat pineal melatonin biosynthesis by N-acetylserotonin. Int. J. Neurosci. **77:** 237–241.

24. OXENKRUG, G.F., S.O. BACHURIN, I.V. PRAKHIE, P.J. REQUINTINA, A. AFANASIEV, B. BEZNOSKO, G. VANKIN, N. LERMONTOVA & T. SERKOVA. 1999. Neurobiological effects of the new indolalkylamine derivatives. Biol. Psychiatry **45:** 92S.

Neuroprotective Action of Bilirubin against Oxidative Stress in Primary Hippocampal Cultures

SYLVAIN DORÉ[a] AND SOLOMON H. SNYDER[b]

Johns Hopkins University, School of Medicine, Department of Neuroscience, 725 North Wolfe Street, Baltimore, Maryland 21205, USA

INTRODUCTION

Bilirubin (BR) elicits substantial antioxidant effects and is probably one of the most abundant endogenous antioxidants in mammalian tissues.[1–3] Very little is known about its role in the nervous system. Heme oxygenase, the enzyme responsible for the synthesis of BR, is highly expressed in the brain, being enriched in the hippocampus.[4] We wondered if BR applied to primary hippocampal neurons would be protective against hydrogen peroxide-induced toxicity.

MATERIALS AND METHODS

We prepared cultures of hippocampal neuronal cells isolated from 17-day-old embryos of timed pregnant Sprague-Dawley rats. Unless stated otherwise, all compounds used for cell culture were from Gibco BRL (Gaithersburg, MD). Neurons were cultured in serum-free conditions with the B-27 supplement, as previously described.[5] Experimental treatments were conducted in the *N*-2 supplement *N*-2-hydroxyethylpiperazine-*N'*-2-ethanesulfonic acid (HEPES)-buffered high glucose neurobasal medium. Following the different treatments, neurons were maintained for an additional period of 24 hr, and their survival was assessed by phase-contrast microscopy with Trypan Blue exclusion assay and quantified using MTT [(3-(4,5-dimethylthiazol-2-yl)-2,5-diphenyl tetrazolium bromide)] colorimetric assay. Survival of control vehicle treated neuronal cells not exposed to H_2O_2 was set at 100%, and treated groups were represented as percentage of control values. All experiments were conducted under a dim light to avoid heme pigment photodegradation. BR (1 mM, Sigma, St-Louis MO) was freshly dissolved in NaOH. Bovine and human serum albumin (Sigma; fraction V) were dissolved in 0.1 M phosphate-buffered saline, pH 7.4 mixed in a ratio of 1:5 as described.[1] Addition of BR to albumin in this way results in binding of the pigment to its primary physiological binding site.[6] All experiments were repeated with at least three separate batches of cultures, and the

[a]Phone, 410/955-3083; fax, 410/614-6249.
e-mail, sdore@welchlink.welch.jhu.edu
[b]Phone, 410/955-3024; fax, 410/955-3623.
e-mail, s.snyder@jhmi.edu

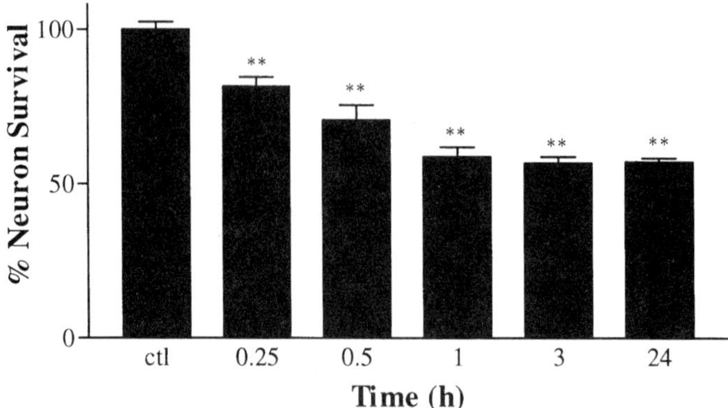

FIGURE 1. Neuronal toxicity induced by hydrogen peroxyde (H_2O_2). Rat primary hippocampal neurons were exposed to H_2O_2 (75 µM) for different periods of time, then replaced with fresh culture medium, and neuron survival was estimated 24 hr after the beginning of the experiment.

data are represented as the mean ± SEM with $*p < 0.05$, $**p < 0.01$ being considered significant.

RESULTS

FIGURE 1 depicts the time course for the influence of H_2O_2 on survival of primary hippocampal neurons estimated after 24 hr of the initial treatment. A significant decrease is observed very rapidly, with only 15 min exposure. This decrease becomes more prominent and reaches a plateau of toxicity at approximately 1 hr. It is known that the effect of H_2O_2 is very rapid, and its half-life in petri dishes is approximately 15 min. Because of the very short half-life of H_2O_2 and the sensitivity of neurons to medium changes, we left the H_2O_2 for the entire experiment.

To ascertain whether BR is neuroprotective, we examined its effects upon neurons treated with H_2O_2 (FIG. 2). As a first step, we tested different concentrations of BR and showed that 25–50 nM were the optimal concentrations for neuroprotection against H_2O_2-induced toxicity (FIG. 2A).

Knowing that BR has low water solubility, estimated as <100 nM at pH 7.4,[6] we coupled it to serum albumin in order to increase it solubility. We first looked at the effect of BR coupled to bovine serum albumin (BSA) and found significant neuroprotection at 10- and 25-nM concentrations (FIG. 2B).

There is a primary and a secondary binding site on albumin for BR. Since human serum albumin (HSA) has higher affinity for those binding sites, we subsequently used BR coupled to HSA and found that as little as 10 nM BR almost completely reverses the neurotoxic actions of H_2O_2 (FIG. 2C), while lesser protection occurs at 1 and 3 nM. The neuroprotective effect diminishes at higher concentrations of BR, presumably because higher levels of BR are themselves neurotoxic. This is suggested by the diminished neuronal survival of control cultures treated with 100 and

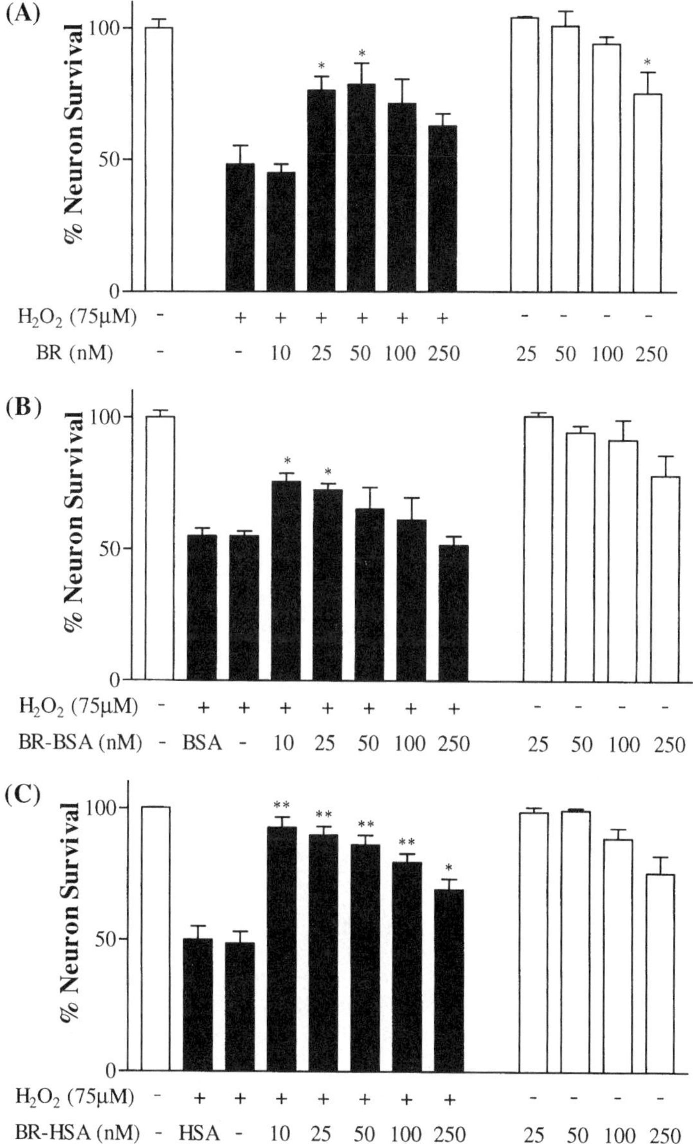

FIGURE 2. Protective effect of bilirubin, BR-BSA, and BR-HSA on H$_2$O$_2$-induced toxicity on neurons. Induction of toxicity by H$_2$O$_2$ (75 µM) started after the addition BR and its complexes. Neuron survival was estimated 24 hr after the beginning of the experiment. Increasing concentrations of free BR (**A**) or BR complexed with bovine serum albumin (BR-BSA) (**B**) or human serum albumin (BR-HSA) (**C**) were added to neurons. Addition of equivalent amounts of albumin alone were without effect. Control experiments were done without H$_2$O$_2$.

250 nM BR-SA. No significant effects are observed with the equivalent concentrations of BSA or HSA alone.

DISCUSSION

Hydrogen peroxide (H_2O_2) is normally detoxified in the cell by catalase and glutathione peroxidase, whose levels do not change after brief application of H_2O_2. The highly reactive hydroxyl radical (in the presence of transition metal cations) can initiate lipid peroxidation and damage proteins and DNA. BR, which is toxic at high concentrations, has antioxidant properties at low concentrations.[1,7] One of the most interesting findings of the present study is the very potent protective effect of BR on primary hippocampal neurons with complete neuroprotection evident at 10 nM. BR actions have been mostly characterized in the high micromolar range where toxic effects also occur. How can nM concentrations of BR protect against higher H_2O_2 concentrations? The most likely explanation is a cycle of oxidation-reduction between BR and biliverdin (BV), the major oxidation product of BR.[8,9] In mediating its antioxidant actions, BR would be transformed to BV. Biliverdin reductase, present in large functional excess in all tissues, would immediately regenerate BR.

BR is one of the most abundant endogenous antioxidants in mammalian tissues, accounting for the majority of the antioxidant activity of human serum.[10] In an extensive series of antioxidants, BR displayed the most potent superoxide and peroxide radical scavenger activity.[11] In the circulation, BR is largely complexed with albumin. We have observed more extensive neuroprotection with BR complexed with HSA compared to BSA, perhaps because human albumin has higher affinity for the primary and secondary binding sites for BR than its bovine homolog. In most cells, BR is stored in a complex with various isoforms of glutathione-*S*-transferase (GST).[12] Thermodynamic parameters for BR dissociation from GST are similar to those for HSA.[13] Binding of BR to these proteins keeps BR in solution and inhibits its efflux from the cell thereby increasing the net accumulation. GSTs play a role in cellular uptake and the intracellular transport of BR.[14] Certain GST isoforms are selectively present in neurons.[15] A GST isoenzyme-specific distribution was also found in cytoplasm, microsome, nuclei and nucleoli suggesting the possibility of scavenging free radicals in different cell compartments.

BR is best known as a potentially toxic agent that accumulates in the serum of neonates to cause jaundice. In high concentrations, BR can deposit in selected brain regions to elicit the neurotoxicity associated with kernicterus.[16] The "physiologic jaundice" of normal neonates with BR levels fairly close to toxic levels has been puzzling. Conceivably, physiologic jaundice has a protective effect. It could represent a transitional antioxidative mechanism in the neonatal circulation. Serum antioxidant activities are selectively associated with BR in neonatal Gunn rats[17] and jaundiced newborn infants.[2] In preterm infants, higher bilirubin levels are associated with a lower incidence of oxygen radical-mediated injury.[18] BR administration protects against retinopathy in premature babies.[19] Moreover, beneficial effects of breast feeding are often accompanied with high BR levels.[20] BR may be particularly important as a cytoprotector for tissues with relatively weak endogenous antioxidant defenses such as the myocardium and the nervous system.[21] Interestingly, a decreased risk for coronary artery disease is associated with mildly elevated serum BR, with a protective effect comparable to that of high-density lipoprotein (HDL)-cholesterol.[3]

Our findings imply that BR affords physiologic neuroprotection. This conclusion is supported by our recent observations that neuronal damage following middle cerebral artery occlusion is substantially worsened in heme oxygenase 2 knockout mice, the rate limiting enzyme for the BR synthesis in the brain.[22]

REFERENCES

1. NEUZIL, J. & R. STOCKER. 1994. Free and albumin-bound bilirubin are efficient co-antioxidants for alpha-tocopherol, inhibiting plasma and low density lipoprotein lipid peroxidation. J. Biol. Chem. **269:** 16712–16719.
2. BÉLANGER, S., J.C. LAVOIE & P. CHESSEX. 1997. Influence of bilirubin on the antioxidant capacity of plasma in newborn infants. Biol. Neonate **71:** 233–238.
3. HOPKINS, P.N., L.L. WU, S.C. HUNT, B.C. JAMES, G.M. VINCENT *et al.* 1996. Higher serum bilirubin is associated with decreased risk for early familial coronary artery disease. Arterioscler. Thromb. Biol. **16:** 250–255.
4. VERMA, A., D.J. HIRSCH, C.E. GLATT, G.V. RONNETT & S.H. SNYDER. 1993. Carbon monoxide: a putative neural messenger. Science **259:** 381–384.
5. DORÉ, S., S. KAR & R. QUIRION. 1997. Insulin-like growth factor I protects and rescues hippocampal neurons against beta-amyloid- and human amylin-induced toxicity. Proc. Natl. Acad. Sci. USA **94:** 4772–4777.
6. BRODERSEN, R. 1979. Bilirubin. Solubility and interaction with albumin and phospholipid. J. Biol. Chem. **254:** 2364–2369.
7. STOCKER, R., Y. YAMAMOTO, A.F. MCDONAGH, A.N. GLAZER & B.N. AMES. 1987. Bilirubin is an antioxidant of possible physiological importance. Science **235:** 1043–1046.
8. MINETTI, M., C. MALLOZZI, A.M. DI STASI & D. PIETRAFORTE. 1998. Bilirubin is an effective antioxidant of peroxynitrite-mediated protein oxidation in human blood plasma. Arch. Biochem. Biophys. **352:** 165–174.
9. DE MATTEIS, F., S.J. DAWSON & A.H. GIBBS. 1993. Two pathways of iron-catalyzed oxidation of bilirubin: effect of desferrioxamine and trolox, and comparison with microsomal oxidation. Free Radical Biol. Med. **15:** 301–309.
10. GOPINATHAN, V., N.J. MILLER, A.D. MILNER & C.A. RICE-EVANS. 1994. Bilirubin and ascorbate antioxidant activity in neonatal plasma. FEBS Lett. **349:** 197–200.
11. FARRERA, J.A., A. JAUMA, J.M. RIBO, M.A. PEIRE, P.P. PARELLADA *et al.* 1994. The antioxidant role of bile pigments evaluated by chemical tests. Bioorg. Med. Chem. **2:** 181–185.
12. BOYER, T.D. 1989. The glutathione *S*-transferases: an update. Hepatology **9:** 486–496.
13. ZUCKER, S.D., W. GOESSLING & J.L. GOLLAN. 1995. Kinetics of bilirubin transfer between serum albumin and membrane vesicles. Insight into the mechanism of organic anion delivery to the hepatocyte plasma membrane. J. Biol. Chem. **270:** 1074–1081.
14. LISTOWSKY, I., M. ABRAMOVITZ, H. HOMMA & Y. NIITSU. 1988. Intracellular binding and transport of hormones and xenobiotics by glutathione-*S*-transferases. Drug Metab. Rev. **19:** 305–318.
15. JOHNSON, J.A., A. EL BARBARY, S.E. KORNGUTH, J.F. BRUGGE & F.L. SIEGEL. 1993. Glutathione *S*-transferase isoenzymes in rat brain neurons and glia. J. Neurosci. **13:** 2013–2023.
16. GOURLEY, G.R. 1997. Bilirubin metabolism and kernicterus. Adv. Pediatr. **44:** 173–229.

17. DENNERY, P.A. & P.A. RODGERS. 1996. Ontogeny and developmental regulation of heme oxygenase. J. Perinatol. **16:** S79–S83.
18. HEGYI, T., E. GOLDIE & M. HIATT. 1994. The protective role of bilirubin in oxygen-radical diseases of the preterm infant. J. Perinatol. **14:** 296–300.
19. HEYMAN, E., A. OHLSSON & P. GIRSCHEK. 1989. Retinopathy of prematurity and bilirubin. N. Engl. J. Med. **320:** 256.
20. SCHNEIDER, A.P. 2d. 1986. Breast milk jaundice in the newborn. A real entity. JAMA **255:** 3270–3274.
21. WU, T.W., J. WU, R.K. LI, D. MICKLE & D. CAREY. 1991. Albumin-bound bilirubins protect human ventricular myocytes against oxyradical damage. Biochem. Cell Biol. **69:** 683–688.
22. DORÉ, S., K. SAMPEI, S. KOEHLER, S. BLACKSHAW, M. TAKAHASHI *et al.* 1998. Neuroprotective role of heme oxygenase-2 on brain damage after focal cerebral ischemia. Soc. Neurosc. Abstr. **24:** 1233.

Protective Effect of L-Carnitine in the Neurotoxicity Induced by the Mitochondrial Inhibitor 3-Nitropropionic Acid (3-NPA)

ZBIGNIEW BINIENDA,[a,c] JOHN R. JOHNSON,[a]
ALEXANDER A. TYLER-HASHEMI,[a] ROBERT L. ROUNTREE,[a]
PHILIP P. SAPIENZA,[b] SYED F. ALI,[a] AND CHUNG S. KIM[b]

[a]*Division of Neurotoxicology, National Center for Toxicological Research/
Food and Drug Administration (NCTR/FDA), Jefferson, Arkansas, USA*

[b]*Division of Toxicological Research, Center for Food Safety and Applied Nutrition/
Food and Drug Administration (CFSAN/FDA), Washington, DC, USA*

INTRODUCTION

The fungal and plant toxin, 3-nitropropionic acid (3-NPA), acts as a competitive suicide substrate for succinate dehydrogenase (SDH), an enzyme present in the Krebs cycle and complex II of the mitochondrial electron transport chain. Studies have shown that irreversible inhibition of SDH by the acute or chronic administration of 3-NPA leads to neurotoxicity, particularly in the striatum but also in the hippocampus, thalamus, cerebral cortex, and cerebellum.[3,10,13] There is a growing body of evidence that a major factor in 3-NPA neurotoxicity is the failure of energy metabolism, i.e., histotoxic hypoxia, followed by secondary excitotoxicity.[14] Additionally, oxidative stress, due to overproduction of reactive oxygen species (ROS), may facilitate 3-NPA-induced brain injury. ROS are physiologically generated as by-products of cellular enzymatic reactions such as mitochondrial respiration, phagocytosis, arachidonate metabolism, etc. ROS are usually deactivated by endogenous antioxidant systems.

We found that acute treatment with 3-NPA was associated with an ubiquitous elevation in brain free fatty acids (FFA).[4] FFA, which are useful markers of cellular membrane degradation, are substrates for the production of ROS. A possible protective role of L-carnitine in 3-NPA neurotoxicity was implied from the results of *in vitro* studies.[12] L-Carnitine may prevent loss of mitochondrial function via enhancement of fatty acid β-oxidation and decreases in ROS formation. The aim of our study was to examine whether pretreatment of rats with L-carnitine would alleviate 3-NPA-induced oxidative stress by assessing the activities of antioxidant enzymes and the concentrations of brain free fatty acids.

[c]Corresponding author: Zbigniew Binienda, D.V.M., Ph.D., FDA/NCTR, Division of Neurotoxicology, HFT-132, 3900 NCTR Road, Jefferson, AR 72079-9502. Phone, 870/543-7920; fax, 870/543-7745.
e-mail, zbinienda@nctr.fda.gov

MATERIALS AND METHODS

Animals

Sprague-Dawley male rats, three months old, obtained from the National Center for Toxicological Research (NCTR) colony were used in the study. Animals were housed under controlled environmental conditions. Food and water were provided *ad libitum.* The rats were divided into five groups and injected with 3-NPA alone (30 mg/kg, subcutaneously (s.c.)) or 3-NPA and either a low (50-mg/kg) or high (100-mg/kg) dose of L-carnitine administered 60 min prior to 3-NPA. Control rats received either 0.1 M phosphate buffer or L-carnitine (high dose). All animals were sacrificed 90 min after 3-NPA treatment. Changes in activities of catalase and superoxide dismutase (SOD) were examined in the frontal cortex (FC), caudate nucleus (CN), and hippocampus (HIP).

Analysis of Antioxidant Enzyme Activities

Brain tissues were sonicated on ice for 10 sec in an ice-cold, 0.32-M sucrose solution (5 mg tissue per ml sucrose solution). The brain homogenates were centrifuged at $10,000 \times g$ for 45 min at 4°C. The supernatant was divided into two portions: one was used immediately for determination of catalase (CAT) activity according to the method of Beers and Sizer,[2] in which the disappearance of the substrate (H_2O_2) was measured spectrophotometrically at 240 nm. Total SOD activity was assayed by a method based on the inhibition of nitrite formation from hydroxylammonium in the presence of O_2· generators.[11] Manganese SOD (Mn-SOD) was differentiated from copper/zinc SOD (CuZn-SOD) using 2 mM KCN in the reaction mixture to selectively inhibit CuZn-SOD. One unit of SOD was defined as that amount needed to produce 50% inhibition of the initial rate of nitrite formation.

Analysis of FFA Concentrations

FFA were isolated from tissue homogenates by column chromatography on acid-washed Florisil as described by Carroll.[6] FFA were derivatized with BF_3/methanol, and the resulting fatty acid methyl esters were quantitated using gas chromatography on a DB-23 capillary column (J and W Scientific, Folsom, CA) using a modification of the procedure described by Dinnauer.[8]

Statistical Analysis

Data were analyzed using one way analysis of variance (ANOVA) followed by the Dunnett correction for multiple comparisons. The level of statistical significance was set at $p < 0.05$.

RESULTS AND DISCUSSION

Administration of 3-NPA at 30 mg/kg, s.c. to rats was previously shown to induce neurobehavioral alterations corresponding with human neurotoxicity.[10] Since in our study the initial metabolic response to 3-NPA was examined, animals were sacri-

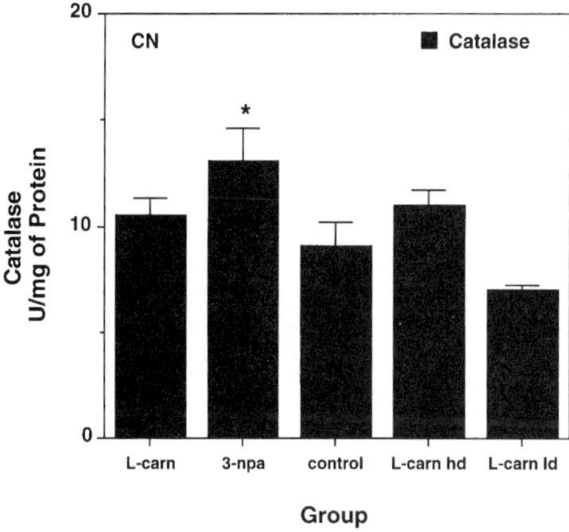

FIGURE 1. Effect of pretreatment with L-carnitine on the activity of catalase (CAT; units per mg of protein) in caudate nucleus (CN) following 3-NPA administration. L-carn = L-carnitine 100 mg/kg; 3-NPA = 3-nitropropionic acid 30 mg/kg, s.c.; control = 0.1 M phosphate buffer; L-carn hd = L-carnitine 100 mg/kg injected 60 min before 3-NPA administration (30 mg/kg, s.c.); L-carn ld = L-carnitine 50 mg/kg injected 60 min before 3-NPA administration (30 mg/kg, s.c.). Mean ± SEM, $n = 3$; *p <0.05 significantly different from control.

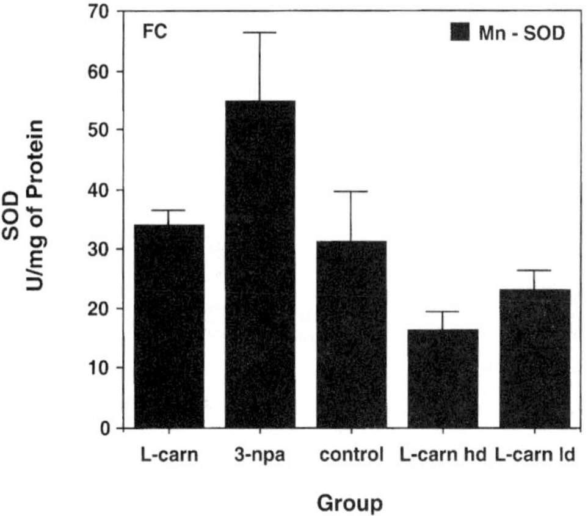

FIGURE 2. Effect of pretreatment with L-carnitine on the activity of manganese superoxide dismutase (Mn-SOD; units per mg of protein) in frontal cortex (FC) following 3-NPA administration. *Abbreviations* of the descriptions are the same as for FIGURE 1. Mean ± SEM, $n = 3$.

ficed earlier than the onset of observable behavioral signs of toxicity. The time-point for animal sacrifice was based on our previously made observations of 3-NPA-induced increases in catalase and Mn-SOD in the hippocampus and caudate nucleus.[5]

Administration of 3-NPA alone was associated with a significant increase in CAT activity in the CN (FIG. 1). Likewise, the activity of CuZn-SOD increased significantly in the FC and HIP (FIGS. 3 and 5). A trend toward higher Mn-SOD activity in the FC and HIP was observed as well (FIGS. 2 and 4). On the other hand, pretreatment with low or high doses of L-carnitine was associated with activities of CAT, Mn-SOD and CuZn-SOD equivalent to or below the level of control values (FIGS. 1–5). A similar effect of L-carnitine pretreatment on the FFA level after 3-NPA administration was not observed (TABLE 1).

The attenuation of the increase in antioxidant enzyme activities induced by exposure to 3-NPA in the presence of L-carnitine suggests the possible protective effect of L-carnitine in 3-NPA-induced neurotoxicity. This corresponds with the *in vitro* observations of the protective actions of L-carnitine.[12] It is of interest that pretreatment

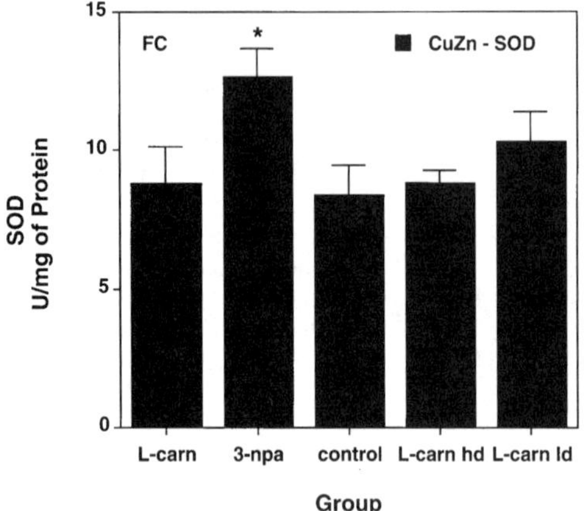

FIGURE 3. Effect of pretreatment with L-carnitine on the activity of copper/zinc superoxide dismutase (Cu/Zn-SOD; units per mg of protein) in frontal cortex (FC) following 3-NPA administration. *Abbreviations* of the descriptions are the same as for FIGURE 1. Mean ± SEM, $n = 3$; *$p < 0.05$ significantly different from control.

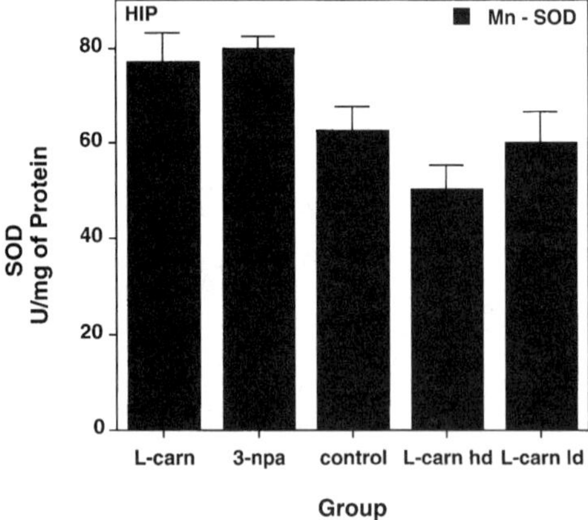

FIGURE 4. Effect of pretreatment with L-carnitine on the activity of manganese superoxide dismutase (Mn-SOD; units per mg of protein) in hippocampus (HIP) following 3-NPA administration. *Abbreviations* of the descriptions are the same as for FIGURE 1. Mean ± SEM, $n = 3$.

with L-carnitine did not prevent the increase in total FFA level observed after 3-NPA. On the contrary, the total FFA level significantly increased after the high dose of L-carnitine. The β-oxidation of FFA involves the formation of long-chain fatty acid esters of acetyl-coenzyme A (CoA) and their transport into the mitochondria. However, L-carnitine may also promote the release of medium and short-chain fatty acids out of mitochondria when oxidation of the long-chain fatty acids is incomplete.[7] This process maintains a ratio of free-to-esterified CoA optimal for oxidative phosphorylation and could result in an increase of total FFA.

Protective actions of L-carnitine in our experimental setting might be conveyed by restoring insufficiency in mitochondrial energy metabolism. However, the beneficial effects could also be mediated via changes in cell membrane viscosity. An increase in the fluidity of brain microsomes and liposomes by acetyl-L-carnitine and L-carnitine was reported.[1] L-Carnitine may also prevent excitotoxicity by decreasing affinity of *N*-methyl-D-aspartate (NMDA) and kainate receptors to glutamate.[9] Additional factors, e.g., conjugation of L-carnitine with 3-NPA and, therefore, elimina-

TABLE 1. Concentrations of total free fatty acids (ng/mg of protein) in frontal cortex (FC) in control and treated rats

Control (FC)	3-NPA	L-Carn.	L-Carn/3-NPA (Low)	L-Carn/3-NPA (High)
993 (58)	1161 (70)	1106 (148)	1278 (105)	1611 (97)*

NOTE: Mean (SEM), $n = 3$; *$p < 0.05$. Treatments: Control = 0.1 M phosphate buffer; 3-NPA = 3-nitropropionic acid 30 mg/kg; L-Carn. = L-carnitine 100 mg/kg; L-Carn/3-NPA (Low) = pretreatment with L-carnitine (50 mg/kg) 60 min before 3-NPA (30 mg/kg) injection; L-Carn/3-NPA (High) = pretreatment with L-carnitine (100 mg/kg) 60 min before 3-NPA (30 mg/kg) injection.

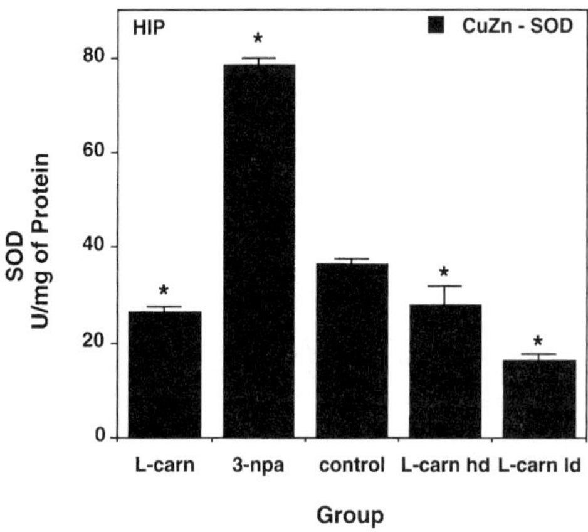

FIGURE 5. Effect of pretreatment with L-carnitine on the activity of copper/zinc superoxide dismutase (Cu/Zn-SOD; units per mg of protein) in hippocampus (HIP) following 3-NPA administration. *Abbreviations* of the descriptions are the same as for FIGURE 1. Mean ± SEM, $n = 3$; *p <0.05 significantly different from control.

tion of 3-NPA's mitochondrial inhibitory effects could play a role and should be investigated.

CONCLUSION

As assessed by the activity of antioxidant enzymes, catalase and SOD, L-carnitine pretreatment in rats injected subsequently with 3-NPA abolished the increase in enzyme activities that otherwise was observed after the 3-NPA alone. The effect of L-carnitine in ameliorating 3-NPA-induced mitochondrial dysfunction and preventing oxidative stress appears to be independent of its effects on FFA concentrations.

REFERENCES

1. ARIENTI, G., M.T. RAMACCI, F. MACCARI, A. CASU & L. CORAZZI. 1992. Acetyl-L-carnitine influences the fluidity of brain microsomes and of liposomes made of rat brain microsomal lipid extracts. Neurochem. Res. **17:** 671–675.
2. BEERS, R.F., JR. & I.W. SIZER. 1952. A spectrophotometric method for measuring the break down of H_2O_2 by catalase. J. Biol. Chem. **195:** 133–140.
3. BINIENDA, Z., D.L. FREDERICK, S.A. FERGUSON, R.L. ROUNTREE, M.G. PAULE, L. SCHMUED, S.F. ALI, W. SLIKKER, JR. & A.C. SCALLET. 1995. The effects of perin-

atal hypoxia on the behavioral, neurochemical, and neurohistological toxicity of the metabolic inhibitor 3-nitropropionic acid. Metab. Brain Dis. **10:** 269–282.

4. BINIENDA, Z. & C.S. KIM. 1997. Increase in levels of total free fatty acids in rat brain regions following 3-nitropropionic acid administration. Neurosci. Lett. **230:** 199–201.

5. BINIENDA, Z., C. SIMMONS, S. HUSSAIN, W. SLIKKER, JR. & S.F. ALI. 1998. Effect of acute exposure to 3-nitropropionic acid on activities of endogenous antioxidants in the rat brain. Neurosci. Lett. **251:** 173–176.

6. CARROLL, K.K. 1976. *In* Column Chromatography of Neutral Glycerides and Fatty Acids. Lipid Chromatographic Analysis. G.V. Marinetti, Ed.: 173–214. Marcel Dekker. New York.

7. BREMER, J. 1983. Carnitine—metabolism and functions. Physiol. Rev. **63:** 1420–1480.

8. DINNAUER, M. 1991. ω-3 highly unsaturated fatty acid methyl esters on DB-23 and DB-WAX. The J and W Separation Times **5:** 10–12.

9. FELIPO, V., M.-D. MINANA, H. CABEDO & S. GRISOLA. 1994. L-Carnitine increases the affinity of glutamate for quisqualate receptors and prevents glutamate neurotoxicity. Neurochem. Res. **19:** 373–377.

10. HAMILTON, B.F. & D.H. GOULD. 1987. Nature and distribution of brain lesions in rats intoxicated with 3-nitropropionic acid: a type of hypoxic (energy deficient) brain damage. Acta Neuropathol. (Berl.) **72:** 286–297.

11. PATTICHIS, K., L. LOUCA & V. GLOVER. 1994. Quantitation of soluble superoxide dismutase in rat striata, based on the inhibition of nitrite formation from hydroxylammonium chloride. Analyt. Biochem. **221:** 428–431.

12. VIRMANI, M.A., R. BISELLI, A. SPADONI, S. ROSSI, N. CORSICO, M. CALVANI, A. FATTOROSSI, C. DE SIMONE & E. ARRIGONI-MARTELLI. 1995. Protective actions of L-carnitine and acetyl-L-carnitine on the neurotoxicity evoked by mitochondrial uncoupling or inhibitors. Pharmacol. Res. **32:** 383–389.

13. WÜLLNER, U., A.B. YOUNG, J.B. PENNEY & M.F. BEAL. 1994. 3-Nitropropionic toxicity in the striatum. J. Neurochem. **63:** 1772–1781.

14. ZEEVALK, G.D., E. DERR-YELLIN & W.J. NICKLAS. 1995. Relative vulnerability of dopamine and GABA neurons in mesencephalic culture to inhibition of succinate dehydrogenase by malonate and 3-nitropropionic acid and protection by NMDA receptor blockade. J. Pharmacol. Exp. Ther. **275:** 1124–1130.

Questions and Answers

QUESTION FOR DR. ABBRACCHIO

From Dr. Youdim

My comment concerns your suggestion that adenosine A_{2A} antagonists may act as antiinflammatory agents in reactive microglia. We have shown recently that adenosine A_{2A} antagonists are neuroprotective in PC12 and neuroblastoma cells where toxicity is induced with H_2O_2 or 6-hydroxydopamine. We do not know their mechanism of action but suspect intracellular calcium mobilization on compartmentalization.

ANSWER: I am glad to hear A_{2A} antagonists are cytoprotective also in your experimental models, because this helps in strengthening the concept that blockade of the actions evoked by this receptor subtype during brain trauma and ischemia may represent a novel strategy to reduce brain damage. As far as the mechanism of action in microglial cells is concerned, previous studies have demonstrated that A_{2A} receptor stimulation upregulates COX-2 expression in microglia;[1] hence, it may be hypothesized that the neuroprotection evoked by A_{2A} antagonists may at least in part reside in their ability to block the pathological induction of an enzyme, whose activity has been associated to inflammation in chronic neurodegenerative events.[2–4] Whether changes of intracellular calcium mobilization or compartmentalization by A_{2A} antagonists play a role in blockade of microglial cell activation is not known at the moment, but certainly represents a likely possibility to be investigated.

QUESTION FOR DRS. ABBRACCHIO AND VON LUBITZ

From Dr. Sobotka

What are the effects of caffeine in terms of neuroprotectant effect?

ANSWER (Abbracchio): Caffeine can both reduce and augment ischemia-associated brain damage simply depending on the protocol of administration.[5] In particular, a chronic caffeine treatment well *before* induction of ischemia greatly ameliorates the ischemic outcome. Caffeine, an adenosine receptor antagonist, induces a continuous blockade of A_1 adenosine receptors, which indeed results in a compensatory upregulation of this adenosine receptor subtype (which has long been known to mediate neuroprotection). Conversely, acute administration of caffeine *during* the ischemic insult results in antagonism of A_1 receptor-mediated neuroprotection, leading to increased damage of brain cells.

QUESTIONS FOR DR. ALI

From Dr. Chiueh

Please give comments on the inhibitory effects of 7-nitroindazole (7-NI) on MAO-B and the bioactiviation of MPTP.

ANSWER: Recently Di Monte *et al.* published a paper in the *Journal of Neurochemistry* where they have shown that 7-NI inhibits the MAO-B and also effects the bioactivation of MPTP.[6]

From Dr. Hall

Have you looked at melatonin effects on methamphetamine loss on nigral cell bodies?
ANSWER: No.

From Dr. Youdim

If melatonin is such a good radical scavenger, why does it not protect again MPTP neurotoxicity of nigro-striatal dopamine neurons? And could it be that it is a very weak antioxidant, and higher concentrations would be neuroprotective. Finally, if it is an important endogenous neuroprotector, why does neural degeneration occur in neurological diseases?
ANSWER: I think the reason it protects against the methamphatamine-induced dopaminergic neurotoxicity but not against the MPTP, is because pretreatment of melatonin protected against methamphetamine-induced hyperthermia. MPTP does not produce hyperthermia, so it could be just a prepherial phenomenon. Also methamphetamine-induced terminal damage, whereas MPTP produced striatal nigral damage by effecting the cell bodies. Therefore, melatonin may just be protecting the terminals rather than cell bodies!

QUESTION FOR DRS. ALI AND SKAPER

From Dr. Lin

The antioxidative property of melatonin is moderate. In Reiter's study, melatonin is 100-fold more potent than vitamin E in scavenging hydroxyl radicals. However, in our experiment, melatonin is 100-fold less potent in inhibiting iron-elevated lipid peroxidation in cortical homogenates.
ANSWER (Ali): I don't know how I can compare Reiter's study with your study. Our study suggests that melatonin acts as an antioxidant and protects against methamphetamine-induced dopaminergic neurotoxicity.
ANSWER (Skaper): Such differences could be due to technical or methodological differences in experimental protocol, e.g., the manner in which lipid peroxation was induced or the oxidative state of the tissue homogenates used in the two studies.

QUESTIONS FOR DR. SKAPER

From Dr. Hall

What is the evidence for melatonin actually scavenging peroxynitrite?

ANSWER: A recent study by Gilad *et al.*[7] describes melatonin as a scavenger of peroxynitrite. The authors demonstrate that melatonin inhibits peroxynitrite-mediated oxidant processes, including the oxidation of dihydrorhodamine 123 by peroxynitrite *in vitro*. In cultured macrophages, melatonin inhibited the development of DNA single strand breaks in response to peroxynitrite and reduced the suppression of mitochondrial respiration.

From Dr. Youdim

Kainate neurotoxicity may be related to its ability to release iron, since iron chelators (e.g., desferol) are protective. Also, the hippocampal neurons of rats made nutritionally iron deficientare resistant to kainate, although the seizure is not altered. The ability of kainate to release iron would explain the depletion of GSH you have shown by kainate and protection by melatonin.

ANSWER: In addition to protecting cultured neurons against kainate neurotoxicity, melatonin prevents injury to hippocampal neurons cultured under conditions where cell loss is caused by excess synaptic activity (Skaper *et al.*[8]). In the latter study, melatonin was neuroprotective when given after termination of the initial insult. In the latter case treatment medium had been removed, so one would expect that any iron released from the cells during that time would no longer be in contact with the neurons. Yet, melatonin was still neuroprotective.

QUESTION FOR DR. VON LUBITZ

From Dr. Manev

Your speculation about the "neurochemical surgery" requires that A3 and A1 receptors co-localize. Is there any evidence for this?

ANSWER: No, there is no such evidence. We do not even know the details of A3 receptor location; their density is rather low, and we do not have sufficiently selective radio ligands to provide unequivocal answers. Electrophysiological work of Dr. Dunwidie *et al.* and Mogul *et al.* indicates that A3 receptors might be located in the vicinity of synaptic regions of neurons. But this is indirect evidence.

QUESTION FOR DRS. ABBRACCHIO AND VON LUBITZ

From Dr. Sobotka

What are the effects of caffeine in terms of neuroprotectant effect?

ANSWER (von Lubitz): Our unpublished data indicate that caffeine given acutely promotes ischemic neuronal damage. Chronic regimen has the reverse effect. Dr. Rudolphi performed a very through study using theophylline-showing aggravation of damage by this nonspecific antagonist. We used a very highly selective A1 receptor antagonist CPX and confirmed the data of Rudolphi *et al.*

QUESTION FOR DR. FADEN

From Dr. Youdim

Are these TRH analogues peptidase resistant, and do they have noradrenaline-releasing properties similar to the peplidose-resistant TRN analogues of Chemie-Gunenthal. The noradenergic action could of paramount importance in the treatment of traumatic brain injury.

ANSWER: The TRH related compounds—they are really not TRH analogs in the traditional sense—are almost certainly resistant to endopeptidases, given their structure and the protective actions with a single bolus injection, but we have not yet studied this issue directly, nor as yet the actions on various neurotransmitter and receptor systems. Such studies are planned, but we have already accumulated convincing evidence that these compounds modulate multiple components of the secondary injury cascade.

REFERENCES

1. FIEBICH, B.L., K. BIBER, K. LIEB, D. VAN CALKER, M. BERGER, J. BAUER & P.J. GEBICKE-HAERTER. 1996. Cyclo-oxygenase-2 expression in rat microglia is induced by adenosine A2A receptors. Glia **18:** 152–160.
2. TOCCO, G., J. FREIRE-MOAR, S.S. SCHREIBER, S.H. SAKHI, P.S. AISEN & G.M. PASINETTI. 1997. Maturational regulation and regional induction of cyclooxygenase-2 in rat brain: implications for Alzheimer's disease. Exp. Neurol. **144:** 339–349.
3. BLOM, M.A.A., M.G. VAN TWILLERI, S.C. DE VRIES, S.F. ENGEL, C.F. FINCH, R. VEERHUIS & P. EIKELENBOOM. 1997. NSAIDS inhibit the IL-1beta-induced IL-6 release from human post-mortem astrocytes: the involvement of prostaglandin E_2. Brain Res. **777:** 210–218.
4. BRAMBILLA, R., G. BURNSTOCK, A. BONAZZI, S. CERUTI, F. CATTABENI & M.P. ABBRACCHIO. 1999. Cyclo-oxygenase-2 mediates P2Y receptor-induced reactive astrogliosis. Br. J. Pharmacol. **126:** 563–567.
5. JACOBSON, K.A., D.K.J.E. VON LUBITZ, J.W. DALY & B.B. FREDHOLM. 1996. Adenosine receptor ligands: differences with acute versus chronic treatment. Trends Pharmacol. Sci. **17:** 108–113.
6. DI MONTE, D.A., J.E. ROYLAND, M.W. JAKOWEC & J.W. LANGATON. 1996. Role of nitric oxide in methamphetamine neurotoxicity: protection by 7-nitroindazole, an inhibitor of neuronal nitric oxide synthase. J. Neurochem. **67:** 2443–2450.
7. GILAD, E., S. CUZZOCREA, B. ZINGARELLI, A.L. SALZMAN & C. SZABO. 1997. Melatonin is a scavenger of peroxynitrite. Life Sci. **60:** PL169–PL174.
8. SKAPER, S.D., B. ANCONA, L. FACCI, D. FRANCESCHINI & P. GIUSTI. 1998. Melatonin prevents the delayed death of hippocampal neurons induced by enhanced excitatory neurotransmission and the nitridergic pathway. FASEB J. **12:** 725–731.

Primary Cultures of Rat Cerebellar Granule Cells as a Model to Study Neuronal 5-Lipoxygenase and FLAP Gene Expression

HARI MANEV[a] AND TOLGA UZ

The Psychiatric Institute, Department of Psychiatry, University of Illinois at Chicago, Chicago, Illinois 60612, USA

ABSTRACT: Aging is associated with chronic neurodegenerative diseases and increased brain vulnerability that may lead to a worse outcome from brain insults in elderly than in young subjects. Inflammation is one of the patholphysiological mechanisms of both chronic and acute neurodegeneration. Leukotrienes are inflammatory lipid mediators whose formation from arachidonic acid is initiated by 5-lipoxygenase (5-LO). 5-LO is also expressed in neurons and can be activated by brain injuries, whereas 5-LO inhibitors can provide neuroprotection. The expression of the 5-LO gene appears to be inhibited by the pineal hormone, melatonin, and stimulated by stress hormone glucocorticoids (e.g., corticosterone and the synthetic glucocorticoid dexamethasone). Melatonin deficiency and hyperglucocorticoidemia frequently develop with aging. We found that old or pinealectomized, i.e., melatonin-deficient rats are more susceptible to kainate-triggered excitotoxic limbic brain injury than the corresponding young or sham-pinealectomized controls, and that pinealectomy, aging, or glucocorticoid treatment result in an enhanced expression of 5-LO in limbic structures. We hypothesize that an aging brain is at a higher risk of neurodegeneration via aging-suppressed melatonin secretion and/or aging-increased glucocorticoid secretion and the resultant upregulation of 5-LO expression. Furthermore, we propose that suppressing the 5-LO expression and/or activity will increase the brain's resistance to injury. The results of our ongoing research are expected to elucidate the role of 5-LO in aging and neurodegeneration and to indicate neuroprotective therapies that would target the 5-LO pathway.

INTRODUCTION

Eicosanoids, the biologically active metabolites of arachidonic acid operative in inflammation, are synthesized by the actions of members of two major enzyme families, lipoxygenases (LO) and cyclooxygenases (COX). Increases in gene expression and in activity of LO and COX have recently been implicated in the pathobiology of neurodegeneration.[1] Moreover, inflammation is being investigated as a possible target for therapeutic approaches to the treatment of neurodegenerative disorders including Alzheimer's disease.[2] Significant progress is being made in developing new

[a]Corresponding author: Hari Manev, M.D., Ph.D., The Psychiatric Institute, University of Illinois at Chicago, 1601 West Taylor Street, MC 912, Chicago, IL 60612. Phone, 312/413-4558; fax, 312/413-4569.

e-mail, HManev@psych.uic.edu

antiinflammatory neuroprotective drugs, particularly the selective COX-2 inhibitors.[3] Of the different known LO types, neurons in the central nervous system have been shown to express 5-LO, the enzyme that leads to synthesis of leukotrienes.[4] No data are currently available, however, to assist in elucidating whether a clinically used 5-LO inhibitor, zileuton, which is utilized for the treatment of asthma,[5] has any effect on neuronal 5-LO.

Particularly high levels of neuronal 5-LO expression have been identified in the cerebellum and in the hippocampus.[4] The gene encoding 5-LO appears to be subject to hormonal regulation,[6–8] and its neuronal expression is remarkably upregulated during aging[9] and in response to glutamate receptor stimulation.[10] Here we demonstrate that 5-LO and a specific cofactor, 5-LO activating protein (FLAP), are expressed in primary cultures of rat cerebellar granule neurons (CGN), and that their expression is affected by neuronal maturation and by changing growth conditions in the culture medium. Thus, we propose that CGN cultures can be used as an *in vitro* model to study the mechanisms regulating neuronal 5-LO and FLAP gene expression.

5-LIPOXYGENASE (5-LO) AND 5-LO ACTIVATING PROTEIN (FLAP)

5-LO catalyses the first part of the two-step lipoxygenation of arachidonic acid in the synthesis of the leukotriene LTA4. 5-LO is an adenosine triphosphate (ATP)-, calcium- and nonheme iron-requiring enzyme. Most of our current knowledge about this enzymatic system is derived from studies in leukocytes, the cell type considered to be the primary site of 5-LO expression. It is believed that for its full enzymatic activity, 5-LO requires the presence of FLAP, a membrane-bound protein. Initially, the localization of FLAP was believed to be at the outer cell membrane, but more recent data indicate that FLAP is associated with the nuclear membrane. This indicates that arachidonic acid released from the nuclear membrane rather than from the outer cell membrane is the primary substrate for leukotriene synthesis.[11] Moreover, recent investigations of how FLAP activates 5-LO propose that 5-LO does not actually bind FLAP but rather that FLAP binds arachidonic acid and presents it to 5-LO in such a manner that 5-LO becomes fully enzymatically active.[11]

Complementary to the classical view that 5-LO is biologically important by virtue of its enzymatic activity is recent evidence suggesting that 5-LO protein may have an additional, nonenzymatic function. This new evidence suggests that 5-LO is capable of binding proteins other than FLAP, and that by doing so, it may influence the tyrosine kinase signaling[12] and/or the processes mediated by the protein termed nuclear factor κB (NF-κB).[13]

5-LO activity is regulated by intracellular calcium and ATP levels, and additionally, the 5-LO gene expression is also subject to complex regulatory mechanisms. This is probably due to the presence of numerous regulatory sites in the 5-LO gene promoter.[6] Several hormones have been identified that may affect 5-LO gene expression, such as melatonin[14] and glucocorticoids.[8] Additional regulatory factors include early-growth response factor-1 (Egr-1), cAMP-response-element-binding-protein-binding protein (CBP) and the CBP-related protein p300.[15] In addition, mutations in the 5-LO gene promoter exist, and they also may influence the rate of 5-LO expression.[16]

5-LO AND FLAP IN CEREBELLAR GRANULE NEURONS (CGN)

Over the years, our laboratory has been using primary rat CGN cultures to study different aspects of neuronal functioning that cannot easily be studied *in vivo*. On the basis of the evidence that *in situ* hybridization detected 5-LO and FLAP mRNAs in the cerebellum of adult rats,[4] we were prompted to verify whether the expression of these mRNAs occurs in primary cultures of rat CGN.

Typically, CGN cultures are prepared from 7-day-old rat pups, and they are grown in medium containing 10% fetal calf serum, whereas the proliferation of non-neuronal cells is prevented by adding 10 µM cytosine arabinofuranoside at about 18 hr after plating.[17] Recently, we developed the reverse-transcription polymerase chain reaction (RT-PCR) assay to study neuronal 5-LO mRNA expression.[9,18] In this study, we used RT-PCR to assay simultaneously 5-LO and cyclophilin (cyc) or FLAP and cyc mRNAs in primary CGN cultures grown in serum-containing medium (FIG. 1). Since cyc is a constitutive gene, its expression can be used as a control when inducible genes are studied.[9,18] We analyzed samples from CGN cultures grown *in vitro* for different periods of time, 1 to 9 days *in vitro* (DIV), and we calculated the ratios of 5-LO or FLAP to cyc RT-PCR products (FIG. 1). Both 5-LO/cyc and FLAP/cyc ratios were higher at 1 DIV than at any subsequent days in culture. By 9 DIV both 5-LO and FLAP mRNA contents were less than 50% of the values observed at the 1 DIV (FIG. 1).

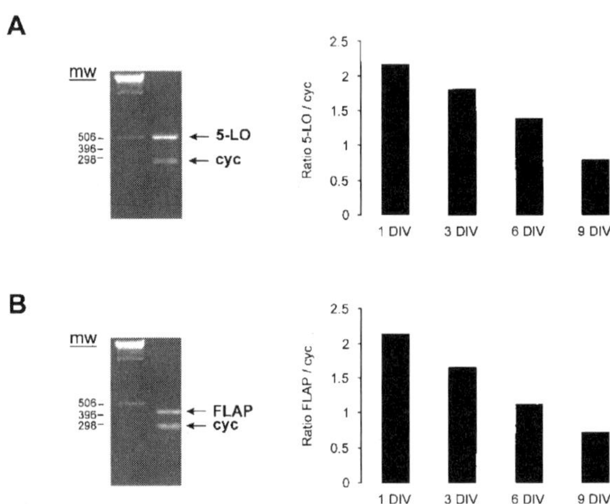

FIGURE 1. Effect of neuronal maturation *in vitro* on the content of 5-LO (**A**) and FLAP (**B**) mRNAs. Cultures were grown in 10-cm dishes (about 10,000,000 cells/dish) containing culture medium with 10% fetal calf serum and 25 mM KCl.[17] RT-PCR was used to assay 5-LO, FLAP, and cyclophilin (cyc) mRNAs; we calculated the ratios of 5-LO or FLAP to cyc RT-PCR products. Since cyc is a constitutive gene, its expression can be used as a control when inducible genes are studied. In order to allow the coamplification of 5-LO and FLAP mRNAs with the more abundant cyclophilin mRNA, pilot studies were conducted to determine the optimal relative primer concentrations and cycle number whereby the PCR would still be within the exponential phase of amplification for all transcripts. Specific 5-

The decrease in 5-LO mRNA during maturation of CGN cultures was accompanied by a similar decrease in content of the 5-LO immunoreactive protein, which we assayed by using 5-LO antiserum and Western blotting (FIG. 2). Although the amount of the constitutive protein β-actin was comparable between samples obtained at different DIV, the signal for 5-LO decreased with increasing DIV, and the 5-LO/β-actin ratio at 9 DIV was about 1/5 of the ratio observed at 3 DIV (FIG. 2).

The expression of various genes and the maturation of neuronal cultures can be affected by the type of the culture medium and the concentration of the serum used in the medium, as well as by the presence of cytosine arabinofuranoside (Ara C), a compound used to prevent cell proliferation. The effect of serum could be due either to the presence of biologically active compounds in the serum (e.g., hormones) or to the action of serum on the so-called "serum response element," which can affect gene expression. For example, serum was shown to be capable of altering 5-LO mRNA expression.[20] A method of growing CGN cultures in a serum-free and Ara C-free medium was recently introduced,[21] and we adopted it to investigate whether the absence of serum and/or Ara C would alter 5-LO and/or FLAP mRNA content. TABLE 1 shows that serum and Ara C have a differential effect on 5-LO and FLAP mRNA content. Namely, while 5-LO mRNA content was lower (by more than 50%) in serum-free than in serum-containing cultures, the content of FLAP mRNA was not affected by serum. On the other hand, Ara C suppressed FLAP expression by about 50%, but it did not significantly affect 5-LO mRNA (TABLE 1).

Thus, our results clearly indicate that both 5-LO and FLAP are expressed by CGN in culture, and that expression of these two genes can be altered by the composition of the growing medium and by neuronal maturation *in vitro*. Although our present data do not suffice to point to the physiological role of the neuronal 5-LO pathway,

---

LO and cyc amplification primers were designed and prepared as described elsewhere;[18] FLAP primers were designed to allow amplification of 113–496 bp of FLAP mRNA.[19] The total RNA isolated from six 10-cm dishes per group was denatured at 80°C for 6 min and then reverse transcribed with cloned Moloney Murine Leukemia Virus (M-MLV) reverse transcriptase (Gibco, BRL; Chagrin Falls, OH, USA; 200 U) in RT buffer containing 50 mM Tris/HCl (pH 8.3), 75 mM KCl, 3 mM MgCl2, 1 mM deoxynucleotide triphosphates (dNTPs) (Gibco, BRL) using random hexamers (Pharmacia Biotech, Piscataway, NJ, USA; 2.5 μM) and ribonuclease inhibitor (HPRI) (Amersham; Arlington Heights, IL, USA; 28 U) in a volume of 20 μl. The RT mixture was incubated at 37°C for 60 min to promote cDNA synthesis. The reaction was terminated by heating the samples at 98°C for 5 min, and the mixture was quick-chilled on ice. After termination of the RT reaction, cDNA aliquots containing reverse transcribed material were amplified with Hot *Tub* DNA polymerase (Amersham). The amplification mixture contained cDNA, 0.5 μM 5-LO- or FLAP- and 0.15 μM cyc-specific primers, 200 μM dNTPs, 1.5 mM MgCl2, 50 mM Tris-HCl (pH 9.0), 20 mM ammonium sulfate, 15 mM KCl, and 1.5 U of Hot *Tub* polymerase in a 100-μl volume. Trace amounts of [^{32}P]dCTP (Amersham; 0.5 μCi/sample) were included during the PCR step for subsequent quantification. The PCR mixture was amplified for 30 cycles with denaturation (94°C, 15 s), annealing (60°C, 30 s), and elongation (72°C, 30 s) amplification steps. The reaction was terminated with a 5-min final elongation step, and products were separated by agarose gel electrophoresis. To quantify the amount of the product corresponding to the amplified mRNA, the ethidium bromide-stained bands (examples are shown on photographs) were excised and the radioactivity was determined by Cerenkov counting. The results (ratios) are presented in arbitrary units. Note that both 5-LO/cyc and FLAP/cyc ratios decrease from 1 day *in vitro* (DIV) to 9 DIV.

TABLE 1. Effect of cytosine arabinofuranoside (Ara C) and serum on 5-LO and FLAP mRNAs in primary culture of rat CGN[a]

	(-) SERUM (-) Ara C	(-) SERUM (+) Ara C	(+) SERUM (+) Ara C
5-LO	100	90	223
FLAP	100	48	47

[a]Cultures were grown in the medium with the B27 supplement (Neurobasal medium; B27 supplement, 10 ml/500 ml medium [Gibco]; 25 mM KCl^{21}) or in this medium supplement with either 10 µM cytosine arabinofuranoside (Ara C),[17] or with both 10 (M Ara C and 10% fetal calf serum. Seven dishes per group (10-cm diameter; about 10,000,000 cells/dish) were used to extract RNA. 5-LO mRNA content was assayed using a quantitative RT-PCR assay with specific internal standards (calculated as attomol 5-LO mRNA per microgram total RNA).[9] FLAP mRNA was assayed as FLAP/cyc mRNA ratios and was calculated as described in FIGURE 1. Results are expressed as % of corresponding control, i.e., cultures grown in the B27 medium without Ara C and serum. Similar results were obtained in one additional experiment.

they demonstrate that primary cultures of CGN can be used as a model to address and study this question.

PUTATIVE FUNCTIONAL IMPLICATIONS OF NEURONAL 5-LO

Recent interest in the involvement of inflammatory mechanisms in the pathobiology of neurodegeneration has also attracted attention to the putative role of the 5-LO pathway. One possibility is that an overexpressed/overactive 5-LO pathway may lead to neurodegeneration by causing lipid peroxidation. For example, it was found that in the neuronal cell line, the gp120 protein of the HIV virus stimulated 5-LO expression and caused lipid peroxidation and cell death that was preventable by a 5-LO inhibitor, caffeic acid.[1] Increased susceptibility to excitotoxic brain injury was found in old rats compared with young ones; old rats also expressed more neuronal 5-LO than did young rats, and protection against excitotoxicity was obtained with caffeic acid.[9] Mobilization and activation of neuronal 5-LO has also been observed in the response of the brain to ischemia.[22]

The above-noted data clearly indicate a possible role of the neuronal 5-LO pathway in neuropathology. A physiological role of neuronal 5-LO was recently proposed in conjunction with its influence on neuronal somatostatin-mediated signaling.[4] Although these, and other, functional implications of the 5-LO pathway usually assume that leukotrienes, which are synthesized by activation of 5-LO, are responsible for the biological effects of 5-LO, it should be stressed that the nonenzymatic action of 5-LO protein may also be functionally relevant. For example, the interaction of 5-LO with the system of tyrosine kinases,[23] which are known to be the receptors for trophic factors, is probably worthy of further exploration. Our observation that 5-LO and FLAP gene expression changes during neuronal culture maturation might involve such a role of 5-LO.

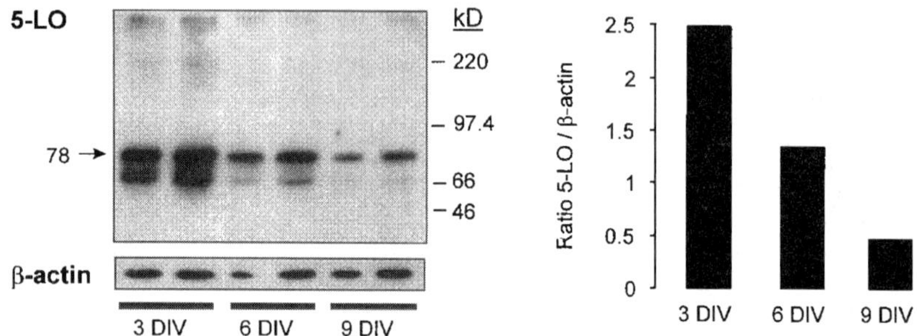

FIGURE 2. Effect of neuronal maturation *in vitro* on the content of 5-LO-immunoreactive protein. Cells from six 10-cm dishes/group were scraped in homogenizing buffer containing 20 mM Tris-HCl, 5 mM EGTA, and 5 mM EDTA. After centrifugation at 14,000 rpm, 30 min, the pellet was resuspended in homogenizing buffer containing 1 mM benzamidine-HCl and 0.5 mg/ml leupeptin. Equal volumes of protein samples (5 and 10 μg protein) and gel loading solution (50 mM Tris-HCl , 8% β-mercaptoethanol, 10% sodium dodecyl-sulfate [SDS], 18% glycerol, and a trace amount of bromphenol blue) were mixed, and the samples were boiled. They were run onto an 7.5% (w/v) acrylamide gel and were subsequently transferred electrophoretically to an ECL nitrocellulose membrane (Amersham). The blots were blocked with 5% (w/v) powdered nonfat milk in TBST, 2 ml nonidet P-40, and 0.02% (w/v) SDS (pH 8.0). They were incubated overnight with the primary anti-5-LO antibody (rabbit polyclonal; gift from Dr. J. Evans, Merck Frosst, Canada) at a dilution of 1:200. The blots were then washed with TBST and incubated with horseradish-peroxidase-linked secondary antibody (anti-rabbit IgG; 1:3000) for 2 hr at room temperature and processed with the Amersham ECL kit (Amersham); blots were then washed with TBST and exposed to ECL film. To normalize our data, we simultaneously measured β-actin immunoreactivity using the monoclonal primary antibody (Sigma, St. Louis, MO, USA; 1:2000 for 2 hr) and anti-mouse IgG (1:3000 for 2 hr) as the secondary antibody. The optical densities of the bands on the autoradiograms (shown is a typical blot; similar results were obtained in one more experiment) were quantified using the Loats Image Analysis System (Westminster, MD, USA), and the optical density of the 5-LO band (78 kD) was corrected by the optical density of the corresponding β-actin band. The values are expressed as arbitrary units. Note that 5-LO/β-actin ratios decrease from 3 day *in vitro* (DIV) to 9 DIV.

CONCLUSION

We have demonstrated that primary cultures of rat cerebellar granule neurons express both 5-LO and its regulatory protein FLAP. The expression of these two genes changes over time during neuronal maturation *in vitro*; in cultures grown in the presence of 10% fetal calf serum, 5-LO and FLAP expression is high on the first day in culture, and decreases markedly by nine days *in vitro*. When cerebellar granule neurons are grown in serum-free and/or Ara C-free conditions, there are differential effects on 5-LO and FLAP mRNA expression; mRNA content of 5-LO increases upon serum exposure and that of FLAP is suppressed by Ara C. These studies establish that primary cultures of cerebellar granule neurons can be used to study the regulation and the functional role of the neuronal 5-LO pathway.

ACKNOWLEDGMENT

This work was in part supported by NIH-NIA grant RO1-AG15347 (H.M.). We thank Dr. Jilly Evans, Merck Frosst, Canada, for the 5-LO antiserum, and Dr. Patrizia Longone for help in assaying the 5-LO immunoblots.

REFERENCES

1. MACCARRONE, M., M. NAVARRA, M.T. CORASANTI, G. NISTICO & A. FINAZZI AGRO. 1998. Cytotoxic effect of HIV-1 coat glycoprotein gp120 on human neuroblastoma CHP100 cells involves activation of arachidonate cascade. Biochem. J. **333:** 45–49.
2. BREITNER, J.C.S. 1996. Inflammatory processes and antiinflammatory drugs in Alzheimer's disease: a current appraisal. Neurobiol. Aging **17:** 789–794.
3. NAKAYAMA, M., K. UCHIMURA, R.L. ZHU, T. NAGAYAMA, M.E. ROSE, R.A. STETLER, P.C. ISAKSON & S.H. GRAHAM. 1998. Cyclooxygenase-2 inhibition prevents delayed death of CA1 hippocampal neurons following global ischemia. Proc. Natl. Acad. Sci. USA **95:** 10954–10959.
4. LAMMERS, C.-H., P. SCHWEITZER, P. FACCHINETTI, J.-M. ARRANG, S.G. MADAMBA, G.R. SIGGINS & D. PIOMELLI. 1996. Arachidonate 5-lipoxygenase and its activating protein: prominent hippocampal expression and role in somatostatin signaling. J. Neurochem. **66:** 147–152.
5. DRAZEN, J. 1998. Clinical pharmacology of leukotriene receptor antagonists and 5-lipoxygenase inhibitors. Am. J. Respir. Crit. Care Med. **157:** S233–S237.
6. HOSHIKO, S., O. RADMAR & B. SAMUELSSON. 1990. Characterization of the human 5-lipoxygenase gene promoter. Proc. Natl. Acad. Sci. USA **87:** 9073–9077.
7. WIESENBERG, I., M. MISSBACH & C. CARLBERG. 1998. The potential role of the transcription factor RZR/ROR as a mediator of nuclear melatonin signaling. Restor. Neurol. Neurosci. **12:** 143–150.
8. RIDDICK, C.A., W.L. RING, J.R. BAKER, C.R. HODULIK & T.D. BIGBY. 1997. Dexamethasone increases expression of 5-lipoxygenase and its activating protein in human monocytes and THP-1 cells. Eur. J. Biochem. **246:** 112–118.
9. UZ, T., C. PESOLD, P. LONGONE & H. MANEV. 1998. Aging-associated up-regulation of neuronal 5-lipoxygenase expression: putative role in neuronal vulnerability. FASEB J. **12:** 439–449.
10. MANEV, H., T. UZ & T. QU. 1998. Early upregulation of hippocampal 5-lipoxygenase following systemic administration of kainate to rats. Restor. Neurol. Neurosci. **12:** 81–85.
11. PETER-GOLDEN, M. 1998. Cell biology of the 5-lipoxygenase pathway. Am. J. Respir. Crit. Care Med. **157:** S227–S232.
12. LEPLEY, R.A. & F.A. FITZPATRICK. 1994. 5-Lipoxygenase contains a functional src homology 3-binding motif that interacts with the src homology 3 domain of Grb2 and cytoskeletal proteins. J. Biol. Chem. **269:** 24163–24168.
13. LEPLEY, R.A. & F.A. FITZPATRICK. 1998. 5-Lipoxygenase compartmentalization in granulocytic cells is modulated by an internal bipartite nuclear localizing sequence and nuclear factor κB complex formation. Arch. Biochem. Biophys. **356:** 71–76.
14. STEINHILBER, D., M. BRUNGS, O. WERZ, I. WIESENBERG, C. DANIELSSON, J.-P. KAHLEN, S. NAYERI, M. SCHRÄDER & C. CARLBERG. 1995. The nuclear receptor for melatonin represses 5-lipoxygenase gene expression in human B lymphocytes J. Biol. Chem. **270:** 7037–7040.
15. SILVERMAN, E.S., J. DU, A.J. WILLIAMS, R. WADGAONKAR, J.M. DRAZEN & T. COLLINS. 1998. CAMP-response-element-binding-protein-binding protein (CBP) and p300 are transcriptional co-activators of early growth response factor-1 (Egr-1). Biochem. J. **336:** 183–189.

16. IN, K.H., K. ASANO, D. BEIER, J. GROBHOLZ, P.W. FINN, E.K. SILVERMAN, E.S. SIL-VERMAN, T. COLLINS, A.R. FISCHER, T.P. KEITH, K. SERINO, S.W. KIM, G.T. DESANCTIS, C. YANDAVA, A. PILLARI, P. RUBIN, J. KEMP, E. ISRAEL, W. BUSSE, D. LEDFORD, J.J. MURRAY, A. SEGAL, D. TINKLEMAN & J.M. DRAZEN. 1997. Naturally occurring mutations in the human 5-lipoxygenase gene promoter that modify transcription factor binding and reporter gene transcription. J. Clin. Invest. **99:** 1130–1137.

17. MANEV, H., M. FAVARON, A. GUIDOTTI & E. COSTA. 1989. Delayed increase of calcium influx elicited by glutamate: role in neuronal death. Mol. Pharmacol. **36:** 106–112.

18. UZ, T., P. LONGONE & H. MANEV. 1997. Increased hippocampal 5-lipoxygenase mRNA content in melatonin-deficient, pinealectomized rats. J. Neurochem. **69:** 2220–2223.

19. DIXON, R.A.F., R.E. DIEHL, E. OPAS, E. RANDS, P.J. VICKERS, J.F. EVANS, J.W. GILLARD & D.K. MILLER. 1990. Requirement of a 5-lipoxygenase-activating protein for leukotriene synthesis. Nature **343:** 282–284.

20. BRUNGS, M., O. RADMARK, B. SAMUELSSON & D. STEINHILBER. 1994. On the induction of 5-lipoxygenase expression and activity in HL-60 cells: effects of vitamin D_3, retinoic acid, DMSO and TGF beta. Biochem. Biophys. Res. Commun. **205:** 1572–1580.

21. BREWER, G.J. 1995. Serum-free B27/neurobasal medium supports differentiated growth of neurons from the striatum, substantia nigra, septum, cerebral cortex, cerebellum, and dentate gyrus. J. Neurosci. Res. **42:** 674–683.

22. OHTSUKI, T., M. MATSUMOTO, Y. HAYASHI, K. YAMAMOTO, K. KITAGAWA, S. OGAWA, S. YAMAMOTO & T. KAMADA. 1995. Reperfusion induces 5-lipoxygenase translocation and leukotriene C4 production in ischemic brain. Am. J. Physiol. **268:** H1249–H1257.

23. LEPLEY, R.A., D.T. MUSKARDIN & F.A. FITZPATRICK. 1996. Tyrosine kinase activity modulates catalysis and translocation of cellular 5-lipoxygenase. J. Biol. Chem. **271:** 6179–6184.

Intraneuronal Ion Distribution during Experimental Oxygen/Glucose Deprivation

Routes of Ion Flux as Targets of Neuroprotective Strategies

RICHARD M. LOPACHIN[a]

Department of Anesthesiology, Albert Einstein College of Medicine, Montefiore Medical Center, Bronx, New York 10467

ABSTRACT: Ischemic neuronal injury appears to be mediated by disruption of subcellular ion distribution and, therefore, prevention of ion relocation might be neuroprotective. X-ray microanalysis was used to measure concentrations of Na, K, Ca and other elements in subcellular compartments (e.g., mitochondria) of CA1 neurons from oxygen/glucose-deprived (OGD) hippocampal slices. Results showed that OGD produced progressive loss of ion regulation in CA1 cells. Post-OGD reperfusion with normal media exacerbated the initial ion deregulation. To study neuroprotective mechanisms, we determined the ability of hypothermia (31°C) or ion channel blockade to retard intraneuronal ion disruption induced by OGD/reperfusion. Whereas Ca^{2+} channel blockade (ω-conotoxin MVIIC, 3 μM) was ineffective, hypothermia and Na^+ channel blockers (tetrodotoxin, TTX, 1 μM; lidocaine, 200 μM) reduced ion deregulation in subneuronal compartments. Blockade of glutamate receptors (AMPA, 10 μM; the non-NMDA receptor antagonist CNQX, 10 μM/100 μM glycine; the NMDA receptor antagonist CCP, 100 μM) during OGD/reperfusion provided nearly complete protection. These findings provide a foundation for identifying potential pharmacotherapeutic approaches and for discerning corresponding mechanisms of neuroprotection

INTRODUCTION

Neuronal function is critically dependent upon proper maintenance of transmembrane Na^+, K^+, Cl^- and Ca^{2+} gradients. These gradients are established and regulated primarily by the activities of adenosine triphosphate (ATP)-dependent membrane ion transport proteins such as Na^+/K^+ ATPase and Ca^{2+} ATPase. However, neuronal ATP production is significantly reduced as an early consequence of the oxygen and glucose deprivation (OGD) associated with ischemic episodes in brain.[1,2] OGD-induced decline in energy production impairs activity of ion regulatory mechanisms and leads to a loss of active ion transport and subsequent collapse of ion gradients with membrane depolarization.[3] Depolarization inhibits neuronal (and glial) glutamate buffering, which increases extracellular levels of this excitatory amino

[a]Address for correspondence: Richard M. LoPachin, Ph.D., Department of Anesthesiology, Montefiore Medical Center, 111 E. 210th St., Bronx, NY 10467. Phone, 718/920-5054; fax, 718/515-4903.

e-mail, lopachin@aecom.yu.edu

acid.[4] Excess glutamate-stimulation of ionotropic receptors (e.g., NMDA, AMPA receptors) promotes Na^+ and Ca^{2+} fluxes, which further contribute to the developing intraneuronal ion deregulation during OGD.[5] *In vivo* brain ischemic or hypoxic events are often transient and are followed by local reperfusion. However, despite restoration of normal extraneuronal oxygen tension and glucose content, reperfusion is paradoxically associated with additional nerve cell injury.[1] Reperfusion injury involves multiple factors (e.g., free radical generation, mitochondrial dysfunction) that promote additional neuronal Na^+ and Ca^{2+} entry.[6,7] Disruption of intraneuronal ion distribution, in particular loss of Ca^{2+} homeostasis, during the initial ischemic insult and subsequent reperfusion is structurally and functionally damaging and can, depending upon conditions (e.g., length of ischemia), initiate an injury cascade that culminates in neuronal cell death.[6] Thus, because transmembrane Na^+, K^+, Cl^- and Ca^{2+} distributions maintain structure, function and viability of nerve cells, loss of ion gradients is considered to be a cardinal event in the pathophysiology of brain ischemia.[2,8]

Despite the apparent importance of disturbed nerve cell ion homeostasis during transient OGD, very little direct information existed regarding the disposition, extent and magnitude of intraneuronal ionic changes. To address this information gap, in a recent study we[9] used electron probe X-ray microanalysis (EPMA) to determine the direct effects of experimental OGD and reoxygenation on subcellular distribution of Na, K, Ca, and other biological elements in CA1 nerve cells of rat hippocampal slices. EPMA is a quantitative electron microscopy technique that simultaneously measures water content and total (free plus bound) concentrations of elements in selected morphological compartments of rapidly frozen tissue.[10] This technique permits optical identification of individual neurons and analyses of respective subcellular compartments such as mitochondria and nuclei.[11] Results showed that OGD produced an early (2 min) loss of evoked synaptic potentials and decreased concentrations of K, Cl, P and Mg in CA1 cell mitochondria, cytoplasm and nuclei. Continued OGD exposure (5 min) caused a negative DC shift in interstitial voltage followed by a general worsening of elemental disruption in cytoplasm and nucleus (5–42 min). Similar elemental changes were noted in mitochondria, except that Ca levels increased during the first 5 min of OGD and then decreased over the remaining experimental period (12–42 min). Post-OGD reperfusion with normal, oxygenated solutions (12 min OGD/30 min reperfusion) was associated with exacerbated Ca accumulation in all compartments, whereas other elemental changes (Na, K, Cl, P, and Mg) resembled those caused by 42 min of OGD. Elemental and electrophysiological changes during OGD/reperfusion occurred in parallel with marked alterations in cellular morphology; i.e., CA1 cells exhibited progressive swelling of perikarya, mitochondria and nuclei with dendritic blebbing. Finally, when hippocampal slices were incubated in mild hypothermic conditions (31°C) during the OGD/reperfusion period, elemental, electrophysiological and morphologic disruptions were minimized.

Thus, *in vitro* OGD/reperfusion of CA1 neurons in rat hippocampal slices caused a collapse of transmembrane Na^+, K^+, Cl^-, and Ca^{2+} gradients, which correlated with synaptic dysfunction and neuropathic changes. We also showed that neuronal dysfunction and elemental deregulation could be partially preserved by mild hypothermic incubation. Although this research represents a detailed characterization of ion disruption during OGD/reperfusion of CA1 neurons, the corresponding pathogenic mechanism remains to be determined. Therefore, using different ion channel blockers (Na$^+$ channel, TTX; AMPA ionophoric receptor, CNQX), we have initiated pharmacologic studies to identify relevant routes of ion flux. The findings presented in this paper represent fundamental information regarding the role of ions in the pathophysiology of experimental OGD/reperfusion. In addition, they provide a foundation for identifying potential pharmacotherapeutic approaches and for discerning respective mechanisms of neuroprotection.

METHODS

Only a brief description of methodology is provided here. For details see Taylor *et al.*[9]

Hippocampal Slice Preparation and Pharmacology

Rat hippocampal slices were prepared according to a modification of Weber and Taylor.[12] Slices were placed in an interface recording chamber (Scientific Systems Design) and incubated at 36°C in artificial cerebrospinal fluid (aCSF). OGD was produced by superfusing slices with D-glucose-deficient aCSF equilibrated with a 95% N_2/5% CO_2 gas mixture. Thus, hippocampal slices ($n = 6$) were exposed to 12 min of OGD followed by 30 min post-OGD perfusion with normal, oxygenated aCSF. For pharmacological identification of ion routes, exposure of slices ($n = 3$–4 per compound) to channel blockers was initiated 30 min prior OGD/reperfusion and then continued throughout the experimental period. As parallel temporal controls (n = 2/time period), slices were incubated in normal, oxygenated aCSF for 0, 12, or 42 min. Respective data did not differ statistically, and results were pooled (see TABLE 1). Pharmacological compounds were as follows: Ca^{2+} channel blocker ω-conotoxin MVIIC (3 μM); Na$^+$ channel blockers lidocaine (200 μM) and tetrodotoxin (TTX, 1 μM); glutamate receptor blockers 6-cyano-7-nitroquinoxaline-2,3-dione (CNQX, 10 μM/100 μM glycine) and 3-(2-carboxypiperazin-4-yl)propyl-1-phosphonic acid (CPP, 100 μM). At the end of each experimental or control period, tissue samples were rapidly removed from the incubation chamber and were immediately quench-frozen by immersion in melting isopentane. Frozen slices were then stored in liquid nitrogen for later analysis.

Cryoultramicrotomy and EPMA

The methodologies for cryomicrotomy and EPMA have been published extensively.[10] Briefly, unfixed, unstained frozen hippocampal slices were sectioned (500 nm) on a cryomicrotome (−55°C). Cryosections were transferred under vacuum to the cold stage (−185°C) of an AMRay 1000 scanning electron microscope. The electron microscope was equipped with a Tracor Northern energy dispersive detector and pulse processor that was connected to a PC-based multichannel analyzer for collection and processing of X-rays.[13] The electron beam (20 kV, 0.4 nA current) was rastered within anatomical boundaries of chosen CA1 cell regions and organelles. X-ray spectra were collected over 100 sec of live counting time. Dry weight elemental mass fractions (milimoles/kilogram of dry weight) for N, K, P, Cl, Mg, and Ca were

TABLE 1. Elemental composition and water content of control incubated hippocampal CA1 nerve cells

	Na	P	Cl	K	Ca	Mg	Water
Cytoplasm	252 ± 11	609 ± 35	265 ± 17	662 ± 32	5 ± 1	25 ± 4	75 ± 1
Mitochondria	321 ± 18	776 ± 70	351 ± 29	739 ± 38	3 ± 1	29 ± 1	63 ± 1
Nucleus	232 ± 22	758 ± 81	254 ± 31	807 ± 75	6 ± 1	31 ± 6	62 ± 1

NOTE: Rat hippocampal slices were prepared as described in text and were allowed to recover in oxygenated, glucose-containing aCSF for approximately 1 hr at 36°C. For timed-control data, slices were incubated in control conditions for 0, 12, or 42 min. Respective data did not differ statistically and results were pooled. Pooled elemental data are expressed as mean (±SEM) mmol element per kilogram dry weight. Pooled compartmental water data are expressed as mean (±SEM) percent water.

determined using software applying the Hall *et al.*[14] method of continuum normalization.[13] Water content (percentage water) of morphological compartments was determined by the method of Bulger *et al.*[15] EPMA does not distinguish ionic versus bound element but rather measures total elemental concentrations. Therefore, symbols for each element are expressed without oxidation state (e.g., K) when corresponding concentrations have been derived by EPMA. Morphological compartments (cytoplasm, nuclei and mitochondria) were visualized and analyzed in dehydrated cryosections using scanning-transmission electron microscopy.

Statistics

Statistical differences ($p < 0.05$) among group means were determined using one-factor ANOVA followed by Dunnett's test modified for unbalanced data.

RESULTS

Elemental Composition and Water Content of Control CA1 Nerve Cell Compartments

TABLE 1 shows that in control incubated neurons, mean (± SEM) dry weight Na, Cl, Mg, and Ca concentrations were similar regardless of compartment examined. Compartments were distinguished by differences in P, K, and water content. Mean P and K concentration were lower in cytoplasm when compared to mitochondria or nucleus, whereas water content of cytoplasm was higher than that of the other compartments (TABLE 1).

Elemental Composition and Water Content of CA1 Nerve Cells Exposed to OGD/Reperfusion at 36°C and 31°C

As we reported previously,[9] post-OGD reperfusion of hippocampal slices with glucose-containing, oxygenated aCSF (36°C) failed to restore normal element and water composition in any CA1 cell morphologic compartment examined (FIGS. 1–3). In fact, the extent of compartmental deregulation caused by 12 min of OGD was

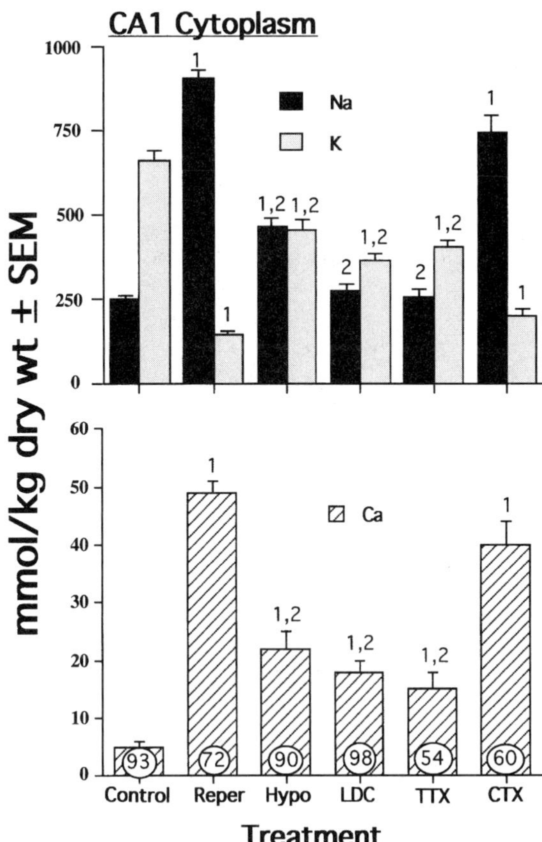

FIGURE 1. Mean (±SEM) dry weight Na, K (*upper panel*), and Ca (*lower panel*) concentrations (millimoles of element per kilogram) in hippocampal CA1 nerve cell cytoplasm. Control data are presented in TABLE 1. Reper = hippocampal slices were exposed to 12 min of oxygen-glucose deprivation (OGD) followed by 30 min reperfusion with oxygenated, glucose-containing aCSF. Hypo = slices were incubated in mild hypothermic conditions (31°C) and exposed to OGD/reperfusion. LDC = slices were incubated with lidocaine (200 μM) 30 min prior to initiating the OGD/reperfusion paradigm. Perfusion with LDC-containing aCSF continued during the experimental period. TTX = slices were incubated with tetrodotoxin (1 μM) 30 min prior to initiating the OGD/reperfusion paradigm. Perfusion with TTX-containing aCSF continued during the experimental period. CTX = slices were incubated with ω-conotoxin MVIIC (3 μM) 30 min prior to initiating the OGD/reperfusion paradigm. Perfusion with CTX-containing aCSF continued during the experimental period. [1]Significantly different ($p < 0.05$) from control data. [2]Significantly different ($p < 0.05$) from reperfusion data.

exacerbated by reperfusion for 30 min; i.e., relative to OGD-induced changes, neuronal Na, Cl and Ca levels increased significantly, whereas concentrations of P, Cl and Mg decreased (see Taylor *et al.*,[9] FIG. 4 for details). However, incubation of slices in mild hypothermic conditions (31°C) provided nearly complete protection

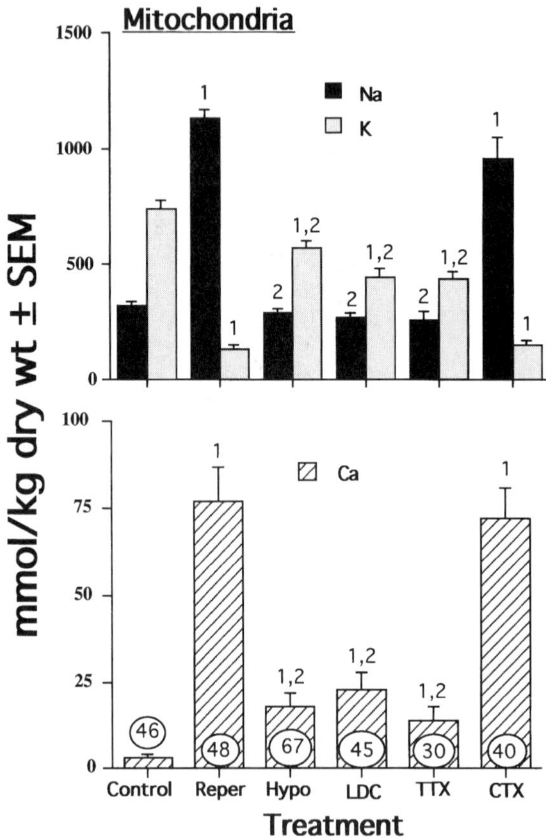

FIGURE 2. Mean (±SEM) dry weight Na, K (*upper panel*), and Ca (*lower panel*) concentrations (millimoles of element per kilogram) in hippocampal CA1 nerve cell mitochondria. Details as in FIGURE 1.

against compartmental elemental disruption produced by OGD/reperfusion (FIGS. 1–3). Preservation of intraneuronal elemental distribution correlates with the well described ability of hypothermia to diminish certain morphologic and electrophysiologic changes associated with experimental ischemia or reperfusion injury.[16,17]

Neuroprotective Effects of Ion Channel Blockade

Sodium channel blockade with either lidocaine or TTX reduced the extent and magnitude of elemental deregulation in CA1 neurons subjected to 12 min of OGD followed by 30 min of reperfusion (FIGS. 1–3). The level of neuroprotection afforded was quantitatively similar to that produced by hypothermia. Both lidocaine (200 μM) and TTX (1 μM) prevented Na buildup in cytoplasm, mitochondria and nuclear areas of CA1 neurons exposed to OGD/reperfusion. Pharmacological block-

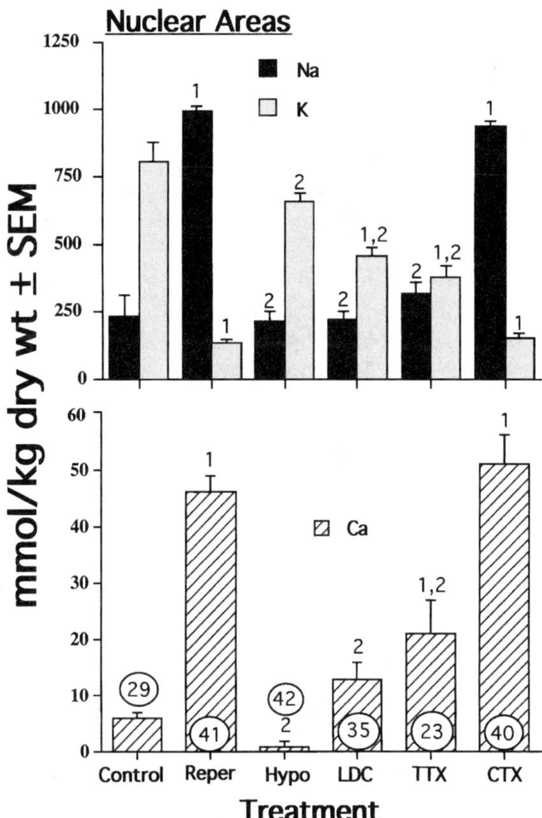

FIGURE 3. Mean (±SEM) dry weight Na, K (*upper panel*), and Ca (*lower panel*) concentrations (millimoles of element per kilogram) in hippocampal CA1 nerve cell nucleus. Details as in FIGURE 1.

ade of Na^+ channels significantly lowered compartmental Ca burden and reduced the loss of neuronal K normally associated with OGD/reperfusion (FIGS. 1–3). Moreover, Na^+ channel blockers minimized the perturbation of Cl, P and Mg levels in OGD/reperfusion-exposed neurons (data not shown). In contrast, blockade of N-type and P-type Ca^{2+} channels with ω-conotoxin MVIIC (3 μM) did not prevent intraneuronal elemental deregulation caused by OGD/reperfusion (FIGS. 1–3).

Perfusion of hippocampal slices with ionotropic glutamate receptor antagonists maintained nearly normal intraneuronal elemental distribution during OGD/reperfusion. Thus, both the non-NMDA receptor antagonist CNQX (10 μM CNQX/100 μM glycine) and the NMDA receptor antagonist CPP (100 μM) prevented compartmental Na and Ca accumulation associated with OGD/reperfusion (FIGS. 4–6). Both blockers also lessened K loss (FIGS. 4–6), although OGD/reperfusion-induced changes in neuronal P, Cl and Mg levels were not affected by either CNQX or CPP (data not shown).

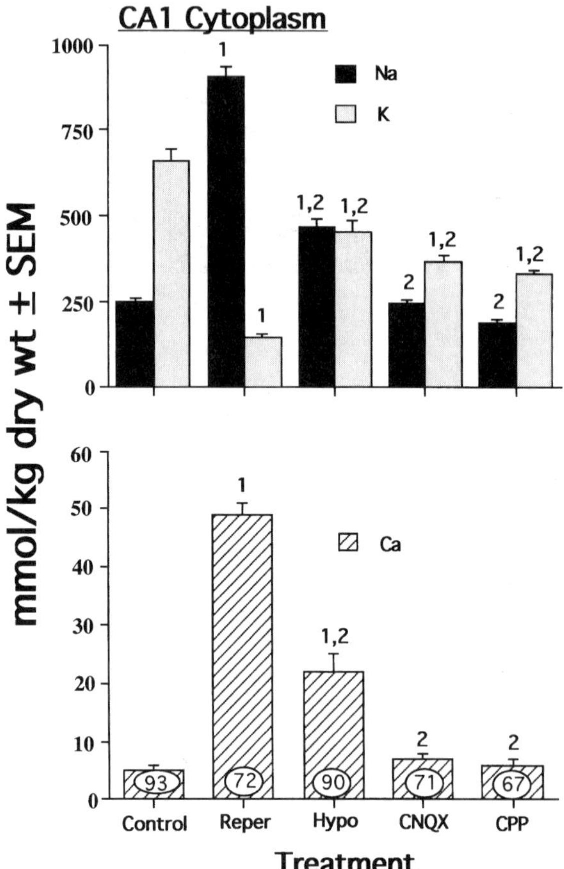

FIGURE 4. Mean (±SEM) dry weight Na, K (*upper panel*), and Ca (*lower panel*) concentrations (millimoles of element per kilogram) in hippocampal CA1 nerve cell cytoplasm. Control data are presented in TABLE 1. Reper = hippocampal slices were exposed to 12 min of oxygen-glucose deprivation (OGD) followed by 30 min reperfusion with oxygenated, glucose-containing aCSF. Hypo = slices were incubated in mild hypothermic conditions (31°C) and exposed to OGD/reperfusion. CNQX = slices were incubated with CNQX (10 μM)/glycine (100 μM) 30 min prior to initiating the OGD/reperfusion paradigm. Perfusion with CNQX-containing aCSF continued during the experimental period. CPP = slices were incubated with CPP (100 μM) 30 min prior to initiating the OGD/reperfusion paradigm. Perfusion with CPP-containing aCSF continued during the experimental period. CTX = slices were incubated with ω-conotoxin MVIIC (3 μM) 30 min prior to initiating the OGD/ reperfusion paradigm. Perfusion with CTX-containing aCSF continued during the experimental period. [1]Significantly different ($p < 0.05$) from control data. [2]Significantly different ($p < 0.05$) from reperfusion data.

DISCUSSION

Our initial studies[9] showed that *in vitro* oxygen-glucose deprivation caused progressive element deregulation in CA1 hippocampal neurons. Post-OGD (12 min) reperfusion with glucose-containing, oxygenated aCSF did not promote recovery and, instead, exacerbated the progression of elemental disruption.[9] We also showed that incubation of hippocampal slices in mild hypothermic conditions offered protection against the disruptive effects of OGD/reperfusion.[9] The present research has demonstrated that, like hypothermia, pharmacologic blockade of CA1 nerve cell Na^+ channels and ionotropic glutamate receptors also modified elemental perturbation associated with OGD/reperfusion.

Previously published evidence indicates that Na^+ channel blockade with, for example, local anesthetics, TTX or phenytoin protects against the structural and functional deficits produced by experimental brain ischemia.[12,18,19] In the present study, we found that both TTX and lidocaine prevented Na^+ accumulation and reduced general ion deregulation in all compartments of CA1 neurons from hippocampal slices exposed to OGD/reperfusion. Our data, in conjunction with earlier evidence, strongly implicate Na^+ loading of neurons via TTX-sensitive, voltage-gated Na^+ channels as a critical event in ischemia-induced neuronal damage.[19,20] Although the exact mechanism of neuroprotection is unknown, decreasing the Na^+ load during ischemia would conserve ATP otherwise consumed by stimulated Na^+/K^+ ATPase-mediated Na^+ transport. ATP conservation has obvious neuroprotective potential, since it could abate or delay the secondary injury cascade initiated by the energy-limiting effects of ischemia.[20] In addition, our study demonstrated that Na^+ channel blockade significantly reduced the compartmental Ca burden associated with OGD/reperfusion. This suggests Ca^{2+} entry might be coupled to Na^+ influx possibly through reverse Na^+-Ca^{2+} exchange.[21] Thus, in addition to promoting ATP retention, Na^+ channel blockade might be neuroprotective by decreasing intraneuronal Ca^{2+} accumulation and lessening the impact of Ca^{2+}-stimulated events in the pathobiochemical cascade.

Although Na^+-dependent Ca^{2+} entry is suggested by our data, other routes of Ca^{2+} entry appear to be involved, since TTX only partially decreased neuronal Ca^{2+} accumulation associated with OGD/reperfusion. Because ω-conotoxin did not affect intraneuronal ionic deregulation, it is unlikely N- or P-type channels mediate Ca^{2+} entry. The role of L-type channels was not assessed in the present study, but existing data are contradictory.[22–25] Our study of glutamate receptor antagonists, CNQX and CPP, suggests that neuronal Na^+ and Ca^{2+} entry during ischemia is mediated by AMPA- and/or NMDA-gated ion channels. Both blockers prevented Na and Ca build-up in CA1 neurons subjected to OGD/reperfusion. Whereas AMPA and NMDA blockade was associated with a similar pattern of intraneuronal elemental preservation, the mechanism of this neuroprotection might be different. According to current understanding of ionotropic glutamate channel operation,[2,5,6] NMDA-gated channels exhibit high permeability to Na^+, K^+ and Ca^{2+}. Blockade by CPP would be expected to stabilize ischemia-induced flux of these ions. Our elemental data are consistent with this expectation (see FIGS. 4–6). AMPA-gated channels mediate Na^+ and K^+ exchange and, as a result, pharmacological receptor antagonism might produce TTX-like protection; i.e., inhibition of Na^+ entry blocks coupled Ca^{2+}

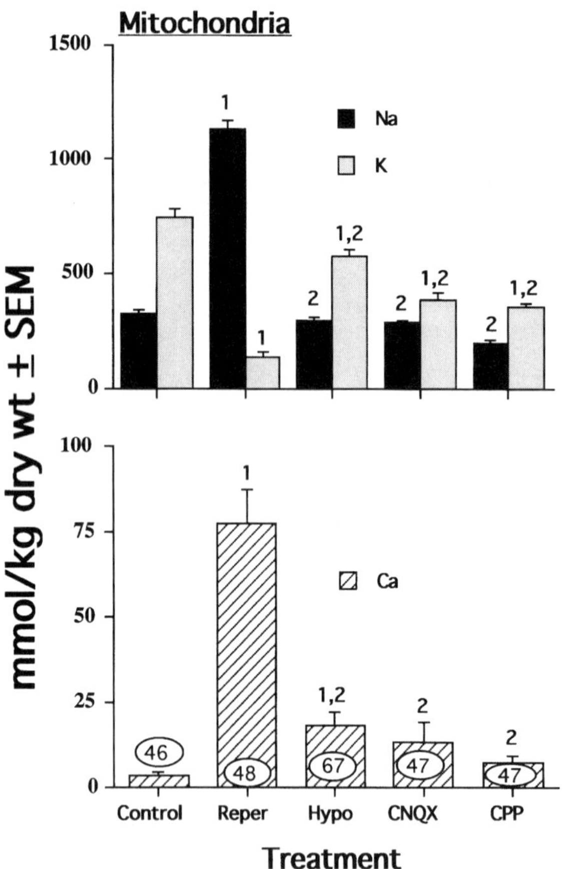

FIGURE 5. Mean (±SEM) dry weight Na, K (*upper panel*), and Ca (*lower panel*) concentrations (millimoles of element per kilogram) in hippocampal CA1 nerve cell mitochondria. Details as in FIGURE 4.

influx via reverse Na^+-Ca^{2+} exchanger operation. Our CNQX data support this potential mechanism of neuroprotection (see FIGS. 4–6).

In conclusion, present findings demonstrate that Na^+ channel blockade and glutamate receptor antagonism offer effective protection against intraneuronal ion disruption caused by an experimental *in vitro* ischemic episode. The magnitude and extent of pharmacologic protection are comparable to that associated with mild hypothermia, which has well documented neuroprotective abilities. These results suggest a complex pathophysiology for transient CNS oxygen-glucose deprivation involving Na^+ entry through voltage-gated Na^+ channels and ionophoric glutamate receptors. Intraneuronal Ca^{2+} influx appears to be mediated by several routes including glutamate-gated channels, reverse Na^+-Ca^{2+} exchanger and possibly L-type Ca^{2+} channels. Our studies of ischemic mechanisms are preliminary and form a basis for

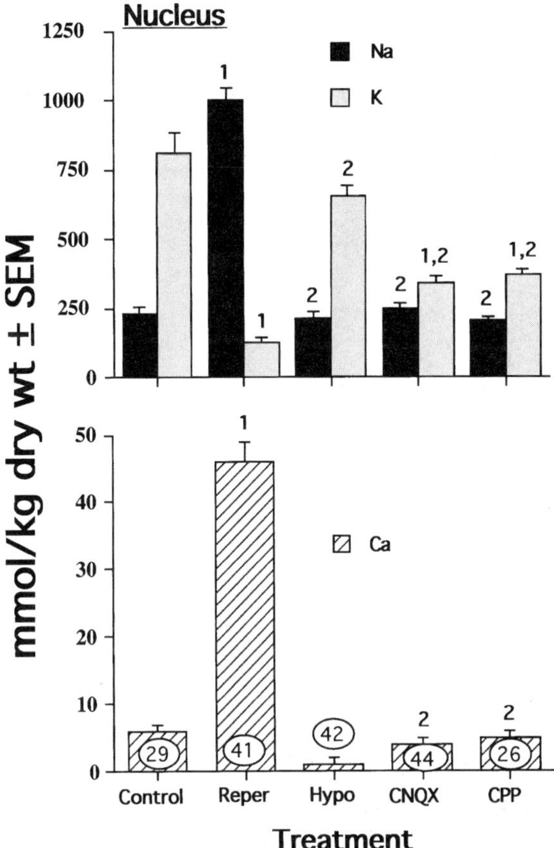

FIGURE 6. Mean (±SEM) dry weight Na, K (*upper panel*), and Ca (*lower panel*) concentrations (millimoles of element per kilogram) in hippocampal CA1 nerve cell nucleus. Details as in FIGURE 4.

more detailed research investigating routes of ion flux. Such research might lead to development of efficacious pharmacotherapies based on routes of neuronal ion movement during brain ischemia.[19,20,26]

ACKNOWLEDGMENTS

The research discussed in this paper was supported by a Research Initiation Grant from the Montefiore Medical Center and by the Parke-Davis Research Division, Ann Arbor, MI.

REFERENCES

1. SIESJO, B.K. 1992. Pathophysiology and treatment of focal cerebral ischemia. Part I: pathophysiology. J. Neurosci. **77:** 169–184.
2. MARTIN, R.L., H.G.E. LLOYD & A.I. COWAN. 1994. The early events of oxygen and glucose deprivation: setting the scene for neuronal death? Trends Neurosci. **17:** 251–257.
3. ERECINSKA, M. & I.A. SILVER. 1994. Ions and energy in mammalian brain. Prog. Neurobiol. **43:** 37–71.
4. BOUVIER, M., M. SZATKOWSKI, A. AMATO & D. ATTWELL. 1992. The glial cell glutamate uptake carrier countertranports pH-changing anions. Nature **360:** 471–474.
5. CHOI, D.W. & S.M. ROTHMAN. 1990. The role of glutamate neurotoxicity in hypoxic-ischemic neuronal death. Annu. Rev. Neurosci. **13:** 171–182.
6. CHOI, D.W. 1995. Calcium: still center-stage in hypoxic-ischemic neuronal death. Trends Neurosci. **18:** 58–60.
7. KRISTIAN, T. & B.K. SIESJO. 1996. Calcium-related damage in ischemia. Life Sci. **59:** 357–367.
8. HANSEN, A.J. 1985. Effects of anoxia on ion distribution in the brain. Physiol. Rev. **65:** 101–148.
9. TAYLOR, C.P., M.L. WEBER, C.L. GAUGHAN, E.J. LEHNING & R.M. LoPACHIN. 1999. Oxygen/glucose deprivation in hippocampal slices: altered intraneuronal elemental composition predicts structural and functional damage. J. Neurosci. **19:** 619–629.
10. LoPACHIN, R.M. 1995. Electron probe X-ray microanalysis as a tool for discerning mechanisms of nerve injury. *In* Neurotoxicology: Approaches and Methods. L. Chang & W. Slikker, Eds.: 445–453. Academic Press. San Diego, CA.
11. LoPACHIN, R.M., J. LOWERY, J. EICHBERG, J.B. KIRKPATRICK, J. CARTWRIGHT & A.J. SAUBERMANN. 1988. Distribution of elements in rat peripheral axons and nerve cell bodies determined by X-ray microprobe analysis. J. Neurochem. **51:** 764–775.
12. WEBER, M.L. & C.P. TAYLOR. 1994. Damage from oxygen and glucose deprivation in hippocampal slices is prevented by tetrodotoxin, lidocaine and phenytoin without blockade of action potentials. Brain Res. **664:** 167–177.
13. FOSTER, M.C. & A.J. SAUBERMANN. 1990. Personal-computer based system for electron beam X-ray microanalysis of biological samples. J. Microsc. **161:** 367–373.
14. HALL, T.A., H.C. ANDERSON & T. APPLETON. 1973. The use of thin specimens for X-ray microanalysis in biology. J. Microsc. **99:** 177–182.
15. BULGER, R.E., R. BEEUWKES & A.J. SAUBERMANN. 1981. Application of scanning electron microscopy to X-ray analysis of frozen-hydrated sections. III. Elemental content of cells in rat renal papillary tip. J. Cell Biol. **88:** 274–280.
16. TAYLOR, C.P. & M.L. WEBER. 1993. Effect of temperature on synaptic function after reduced oxygen and glucose in hippocampal slices. Neuroscience **52:** 555–562.
17. MORIKAWA, E., M.D. GINSBERG, W.D. DIETRICH, R.C. DUNCAN, S. KRAYDIEH, M.Y.-T. GLOBUS & R. BUSTO. 1992. The significance of brain temperature in focal cerebral ischemia: histopathological consequence of middle cerebral atrery occlusion in the rat. J. Cereb. Blood Flow Metab. **12:** 380–389.
18. XIE, Y., K. DENGLER, E. ZACHARIAS, B. WIFFERT & F. TEGTMEIER. 1994. Effects of the sodium channel blocker tetrodotoxin (TTX) on cellular ion homeostasis in rat brain subjected to complete ischaemia. Brain Res. **652:** 216–224.
19. URENJAK, J. & T.P. OBRENOVITCH. 1996. Pharmacological modulation of voltage-gated Na channels: a rational and effective strategy against ischemic brain damage. Pharmacol. Rev. **48:** 21–67.
20. TAYLOR, C.P. & B.S. MELDRUM. 1995. Na$^+$ channels as targets for neuroprotective drugs. Trends Neurosci. **16:** 309–316.

21. Stys, P.K. & R.M. LoPachin. 1998. Mechanisms of calcium and sodium fluxes in anoxic myelinated central nervous system axons. Neuroscience **82:** 21–32.
22. Goldberg, M.P. & D.W. Choi. 1993. Combined oxygen and glucose deprivation in cortical cell culture: calcium-dependent and calcium-independent mechanisms of neuronal injury. J. Neurosci. **13:** 3510–3524.
23. Takakura, S., K. Sogabe, H. Satoh, J. Mori, T. Fujiwara, Z. Totsuka, Y. Tokuma & M. Kohsaka. 1992. Nilvadipine as a neuroprotective calcium entry blocker in a rat model of global cerebral ischemia. A comparative study with nicardipine hydrochloride. Neurosci. Lett. **141:** 199–202.
24. Kimura, M., K. Sawada, T. Miyagawa, M. Kuwada, K. Katayama & Y. Nishizawa. 1998. Role of glutamate receptors and voltage-dependent calcium and sodium channels in the extracellular glutamate/aspartate accumulation and subsequent neuronal injury induced by oxygen/glucose deprivation in cultured hippocampal neurons. J. Pharmacol. Exp. Ther. **285:** 178–185.
25. Bickler, P.E. & B.M. Hansen. 1994. Causes of calcium accumulation in rat cortical brain slices during hypoxia and ischemia: role of ion channels and membrane damage. Brain Res. **669:** 269–276.
26. Dorman, P.J., C.E. Counsell & A.G. Sandercock. 1996. Recently developed neuroprotective therapies for acute stroke: a qualitative systematic review of clinical trials. CNS Drugs **5:** 457–474.

Matrix Remodeling after Stroke

De Novo Expression of Matrix Proteins and Integrin Receptors

JULIE A. ELLISON, FRANK C. BARONE, AND GIORA Z. FEUERSTEIN[a]

Department of Cardiovascular Pharmacology, SmithKline Beecham Pharmaceuticals, Philadelphia, Pennsylvania, USA

ABSTRACT: Following an ischemic insult to the central nervous system a reorganization of cells and tissue takes place as the surrounding cells attempt to limit the injury, repair the damage, and restore normal architecture of the brain. This tissue remodeling requires *de novo* synthesis of genes and proteins which enables cells to actively change their relationship with the existing extracellular matrix and with other cells to reorganize the damaged tissue. We have identified two key molecular components of the matrix remodeling process after focal ischemia: osteopontin (OPN) and its integrin receptor $\alpha_v\beta_3$ ($\alpha_v\beta_3$). OPN is initially expressed by activated macrophages and microglia in the periinfarct region (24–48 hr) and at later times (5–15 days) in the core infarct. After focal stroke the $\alpha_v\beta_3$ was upregulated by astrocytes in the periinfarct region. Spatial and temporal analyses demonstrated that at 5 days after injury the $\alpha_v\beta_3$-positive astrocytes were at a distance from the osteopontin-expressing macrophages; by 15 days the $\alpha_v\beta_3$-expressing astrocytes were localized within an osteopontin-rich matrix. *In vitro* OPN was shown to induce migration of astrocytes in a Boyden chamber system. These data suggest that OPN derived from microglia at the infarct border zone (and possible macrophages in the infarct core) may serve as an "astrokine" (suggested term for astrocyte chemoattractant) to organize the astrocyte scar after focal stroke. Our data demonstrate profound changes in brain matrix remodeling after focal ischemic stroke, including the synthesis and release of matrix proteins alien to the normal brain, the expresion of integrin receptors that ligate these proteins, and possibly a novel function for microglial-derived OPN in astrocyte migration after focal ischemia that may drive glial activation, organization, and repair functions.

INTRODUCTION

Inflammation is a cellular response following injury to a vascularized tissue. After an ischemic insult to the brain the injured endothelium, glia, and neurons release cytokines and chemokines that recruit activated peripheral immune cells to the site of injury. Subsequently these immune cells secrete inflammatory mediators that generate the classic brain response to injury characterized by astrocytic gliosis[1–5] and

[a]Address for correspondence: Giora Z. Feuerstein, M.D., MS.c., Senior Director of Cardiovascular Research, Dupont Pharmaceuticals, Experimental Station E400/3255, Route 141 and Henry Clay Road, Wilmington, DE 19880-0400. Phone, 302/695-1840; fax, 302/695-4162.
e-mail, giora.z.feuerstein@dupontpharma.com

microglial activation.[6,7] Investigations of inflammation after brain ischemia have focused upon the acute sequelae of inflammation documenting a cascade of novel gene expression associated with cell activation and recruitment to the site of injury. Little attention has been given to the initial inflammatory signals that are responsible for restoring the cellular homeostasis and tissue integrity. While the initial recruitment of leukocytes to the injured brain can be viewed negatively, in fact macrophages are critical for establishing the milieu necessary for debridement and repair of the injured tissue.[8] Thus it might be argued that the purpose of the inflammatory response after focal stroke is to activate and recruit cells to mediate the repair of brain injury by: 1) activation of glia in the periinfarct region; 2) compartmentalization of the injured cells; 3) removal of the infarcted tissue debris by phagocytes; 4) stimulation of angiogenesis and 5) establishment of a new glial-pial boundary if necessary.

Comparison of the inflammatory response in the brain with that seen in peripheral organs supports the idea that the brain inflammatory response uses the same effector molecules to generate the acute response. Studies have revealed that the de novo synthesis of cytokines, chemokines, and adhesion molecules occurs in the brain as in the periphery in response to injury.[9] However very little work has been conducted to understand the late resolution phase of the inflammatory reaction. While attenuating the early inflammatory response appears to be important, it is the wound healing response that ultimately confines the injury and remodels the cellular and structural elements to restore homeostasis thus permitting an environment conducive to regeneration. Wound healing after injury to the central nervous system is generally considered within the broad context of gliosis, which for decades has been portrayed in an entirely negative context: gliosis is the barrier to regeneration. This focus solely upon astrocytes, gliosis and scar formation as negative elements has skewed our perception of wound healing in the central nervous system (CNS). In fact recent studies present a much more complex picture of wound healing after brain injury as a cellular response that limits and contains the injury, and potentially can provide a positive environment for regeneration.[3,10–12]

In this review we will briefly present key aspects of the acute inflammatory response after focal brain ischemia. The cascade of new gene expression that unfolds following focal stroke will be outlined. Furthermore the roles of two key cytokines, tumor necrosis factor alpha (TNFα) and interleukin-1 beta (IL-1β), and the cooperative actions of adhesion molecules in the acute inflammatory response will be discussed. The main focus of the review will be upon the late matrix remodeling and wound healing process initiated in response to the ischemic insult. Although often considered as a single event, inflammation and wound healing can be considered as two responses to injury; the inflammation occurs early (hours, days) after the injury while the wound healing occurs later (days, weeks) after the insult. Recent data concerning the complex wound healing response of the brain will be presented with data from our laboratory illustrating the need to consider wound healing as a necessary aspect of restoring homeostasis after injury.

NEW GENE EXPRESSION AFTER FOCAL STROKE

Focal ischemia is a powerful stimulus to elicit genomic responses in the brain. The pattern of gene expression induced by ischemia is exhibited as "waves" of sequential genes expressed over different time points. FIGURE 1 illustrates that in response to ischemia many genes exhibit an increased expression. Transcription factors (immediate early genes; IEG) are the first "wave" as shown by members of the fos and jun families that are rapidly and transiently upregulated.[13–17] A second "wave" consists of the heat shock proteins (HSPs). Heat shock protein mRNA is usually expressed within 1–2 hours and then downregulated by 1–2 days.[13,15] Of great interest is the third "wave," which initially was charaterized by the initiation of the classic inflammatory gene expression cascade but has now been expanded to include expression of neurotrophic factors and cell death mediators. Genes induced in the inflammatory cascade include TNFα and IL-1β,[18–20] IL-6,[17] IL-8 and monocyte chemoattractant protein 1 (MCP-1).[21,22] This third "wave" is likely to play a significant role in the initiation of endothelial priming prior to neutrophil and monocyte infiltration. In addition to cytokine gene induction, adhesion molecule expression such as intercellular adhesion molecule 1 (ICAM-1), endothelial leukocyte adhesion molecule 1 (ELAM-1) and P-selectin is also increased.[23–25] These adhesion molecules are crucial for leukocyte adhesion to the endothelium prior to infiltration. Several neurotrophic factor genes are induced after ischemia. In several models of ischemic insult to the brain, brain-derived neurotropic factor (BDNF), nerve growth factor (NGF) and basic fibroblast growth factor (bFGF) increase within the first 24 hours after injury.[16,26–29] More recently, we have identified a fourth "wave" of new gene expression that may well be associated with the acute inflammatory reaction to brain ischemia. This fourth "wave" includes proteolytic enzymes (metalloproteinases; Col9/2) implicated in damage to extracellular matrix,[26,30] and their endogenous protease inhibitors after focal stroke. The expression of these genes in stroke appears to be related to the influx of inflammatory cells and is associated with secondary brain injury and repair processes after stroke. The fifth "wave" of new gene expression includes mediators such as transforming growth factor beta (TGF-β) and osteopontin, which may be important in tissue remodeling.

INFLAMMATION, TNFα, IL-1β AND BRAIN ISCHEMIA

The response to injury in peripheral organs is manifested by the rapid production of a wide array of inflammatory mediators that initiate inflammatory processes. A key mediator of this response is TNFα, which may act as a pleiotropic peptide to elicit the production of other cytokines (e.g., IL-1β, IL-6 and IL-8), endothelial cell adhesion molecules (e.g., ELAM-1, ICAM-1, and vascular cell adhesion molecule 1 (VCAM-1)), and surface adhesion ligands on neutrophils and monocytes (e.g., very late antigen 4 (VLA-4), leukocyte function-associated antigen 1 (LFA-1) and Mac-1 integrins; for reviews see Refs. 27–34). The resultant activation of endothelial-cell adhesion molecules promotes neutrophil adherence to activated endothelium—a key event in the inflammatory reaction. The initiation of the inflammatory response in the brain is believed to be triggered by TNFα, the mRNA and protein both increasing after brain ischemia.[19,20,31,35] After middle cerebral artery occlusion (MCAO) TNFα mRNA is elevated in the infarcted zone as early as 1 hour post-occlusion with peak expression at 12 hours and persistent expression for about 5 days. The early expression of TNFα mRNA prior to leukocyte infiltration suggests that TNFα may be involved in this response. TNFα has been localized to neurons and astrocytes.[19] The functional significance of TNFα expression in the brain was studied by microinjection of TNFα into the rat cortex; TNFα induced leukocyte adhesion to the capillary endothelium, but no evidence for neurotoxicity at the site of injection was found. Therefore, TNFα may exert a primary effect on microvascular inflammatory response as reflected by neutrophil adhesion to brain capillary endothelium. The injection of TNFα into the cerebroventricular space prior to injury exacerbated the ischemic injury.[32,36] Additional evidence for the effect of TNFα comes from *in vitro* studies demonstrating that addition of TNFα to endothelial cells cause a cytoskeletal rearrangement of endothelial cells such that a sheet of endothelial cells has long-lasting increases in permeability.[33,37] These data suggest that TNFα may prime the brain for subsequent damage by activating capillary endothelium to a "partial," proadhesive state possible through the upregulation of surface endothelial adhesion molecules, and by contributing to vascular leakiness essential for leukocyte diapedesis.[34,38]

The early accumulation of neutrophils after ischemic brain damages has been clearly demonstrated based upon histological,[3,35–44] biochemical (increased myeloperoxidase activity[41–43,45–47] and ^{111}In-labeled leukocyte studies.[44,48] It is postulated that neutrophils induce tissue damage due to their vascular plugging and rheologic effects, and by their generation and release of oxygen radicals and cytotoxic products as they are activated in ischemic tissue.[40,44–52]

IL-1β, like TNFα, is one of the initiating molecules in the inflammatory process. IL-1β is a cytokine with multiple proinflammatory and cell-growth modulatory actions.[49,53] Like TNFα, IL-1β modulates endothelial permeability.[27,31,33,.37] After focal stroke IL-1β mRNA is rapidly upregulated within 3–6 hours, peaks at 12 hours, and returns to basal levels at 5 days, mimicking the profile of TNFα.[18,20] Evidence that IL-1β may play a deleterious role after focal stroke is found in several studies utilizing overexpression of IL-1β or its endogenous antagonist IL-1 receptor antagonist (IL-1ra). Intracerebroventricular (ICV) injections of IL-1β enhances brain edema, increases the number of neutrophils in ischemic areas and increases neutrophil-endothelial cell adhesion.[50,54] Furthermore, ICV injections of IL-1β exacerbate the degree of infarction after MCAO,[51,55] whereas injections of IL-1ra and IL-1β antagonists reduce infarct size.[51–58]

As stated previously a cascade of de novo gene expression manifests the inflammatory response. Prominent in this response is the induction of adhesion molecules required for leukocyte infiltration by cytokines. Temporally the *in vivo* expression of cytokines precedes the expression of adhesion molecules (see above). *In vitro* studies have directly demonstrated induction of adhesion molecule expression by both TNFα and IL-1β. Endothelial cells exposed to TNFα and IL-1β had increased expression of ICAM-1.[55,59] Astrocytes exposed to TNFα and IL-1β increased expression of ICAM-1, VCAM-1, and E-selectin.[56–58,60–62] Microglia exposed to TNFα and IL-1β had increased expression of ICAM-1, VCAM-1, and β1 and β2 integrins.[59,63] *In vivo* after MCAO, ICAM-1 is upregulated in microvessels as early as 1 hour after injury.[24,60,64] At 24 hours, when leukocytes are entering the brain in increasing numbers, these cell populations expressed ICAM-1 and continued to express this adhesion molecule for 7 days. In the nonhuman primate MCAO model P-selectin and ICAM-1 were shown to be upregulated and similarly localized to the endothelium.[23] While the expression of adhesion molecules associated with leukocyte trafficking into the brain after injury appears to be well documented, the expression of adhesion molecules and associated matrix molecules that mediate matrix remodeling and regeneration within the brain parenchyma is just beginning to be mapped out.

WOUND HEALING IN THE BRAIN

Following an ischemic insult to the central nervous system a massive reorganization of cells and tissue takes place as the surrounding cells attempt to limit the injury, repair the damage and restore the normal architecture of the brain. This tissue remodeling requires de novo synthesis of proteins (largely via gene transcription), which enable cells to actively change their relationship with the existing extracellular matrix (ECM) and with other cells to reorganize the damaged tissue. The induced genetic response to effect matrix remodeling falls into three general categories: matrix proteases, extracellular matrix molecules, and integrins. Together these three categories of molecules enable cells to initiate a classic wound healing response as dead cells are removed and the remaining tissue is remodeled to form scar tissue.

Both astrocytes and microglia must alter their association with the ECM as a precursor to changes in cell shape, proliferation and migration. This is accomplished by altering the presentation of integrin receptors coupled with synthesis and secretion of new ECM and matrix proteases to degrade and reformat existing cell-matrix associations. Integrin receptor couple intracellular cytoskeletal elements and associated signaling molecules such as those found at focal adhesion sites with ECM molecules. Once thought to simply anchor the cell to the matrix, recent studies have demonstrated a dynamic role for integrin receptors that transduce signals in both an outside-in and inside-out direction.[61,65] In addition to synthesizing a set of integrin receptors specifically for matrix remodeling, cells synthesize provisional extracellular matrix molecules, which allow for the dynamic adherence and attachment required for changes in cell shape, proliferation and migration.

The central nervous system contains very few of the classic extracellular matrix molecules that are found in the peripheral tissues. Only two sites in the brain, the blood vessels and the glial limitans at the pial surface, have basal lamina containing classic basal lamina molecules,[62,66] such as collagen, thrombospondin, fibronectin, laminin and vitronectin.[63–65,67–69] Within the interstitial matrix of the adult brain the predominant ECM components are hyaluronan, hyaluronan-binding proteoglycans such as members of the aggrecan family, versican and brevican and glycoproteins such as members of the tenascin family.[66–68,70–72] During the development of the brain the molecular composition of the chondroitin-sulfate proteoglycans change dramatically to reflect the maturation of synaptic contacts[67,71] concomitant with a decreasing extracellular space that exists in the adult brain.[69,70,73,74] The extracellular space of the adult nervous system is not permissive for the type of proliferation and migration that occurs after an ischemic insult.[71,75] Thus after an insult to the adult nervous system the ECM must be modified though de novo synthesis of key matrix proteases, ECM components and integrin receptors to allow microglia, astrocytes, and exogenous leukocytes the space to migrate and repair the injured tissue.

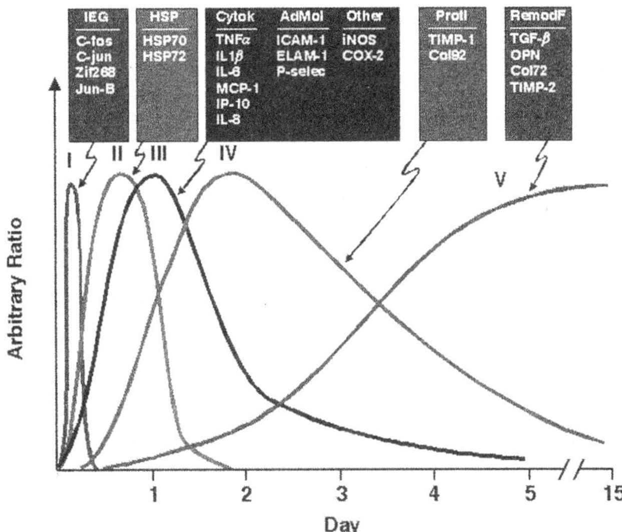

FIGURE 1. Time course of gene expression after focal ischemia in the rat cortex induced by middle cerebral artery occlusion. Five waves of gene expression include a broad range of upregulated transcription factors (phase 1); heat-shock proteins (phase 2); proinflammatory mediators including cytokines, chemokines, adhesion molecules, and growth factors (phase 3); protease and protease inhibitor gene expression (phase 4); and delayed remodeling of proteins involved in resolution of the tissue injury (phase 6).

OSTEOPONTIN, A PROVISIONAL MATRIX MOLECULE

Many matrix molecules that are upregulated after brain injury are also expressed during the development of the nervous system.[10,72,76] Their expression after injury is presumed to recapitulate the remodeling processes that formed the cytoarchitecture initially. We have recently identified expression of matrix protein, osteopontin (OPN) that does not appear to be expressed as a matrix protein during nervous system development, but is upregulated after focal stroke.

Osteopontin, an integrin ligand, is an acidic, secreted 41-kDa phosphoprotein containing an arginine-glycine-aspartate (RGD) recognition site, was originally identified as a bone matrix protein and was subsequently localized to kidney, placenta, and blood vessels.[73,74,77,78] OPN interacts with multiple integrin receptors to effect cell adhesion, migration, and phagocytosis depending upon the specific integrin receptor. The functions of OPN have been extensively studied in peripheral smooth muscle cells, endothelial cells and macrophages. Functionally, OPN has chemotactic activity for smooth muscle cells and endothelial cells[75,76,79,80] regulating cell adhesion and migration[77,81] by interacting with three different integrin receptors $\alpha_v\beta_1$, $\alpha_v\beta_3$, and $\alpha_v\beta_5$. Cell adhesion is mediated by integrin receptors $\alpha_v\beta_1$ and

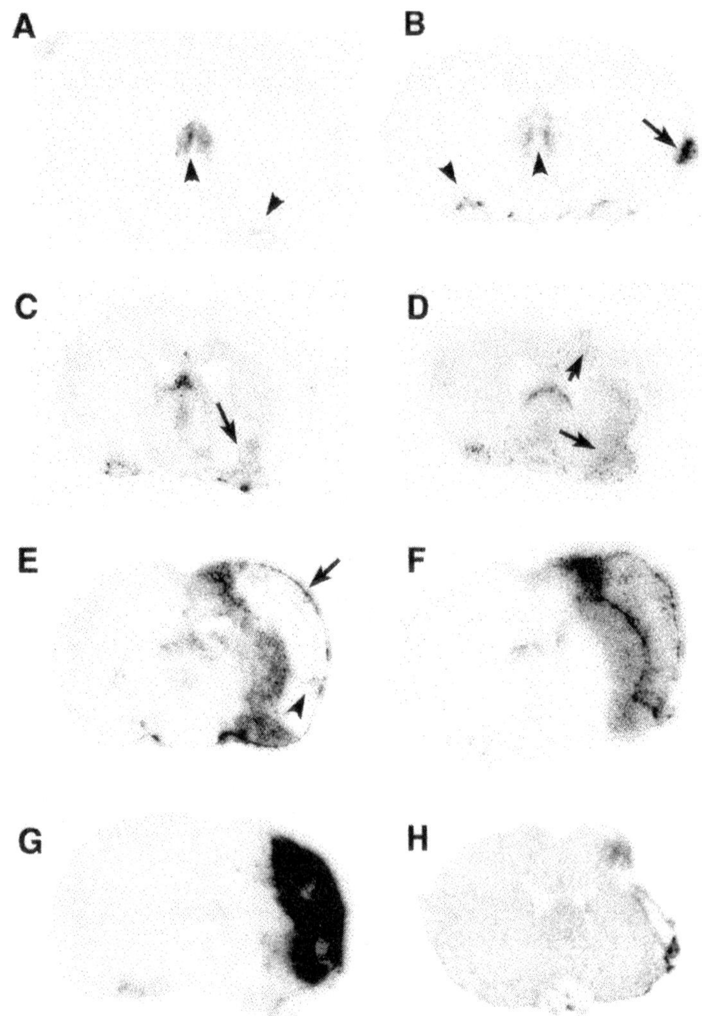

FIGURE 2. OPN gene expression after focal stroke. By *in situ* hybridization OPN mRNA expression is constitutively expressed in the septal nucleus and in ventral brain nuclei (**A**, *arrowheads*). In sham animals OPN mRNA was induced at the surgery site (**B**, *arrow*). At 3 hours (**C**) and 6 hours (**D**) OPN mRNA was induced in cells initially at the ventromedial aspect (C, *arrow*) and continuing to the dorsomedial aspect (D, *arrows*) of the infarct. At 24 hours cells expressing OPN mRNA are still largely confined to the periinfarct region (**E**) with expression at the pial surface (*arrow*) and by a few cells in the infarct (*arrowhead*). At 48 hours (**F**) more cells within the infarct expressed OPN mRNA; by 5 days (**G**) the majority of cells expressing OPN mRNA are within the infarct with little expression in the periinfarct region. At 15 days (**H**) mRNA levels returned to those found in naive rats.

$\alpha_v\beta_5$,[78,82] while integrin receptor $\alpha_v\beta_3$ mediates cell migration.[77,81] Two inflammatory cytokines, IL-1β and TNFα, upregulate expression of OPN in macrophages[83] and in osteoblasts,[84] demonstrating that cytokine expression can initiate the wound healing process. OPN expression has been associated with a number of disease processes involving extensive matrix remodeling including neointima formation in carotid arteries subjected to balloon angioplasty,[79,80,85,86] human atherosclerotic plaques,[79–81,87] myocardial injury[82,88] and renal tubulointerstitial fibrosis.[83,84,89,90] Furthermore, mice lacking a functional OPN gene display significantly decreased levels of debridement and greater disorganization of matrix during healing of an incisional skin wound.[91] Since extensive matrix remodeling occurs after focal ischemia in the brain, we considered that OPN might be upregulated following this insult.[12,92]

Our studies demonstrated that OPN mRNA was maximally expressed at 5 days postischemia (FIG. 1). Initial expression was seen at 3 hours after stroke; and by *in situ* hybridization was localized to the ventral medial aspect of the periinfarct border. With time OPN mRNA increased in the periinfarct region such that by 24 hours the core infarct was delineated by the surrounding cells expressing this mRNA. At 24 hours OPN protein is initially seen in quiescent microglia at the infarct border (FIG. 2) and during 2–5 days after injury is seen within activated macrophages and secreted into the extracellular space (FIG. 2). OPN protein was expressed at very high levels by macrophages in the infarct core at 5 days after focal stroke, and by 15 days levels had decreased significantly with expression restricted to an area of tissue adjacent to the newly formed pial surface.

To establish a functional role for the secreted OPN we conducted a migration assay using OPN and found that OPN had the capacity to induce directed migration of astrocytes.[92] In other models[82,86,88,93] where OPN expression was seen in conjunction with matrix modeling, the integrin receptor $\alpha_v\beta_3$ appeared to be one of the receptors modulating cell-OPN interactions. Moreover, upregulation of $\alpha_v\beta_3$ has been reported to be essential for endothelial transformation to an angiogenic phenotype[87,94] and for migration toward an OPN gradient.[74,78]

EXPRESSION OF INTEGRIN RECEPTORS AFTER BRAIN ISCHEMIA

Integrins are a family of transmembrane glycoprotein receptors that couple intracellular cytoskeletal elements with extracellular matrix molecules. Integrins exist as $\alpha\beta$ heterodimers that associate at their extracellular domains. Both the α and β subunit contribute to the ligand binding domain. Integrin receptors can recognize more than one ligand and likewise individual ligands can recognize and bind more than one integrin. One of the classic recognition sites in ECMs such as fibronectin, vitronectin, osteopontin is the Arg-Gly-Asp (RGD) sequence.[61,65]

Research into integrin receptor and associated ligand expression after focal stroke is in its infancy. Most of the work to date has focused upon the role of integrin receptors in modulating early events associated with vascular changes after an ischemic insult. Two integrins receptors, $\alpha_v\beta_3$ and $\alpha_6\beta_4$ have been suggested to play a role in vascular integrity and remodeling following focal ischemia within the infarcted area.[88,89,95,96] In a nonhuman primate model of transient forebrain ischemia the integrin receptor $\alpha_v\beta_3$ was upregulated early (hours) in the ischemic event concomitant with an increase in one of its ligands, fibrinogen. Conversely in another study,

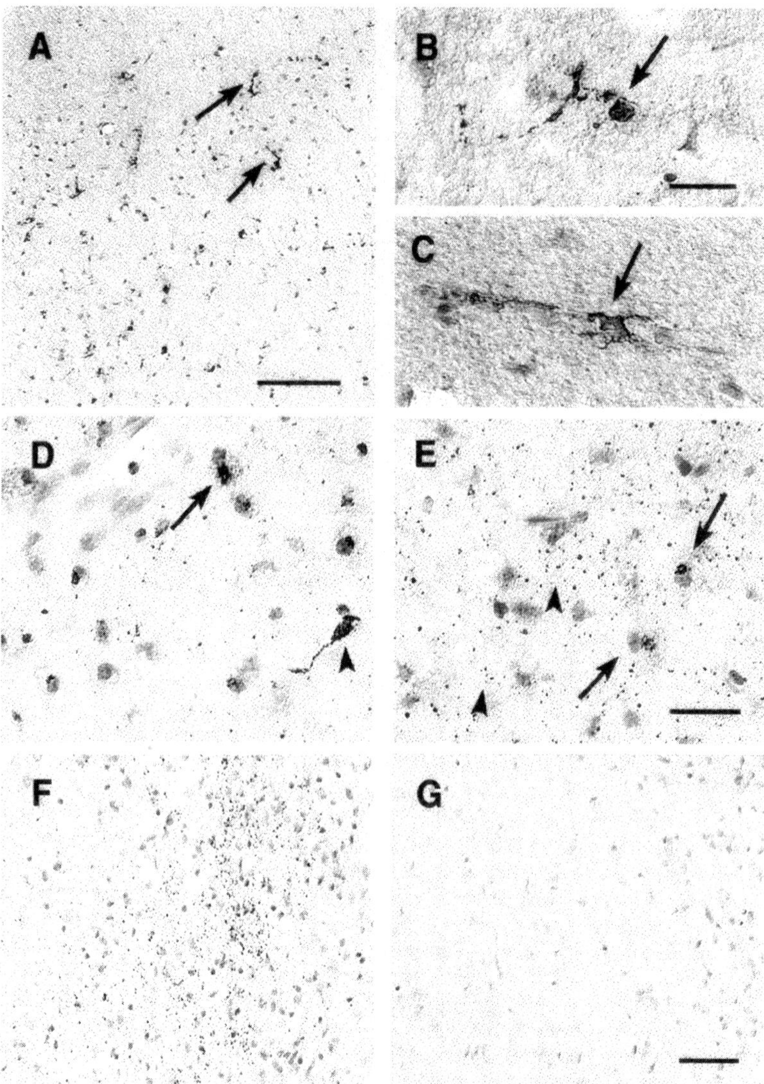

FIGURE 3. OPN protein expression in microglia and macrophages. At 24 hours OPN was expressed by microglia in the periinfarct region (**A**, *arrows*); the microglia have a ramified appearance (**B,C**, *arrows*) and do not appear activated. At 48 hours, occasional microglia (**D**, *arrowhead*) expressing OPN are seen with the majority of OPN expressed by macrophages (D, *arrow*). By 5 days OPN was seen in a perinuclear location intracellularly (**E**, *arrows*) and in the extracellular matrix (E, *arrowheads*). At 15 days OPN expression was restricted to a thin area adjacent to the pial surface (**F**). No immunoperoxidase reaction was detected in the absence of primary antibody at any timepoint (**G**). Scale bar for (A) is 100 μm; (B,C) is 20 μm; (D,E) is 40 μm; (F,G) is 100 μm.

the expression of integrin receptor $\alpha_6\beta_4$ and one of its ligands, laminin were both shown to decrease following ischemia.

Given the potential role of integrin receptors in matrix remodeling of the interstitial brain matrix at sites distal to the vasculature we undertook a study to determine the expression of integrin receptor $\alpha_v\beta_3$ after focal stroke.[12] The OPN receptor, integrin $\alpha_v\beta_3$ is expressed by astrocytes at 5 days and 15 days postischemia (FIG. 3). These timepoints were chosen to identify potential cell populations that could interact with the OPN in the extracellular matrix. At 5 days postischemia astrocytes expressing integrin receptor $\alpha_v\beta_3$ are dispersed in the periinfarct region; by 15 days these cells have reformed the glial limitans at the pial surface lost initially due to tissue injury following focal stroke. These data were intriguing as astrocytes *in vitro* express $\alpha_v\beta_3$[90,97] and radial glial of the developing nervous system have been reported to express integrin α_v.[91,98] Hirsch and colleagues[91,98] suggest that this integrin might be involved in the formation and orientation of the glial fibers that extend from

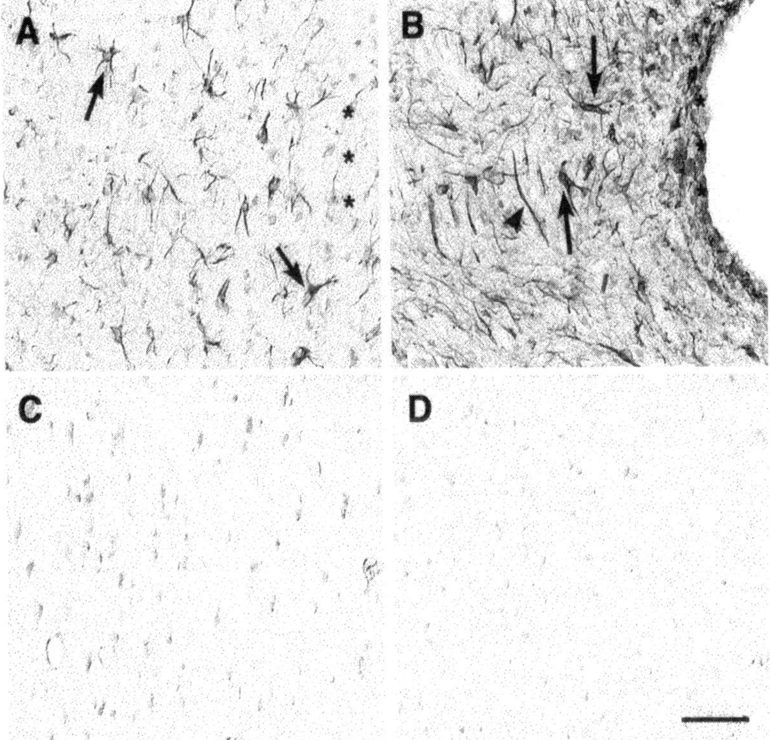

FIGURE 4. Integrin $\alpha_v\beta_3$ expression at 5 and 15 days post occlusion. The integrin $\alpha_v\beta_3$ was upregulated at 5 days in the ipsilateral cortex (**A**) as compared to the contralateral cortex (**C**). Integrin $\alpha_v\beta_3$ was expressed by cells (A, *arrows*) adjacent to the infarct (periinfarct/infarct border identified by *asterisks*). By 15 days cells expressing integrin $\alpha_v\beta_3$ (**B**, *arrows*) had elongated cells processes (B, *arrowhead*) and were found adjacent to and at the glial-pial boundary (identified by *asterisks*). Scale bar for (A,B) is 100 μm; for (C,D) is 40 μm.

the ventricular zone to the cortical plate. Similarly, the astrocytes expressing $\alpha_v\beta_3$ following focal ischemia reorganize from a stellate morphology to the more bipolar morphology characteristic of astrocytes of the glial limitans. These results presented demonstrate the diverse role integrin receptors might have in tissue remodeling. In addition to a role in vascular remodeling seen early following focal stroke[88,89,95,96] these findings suggest that integrin receptor $\alpha_v\beta_3$ participates in nonvascular remodeling associated with formation of a glial scar, which occurs late in the resolution of the ischemic insult.

INTERACTION OF OSTEOPONTIN WITH INTEGRIN RECEPTOR $\alpha_v\beta_3$

To explore potential functional aspects of the interaction between OPN and integrin receptor $\alpha_v\beta_3$ we established the timing of receptor-ligand interaction (FIG. 4). The spatial-temporal interaction of extracellular OPN ligand and integrin receptor $\alpha_v\beta_3$ is at a distance at 5 days. However, by 15 days the astrocytes are localized within a matrix of OPN, suggesting that OPN may act as a chemotactic factor for astrocytes. This *in vivo* demonstration of an OPN gradient at a distance from astrocytes early in the formation of the glial scar followed by localization of astrocytes within an OPN-rich extracellular region suggests the findings of OPN as a chemotactic factor, an "astrokine," *in vitro* may also be true *in vivo*.

How might OPN act to stimulate astrocyte process elongation and migration via the integrin receptor $\alpha_v\beta_3$? Ligation of integrin receptor $\alpha_v\beta_3$ by OPN ligand results in the rapid production of phosphoinositides.[92,99] Astrocytic hypertrophy and migration are dependent upon glial fibrillary acidic protein (GFAP), the predominant intermediate filament expressed by these cells. The assembly/disassembly of GFAP is Ca^{2+} dependent,[93,100] and inositol-1,4,5-triphosphate (IP$_3$)-induced Ca^{2+} release in astrocytes is directed by the type 3-inositol-1,4,5-trisphosphate receptor.[94,101] Thus OPN ligand binding to integrin receptor $\alpha_v\beta_3$ could stimulate release of intracellular Ca^{2+} stores causing a subsequent reorganization of the GFAP filament network.

Ligation of integrin receptors also mediates changes in gene expression. For instance, signaling through the fibronection and tenascin integrin receptors upregulated synthesis of matrix proteases in fibroblast.[95,102] In endothelial cells integrin ligation promoted cell survival by suppressing p53 activity, and by increasing the bcl-2/bax ratio.[96,103] Although no datum exists regarding integrin-mediated gene induction in astrocytes, the activation of astrocytes, their transformation to migratory cells and subsequent acquisition of a pial astrocyte phenotype strongly suggests that a change in gene expression does occur.

MULTIFUNCTIONAL ROLES OF OSTEOPONTIN
AFTER ISCHEMIC INJURY

The OPN gene is induced within 3 hours of an ischemic insult to the brain. This early gene expression suggests OPN might function as a stress response gene following focal ischemia. An acute phase response element has been identified within the promoter region of the OPN gene.[97,104] *In vitro* cells adhered to OPN have enhanced

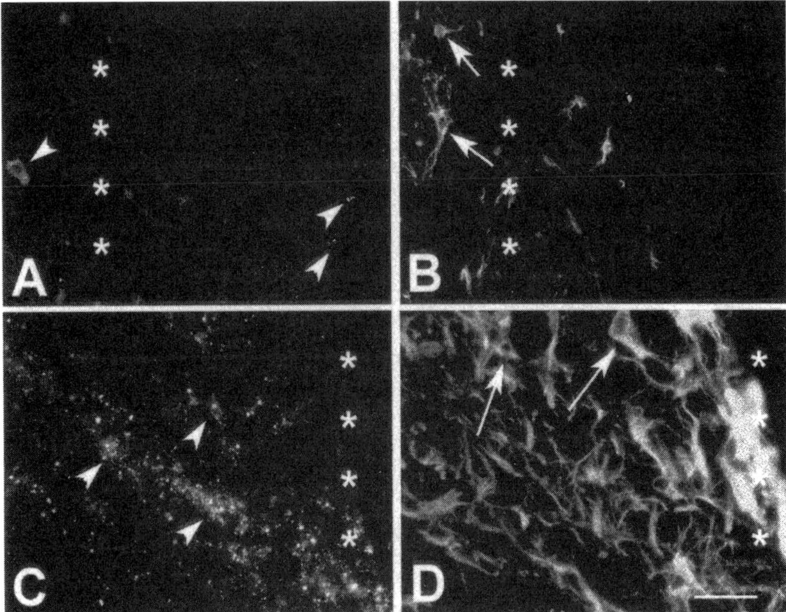

FIGURE 5. Timing of OPN-integrin $\alpha_v\beta_3$ interaction. Double immunofluorescence at 5 **(A,B)** and 15 **(C,D)** days demonstrated that at 5 days GFAP + astrocytes (B, *arrows*) were at a distance from extracellular OPN (A, *arrowheads*) which was localized to the core infarct (to the right of the *asterisks*). By 15 days GFAP + astrocytes (C, *arrowheads*) were found within a matrix of OPN (D, *arrows*). The medial periinfarct/infarct border with a large infarct region to the right (A,B), and the glial-pial boundary (C,D) are indicated by *asterisks*. Scale bar is 20 μm.

expression of heat shock proteins, and display a greater resistance to heat shock injury[98,105] Furthermore, OPN confers cellular resistance to the damaging effects of nitric oxide and oxidative burst associated with inflammation by inhibiting induction of nitric oxide synthase,[99,106] suggesting that in addition to mediating cell attachment and migration OPN has protective roles.[100,107] An inflammatory response after focal stroke has been clearly demonstrated;[9] thus it is not inconsistent that the cells responsible for clearing tissue debris and remodeling the matrix require protection from the toxic environment of the ischemic region.

SUMMARY

The glial cell (astrocyte and microglia) response to brain injury is complex. One of the best understood responses is a classic wound healing response[3] with formation of a barrier between the injured and healthy tissue.[10,101,102] Historically the glial scar has been considered the singular barrier that must be prevented for restoration of normal brain function. However, many recent studies have suggested that the formation of a glial scar contrigutes to the walling off of the injury zone from the uninjured tissue, thus protecting healthy cells from death as a result of the injury spreading.[10,12,101] Indeed in our model of focal stroke the glial scar formed in the early stages of an injury develops into a new glial limitans reestablishing the interface of the glial-pial boundary. Without this type of matrix remodeling the injury might increase in size, and the surface of the brain remain exposed.

These early events (hours, days) can probably be distinguished from later regenerative events (weeks, months) related to reestablishment of axonal connections and restoration of the normal cytoarchitecture of the brain. It is at this later time once the acute injury has been confined that these provisional matrix proteins, matrix enzymes and integrin receptors might possibly prevent the regeneration. Taken together, our data demonstrate profound changes in brain matrix remodeling following focal ischemic stroke, including the synthesis and release of matrix proteins alien to the normal brain, the expression of integrin receptors that ligate these proteins, and possibly a novel function for microglial-derived OPN in astrocyte migration following focal ischemia that may drive glial activation, organization and repair functions.

REFERENCES

1. PERRY, V.H. & S. GORDON. 1991. Macrophages and the nervous system. Int. Rev. Cytol. **125:** 203–244.
2. PETITO, C.K., S. MORGELLO, J.C. FELIX & M.L. LESSER. 1990. The two patterns of reactive astrocytosis in postischemic rat brain. J. Cereb. Blood Flow Metab. **10**(6): 850–859.
3. CLARK, R.K., E.V. LEE, C.J. FISH, R.F. WHITE, W.J. PRICE, Z.L. JONAK, G.Z. FEUERSTEIN & F.C. BARONE. 1993. Development of tissue damage, inflammation and resolution following stroke: an immunohistochemical and quantitative planimetric study. Brain Res. Bull. **31:** 565–572.
4. GARCIA, J.H., Y. YOSHIDA, H. CHEN, Y. LI, Z.G. ZHANG, J. LIAN, S. CHEN & M. CHOPP. 1993. Progression from ischemic injury to infarct following middle cerebral artery occlusion in the rat. Am. J. Pathol. **142**(2): 623–535.
5. LI, Y., M. CHOPP, Z.G. ZHANG & R.L. ZHANG. 1995. Expression of glial fibrillary acidic protein in areas of focal cerebral ischemia accompanies neuronal expression of 72-kDa heat shock protein. J. Neurol. Sci. **128**(2): 134–142.
6. GEHRMANN, J., P. BONNEKOH, T. MIYAZAWA, K.A. HOSSMANN & G.W. KREUTZBERG. 1992. Immunocytochemical study of an early microglial activation in ischemia. J. Cereb. Blood Flow Metab. **12**(2): 257–269.
7. KATO, H., K. KOGURE, T. ARAKI & Y. ITOYAMA. 1995. Graded expression of immunomolecules on activated microglia in the hippocampus following ischemia in a rat model of ischemic tolerance. Brain Res. **694:** 85–93.
8. LEIBOVICH, S.J. & R. ROSS. 1975. The role of the macrophage in wound repair. Am. J. Pathol. **78:** 71–100.
9. FEUERSTEIN, G.Z., X.K. WANG & F.C. BARONE. 1996. Inflammation-related gene expression and stroke: implications for new therapeutic targets. *In* Pharmacology of Cerebral Ischemia. J. Krieglestein, Ed.: 405–419. MedPharm Scientific Publishers. Stuttgart.
10. FITCH, M.T. & J. SILVER. 1997. Activated macrophages and the blood-brain barrier: inflammation after CNS injury leads to increases in putative inhibitory molecules. Exp. Neurol. **148:** 587–603.
11. LEHRMANN, E., T. CHRISTENSEN, J. ZIMMER, N.H. DIEMER & B. FINSEN. 1997. Microglial and macrophage reactions mark progressive changes and define the penumbra in the rat neocortex and striatum after transient middle cerebral artery occlusion. J. Comp. Neurol. **386:** 461–476.

12. ELLISON, J.A., J.J. VELIER, P. SPERA, Z.L. JONAK, X. WANG, F.C. BARONE & G.Z. FEUERSTEIN. 1998. Osteopontin and its integrin receptor $\alpha_v\beta_3$ are upregulated during formation of the glial scar after focal stroke. Stroke **29:** 1698–1706.

13. NOWAK, T.S., JR, J. IKEDA & T. NAKAJIMA. 1990. 70 kDa heat shock protein and c-fox gene expression after transient ischemia. Stroke **21**(Suppl. III)**:** 107–111.

14. UEMURA, Y., N.W. KOWALL & M.A. MOSKOWITZ. 1991. Focal ischemia in rats causes time-dependent expression of c-fox protein immunoreactivity in widespread regions of ipsilateral cortex. Brain Res. **552:** 99–105.

15. WELSH, F.A., D.J. MOYER & V.A. HARRIS. 1992. Regional expression of heat shock protein 70 mRNA and c-fos mRNA following focal ischemia in rat brain. J. Cereb. Blood Flow Metab. **12:** 204–212.

16. HSU, C.Y., G. AN, J.S. LIU, J.J. XUE, Y.Y. HE & T.N. LIN. 1993. Expression of immediate early gene and growth factor mRNAs in a focal cerebral ischemia model in the rat. Stroke **24:** I-78–I-81.

17. WANG, X.K., T.-L. YUE, P.R. YOUNG, F.C. BARONE & G.Z. FEUERSTEIN. 1995. Expression of interleukin-6, c-fox and zif268 mRNA in rat ischemic cortex. J. Cereb. Blood Flow Metab. **15:** 166–171.

18. LIU, T., P.C. MCDONNELL, P.R. YOUNG, R.F. WHITE, A.L. SIREN, F.C. BARONE & G.Z. FEUERSTEIN. 1993. Interleukin-1β mRNA expression in ischemic rat cortex. Stroke **24:** 125–128.

19. LIU, T., R.F. CLARK, P.C. MCDONNELL, P.R. YOUNG, R.F. WHITE, F.C. BARONE & G.Z. FEUERSTEIN. 1994. Tumor necrosis factor a expression in ischemia neurons. Stroke **25:** 1481–1488.

20. WANG, X.K., T.-L. YUE, F.C. BARONE, R.F. WHITE, P.R. YOUNG, P.C. MCDONNELL & G.Z. FEUERSTEIN. 1994. Concomitant cortical expression of TNFα and IL-1β mRNA following transient focal ischemia. Mol. Chem. Neuropathol. **23:** 103–114.

21. LIU, T., P.R. YOUNG, P.C. MCDONNELL, R.F. WHITE, F.C. BARONE & G.Z. FEUERSTEIN. 1993. Cytokine-induced neutrophil chemoattractant mRNA expressed in cerebral ischemia. Neurosci. Lett. **164:** 125–128.

22. WANG, X.K., T.-L. YUE, F.C. BARONE & G.Z. FEUERSTEIN. 1995. Monocyte chemoattractant protein-1 (MCP-1) mRNA expression in rat ischemic cortex. Stroke **26:** 661–666.

23. OKADA, Y., B.R. COPELAND, E. MORI, M.M. TUNG, W.S. THOMAS & G.J. DEL ZOPPO. 1994. P-selectin and intercellular adhesion molecule-1 expression after focal brain ischemia and reperfusion. Stroke **25:** 202–211.

24. WANG, X., A.-L. SIREN, Y. LIU, F.C. BARONE & G.Z. FEUERSTEIN. 1994. Upregulation of intercellular adhesion molecule 1 (ICAM-1) on brain microvascular endothelial cells in rat ischemia cortex. Mol. Brain Res. **26:** 61–68.

25. WANG, X.K., T.-L. YUE, F.C. BARONE & G.Z. FEUERSTEIN. 1995. Demonstration of increased endothelial-leukocyte adhesion molecule 1 mRNA expression in rat ischemic cortex. Stroke **26:** 1665–1669.

26. LINDVALL, O., P. ERNFORS, J. BENGZON, Z. KOKAIA, M.L. SMITH, B.K. SIESGO & H. PERSSON. 1992. Differential regulation of mRNAs for nerve growth factor, brain-derived neurotrophic factor, and neurotrophin 3 in the adult rat brain following cerebral ischemia and hypoglycemic coma. Proc. Natl. Acad. Sci. USA **89:** 648–652.

27. TAKEDA, A., H. ONODERA, A. SUGIMOTO, K. KOGURE, M. OBINATA & S. SHIBAHARA. 1993. Coordinated expression of messenger RNAs for nerve growth factor, brain-derived neurotrohic factor and neurotrophin-3 in the rat hippocampus following transient forebrain ischemia. Neuroscience **55:** 23–31.

28. LIN, T.N., J. TE, M. LEE, G.Y. SUN & C.Y. HSU. 1997. Induction of basic fibroblast growth factor (bFGF) expression following focal cerebral ischemia. Brain Res. Mol. Brain Res. **49:** 255–265.

29. FERRER, I., E. LOPEZ, E. POZAS, J. BALLABRIGA & E. MARTI. 1998. Multiple neurotrophic signals converge in surviving CA1 neurons of the gerbil hippocampus following transient forebrain ischemia. **394:** 416–430.
30. ROSENBERG, G.A., M. NAVRATIL, F.C. BARONE & G.Z. FEUERSTEIN. 1996. Proteolytic cascade enzymes increase in focal cerebral ischemia in rat. J. Cereb. Blood Flow Metab. **16:** 360–366.
31. POBER, J.S. & R.S. COTRAN. 1990. Cytokines and endothelial cell biology. Physiol. Rev. **70:** 427–451.
32. ZIMMERMAN, G.A., S.M. PRESCOTT & T. M. MCINTYRE. 1992. Endothelial cell interaction with granulocytes: tethering and signaling molecules. Immunol. Today **13:** 93–100.
33. TRACEY, K.J. & A. CERAMI. 1993. Tumor necrosis factor, other cytokines and disease. Annu. Rev. Cell Biol. **9:** 317–343.
34. HOPKINS, S.J. & N.J. ROTHWELL. 1995. Cytokines and the nervous system. I: Expression and recognition. Trends Neurosci. **18:** 83–88.
35. SAITO, K., K. SUYAMA, K. NISHIDA, Y. SEI & A.S. BASILE. 1996. Early increases in TNF-α and IL-1β levels following transient cerebral ischemia in gerbil brain. Neurosci. Lett. **206:** 149–152.
36. BARONE, F.C., B. ARVIN, R.F. WHITE, A. MILLER, C.L. WEBB, R.N. WILLETTE, P.G. LYSKO & G.Z. FEUERSTEIN. 1997. Tumor necrosis factor α: a mediator of focal ischemic brain injury. Stroke **28**(6): 1233–1244.
37. STOLPEN, A.H., E.C. GUINAN, W. FIERS & J.A. POBER. 1986. Recombinant tumor necrosis factor and immune interferon act single and in combination to reorganize human vascular endothelial cell monolayers. Am. J. Pathol. **123:** 16–24.
38. YI, E.S. & T.R. ULICH. 1992. Endotoxin, interleukin-1 and tumor necrosis factor cause neutrophil dependent microvascular leakage in postcapillary venules. Am. J. Pathol. **140:** 659–663.
39. GARCIA, J.H. & KAMIJYO. 1974. Cerebral infarction: evolution of histopathological changes after occlusion of a middle cerebral artery in primates. J. Neuropathol. Exp. Neurol. **33:** 409–421.
40. POZZILLI, C., G.L. LENZI, C. ARGENTINO, A. CAROLEI, M. RASURA, A. SIGNOR, L. BOZZAO & P. POZZILLI. 1985. Imaging of leukocytic infiltration in human cerebral infarcts. Stroke **16:** 251–255.
41. HALLENBECK, J.M., A.J. DUTKA, T. TANISHIMA, P.M. KOCHANEK, K.K. KUMAROO, C.B. THOMPSON, T.P. OBRENOVITCH &. T.J. CONTRERAS. 1986. Polymorphonuclear leukocyte accumulation in brain regions with low blood flow during the early postischemic period. Stroke **17:** 246–253.
42. CHEN, H., M. CHOPP & G. BODZIN. 1992. Neutropenia reduces the volume of cerebral infarct after transient middle cerebral artery occlusion in the rat. Neurosci. Res. Commun. **11:** 93–99.
43. DERESKI, M.O., M. CHOPP, R.A. KNIGHT, H. CHEN & J.H. GARCIA. 1992. Focal cerebral ischemia in the rat: temporal profile of neutrophil responses. Neurosci. Res. Commun. **11:** 179–186.
44. ZHANG, R.L., M. CHOPP, H. CHEN & J.H. GARCIA. 1994. Temporal profile of ischemic tissue damage, neutrophil response, and vascular plugging following permanent and transient (2H) middle cerebral artery occlusion in the rat. J. Neurol. Sci. **125:** 3–10.
45. BARONE, F.C., L.M. HILLEGASS, W.J. PRICE, R.F. WHITE, E.V. LEE, G.Z. FEUERSTEIN, H.M. SARAU, R.K. CLARK & D.E. GRISWOLD. 1991. Polymorphonuclear leukocyte infiltration into cerebral focal ischemic tissue: myeloperoxidase activity assay and histologic verification. J. Neurosci. Res. **29:** 336–345.
46. BARONE, F.C., D.B. SCHMIDT, W.J. PRICE, R.F. WHITE, G.Z. FEUERSTEIN, R.K. CLARK, E.V. LEE, D.E. GRISWOLD & H.M. SARAU. 1992. Reperfusion increases

neutrophils and LTB4 receptor binding in rat focal ischemia. Stroke **23:** 1337–1348.

47. BARONE, F.C., L.M. HILLEGASS, M.N. TZIMAS, D.B. SCHMIDT, J.J. FOLEY, R.F. WHITE, W.J. PRICE, G.Z. FEUERSTEIN, R.K. CLARK, D.E. GRISWOLD & H.M. SARAU. 1995. Time-related changes in myeloperoxidase activity and leukotriene B4 receptor binding reflect leukocyte influx in cerebral focal stroke. Mol. Chem. Neuropathol. **24:** 13–30.

48. DUTKA, A.J., P.M. KOCHANEK & J.M. HALLENBECK. 1989. Influences of granulocytopenia on canine cerebral ischemia induced by an embolism. Stroke **20:** 390–395.

49. HALLENBECK, J.M. & A.J. DUTKA. 1990. Background review and current concepts of reperfusion injury. Arch. Neurol. **47:** 1245–1254.

50. DEL ZOPPO, G.J., G.W. SCHMID-SCHONBEIN, E. MORI, B.R. COPELAND & C.M. CHANG. 1991. Polymorphonuclear leukocytes occlude capillaries following middle cerebral artery occlusion and reperfusion in baboons. Stroke **22:** 1276–1283.

51. GRAU, A.J., E. BERGER, K.-L. SUNG & P. SCHMID-SCHONBEIN. 1992. Granulocyte adhesion, deformability, and superoxide formation in acute stroke. Stroke **23:** 33–39.

52. KOCHANEK, P.M. & J.M. HALLENBECK. 1992. Polymorphonuclear leukocytes and monocytes/macrophages in the pathogenesis of cerebral ischemia and stroke. Stroke **23:** 1367–1379.

53. DINARELLO, C.A. 1988. Biology of interleukin-1. FASEB J. **2:** 108–115.

54. YAMASAKI, Y., N. MATSUURA, H. SHOZUHARA, H. ONODERA, Y. ITOYAMA & K. KOGURE. 1995. Interleukin-1 as a pathogenetic mediator of ischemic brain damage in rats. Stroke **26:** 676–681.

55. LODDICK, S.A. & N.J. ROTHWELL. 1996. Neuroprotective effects of human recombinant interleukin-1 receptor antagonist in focal cerebral ischemia in the rat. J. Cereb. Blood Flow Metab. **16:** 932–940.

56. RELTON, J.K. & N.J. ROTHWELL. 1992. Interleukin-1 receptor antagonists inhibit ischemic and excitotoxic neuronal damage in the rat. Brain Res. Bull. **29:** 243–246.

57. RELTON, J.K., D. MARTIN, R.C. THOMPSON & D.A. RUSSELL. 1996. Peripheral administration of interleukin-1 receptor antagonist inhibits brain damage after focal cerebral ischemia in the rat. Exp. Neurol. **138:** 206–213.

58. GARCIA, J.H., K.-F. LIU & J.K. RELTON. 1995. Interleukin-1 receptor antagonist decreases the number of necrotic neurons in rats with middle cerebral artery occlusion. Am. J. Pathol. **147:** 1477–1486.

59. FABRY, Z., M.M. WALDSCHMIDT, D. HENDRICKSON, J. KEINER, L. LOVE-HOMAN, F. TAKEI & M.N. HART. 1992. Adhesion molecules on murine brain microvascular endothelial cells: expression and regulation of ICAM-1 and LGp 55. J. Neuroimmunol. **36:** 1–11.

60. SATOH, J., L.F. KASTRUKOFF & S.U. KIM. 1991. Cytokine-induced expression of intercellular adhesion molecule-1 (ICAM-1) in cultured human oligodendrocytes and astrocytes. J. Neuropathol. Exp. Neurol. **50:** 215–216.

61. ALOISI, F., G. BORSELLINO, P. SAMOGGIA, U. TESTA & C. CHELUCCI. 1992. Astrocytes cultures from human embryonic brain: characterization and modulation of surface molecules by inflammatory cytokines. J. Neurosci. Res. **32:** 494–506.

62. HURWITZ, A.A., W.D. LYMAN, M.P. GUIDA, T.M. CALDERON & J.W. BERMAN. 1992. Tumor necrosis factor alpha induces adhesion molecule expression on human fetal astrocytes. J. Exp. Med. **176:** 1631–1636.

63. SEBIRE, G., C. HERY, S. PEUDENIER & M. TARDIEU. 1993. Adhesion proteins on human microgial cells and modulation of their expression by IL-1α and TNFα. Res. Virol. **144:** 47–52.

64. CLARK, W.M., J.D. LAUTEN, N. LESSOV, W. WOODWARD & B.M. COULL. 1994. Time course of ICAM-1 expression and leukocyte subset infiltration in rat forebrain

ischemia. Mol. Chem. Neuropathol. **26:** 213–230.

65. HYNES, R.O. 1992. Integrins: versatility, modulation, and signaling in cell adhesion. Cell **69:** 11–25.

66. FERINGA, E.R., T.F. KOWALSKI & H.L. VAHLSING. 1980. Basal lamina formation at the site of spinal cord transection. Ann. Neurol. **8:** 148–154.

67. ESIRI, M.M. & C.S. MORRIS. 1991. Immunocytochemical study of macrophages and microglial cells and extracellular matrix components in human CNS disease. 2. Non-neoplastic diseases. J. Neurol. Sci. **101:** 59–72.

68. NAG, S. 1996. Immunohistochemical localization of extracellular matrix proteins in cerebral vessels in chronic hypertension. J. Neuropathol. Exp. Neurol. **55:** 381–388.

69. SEIFFERT, D., G.M. BORDIN & D.J. LOSKUTOFF. 1996. Evidence that extrahepatic cells express vitronectin mRNA at rates approaching those of hepatocytes. Histochem. Cell Biol. **105:** 195–201.

70. VENSTROM, K.A. & L.F. REICHARDT. 1993. Extracellular matrix 2: role of extracellular matrix molecules and their receptors in the nervous system. FASEB J. **7:** 996–1003.

71. KOPPE, G., G. BRUCKNER, K. BRAUER, W. HARTIG & V. BIGL. 1997. Developmental patterns of proteoglycan-containing extracelullar matrix in perineuronal nets and neuropil of the postnatal rat brain. Cell Tissue Res. **288:** 33–41.

72. RAUCH, U. 1997. Modeling an extracellular environment for axonal pathfinding and fasciculation in the central nervous system. Cell Tissue Res. **290:** 349–356.

73. VAN HARREVELD, A. 1972. The extracellular space in the vertebrate central nervous system. *In* Structure and Function of Nervous Tissue. Vol. 4. G.H. Bourne, Ed.: 447–511. Academic Press. New York.

74. LEHMENKUHLER, A., E. SYKOVA, J. SVOBODA, K. ZILLES & C. NICHOLSON. 1993. Extracellular space parameters in the rat neocortex and subcortical white matter during postnatal development determined by diffusion analysis. Neuroscience **55:** 339–351.

75. NICHOLSON, C. & E. SYKOVA. 1998. Extracellular space structure revealed by diffusion analysis. Trends Neurosci. **21:** 207–215.

76. LAYWELL, E.D., U. DORRIES, U. BARTSCH, A. FAISSNER, M. SCHACHNER & D.A. STEINDLER. 1992. Enhanced expression of the developmentally regulated extracellular matrix molecule tenascin following adult brain injury. Proc. Natl. Acad. Sci. USA **89:** 2634–2638.

77. BUTLER, W.T. 1989. The nature and significance of osteopontin. Connect. Tissue Res. **23:** 123–126.

78. GIACHELLI, C.M., L. LIAW, C.E. MURRY, S.M. SCHWARTZ & M. ALMEIDA. 1995. Osteopontin expression in cardiovascular diseases. Ann. N.Y. Acad. Sci. **760:** 109–126.

79. LIAW, L., M. ALMEIDA, C.H. HART, S.M. SCHWARTZ & C.M. GIACHELLI. 1994. Osteopontin promotes vascular cell adhesion and spreading and is chemotactic for smooth muscle cells *in vitro*. Circ. Res. **74:** 214–224.

80. YUE, T.-L., P.J. MCKENNA, E.H. OHLSTEIN, M.C. FARACH-CARSON, W.T. BULTER, K. JOHANSON, P. MCDEVITT, G.Z. FEUERSTEIN & J.M. STADEL. 1994. Osteopontin-stimulated vascular smooth muscle cell migration is mediated by β_3 integrin. Exp. Cell Res. **214:** 459–464.

81. WEINTRAUB, A.S., C.M. GIACHELLI, R.S. KRAUSS, M. ALMEIDA & M.B. TAUBMAN. 1996. Autocrine secretion of osteopontin by vascular smooth muscle cells regulates their adhesion to collagen gels. Am. J. Pathol. **149:** 259–272.

82. LIAW, L., M.P. SKINNER, E.W. RAINES, R. ROSS, D.A. CHERESH, S.M. SCHWARTZ & C.M. GIACHELLI. 1995. The adhesive and migratory effects of osteopontin are mediated via distinct cell surface integrins: role of smooth muscle cell migration to osteopontin *in vitro*. J. Clin. Invest. **95:** 713–724.

83. MIYAZAKI, T., T. TASHIRO, Y. HIGUCHI, M. SETOGUCHI, S. YAMAMOTO, H. NAGAI, M. NASU & P. VASSALLI. 1995. Expression of osteopontin in a macrophage cell line and in transgenic mice with pulmonary fibrosis resulting from the lung expression of a tumor necrosis factor-alpha transgene. **760:** 334–341.

84. JIN, C.H., C. MIYAURA, Y. ISHIMI, M.H. HONG, T. SATO, E. ABE & T. SUDA. 1990. Interleukin 1 regulates the expression of osteopontin mRNA by osteoblasts. **74:** 221–228.

85. GIACHELLI, C.M., N. BAE, M. ALMEIDA, D.T. DENHARDT, C.E. ALPERS & S.M. SCHWARTZ. 1993. Osteopontin is elevated during neointima formation in rat arteries and is a novel component of human atherosclerotic plaques. J. Clin. Invest. **92:** 1686–1696.

86. WANG, X.K., C. LOUDEN, E.H. OHLSTEIN, J.M. STADEL, J.-L. GU & T.-L. YUE. 1996. Osteopontin expression in platelet-derived growth factor stimulated vascular smooth muscle cells and carotid artery after balloon angioplasty. Arterioscler. Thromb. Vasc. Biol. **16:** 1365–1372.

87. O'BRIEN, E.R., M.R. GARVIN, D.K. STEWART, T. HINOHARA, J.B. SIMPSON, S.M. SCHWARTZ & C.M. GIACHELLI. 1994. Osteopontin is synthesized by macrophage, smooth muscle, and endothelial cells in primary and restenotic human coronary atherosclerotic plaques. Arterioscler. Thromb. **14:** 1648–1656.

88. MURRY, C.E., C.M. GIACHELLI, S.M. SCHWARTZ & R. VRACKO. 1994. Macrophages express osteopontin during repair of myocardial necrosis. Am. J. Pathol. **145:** 1450–1462.

89. GIACHELLI, C.M., R. PICHLER, D. LOMBARDI, D.T. DENHARDT, C.E. ALPERS, S.M. SCHWARTZ & R.J. JOHNSON. 1994. Osteopontin expression in angiotensin II-induced tubulointerstitial nephritis. Kidney Int. **45:** 515–524.

90. PICHLER, R., C.M. GIACHELLI, D. LOMBARDI, J. PIPPIN, K. GORDON, C.E. APLERS, S.M. SCHWARTZ & R.J. JOHNSON. 1994. Tubulointerstitial disease in glomerulonephritis: potential role of osteopontin (uropontin). Am. J. Pathol. **144:** 915–926.

91. LIAW, L., D.E. BIRK, C.B. BALLAS, J.S. WHITSITT, J.M. DAVIDSON & B.L. HOGAN. 1998. Altered wound healing in mice lacking a functional osteopontin gene (suppl.). J. Clin. Invest. **101:** 1468–1478.

92. WANG, X.K., C. LOUDEN, T.-L. YUE, J.A. ELLISON, F.C. BARONE, H.A. SOLLEVELD & G.Z. FEUERSTEIN. 1998. Regulation of osteopontin expression in brain ischemia: implication for matrix remodeling and astrocyte function. J. Neurosci. **18:** 2075–2083.

93. PANDA, D., G.C. KUNDU, B.I. LEE, A. PERI, D. FOHL, I. CHACKALAPARAMPIL, B.B. MUKHERJEE, X.D. LI, D.C. MUKHERJEE, S. SEIDES, J. ROSENBERG, K. STARK & A.B. MUKHERJEE. 1997. Potential roles of osteopontin and alpha v beta 3 integrin in the development of coronary artery restenosis after angioplasty. Proc. Natl. Acad. Sci. USA **94:** 9308–9313.

94. BROOKS, P.C., R.A.F. CLARK & D.A. CHERESH. 1994. Requirement for vascular integrin alpha v beta 3 for angiogenesis. Science **264:** 569–571.

95. OKADA, Y., B.R. COPELAND, G.F. HAMANN, J.A. KOZIOL, D.A. CHERESH & G.J. DEL ZOPPO. 1996. Integrin alpha v beta 3 is expressed in selected microvessels after focal cerebral ischemia. Am. J. Pathol. **149:** 37–44.

96. WAGNER, S., M. TAGAYA, J.A. KOZIOL, V. QUARANTA & G.J. DEL ZOPPO. 1997. Rapid disruption of an astrocyte interaction with the extracellular matrix mediated by integrin alpha 6 beta 4 during focal cerebral ischemia/reperfusion. Stroke **28:** 858–865.

97. TAWIL, N.J., P. WILSON & S. CARBONETTO. 1994. Expression and distribution of functional integrins in rat CNS glia. J. Neurosci. Res. **39:** 436–447.

98. HIRSCH, E.M., D. GULLBERG, F. BALZAC, F. ALTRUDA, L. SILENGO & G. TARONE. 1994. α_v integrin subunit is predominantly located in nervous tissue and skeletal

muscle during mouse development. Dev. Dyn. **201:** 108–120.

99. HRUSKA, K.A., F. ROLNICK, M. HUSKEY, U. ALVAREZ & D. CHERESH. 1995. Engagement of the osteoclast integrin alpha v beta 3 by osteopontin stimulates phosphatidylinositol 3-hydroxyl kinase activity. Endocrinology **136:** 2984–2992.

100. BIANCHI, R., M. GARBUGLIA, M. VERZINI, I. GIAMBANCO, A. SPRECA & R. DONATO. 1995. S-100 protein and annexin II2-p11(2) (calpactin I) act in concert to regulate the state of assembly of GFAP intermediate filaments. Biochem. Biophys. Res. Commun. **208:** 910–918.

101. YAMAMOTO-HINO, M., A. MIYAWAKI, H. KAWANO, T. SUGIYAMA, T. FURUICHI, M. HASEGAWA & K. MIKOSHIBA. 1995. Immunohistochemical study of inositol 1,4,5-trisphosphate receptor type 3 in rat central nervous system. Neuroreport **6:** 273–276.

102. TREMBLE, P., R. CHIQUET-EHRISMANN & Z. WERB. 1994. The extracellular matrix ligands fibronectin and tenascin collaborate in regulating collagenase gene expression in fibroblasts. Mol. Biol. Cell **5:** 439–453.

103. STROMBLAD, S., J.C. BECKER, M. YEBRA, P.C. BROOKS & D.A. CHERESH. 1996. Suppression of p53 activity and p21WAF1/IP1 expression by vascular cell integrin alpha v beta 3 during angiogenesis. J. Clin. Invest. **98:** 426–433.

104. KIMBRO, K.S. & R.A. SAAVEDRA. 1995. The puerap motif in the promoter of the mouse osteopontin gene. Ann. N.Y. Acad. Sci. **760:** 319–320.

105. Sauk, J.J., C.L. Van Kampen, K. Norris, R. Foster & M.J. Somerman. 1990. Expression of constitutive and inducible HSP70 and HSP47 is enhanced in cells persistently spread on opn or collagen. Biochem. Biophys. Res. Commun. **2:** 135–142.

106. HWANG, S.-M., C.A. LOPEZ, D.E. HECK, C.R. GARDNER, D.L. LASKIN, J.D. LASKIN & D.T. DENHARDT. 1994. Osteopontin inhibits induction of nitric oxide synthase gene expression by inflammatory mediators in mouse kidney epithelial cells. J. Biol. Chem. **269:** 711–715.

107. DENHARDT, D.T. & A.F. CHAMBERS. 1994. Overcoming obstacles to metastasis—defenses against host defenses: osteopontin (opn) as a shield against attack by cytotoxic host cells. J. Cell. Biochem. **56:** 48–51.

108. IDE, C.F., J.L. SCRIPTER, B.W. COLTMAN, R.S. DOTSON, D.C. SNYDER & A. JELASO. 1996. Cellular and molecular correlates to plasticity during recovery from injury in the developing mammalian brain. Prog. Brain Res. **108:** 365–377.

109. REIER, P.J. 1986. Gliosis following CNS injury: the anatomy of astrocytic scars and their influences on axonal elongation. *In* Cell Biology and Pathology of Astrocytes. S. Fedoroff & A. Vernadiakis, Eds.: 263–324. Academic Press. New York.

Metallothioneins Attenuate Methylmercury-Induced Neurotoxicity in Cultured Astrocytes and Astrocytoma Cells

CHANG PING YAO, JEFFREY W. ALLEN, AND MICHAEL ASCHNER[a]

Department of Physiology and Pharmacology, Wake Forest University School of Medicine, Winston-Salem, North Carolina 27157-1083

ABSTRACT: Metallothionein-I (MT-I) was expressed in neonatal rat primary astrocyte cultures and an astrocytoma cell line by pGFAP-MT-I plasmid transfection under the control of the astrocyte-specific glial fibrillary acidic protein (GFAP) promoter. Following transient transfection of the pGFAP-MT-I plasmid, MT-I mRNA and MT-I protein levels were determined by Northern blot and immunoprecipitation analyses, respectively. The ability of cells overexpressing MT-I to withstand acute methylmercury (MeHg) treatment was measured by the release of preloaded $Na_2{}^{51}CrO_4$, an indicator of membrane integrity. Transfection with the pGFAP-MT-I plasmid led to increased mRNA (2.5-fold in astrocytes and 7.4-fold in astrocytomas) and MT-I protein (2.4-fold in astrocytes and 4.0-fold in astrocytomas) levels compared with their respective controls. Increased expression of MT-I was associated with attenuated release of $Na_2{}^{51}CrO_4$ upon MeHg (5 μM) treatment. These results demonstrate that MT-I can be highly expressed both in primary astrocyte cultures and astrocytomas by pGFAP-MT-I plasmid transfection, and lend credence to the hypothesis that increased expression of MT-I affords protection against the cytotoxic effects of MeHg. Taken together, the data suggest that MTs offer effective cellular adaptation to MeHg cytotoxicity.

Metallothioneins (MTs) are cysteine containing, low-molecular weight proteins with widespread phylogenic and cellular expression from bacteria, fungi, and plants, to eukaryotic species. MTs' preponderant distribution in all tissues, and their synthesis, both in regeneration and development, point to their pivotal roles in metal-related cell homeostasis. Although not fully elucidated, MTs are believed to function[1] in the sequestration of metal ions.[2] As homeostatic mediators that regulate the biosynthesis and activity of zinc metalloproteins, most notably zinc-dependent transcription factors.[3] As cytoprotectants against the damaging effects of reactive oxygen species, ionizing radiation, electrophilic anticancer drugs and mutagens, as well as metals.[1–8,11]

[a]Corresponding author: Michael Aschner, Ph.D., Department of Physiology and Pharmacology, Wake Forest University School of Medicine, Medical Center Boulevard, Winston-Salem, NC 27157-1083. Phone, 336/716-8530; fax, 336/716-8501.
e-mail, maschner@bgsm.edu

In contrast to the previously emphasized support roles of astrocytes for neurons, today, the role of astrocytes extends well beyond passive structural support and sensitivity to axon commands. In fact, astrocytes and neurons establish a highly dynamic reciprocal relationship that influences subsequent nervous tissue growth, morphology, behavior and repair. The preferential distribution of MT-I and MT-II isoforms within astrocytes remains a subject for speculation, but likely reflects differing roles and compartmentalization of metals between the various cell types within the CNS, analogous to the distribution of iron and its binding proteins.[14] The preponderance of astrocytic MTs was also postulated to serve a distinct function in regulating the intracellular concentration of zinc that is needed for activation of some enzymes or transcription factors that are particularly abundant in astrocytes.[14]

Astrocytes are a known "sink" for brain methylmercury (MeHg). Although the significance of its accumulation in astrocytes remains elusive, neurotoxicity may be indirectly mediated because of the inability of MeHg-treated astrocytes to maintain proper control of the extracellular fluid microenvironment. Since MTs form high-affinity thiolate clusters with several metals, they are likely to reduce the ability of MeHg to react with other endogenous targets, keeping them in a relatively nontoxic form within the astrocytes. Whereas, high levels and chronic exposure to heavy metals can short circuit astrocytic function, at low concentrations, MTs may serve to attenuate toxicity, protecting the vulnerable astrocytic -SH group. Once MT induction mechanisms are overwhelmed, pervasive astrocytic dysfunction may lead to failure to control the extracellular environment. We have recently postulated that the preponderance of astrocytic MTs may also serve to attenuate the neurotoxicity of MeHg.

Cultured astrocytes induced to overexpress MT-I and MT-II levels by pretreatment with cadmium (Cd)[10] were shown to be resistant to the cytotoxic effects of MeHg. Increased astrocytic MT-I complement completely reversed the inhibitory effect of MeHg on D-aspartate uptake that occurs in MeHg-treated astrocytes with constitutive MT levels.[12] The inhibition of regulatory volume decrease (RVD) upon MeHg-induced swelling was also shown to progressively reverse by the induction of MTs in astrocytes preexposed to $CdCl_2$ for 72, 96, and 120 hours. Consistent with this effect, $CdCl_2$ preexposure was also associated with a partial reversal of MeHg inhibited ^{3}H-taurine release at 72 hour preexposure, and complete reversal by 96 hour preexposure.[12] Hence, as intracellular MT levels increased, the astrocytes appeared to volume regulate more efficiently. Most recently we have undertaken studies to determine (1) whether neonatal rat primary astrocytes and astrocytomas can be induced to express high levels of the MT-I cDNA gene under the control of the astrocyte-specific glial fibrillary acidic protein (GFAP) promoter, and (2) to test the hypothesis that increased astrocytic MT-I protein expression confers cytoprotection against MeHg-induced cytotoxicity.

By recombining MT-I cDNA with the pGFAP plasmid,[13] we developed an astrocyte-specific MT-I expression system. An astrocyte-specific MT-I plasmid was constructed by excising the LacZ gene and replacing it with MT-I cDNA, so that the transcription of MT-I mRNA could be driven under the GFAP promoter. Since the mp-I gene in pGFAP plasmids supplied an intron, stabilizing 3′ UTR and a polyadenylation signal, we retained it in this recombinant pGFAP-MT-I plasmid. The pGFAP-MT-I plasmid was transfected into neonatal rat primary astrocyte cultures and astrocytomas, and twenty-four hours after the transfection, the transcription of MT-I mRNA was analyzed by northern blot analysis. MT-I mRNA levels in pGFAP-MT-I transfected astrocytes and astrocytomas were significantly greater compared with MT-I mRNA levels in plasmid controls and cell controls. The relative content of newly synthesized MT-I in the extracts of the two cell types was also evaluated by immunoprecipitation. The expression of MT-I protein in pGFAP-MT-I transfected astrocytes and astrocytomas were greater compared with their respective control groups.

To determine the relationship between the cytotoxicity of MeHg and the relative abundance of MT expression, $Na_2^{51}CrO_4$ efflux measurement were carried out. In order to distinguish between cell loss or cell lysis and authentic release of intracellular molecules, one could simultaneously examine the compound that one is studying and the release of intracellular ^{51}Cr. The labeling of cells with ^{51}Cr sodium chromate, a compound routinely applied in studies of cell lysis or death in immunological interactions, was shown to be an effective way for distinguishing between cell lysis and authentic release.[9] As expected, MeHg induced a dose-dependent increase in the fractional release of ^{51}Cr as its concentration in the perfusion buffer increased. The release of ^{51}Cr in the MT-I transfected groups was lower in pGFAP-MT-I-transfected astrocytomas compared to their respective controls. The results of the ^{51}Cr efflux measurements support the hypothesis that intracellular MT levels confer resistance to MeHg toxicity. ^{51}Cr release in response to MeHg treatment was attenuated in cells overexpressing MT-I compared to their respective controls, but this effect attained statistical significance only in the 5-μM MeHg treatment group. The absence of a significant decrease in ^{51}Cr release in pGFAP-MT-I plasmid transfected astrocytoma at 2 μM MeHg suggests that MT-I protein levels in controls are sufficiently high to mitigate the effect of MeHg taken up by these cells. The absence of a significant decrease in ^{51}Cr release in pGFAP-MT-I plasmid transfected astrocytoma at 10 μM MeHg was rather surprising, and at present we can only speculate on the mechanisms which may account for this observation. One such mechanism likely represents the limited capacity of these cells to synthesize MT-I, such that its intracellular levels do not attain a sufficiently high concentration to buffer incoming MeHg. Since the mechanism of MT-I gene expression in primary astrocytes is at present unclear, further work is required to optimize conditions that would allow for a greater increase MT-I expression in primary astrocytes or astrocytomas. This can be potentially achieved by setting up more efficient astrocyte-specific expression systems or by performing MT-I transfection in astrocytes with basal expression of MT-I levels decreased by contemporary knockout techniques.

In summary, the MT-I protein can be efficiently expressed both in primary astrocyte cultures and the astrocytoma cell line by MT-I gene transfection under the control of the astrocyte-specific glial fibrillary acidic protein (GFAP) promoter. MT-I gene transfection leads to a 2.4- and 4-fold increase in the basal levels of MT proteins in primary astrocyte cultures and astrocytomas, respectively.[13] Furthermore, *in vitro* MT enrichment in astrocytomas confers resistance against the cytotoxicity of MeHg. This interpretation is consistent with our previous observations that resistance to heavy metal toxicity is closely related to MT levels.[10,12] It is noteworthy that in cells exposed to highly toxic metals, such as MeHg and Cd,[10] cytotoxicity appears at metal concentrations higher than those at which MT induction is saturated. This might reflect the toxicity exerted by free heavy metal ions in excess of the metal-binding capacity of induced MTs. This interpretation is consistent with the observation that resistance to heavy metal toxicity is closely related to their ability to synthesize MTs, and raises interesting questions regarding the potential involvement of heavy metals in neurodegeneration under conditions of compromised MT synthesis.

ACKNOWLEDGMENTS

This study was supported in part by PHS grants NIEHS 07331 and NIAA11617 awarded to M.A. J.W.A. was supported by a NIAAA training grant (T32 AA07565).

REFERENCES

1. BREMNER, I. 1987. Interactions between metallothionein and trace elements. Prog. Food Nutr. Sci. **11:** 1–37.
2. DUNN, M.A., T.L. BLALOCK & R.J. COUSINS. 1987. Metallothionein. Proc. Soc. Exp. Biol. Med. **185:** 107–119.
3. DURNAM, D.M. & R.D. PALMITER. 1984. Induction of metallothionein-I mRNA in cultured cells by heavy metals and iodoacetate: evidence for gratuitous inducers. Mol. Cell. Biol. **4:** 484–491.
4. HAGER, L.G. & R.D. PALMITER. 1981. Transcriptional regulation of mouse liver metallothionein-I gene by glucocorticoids. Nature **291:** 340–342.
5. HAMER, D.H. 1986. Metallothionein. Annu. Rev. Biochem. **55:** 913–951.
6. KÄGI, J.H.R. & Y. KOJIMA. 1987. Chemistry and biochemistry of metallothionein. Experientia (Suppl.) **52:** 25–61.
7. KÄGI, J.H.R. & A. SCHÄFFER. 1988. Biochemistry of metallothionein. Biochemistry **27:** 8509–8515.
8. KÄGI, J.H.R. 1991. Overview of metallothionein. *In* Methods in Enzymology. Vol. 205. Metallobiochemistry. Part B. Metallothionein and Related Molecules. J.F. Riordan & B.L. Vallee, Eds.: 613–626. Academic Press. New York.
9. KIMELBERG, H.K., D.J. BONVILLE & S.K. GODERIE. 1993. Use of ^{51}Cr cell labeling to distinguish between release of radiolabeled amino acids from primary astrocyte cultures being due to efflux or cell damage. Brain Res. **622:** 237–242.
10. RISING, L., D. VITARELLA, H.K. KIMELBERG & M. ASCHNER. 1995. Metallothionein induction in neonatal rat primary astrocyte cultures protects against methylmercury cytotoxicity. J. Neurochem. **65:** 1562–1568.
11. VALLEE, B.L. & V. MARET. 1993. The functional and potential functions of metallothioneins: a personal perspective. *In* Metallothionein III: Biological Roles and Medical Implications. K.T. Suzuki, N. Imura & M. Kimura, Eds.: 1–27. Birkhäuser Verlag. Berlin.
12. VITARELLA, D., D.R. CONKLIN, H.K. KIMELBERG & M. ASCHNER. 1996. Metallothionein induction protects swollen rat primary astrocyte cultures from methylmercury-induced inhibition of regulatory volume decrease. Brain Res. **738:** 213–221.
13. YAO, C.P., J.W. ALLEN, D.R. CONKLIN & M. ASCHNER. 1999. Transfection and overexpression of metallothionein-I in neonatal rat primary astrocyte cultures and in astrocytoma cells increases their resistance to methylmercury-induced cytotoxicity. Brain Res. In press.
14. YOUNG, J.K. 1994. Glial metallothionein. Biol. Signals **3:** 169–175.

Implication of Poly(ADP-Ribose) Polymerase (PARP) in Neurodegeneration and Brain Energy Metabolism

Decreases in Mouse Brain NAD$^+$ and ATP Caused by MPTP Are Prevented by the PARP Inhibitor Benzamide

CRISTINA COSI[a] AND MARC MARIEN

Divisions of Neurobiology I and II, Centre de Recherche Pierre Fabre,
17 Avenue Jean Moulin, Castres 81106, France

ABSTRACT: Poly(ADP-ribose) polymerase (PARP) is a DNA binding protein that uses nicotinamide adenine dinucleotide (NAD$^+$) as a substrate. Evidence from *in vitro* studies on nonneuronal cells in culture have shown that when fully activated by free radical-induced DNA damage, PARP depletes cellular NAD$^+$ and consequently adenosine triphosphate (ATP) levels within a matter of minutes, and that this depletion is associated with a cell death that can be prevented by PARP inhibitors. The present *in vivo* study utilized the 1-methyl-4-phenyl-1,2,3,6-tetrahydropyridine (MPTP)-treated mouse, a model of central nigrostriatal dopamine neurotoxicity that recapitulates certain features of Parkinson's disease (PD), and one in which we have previously shown PARP inhibitors to be protective,[6] to examine whether MPTP acutely caused region- and time-dependent changes in levels of NAD$^+$ and ATP in the brain *in vivo* and whether such effects were modified by treatments with neuroprotective doses of the PARP inhibitor benzamide. The results confirm that MPTP reduces striatal ATP levels, as previously reported by Chan *et al.*,[4] show that MPTP causes a regionally-selective (striatal and midbrain) loss of NAD$^+$, and indicate that the PARP inhibitor benzamide can prevent these losses without interfering with MPTP-induced striatal dopamine release. These findings suggest an involvement of PARP in the control of brain energy metabolism during neurotoxic insult, provide further evidence in support of the participation of PARP in MPTP-induced neurotoxicity *in vivo* and suggest that PARP inhibitors might be beneficial in the treatment of PD.

INTRODUCTION

Poly(ADP-ribose) polymerase (PARP) is a DNA binding protein that uses nicotinamide adenine dinucleotide (NAD$^+$) as a substrate. PARP has been shown to be involved in DNA plasticity-related phenomena, such as DNA repair, and to regulate

[a]Corresponding author: Dr. Cristina Cosi, Division de Neurobiologie II, Centre de Recherche Pierre Fabre, 17, avenue Jean Moulin, Castres 81106, France. Phone, +33 5-63-71-42-86; fax, +33 5-63-71-43-63.
e-mail, cristina.cosi@pierre-fabre.com

the activity of histones, topoisomerases, DNA and RNA polymerases, DNA ligases and Ca^{2+}/Mg^{2+}-dependent endonucleases. PARP is activated by nicks in the DNA molecule induced by different damaging agents, including free radicals.

At steady state, nuclear NAD^+, which is in equilibrium with cytoplasmic NAD^+, is catabolized to allow poly(ADP-ribosyl)ation of nuclear proteins. In this reaction, nicotinamide (Nam) is formed and can be then either methylated (meNam) and excreted or converted to nicotinamide mononucleotide (NMN) and subsequently back to NAD^+. This regeneration of NAD^+ consumes adenosine triphosphate (ATP) and phosphoribosyl pyrophosphate (PRPP). Since the polymers of ADP-ribose are rapidly degraded by the specific glycohydrolase (half-life of 1 min), NAD^+ is continuously catabolized. An extreme activation of PARP by free radical damage of the DNA molecule would increase the consumption of NAD^+, disrupting the equilibrium of pyridine nucleotide metabolism and causing a depletion of the cellular ATP pool, with the consequence of the disruption of energy-dependent cellular functions that eventually culminates in cell death[1] (FIG. 1). Studies with nonneuronal cells in culture confirmed this hypothesis and showed that 3-aminobenzamide, a selective PARP inhibitor and close derivative of benzamide, was able to block these events and prevent cell death.[2,3]

Cellular energy impairment appears to play an important part in 1-methyl-4-phenyl-1,2,3,6-tetrahydropyridine (MPTP)-induced neurotoxicity. Striatal levels of ATP were decreased by 10–27% within 90 min after a single subcutaneous injection of MPTP (40 mg/kg) in C57BL/6 mice, when measured after rapid fixation of the brain *in situ* by focused microwave irradiation.[4,5] This partial loss of ATP appeared to be selective for both the striatum (nigrostriatal dopaminergic terminal field) and the ventral mesencephalon (including the dopaminergic nuclei within the substantia ni-

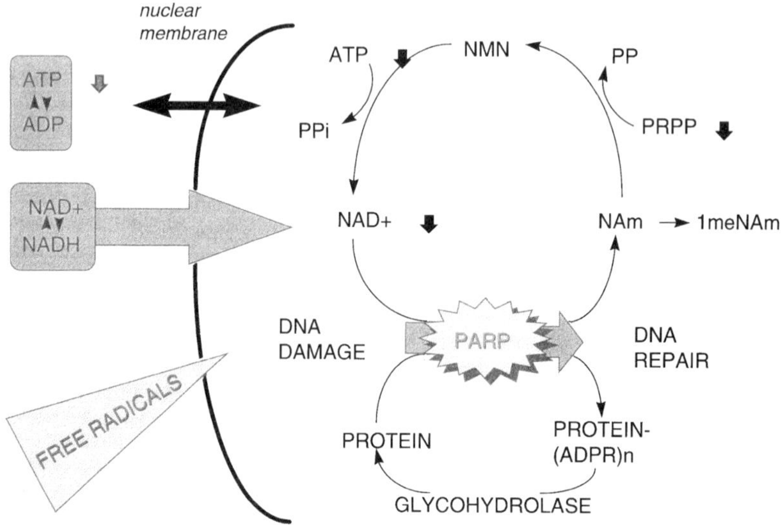

FIGURE 1. The central role of PARP in the control of cellular energy metabolism in response to DNA damage. See Introduction for detailed explanation of the diagram. (Taken in part from Gaal *et al.*[1])

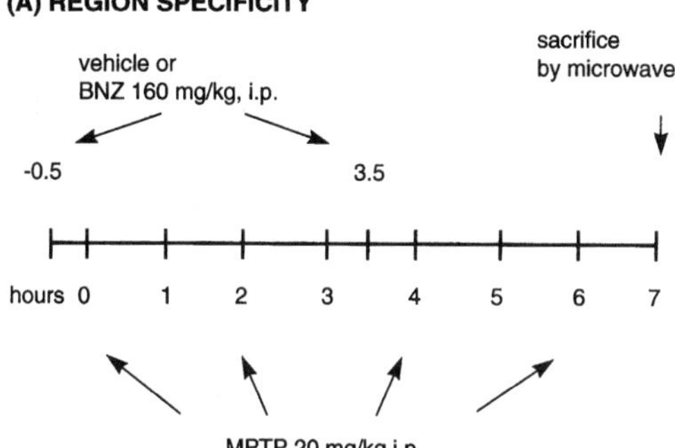

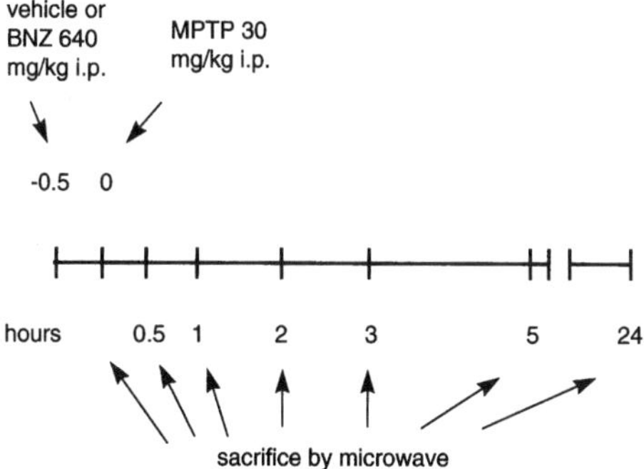

FIGURE 2. Drug treatment protocols. **(A)** Region specificity. A total of 4 experimental groups of C57 Bl/6N mice (7 per group) were used in this study (FIGS. 3–5 and TABLE 1). In two groups, mice received a total of 80 mg/kg MPTP, divided into 4 i.p. injections of 20 mg/kg, each administered at 2-h intervals; the two other groups received injections of the vehicle according to the same schedule. Benzamide (BNZ, 160 mg/kg) or its vehicle was administered i.p. to the above groups at 30 min before the first and third injections of MPTP (or its vehicle). Using this protocol, each group thus received the same total number, volume and timing of multiple i.p. injections. At 1 h after the last injection, mice were killed by head-focused microwave irradiation (3.2 kW, 2450 MHz, 1.1 sec; Sacron™ Model 8000, SAIREM, Vaulx-en-Velin, France). This method of sacrifice was essential for rapid and effective fixation (heat inactivation of enzymes) of the brain *in situ*, such that accurate determinations of analytes that are susceptible to major postmortem changes, including dopamine metabolites[17] and adenine nucleotides (ATP and derivatives),[4] could be made. Brains were then removed, and the striatum, ventral midbrain and frontal cortex were dissected, weighed, and frozen until used for HPLC analysis. **(B)** Time course. A total of 14 experimental groups of mice (6–8 per group) were used in this part of the study. Seven groups were pretreated with BNZ (640 mg/kg i.p.) and 7 groups with vehicle. One vehicle and one BNZ group were killed 30 min later (t = 0 in FIGS. 6–8); at that time, all of the remaining groups received a single i.p. injection of MPTP (30 mg/kg i.p.) and were killed at various times later (0.5, 1.0, 2.0, 3.0, 5.0 and 24 h), as indicated in FIGURES 6–8. Additional groups of mice (12 groups, 6 mice per group) were used in a parallel time-course study to examine the effect of

gra and ventral tegmental areas), and was potentiated by cotreatment with the glucose metabolism inhibitor, 2-deoxyglucose.[4,5]

We have previously shown that a number of currently available and structurally diverse PARP inhibitors, including benzamide (BNZ), were able to protect against MPTP-induced catecholamine neurotoxicity (i.e., the long-lasting depletions of striatal dopamine and cortical noradrenaline) in the C57BL/6N mouse brain, and from these results a role for PARP activation in MPTP neurotoxicity *in vivo* was proposed.[6] Here, we investigated *in vivo* whether MPTP acutely caused region- and time-dependent changes in brain levels of NAD^+, ATP, adenosine diphosphate (ADP) and adenosine monophosphate (AMP) in C57BL/6N mice killed by head-focused microwave irradiation, and whether such effects were modified by treatments with neuroprotective doses of benzamide.

RESULTS AND DISCUSSION

Animals were handled and cared for in accordance with the *Guide for the Care and Use of Laboratory Animals*[7] and the European Directive No. 86/609. Male C57BL/6N CrlDR mice (Charles River, Elbeuf, France) were treated with MPTP and BNZ according to the protocol shown in FIGURE 2. Brain regional levels of NAD^+, ATP, ADP and AMP, and of MPTP, $MPDP^+$, 1-methyl-4-phenylpyridinium (MPP^+) and BNZ were measured using high-performance liquid chromatography (HPLC) with UV detection, as described previously.[8] Dopamine and 3-methoxytyramine (3-MT) were measured using HPLC with electrochemical detection as previously reported.[9]

MPTP-Induced Changes in Brain Regional Levels of ATP, ADP, AMP and NAD^+: Effects of Benzamide

In the present study we confirm that neurotoxic doses of MPTP cause a rapid decrease in striatal ATP,[4,5] that this effect is associated with acute and concomitant decreases in striatal and ventral midbrain levels of NAD^+ *in vivo*, and that both of these changes are prevented by treatment with neuroprotective doses of benzamide.

Brain regional levels of NAD^+, ATP, ADP and AMP were differentially affected following the multiple injections of MPTP. In the striatum and frontal cortex, the ATP/ADP ratio was decreased by 10% and 32%, respectively (FIGS. 3 and 5), while AMP was increased by 32% in the striatum and by 127% in the frontal cortex (TABLE 1). However, no changes in ATP, ADP, AMP or the ATP/ADP ratio were observed in the ventral midbrain (FIG. 4), suggesting that the early impairment of ATP metabolism is more pronounced at the level of catecholaminergic terminals, i.e., in those brain regions where MPP^+ uptake is relatively much higher.[10] In contrast, NAD^+ levels were significantly decreased within both the striatum and the ventral midbrain, by 11% and 13%, respectively (FIGS. 3 and 4), but not within the frontal cortex. Thus,

---

benzamide alone. Six groups received a single i.p. injection of benzamide (640 mg/kg), and six groups received a single injection of vehicle. One vehicle and one benzamide group were killed at 0.5, 1.0, 1.5, 2.5, 3.5 and 5.5 h later, all by head-focused microwave irradiation. Brains were then removed, and the striata were dissected, weighed, and frozen until used for HPLC analysis.

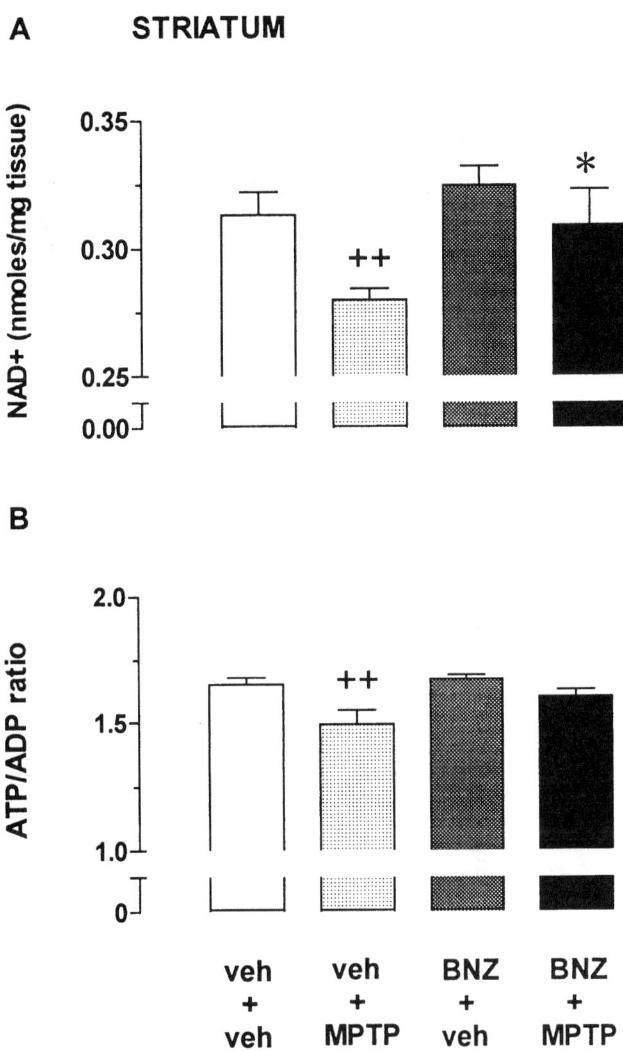

FIGURE 3. Acute effects of MPTP (4×20 mg/kg i.p.), benzamide (BNZ; 2×160 mg/kg i.p.) and cotreatments on the levels of NAD^+ and ATP/ADP ratios in the striatum of C57BL/6N mice. MPTP (or vehicle) injections were separated by 2-h intervals. BNZ (or vehicle) was administered i.p. at 30 min before the first and third injections of MPTP (or vehicle). Mice were killed by head-focused microwave irradiation at 1 h after the last i.p. injection. Brain regions were dissected, and perchloric acid extracts were prepared and analyzed for adenine nucleotide levels by HPLC-UV (see Methods). *Abbreviation*: veh, vehicle. [++]p <0.01 vs [veh + veh] group; [*]p <0.05 vs [veh + MPTP] group (Kruskal-Wallis ANOVA + Mann-Whitney U-test, 7 mice per treatment group). (From Cosi and Marien.[8] Reprinted by permission from *Brain Research*).

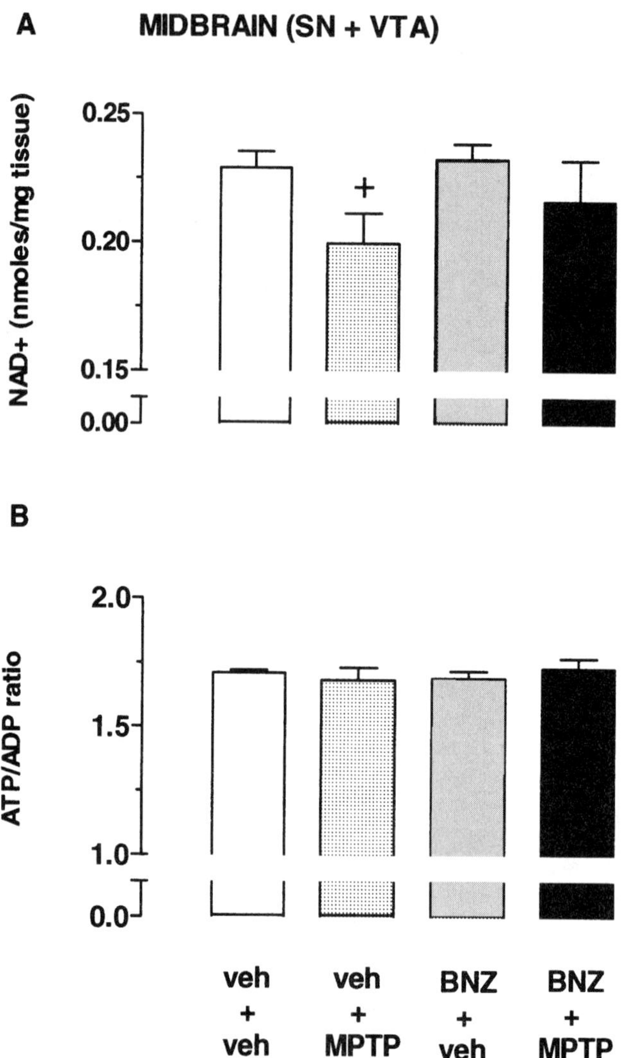

FIGURE 4. Acute effects of MPTP (4×20 mg/kg i.p.), benzamide (BNZ; 2×160 mg/ kg i.p.) and cotreatments on the levels of NAD^+ and the ATP/ADP ratios in the ventral midbrain (including the substantia nigra and ventral tegmental areas) of C57BL/6N mice. Mice were killed by head-focused microwave irradiation at 1 h after the last i.p. injection. See legend to FIGURE 1 and Methods section for experimental details. ^+p <0.05 vs [veh + veh] group (Kruskal-Wallis ANOVA + Mann-Whitney U-test, 7 mice per treatment group). (From Cosi and Marien.[8] Reprinted by permission from *Brain Research*).

the MPTP-induced NAD^+ loss observed here appears to be selectively associated with those regions containing the mesostriatal dopamine system, and appears not to

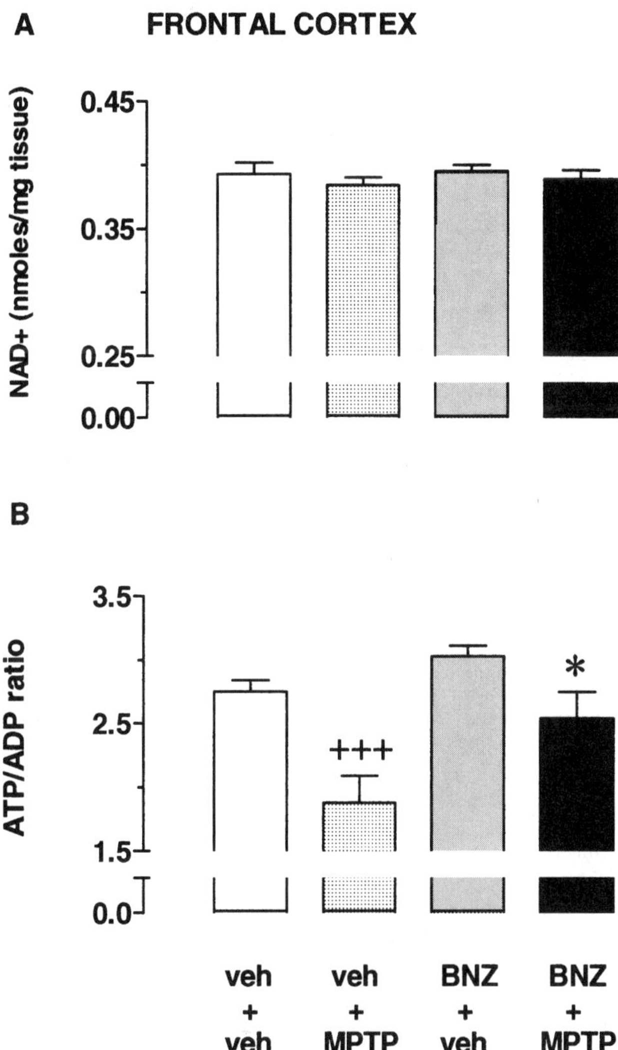

FIGURE 5. Acute effects of MPTP (4×20 mg/kg i.p.), benzamide (BNZ; 2×160 mg/kg i.p.,) and cotreatments on the levels of NAD^+ and the ATP/ADP ratios in the frontal cortex of C57BL/6N mice. Mice were killed by head-focused microwave irradiation at 1 h after the last i.p. injection. See legend to FIGURE 1 and Methods section for details. [+++]$p < 0.001$ vs [veh + veh] group; [*]$p < 0.05$ vs [veh + MPTP] group (Kruskal-Wallis ANOVA + Mann-Whitney U-test, 7 mice per treatment group). (From Cosi and Marien.[8] Reprinted by permission from *Brain Research*).

be secondarily dependent on ATP depletion (e.g., in cortex). Benzamide prevented all of these changes, when administered in the same dosage and injection protocol

TABLE 1. Acute effects of MPTP (4 × 20 mg/kg i.p.), benzamide (2 × 160 mg/kg i.p.) and cotreatments on brain regional levels of ATP, ADP and AMP in C57BL/6N mice

	nmol/mg protein (mean ± SEM)		
	ATP	ADP	AMP
Striatum			
veh + veh	19.751 ± 0.491	11.962 ± 0.111	1.798 ± 0.015
veh + MPTP	18.753 ± 0.723	12.576 ± 0.281	2.382 ± 0.204[++]
BNZ + veh	21.123 ± 0.410	12.641 ± 0.275	1.812 ± 0.056
BNZ + MPTP	19.450 ± 1.643	12.069 ± 0.880	1.771 ± 0.106[**]
Ventral midbrain (SN + VTA)			
veh + veh	14.374 ± 0.451	8.404 ± 0.229	1.333 ± 0.047
veh + MPTP	13.348 ± 0.861	7.907 ± 0.388	1.267 ± 0.041
BNZ + veh	14.638 ± 0.419	8.676 ± 0.239	1.372 ± 0.053
BNZ + MPTP	14.218 ± 1.123	8.211 ± 0.591	1.241 ± 0.106
Frontal cortex			
veh + veh	28.573 ± 0.467	10.434 ± 0.262	2.574 ± 0.176
veh + MPTP	22.478 ± 1.859[++]	10.785 ± 1.578	5.833 ± 0.999[++]
BNZ + veh	30.148 ± 0.454[+]	9.995 ± 0.275	2.614 ± 0.098
BNZ + MPTP	27.572 ± 1.038[*]	11.093 ± 0.499	2.792 ± 0.250[**]

NOTE: MPTP (or vehicle) injections were separated by 2-h intervals. Benzamide (or vehicle) was administered i.p. at 30 min before the first and third injections of MPTP (or vehicle). At 1 h after the last i.p. injection, mice (7 per group) were killed by head-focused microwave irradiation. Brain regions were dissected, and perchloric acid extracts were prepared and analyzed for adenine nucleotide levels by HPLC-UV (see Methods). *Abbreviations*: BNZ, benzamide; veh, vehicle; SN, substantia nigra; VTA, ventral tegmental area. [+,++]p <0.05, 0.01 vs [veh + veh] group; [*,**]p <0.05, 0.01 vs [veh + MPTP] group (Kruskal-Wallis ANOVA plus Mann-Whitney U-test). (From Cosi and Marien.[8] Reprinted by permission from *Brain Research*).

that we showed to be partially protective against the long-lasting striatal dopamine depletion induced by MPTP in C57Bl/6N mice,[6] and had no effect by itself.

The striatal ATP concentrations measured in the present study were similar to those reported by Chan *et al.*[4,5,11] in C57BL/6 mice. The earlier finding[5] that MPTP induces a decrease of striatal ATP levels is also observed here. Some of the decreases in ATP and NAD$^+$ are small but statistically significant. These effects may be "diluted" by ATP and NAD$^+$ levels in nonaffected cells within the same dissected brain region;[4] that is, assuming that the MPTP-induced depletions of ATP and NAD$^+$ specifically involve dopamine neurons (terminals or cell bodies), and that these components constitute only a minor proportion of the total mass of the dissected brain region, a 10–13% decrease in total tissue ATP or NAD$^+$ conceivably represents a major perturbation of energy metabolism within the dopaminergic elements of that region.

Time-Course of Changes in ATP, ADP, AMP and NAD$^+$ Levels and MPTP, and Dopamine Metabolism in the Mouse Striatum: Effects of Benzamide

In a time-course study, a single dose of MPTP (30 mg/kg intraperitoneally (i.p.)) resulted in maximal and transient increases in striatal levels of MPP$^+$ and 3-methoxytyramine (+540%) at 0.5–2 h (FIGS. 7 and 8), followed by maximal and coincidental

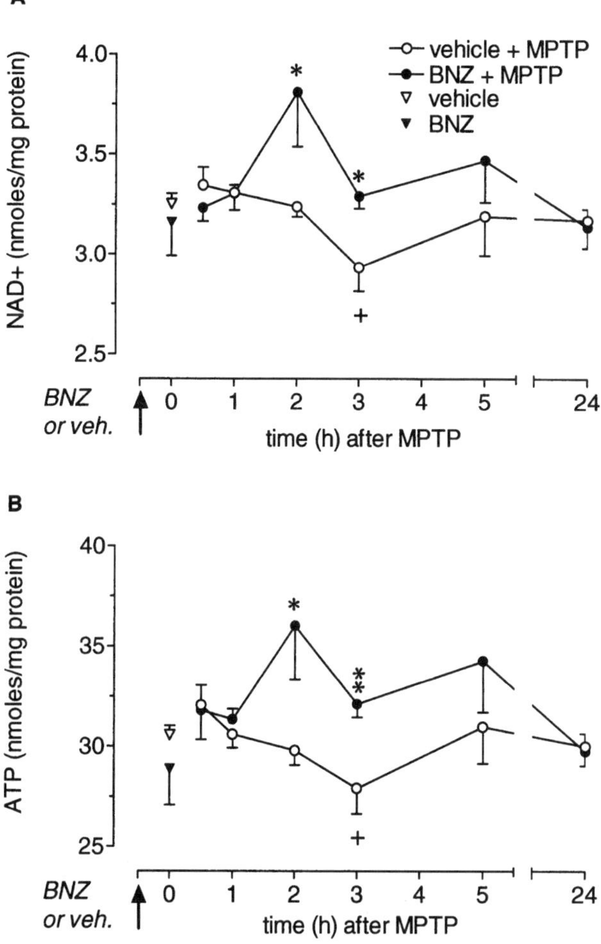

FIGURE 6. Time-course of striatal levels of (**A**) NAD^+ and (**B**) ATP, following a single injection of MPTP (30 mg/kg i.p.): effect of pretreatment with benzamide (BNZ). Seven groups of mice (6–7 per group) were pretreated with BNZ (640 mg/kg i.p.) and 7 groups with vehicle. One vehicle and one BNZ group were killed 30 min later (t = 0 in figure); at that time, all of the remaining groups received a single i.p. injection of MPTP (30 mg/kg i.p.) and were killed at various times later (0.5, 1.0, 2.0, 3.0, 5.0 and 24 h), as indicated. All mice were killed by head-focused microwave irradiation. Striata were dissected, and perchloric acid extracts were prepared and analyzed for NAD^+ and ATP levels by HPLC-UV (see Methods). [+]p <0.05 vs vehicle group at t = 0; [*],[**]p <0.05, 0.01 vs [veh + MPTP] group at corresponding time point (Kruskal-Wallis ANOVA + Mann-Whitney U-test). (From Cosi and Marien.[8] Reprinted by permission from *Brain Research*).

decreases in NAD^+ (−10%), ATP (−11%) and dopamine content (−39%) at 3 h (FIGS. 6 and 7). Benzamide (1 × 640 mg/kg i.p., 30 min before MPTP) partially reduced MPP^+ levels by 30% (FIG. 8) with little or no effect on MPTP or $MPDP^+$ levels. Al-

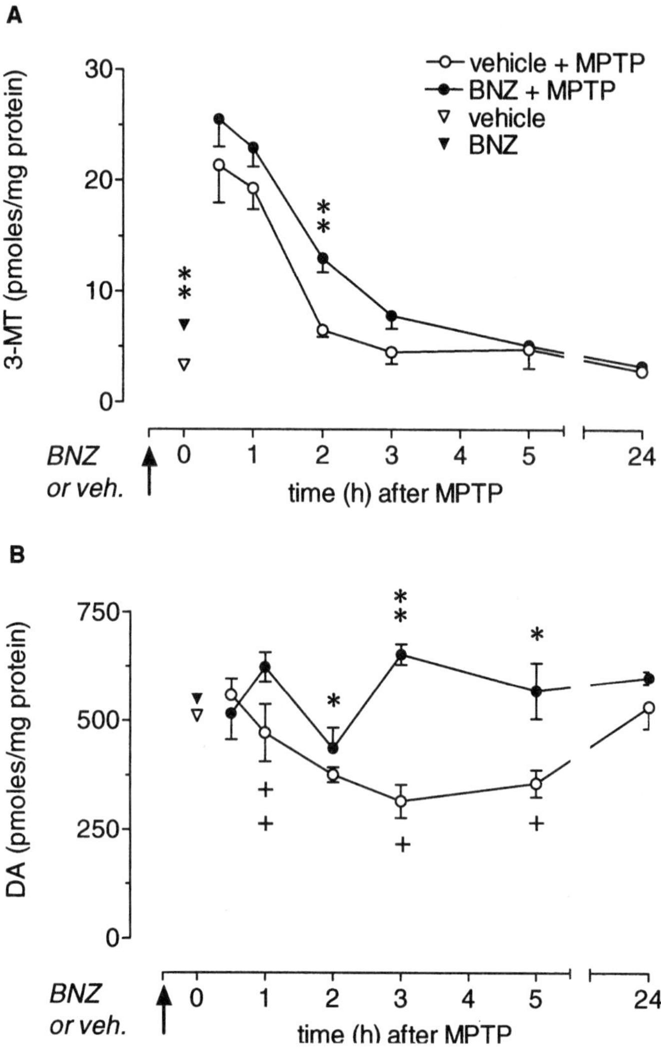

FIGURE 7. Time-course of striatal levels of (**A**) 3-methoxytyramine (3-MT) and (**B**) dopamine, following a single injection of MPTP (30 mg/kg i.p.): effect of pretreatment with benzamide (BNZ; 1 × 640 mg/kg i.p., 30 min prior to MPTP). See legend to FIGURE 4 and Methods section for experimental details. Levels of monoamines and metabolites were measured by HPLC with electrochemical detection in aliquots from the same tissue samples as those analysed in FIGURE 4. [+,++]p <0.05, 0.01 vs vehicle group at t = 0; [*,**]p <0.05, 0.01 vs [veh + MPTP] group at corresponding time point (Kruskal-Wallis ANOVA + Mann-Whitney U-test). (From Cosi and Marien.[8] Reprinted by permission from *Brain Research*).

though this latter finding suggests a possible partial action of benzamide at the level of MPTP biotransformation, it is not completely coherent with a monoamine oxidase

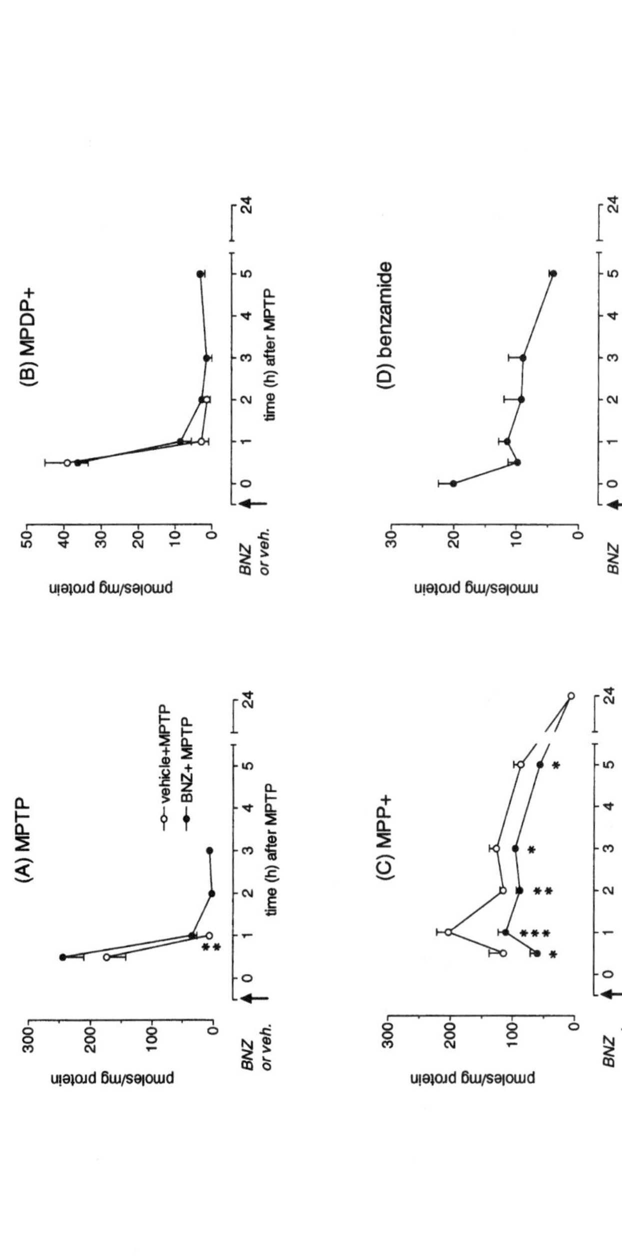

FIGURE 8. Time-course of striatal levels of (**A**) MPTP, (**B**) MPDP+ and (**C**) MPP+ benzamide following a single i.p. injection of MPTP (30 mg/kg i.p.): effect of pretreatment with benzamide (BNZ; 640 mg/kg i.p., 30 min prior to MPTP). See legend to FIGURE 4 and Methods section for experimental details. (**D**) Time-course of benzamide levels in the BNZ-treated group. Levels of MPTP and metabolites, and benzamide, were measured by HPLC-UV in aliquots from the same tissue samples as those analyzed in FIGURES 4 and 5. *, **,*** $p < 0.05, 0.01, 0.001$ vs corresponding vehicle pretreatment group (Kruskal-Wallis ANOVA + Mann-Whitney U-test). (From Cosi and Marien.[8] Reprinted by permission from *Brain Research*).

(MAO) inhibitory activity that would typically result in higher residual levels of MPTP and lower levels of MPDP$^+$.[12,13]

Benzamide completely prevented the losses in striatal NAD$^+$, ATP and dopamine content without by itself causing any changes in these latter parameters in control mice (FIGS. 6 and 7), indicating that the compound did not "rescue" NAD$^+$ levels in MPTP-treated animals by providing an additional source of or promoting an accumulation of the PARP substrate, but that its effect was specific to a mechanism(s) triggered during the early phase of MPTP toxicity. Striatal levels of benzamide (in nmoles/mg protein) were highest at 30 min postinjection (20.1), remained relatively stable at half this concentration (8.9–11.5) at 1–3 h, declined to 4.1 by 5 h, and were not detectable at 24 h; the maximal level at 30 min represents a theoretical concentration in brain water of 2.75 mM, and is consistent with our estimates in a previous study[6] (2.56 mM) (FIG. 8).

The massive and rapid increase in extracellular dopamine and 3-methoxytyramine following MPTP treatment has been interpreted to be a consequence of a rapid disruption or destruction of dopamine nerve terminal function.[14,15] Sustained dopamine overflow is proposed to lead to the generation of cytotoxic free radicals,[16] which might represent an important initial step in the sequence of events that determines MPTP neurotoxicity. Benzamide did not reduce, and if anything tended to increase the MPTP-induced elevations in striatal 3-methoxytyramine, an index of dopamine release.[17] This finding supports the notion that its protective effect against the long-lasting dopamine deficits caused by MPTP after 1 week[6] is due to actions exerted "downstream" to the early massive release of dopamine induced by MPTP.

Based on the above findings, the following hypothesis can be proposed: MPP$^+$ formation and/or the massive increase in dopamine release leads to an early activation of PARP (possibly via free radical-induced DNA damage) with an increased utilization of NAD$^+$ and consequent ATP depletion, which together with impaired mitochondrial respiration caused by MPTP will lead to the energy deficit, disruption of dopamine neuronal homeostasis (e.g., incapacity to maintain transmitter stores), and eventual cell death. Possible additional involvement of PARP at later times, during the gradual course of dopamine axon terminal degeneration and cell body loss, remains to be studied and cannot yet be excluded.

These results (i) confirm that MPTP reduces striatal ATP levels,[4] (ii) show that MPTP causes a regionally-dependent (striatal and midbrain) loss of NAD$^+$, (iii) indicate that the PARP inhibitor benzamide can exert its protective effects[8] in part by preventing these losses and without interfering with MPTP-induced striatal dopamine release, (iv) suggest an involvement of PARP in the control of brain energy metabolism during neurotoxic insult, and (v) provide further evidence in support of the participation of PARP in MPTP-induced neurotoxicity *in vivo*.

ACKNOWLEDGMENTS

The authors gratefully acknowledge the excellent assistance of V. Nguyen, F. Servel, J. Floutard, M. Calmettes, R. Deceuninck, and Dr. A.-D. Degryse, and Dr. F. Colpaert for critical reading of the manuscript.

REFERENCES

1. GAAL, J.C., K.R. SMITH & C.K. PEARSON. 1987. Cellular euthanasia mediated by a nuclear enzyme: a central role for nuclear ADP-ribosylation in cellular metabolism. Trends Biochem. Sci. **12:** 128–129.
2. CARSON, D.A., S. SETO, D.B. WASSON & C.J. CARRERA. 1986. DNA strand breaks, NAD metabolism, and programmed cell death. Exp. Cell Res. **164:** 273–281.
3. SCHRAUFSTATTER, I.U., P.A. HYSLOP, D.B. HINSHAW, R.G. SPRAGG, L.A. SKLAR & C.G. COCHRANE. 1986. Hydrogen peroxide-induced injury of cells and its prevention by inhibitors of poly(ADP-ribose) polymerase. Proc. Natl. Acad. Sci. USA **83:** 4908–4912.
4. CHAN, P., L.E. DELANNEY, I. IRWIN, J.W. LANGSTON & D.A. DI MONTE. 1991. Rapid ATP loss caused by 1-methyl-4-phenyl-1,2,3,6-tetrahydropyridine in mouse brain. J. Neurochem. **57:** 348–351.
5. CHAN, P., J.W. LANGSTON, I. IRWIN, L.E. DELANNEY & D.A. DI MONTE. 1993. 2-Deoxyglucose enhances 1-methyl-4-phenyl-1,2,3,6,-tetrahydropyridine-induced ATP loss in the mouse brain. J. Neurochem. **61:** 610–616.
6. COSI, C., F. COLPAERT, W. KOEK, A. DEGRYSE & M. MARIEN. 1996. Poly(ADP-ribose)polymerase inhibitors protect against MPTP-induced depletions of striatal dopamine and cortical noradrenaline in C57Bl/6 mice. Brain Res. **729:** 264–269.
7. NRC (National Research Council). 1996. Guide for the Care and Use of Laboratory Animals. National Academy Press. Washington, DC.
8. COSI, C. & M. MARIEN. 1998. Decreases in mouse brain NAD$^+$ and ATP induced by 1-methyl-4-phenyl-1,2,3,6-tetrahydropyridine (MPTP): prevention by the poly (ADP-ribose) polymerase inhibitor, benzamide. Brain Res. **809:** 58–67.
9. MARIEN, M.R., M. BRILEY & F. COLPAERT. 1993. Noradrenaline depletion exacerbates MPTP-induced striatal dopamine loss in mice. Eur. J. Pharmacol. **236:** 487–489.
10. ALTAR, C.A., R.E. HEIKKILA, L. MANZINO & M.R. MARIEN. 1986. 1-methyl-4-phenylpyridine (MPP$^+$): regional dopamine neuron uptake, toxicity, and novel rotational behaviour following receptor proliferation. Eur. J. Pharmacol. **131:** 199–209.
11. CHAN, P., D.A. DI MONTE, J.J. LUO, L.E. DELANNEY, I. IRWIN & J.W. LANGSTON. 1994. Rapid ATP loss caused by methamphetamine in the mouse striatum: relationship between energy impairment and dopaminergic toxicity. J. Neurochem. **62:** 2484–2487.
12. CASTAGNOLI, K., S. PALMER, A. ANDERSON, T. BUETERS & N. CASTAGNOLI, JR. 1997. The neuronal nitric oxide synthase inhibitor 7-nitroindazole also inhibits the monoamine oxidase-B-catalyzed oxidation of 1-methyl-4-phenyl-1,2,3,6-tetrahydropyridine. Chem. Res. Toxicol. **10:** 364–368.
13. MARKEY, S.P., J.N. JOHANNESSEN, C.C. CHIUEH, R.S. BURNS & M.A. HERKENHAM. 1984. Intraneuronal generation of a pyridinium metabolite may cause drug-induced parkinsonism. Nature **311:** 464–466.
14. GIOVANNI, A., P.K. SONSALLA & R.E. HEIKKILA. 1994. Studies on species sensitivity to the dopaminergic neurotoxin 1-methyl-4-phenyl-1,2,3,6-tetrahydropyridine. Part 2: Central administration of 1-methyl-4-phenylpyridinium. J. Pharmacol. Exp. Ther. **270:** 1008–1014.
15. WESTERINK, B.H.C., J. TUNTLER, G. DAMSMA, H. ROLLEMA & J.B. DE VRIES. 1987. The use of tetrodotoxin for the characterization of drug-enhanced dopamine release in conscious rats studied by brain dialysis. Naunyn-Schmiedebergs Arch. Pharmacol. **336:** 502–507.
16. CHIUEH, C.C., H. MIYAKE & M.-T. PENG. 1993. Role of dopamine autoxidation, hydroxyl radical generation, and calcium overload in underlying mechanisms involved in MPTP-induced parkinsonism. Adv. Neurol. **60:** 251–258.
17. WOOD, P.L. & C.A. ALTAR. 1988. Dopamine release *in vivo* from nigrostriatal, mesolimbic and mesocortical neurons: utility of 3-methoxytyramine measurements. Pharmacol. Rev. **40:** 163–187.

Neuroprotection against Ischemia by Metabolic Inhibition Revisited

A Comparison of Hypothermia, a Pharmacologic Cocktail and Magnesium Plus Mexiletine

KENNETH I. MAYNARD,[a] ALFREDO QUIÑONES-HINOJOSA, AND JUNAID Y. MALEK

Neurophysiology Laboratory, Neurosurgical Service, Massachusetts General Hospital and Harvard Medical School, Boston. Massachusetts, USA

ABSTRACT: Previous studies have suggested that metabolic inhibition is neuroprotective, but little evidence has been provided to support this proposal. Using the *in vitro* rabbit retina preparation as an established model of the central nervous system (CNS), we measured the rate of glucose utilization and lactate production, and the light-evoked compound action potentials (CAPs) as indices of neuronal energy metabolism and electrophysiologic function, respectively. We examined the effect of three (3) treatments options: hypothermia (i.e., 33°C and 30°C), a six-member pharmacologic "cocktail" (tetrodotoxin (0.1 μM), 2-amino-4-phosphonobutyric acid (20 μM), 2-amino-5-phosphonovaleric acid (1 mM), amiloride (1 mM), magnesium (10 mM) and lithium (10 mM)) and the combination of magnesium (Mg^{2+} 1 mM) and mexiletine (Mex, 300 μM) on *in vitro* rabbit retinas, to see if there is a correlation between neuronal energy metabolism during ischemia (simulated by the reduction of oxygen from 95% to 15% and glucose from 6 mM to 1 mM), and the subsequent recovery of function. Hypothermia and the "cocktail" significantly inhibited both the rate of glucose utilization and lactate production, whereas Mg^{2+} and/or Mex showed only a nonsignificant tendency toward a reduction, compared to control retinas. Recovery of light-evoked CAPs was significantly improved in hypothermia- and cocktail-treated retinas, as well as with retinas exposed to the combination of Mg^{2+} plus Mex, but not with Mg^{2+} or Mex alone, relative to control retinas. A linear regression analysis of the % recovery of function versus the % reduction in the rate of glucose utilization during ischemia showed a significant correlation ($r^2 = 0.80$, correlation coefficient = 0.9, $p < 0.05$) between these two parameters. This and other data discussed provide convincing evidence that there is a correlation between metabolic inhibition, achieved during ischemia, and neuroprotection.

INTRODUCTION

The initial pathophysiological event that leads to ischemic injury is energy depletion.[1–4] The reduction in the supply of oxygen and glucose to the tissue eventually

[a]Corresponding author: Dr. Kenneth I. Maynard, Neurophysiology Laboratory, Edwards 414, Neurosurgical Service, Massachusetts General Hospital and Harvard Medical School, 55 Fruit Street, Boston, MA 02114. Phone, 617/726-3782; fax, 617/726-3926.
e-mail, Maynard@helix.mgh.harvard.edu

leads to adenosine triphosphate (ATP) depletion, resulting in various ischemia-induced cascades, including, but not limited to the loss of ion gradients, membrane depolarization and destabilization.[2,3,5] massive release of multiple neurotransmitters (e.g., glutamate[6] and adenosine[7]), calcium overload,[8] acidosis,[9] free radical generation,[10] nitric oxide overproduction,[11] stress gene activation[12] and activation of caspases,[13] each of which may eventually lead to tissue infarction. Current research in cerebral ischemia generally focuses on protecting against one of the many aforementioned cascades, for example, by using glutamate receptor antagonists, calcium antagonists, free radical scavengers, nitric oxide synthase inhibitors or anti-apoptotic agents, to name a few.[6–18] We maintain that although these approaches attenuate the ischemic injury, each is target-specific and therefore limited in preventing irreversible tissue injury, since each of the other nontargeted, deleterious cascades may also lead to ischemic infarction.

We propose that rather than trying to protect against the myriad consequences of ischemia, a more direct and comprehensive approach would be to rectify (or prevent) the initial energy imbalance that results from the reduced energy supply (e.g., due to hypoperfusion) and the high energy demand of the "tissue at risk." In the central nervous system (CNS) this can be achieved either by reducing the neuronal energy demands (e.g., as with hypothermia), or by improving the neuronal energy reserve (e.g., as with reperfusion, *in vivo*). In the following studies, we have concentrated on the former option. We tested three (3) experimental interventions, hypothermia[19] (as a gold-standard for comparison in our experimental paradigm), a six-member pharmacologic combination of agents[20,21] (cocktail), and the combination of magnesium (Mg^{2+}) and mexiletine (Mex).[22] Each treatment was designed to prevent ischemic injury by reducing the neuronal energy demand, by temporarily blocking nonvital neuronal functions. Hypothermia is well known to inhibit neuronal metabolism,[23–25] and this has also been shown to be true of each of the agents used in the six-member cocktail,[26] as well as with Mg^{2+} [26] and Mex.[27] Interestingly, hypothermia,[28–30] four of the six agents used in the cocktail,[20] Mg^{2+} [31,32] and Mex[33,34] have also been reported to provide neuroprotection.

The aforementioned interventions have been tested using the *in vitro* rabbit retina preparation established in our laboratory.[19,20,22,35–37] For each treatment, we have measured the rate of glucose utilization and lactate production as an index of neuronal energy metabolism, and the light-evoked compound action potentials as an indicator of electrophysiologic neuronal function. Some of the findings presented here have been previously reported.[19,20,22]

MATERIALS AND METHODS

The In Vitro *Rabbit Retina Preparation*

All procedures performed on the animals in this study were approved by the Subcommittee on Research Animal Care of the Massachusetts General Hospital, whose standards meet those of the Federal (NIH) and State (Massachusetts) reviewing organizations.

As previously described, retinas with 4–5 mm of optic nerve attached were isolated from dark-adapted, anesthetized (70 mg kg^{-1} ketamine and 25 mg kg^{-1} xylazine, intramuscularly (i.m.)) New Zealand White male (2–3.5 kg) rabbits.[19,20,22,35-37]

Biochemical Assays

Isolated rabbit retinas were placed in glass boats, maintained at 36.5 ± 0.5°C and rocked at about 1 Hz along their longitudinal axes to allow for an exchange of the gas (95% O_2 and 5% CO_2) and artificial cerebrospinal fluid (Ames' medium, Sigma Chemical Co.) for 1-hr equilibration. The retinas were then incubated in 5 ml of Ames' medium alone ("control") for 1 hr followed by 2 hr of ischemia (see below) and 3 hr of "return-to-control" (see below) conditions. Throughout the experiment the incubation medium was sampled before and after each incubation period. At the end of each experiment, retinas were removed from the medium and weighed (wet weight). Glucose (Glucose/HK, Boehringer Mannheim Corp.) and lactate (Lactate Reagent, Sigma Chemical Co.) levels in the incubation medium were obtained using standard enzymatic determination reaction kits.

Electrophysiology

Each retina was placed in an incubation chamber containing Ames' medium maintained at 36–37.5°C, and gassed with 95% O_2 and 5% CO_2. Light-evoked compound action potentials (CAPs) consisting of "On" and "Off" responses were elicited by a dim 1-sec light flash every 5–30 min, and recorded from the optic nerve using a Gould pen amplifier/recorder (Model 2200) or an AstroMed/Grass Amplifier (CP511). After recording the responses under control conditions, subsequent responses were recorded as the retinas underwent 1, 2 or 3 hr of ischemia (see below) followed by 3–4 hr of "return-to-control" (see below) conditions.

Ischemia and "Return-to-Control" Conditions

Ischemia was induced by the reduction of glucose from 6 mM to 1 mM and O_2 from 95% to 15%. During the period of ischemia the control retinas remained at 36°C without drugs, and the treated retinas were subjected either to hypothermia (i.e., 33°C or 30°C); the six-member cocktail (tetrodotoxin (0.1 μM), 2-amino-4-phosphonobutyric acid (20 μM), 2-amino-5-phosphonovaleric acid (1 mM), amiloride (1 mM), magnesium (10 mM) and lithium (10 mM)), magnesium sulfate (Mg^{2+}, 1 mM) (Sigma Chemical Co.), Mex (300 μM) (Boehringer Ingelheim Pharmaceutical, Inc., CT, USA), or the combination of Mg^{2+} plus Mex. "Return-to-control" conditions returned the retina to preischemic control (i.e., no drugs and normothermic) conditions. The incubation (Ames') medium already contains Mg^{2+} (1.2 mM), therefore the total concentration of Mg^{2+} present when Mg^{2+} (1 mM) was added was 2.2 mM.

Data Calculation and Analysis

Glucose utilization and lactate production were calculated as μmol/min/g wet weight of the retina with the optic nerve removed. The electrophysiologic data were calculated as a percentage of the control light-evoked CAPs (100%) for each retina. Control responses were calculated as the average of three readings of the light-evoked

CAPs prior to introducing ischemic conditions. The amplitudes of the light-evoked "On" and "Off" CAPs were averaged to simplify the calculation. This averaging was justified, since neither ischemia nor treatment conditions selectively impaired the recovery of either the "On" or "Off" light-evoked CAPs.[19,20,22,35–37] During ischemic and "return-to-control" conditions, the analyses were performed using repeated measures analysis of variance (ANOVA) followed by either Fisher's protected least significant difference (LSD) or Student-Newman-Keuls post hoc test, as appropriate, since data were collected from each retina over time throughout the entire procedure. The correlation between the "% recovery" and the "% glucose inhibition" (FIG. 7) was performed using a simple regression analysis. Throughout the text, all data are presented as mean ± standard error of the mean.

RESULTS

The data reported here represent a combination of original data not previously published (i.e., the effect of the 3 different interventions on glucose utilization and lactate production during ischemia), data previously communicated in preliminary form (i.e., all the hypothermia data), and data previously published (i.e., light-evoked CAPs during "return-to-control" conditions for the six-member cocktail, Mg^{2+} and/ or Mex), but which now appear in a different form from its original publication. Only data relevant to the thesis of this paper, and not for the entire experimental protocol

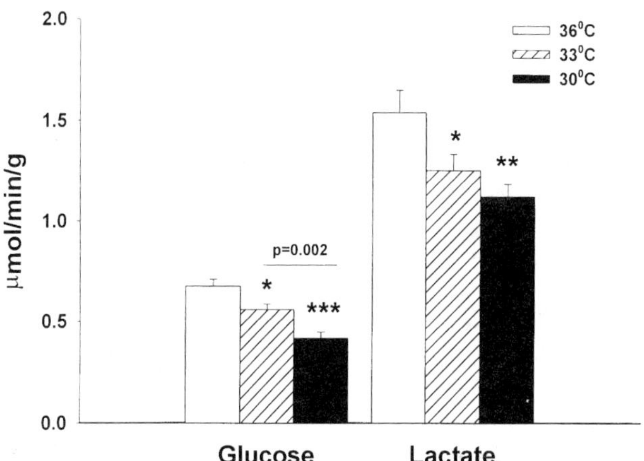

FIGURE 1. Histogram showing the rate of glucose utilization and lactate production during 2 hr of ischemia (simulated by the reduction of oxygen from 95% to 15% and glucose from 6 mM to 1 mM) using the *in vitro* rabbit retina preparation. Retinas treated with mild (33°C, $n = 6$) and moderate (30°C, $n = 6$) hypothermia exhibited significant reductions in both glucose and lactate metabolism compared with control retinas during ischemia (36°C, $n = 6$). In addition, glucose metabolism was also significantly reduced in retinas treated with moderate hypothermia (30°C) compared to those treated with mild hypothermia (33°C). The data are represented as the mean ± standard error of the mean, and were analyzed using the repeated measures ANOVA followed by Student-Newman-Keuls post hoc test. $*p < 0.05$, $**p < 0.01$ and $***p < 0.001$.

described in the Materials and Methods, are reported. Readers are referred to other publications[19,20,22] for a complete account of the excluded data.

Across all the groups of retinas tested the initial rates of glucose utilization and lactate production, and the amplitudes of "On" and "Off" CAPs were similar (data not shown).[19,20,22]

Hypothermia

Glucose Utilization and Lactate Production

There was a significant, temperature-dependent reduction in both glucose utilization and lactate production in retinas treated with 33°C and 30°C during ischemia, compared to those treated with 36°C (i.e., control retinas) (FIG. 1).

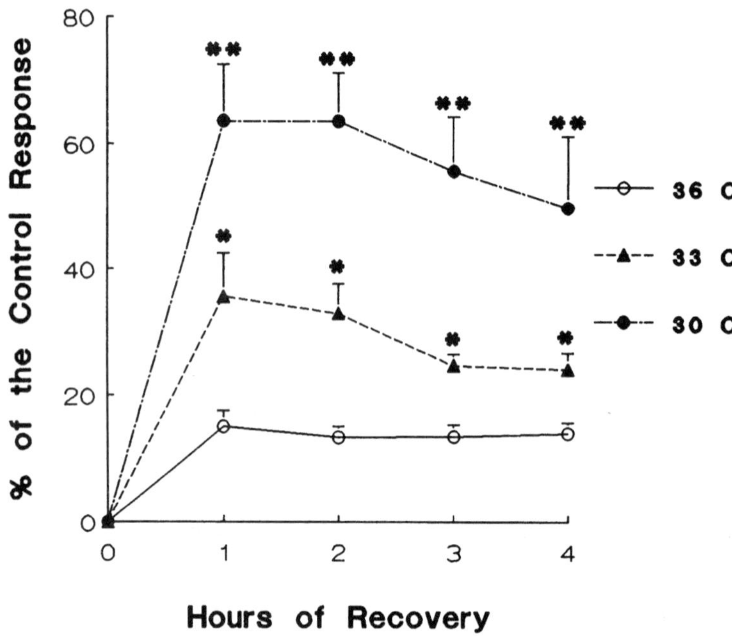

FIGURE 2. Recovery of the light-evoked compound action potentials (CAPs) represented as the "% of the control response" when the retinas were subjected to the "return-to-control" conditions following 1 hr of ischemia (simulated by the reduction of oxygen from 95% to 15% and glucose from 6 mM to 1 mM) using the *in vitro* rabbit retina preparation. During ischemia, exposure to 30°C ($n = 5$) significantly improved the subsequent recovery of function relative to retinas exposed to either 33°C ($n = 6$), or control (36°C-treated) retinas ($n = 6$). The data are represented as the mean ± standard error of the mean, and were analyzed using the repeated measures ANOVA followed by Student-Newman-Keuls post hoc test. *$p < 0.05$ and **$p < 0.01$.

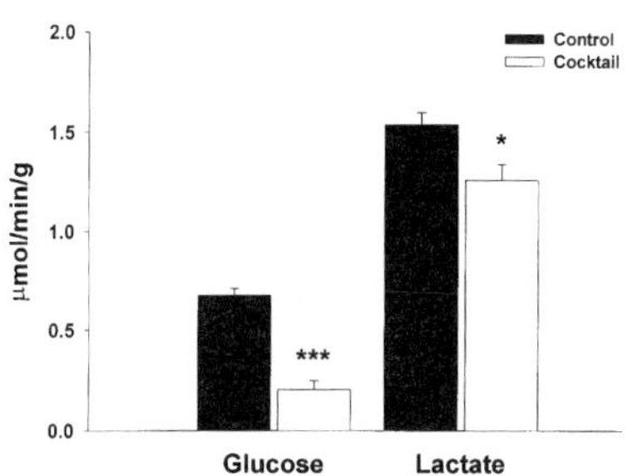

FIGURE 3. Histogram showing the rate of glucose utilization and lactate production during 2 hr of ischemia (simulated by the reduction of oxygen from 95% to 15% and glucose from 6 mM to 1 mM) using the *in vitro* rabbit retina preparation. Retinas treated with the six-member cocktail ($n = 4$) (tetrodotoxin (0.1 µM), 2-amino-4-phosphonobutyric acid (20 µM), 2-amino-5-phosphonovaleric acid (1 mM), amiloride (1 mM), magnesium (10 mM) and lithium (10 mM)), exhibited a marked reduction in both glucose and lactate metabolism compared with control (untreated) retinas during ischemia ($n = 6$). The data are represented as the mean ± standard error of the mean, and were analyzed using the repeated measures ANOVA followed by Student-Newman-Keuls post hoc test. *$p < 0.05$ and ***$p < 0.001$.

Light-Evoked Compound Action Potentials

There was a significant, temperature-dependent improvement in the recovery of light-evoked CAPs in the 33°C- and 30°C-treated versus control (36°C-treated) retinas, following 1 hr of ischemia (FIG. 2).

Six-Member Pharmacologic Cocktail

Glucose Utilization and Lactate Production

The six-member cocktail markedly reduced both the glucose utilization and lactate production in retinas during ischemia, compared to control (untreated) retinas (FIG. 3).

Light-Evoked Compound Action Potentials

Untreated (control) retinas that been exposed to 3 hr of ischemia showed no recovery of light-evoked CAPs during the "return-to-control" conditions. Remarkably, retinas treated with the six-member cocktail during the 3-hr period of ischemia each showed full recovery of the light-evoked CAPs after 3–4 hr of "return-to-control" conditions (FIG. 4).

Magnesium and Mexiletine

Glucose Utilization and Lactate Production

Although there was a tendency, neither the glucose utilization nor the lactate production was significantly reduced during ischemia in retinas in which either Mg^{2+} and/or Mex was present (FIG. 5).

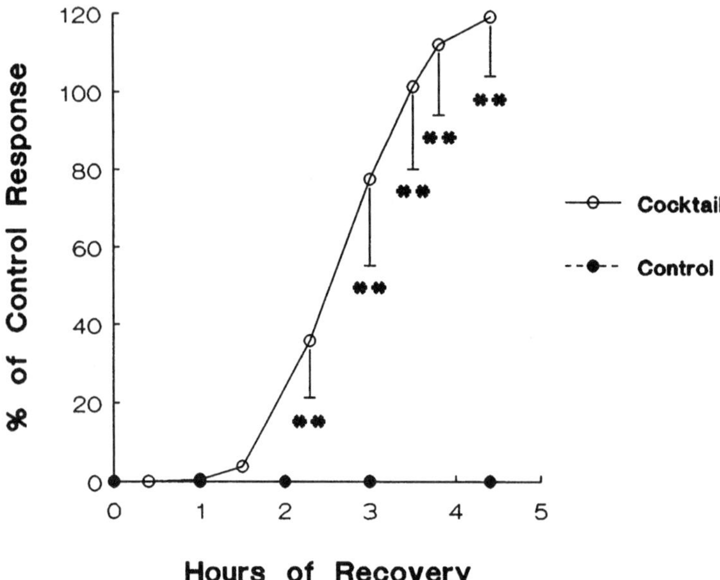

Hours of Recovery

FIGURE 4. Recovery of the light-evoked compound action potentials (CAPs) represented as the "% of the control response" when the retinas were subjected to the "return-to-control" conditions following 3 hr of ischemia (simulated by the reduction of oxygen from 95% to 15% and glucose from 6 mM to 1 mM) using the *in vitro* rabbit retina preparation. Retinas treated with the six-member cocktail ($n = 3$) (tetrodotoxin (0.1 µM), 2-amino-4-phosphonobutyric acid (20 µM), 2-amino-5-phosphonovaleric acid (1 mM), amiloride (1 mM), magnesium (10 mM) and lithium (10 mM)), during ischemia, showed marked recovery of function relative to control (untreated) retinas ($n = 3$). The data are represented as the mean ± standard error of the mean, and were analyzed using the repeated measures ANOVA followed by Fisher LSD (protected) post hoc test. **p <0.01.

Light-Evoked Compound Action Potentials

Following "return-to-control" conditions there was a partial recovery of the light-evoked CAPs in each of the groups of retinas studied. Only the retinas that were treated with the combination of Mg^{2+} plus Mex, however, resulted in significant recovery of light-evoked CAPs (FIG. 6).

Correlation between % Recovery of Function and % Glucose Inhibition

In order to test whether there exists a relationship between the degree of neuronal metabolic inhibition achieved during ischemia, and recovery of neuronal function, we calculated the average recovery of function (i.e., the average of the amplitudes of the "On" and "Off" light-evoked CAPs over the 3–4 hr of "return-to-control" conditions), as a percentage of the preischemic responses for each retina. This is referred to as the "% recovery of function." The latter was then plotted against the % reduction in the glucose utilization obtained during ischemia for each condition in the above interventions (i.e., 33°C, 30°C, six-member cocktail, Mg^{2+}, Mex, Mg^{2+} plus Mex), relative to

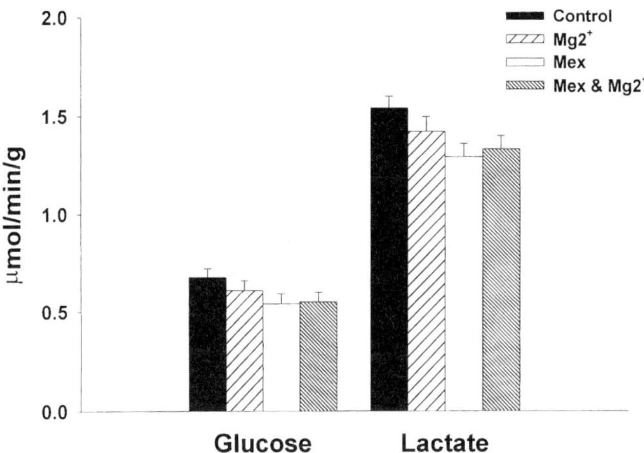

FIGURE 5. Histogram showing the rate of glucose utilization and lactate production during 2 hr of ischemia (simulated by the reduction of oxygen from 95% to 15% and glucose from 6 mM to 1 mM) using the *in vitro* rabbit retina preparation. Retinas treated with magnesium (Mg^{2+}, 1 mM, $n = 4$) mexiletine (Mex, 300 mM, $n = 5$) or Mg^{2+} plus Mex ($n = 5$) showed a nonsignificant trend toward a reduction in glucose and lactate metabolism relative to control (untreated, $n = 6$) retinas. The data are represented as the mean ± standard error of the mean, and were analyzed using the repeated measures ANOVA.

the control (36°C) retinas during ischemia. The analyzed results show that regardless of the length of time of the ischemic insult (which varied from 1 hr with hypothermia, to 2 hr with Mg^{2+} and/or Mex, to 3 hr with the six-member cocktail), there is a significant correlation between the % glucose inhibition during ischemia and the % recovery of function. Specifically, the data indicate that the recovery of function from ischemia is improved with greater glucose utilization inhibition during ischemia (FIG. 7).

DISCUSSION

We have established the use of the *in vitro* rabbit retina preparation as a model of the CNS,[38] for the measurement of both metabolic and electrophysiologic parameters, under normal conditions and simulated ischemia.[19,20,22,35–37] Given the lack of a blood-brain barrier in this preparation, drug treatments have optimal conditions for acting directly on the cells in the retina. Thus, in considering the mechanism of the neuroprotective action observed in these three experimental interventions, i.e., hypothermia, the six-member cocktail and Mg^{2+} and Mex, it is clear that the effect must be based on a direct action on the neurons (and glial cells) of the retina, and not on an indirect effect such as changes in blood flow, which is not a consideration in this preparation.

In the retinas exposed to hypothermia, there appears to be a causal relationship between the reduction in neuronal energy metabolism during ischemia, as measured by the glucose utilization and lactate production, and the recovery of neuronal function,

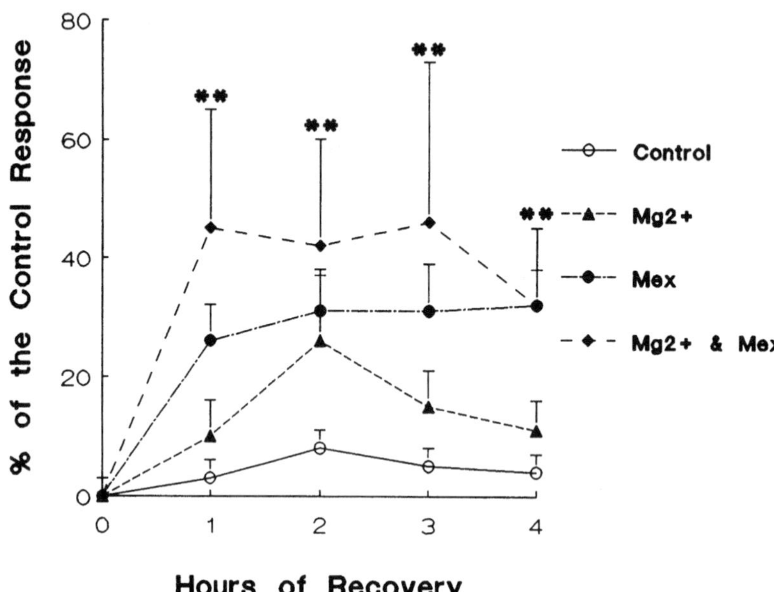

FIGURE 6. Recovery of the light-evoked compound action potentials (CAPs) represented as the "% of the control response" when the retinas were subjected to the "return-to-control" conditions following 2 hr of ischemia (simulated by the reduction of oxygen from 95% to 15% and glucose from 6 mM to 1 mM) using the *in vitro* rabbit retina preparation. Although exposure to either magnesium (Mg^{2+}, 1 mM, $n = 6$) or mexiletine (Mex, 300 mM, $n = 7$) tended to improve the recovery of function, the light-evoked CAPs were not significantly improved until both Mg^{2+} and Mex were combined ($n = 7$), relative to the control (untreated) retinas ($n = 4$). The data are represented as the mean ± standard error of the mean, and were analyzed using the repeated measures ANOVA followed by Fisher LSD (protected) post hoc test. **$p < 0.01$.

as measured by the light-evoked CAPs. We have previously shown that both the six-member cocktail[21] and Mg^{2+} and Mex combined[22] inhibit neuronal metabolism under normal, nonischemic conditions as measured by glucose utilization and lactate production in *in vitro* rabbit retina preparations. In the present experiments, however, we now show that the six-member cocktail, but not the Mg^{2+}- and/or Mex-treated retinas, also significantly inhibit neuronal energy metabolism during ischemia. Examined together, the data from the 3 treatment paradigms show a strong correlation between the % recovery of function and the degree of neuronal metabolic inhibition achieved during ischemia. This significant correlation illustrates that, independent of the duration of ischemia, functional neuroprotection is improved with increasing neuronal energy metabolism inhibition during ischemia. This therefore provides convincing evidence for the proposal that metabolic inhibition during ischemia is a sound neuroprotective strategy.

The experimental outcome using the six-member cocktail further supports the proposal that reducing the neuronal energy demands of the tissue at risk can prevent ir-

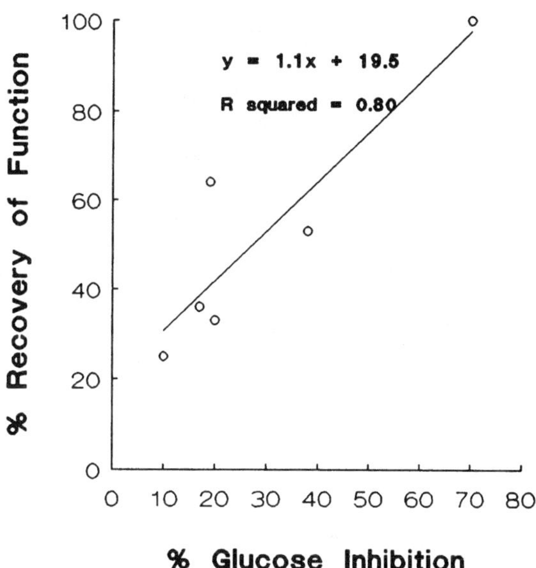

FIGURE 7. "% Recovery" (i.e., the recovery of the light-evoked compound action potentials of the retinas relative to their control responses) versus the "% glucose inhibition" (i.e., the % reduction of the rate of glucose utilization). Retinas were exposed to the following conditions during ischemia, 36°C (control), 33°C, 30°C, the six-member cocktail (tetrodotoxin (0.1 mM), 2-amino-4-phosphonobutyric acid (20 μM), 2-amino-5-phosphonovaleric acid (1 mM), amiloride (1 mM), magnesium (10 mM) and lithium (10 mM)), Mg^{2+} (1 mM), Mex (300 mM), and Mg^{2+} plus Mex. Simple regression analysis revealed a correlation coefficient of 0.90, a regression ANOVA of $F = 16.41$, $p = 0.02$).

reversible injury due to ischemia. We have established that the time at which irreversible functional damage virtually occurs in this preparation is 2 hr.[20,22,37] Yet, treatment with the six-member cocktail led to 100% recovery of function in each retina to which it was exposed, despite the fact that the period of ischemia was 3 hr.[20] Thus we have been able to extend the duration of the ischemia by 1 hr and still achieve 100% recovery of function. We suggest that this may only be possible if there was indeed a rectification of the energy imbalance between the reduced energy supply induced by ischemia, and the temporary reduction in energy demand achieved by blocking numerous functions using the six-member cocktail. Of note is that the six-member cocktail achieved the greatest reduction in neuronal energy demands during ischemia (70%), more so than 30°C hypothermia (38%), and likewise it resulted in the best functional neuroprotection observed (100% versus 53% recovery).[19,20]

Data not reported here show that along with the recovery of neuronal electrophysiologic function is a similar improvement in the rate of glucose utilization and lactate production[19,22] during the "return-to-control" conditions. This neuronal metabolic recovery may represent a tendency to resume normal function of the protected neurons, after washout of the drugs, which temporarily blocked nonvital neuronal functions.

Protecting the brain from ischemia by metabolic inhibition through pharmacological intervention is not a novel strategy.[39–42] Hypothermia, which is the most reproducible and potent neuroprotective strategy[28,29] is thought to achieve neuroprotection via this,[40,41,43–49] as well as other mechanisms, including but not limited to slowing ion leakage,[50] attenuating apoptosis,[51] mediating postischemic metabolic recovery,[52] and delaying the time to ischemia-induced depolarization.[53] Anesthetics,[41,54–56] including barbiturates[57–59] have been used to reduce tissue energy requirements and shown to protect against ischemia. This strategy was reevaluated,[60] however, since it became clear that barbiturates are not as effective as hypothermia.[48,57,60] We propose that previous pharmacologic attempts at reducing energy requirements have not been more successful probably because the degree of metabolic inhibition achieved was insufficient, e.g., less than with hypothermia. In the *in vitro* retina, for example, although the barbiturate, thiopental (340 mM), blocked retinal function, it marginally reduced oxygen and glucose consumption compared with hypothermia.[26] Moreover, barbiturates at toxic levels in humans only decrease oxygen consumption by 25–30%.[61] Thus, although barbiturates block neurotransmission, they do not markedly reduce energy metabolism.[39] This may explain why barbiturates are less likely to be neuroprotective under severe ischemic conditions,[60,62] such as with global ischemia where the energy deficit is large, but may work under conditions of partial focal ischemia,[57–60] where the energy imbalance is less severe for neurons in the penumbra areas. It was for this reason that we used a six-member cocktail, so that multiple nonvital, functional processes could be temporarily blocked in order to achieve a marked reduction in neuronal energy demands that is necessary to counter the effects of a significant reduction in blood flow.

Recently the concept of metabolic inhibition (or reducing energy demands) as a rational approach for protecting against ischemia has been receiving renewed favor.[19–22,24,25,63–66] Given the number of detrimental cascades induced by ischemia, preventing irreversible injury by markedly reducing energy demands may be a more effective means of protection, rather than targeting just one of many lethal pathways. As our data show, metabolic inhibition will probably be more effective using a combination of drugs to achieve profound reduction in neuronal energy demands, by temporarily blocking numerous nonvital neuronal functions.

Use of a combination of drugs in the prevention of stroke has been suggested by us[20–22,63] and others,[15,17,18,67] but this is the first study of which we are aware in which such a strategy is used to show a strong correlation between the combination of agents achieving marked neuronal metabolic inhibition, and the subsequent remarkable recovery of neuronal function. Moreover, we have shown that the six-member cocktail is as profoundly neuroprotective *in vivo* in a model of focal cerebral ischemia in the rabbit,[21] as it is *in vitro* using the rabbit retina preparation.[20] Thus we believe that the approach of metabolic inhibition has great potential to be neuroprotective *in vivo* as well as *in vitro*.

In this study we have shown that under three different treatment interventions, hypothermia, use of a six-member pharmacologic cocktail, and the combination of Mg^{2+} and Mex, functional neuroprotection was achieved. Moreover, we uniquely demonstrate a strong correlation between the reduction in glucose utilization during ischemia and the recovery of light-evoked CAPs from *in vitro* rabbit retinas. Further studies are needed to provide more direct evidence supporting a causal relationship between profound metabolic inhibition during ischemia leading to marked functional neuroprotection *in vivo*.

ACKNOWLEDGMENTS

The authors would like to thank Dr. Christopher S. Ogilvy for his generous support throughout the period during which these experiments were conducted, Dr. Adelbert Ames III for many instructive conversations on the topic and for comments on the manuscript, and Boehringer Ingelheim Pharmaceuticals Inc. for providing the mexiletine. K.I.M. is an American Heart Association, Minority Scientist Development Awardee, and A.Q.-H. is a Howard Hughes Medical Institute, Medical Student Research Training Fellow.

REFERENCES

1. SIESJÖ, B.K. 1992. Pathophysiology and treatment of focal cerebral ischemia. Part I: Pathophysiology. J. Neurosurg. **77:** 169–184.
2. CAFÉ, C., C. TORRI & F. MARZATICO. 1993. Cellular and molecular events of ischemic brain damage. Funct. Neurol. **8:** 121–133.
3. MARTIN, R.L., H.G.E. LLOYD & A.I. COWAN. 1994. The early events of oxygen and glucose deprivation: setting the scene for neuronal death? Trends Neurosci. **17:** 251–257.
4. W. PULSINELLI. 1995. The ischemic penumbra in stroke. Sci. Am. Sci. Med. Jan/Feb: 16–25.
5. CALABRESI, P., G.A. MARFIA, D. CENTONZE *et al.* 1999. Sodium influx plays a major role in the membrane depolarization induced by oxygen and glucose deprivation in rat striatal spiny neurons. Stroke **30:** 171–179.
6. OBRENOVITCH, T.P. & J. URENJAK. 1997. Altered glutamatergic transmission in neurological disorders: from high extracellular glutamate to excessive synaptic efficacy. Prog. Neurobiol. **51:** 39–87.
7. SWEENEY, M.I. 1997. Neuroprotective effects of adenosine in cerebral ischemia: window of opportunity. Neurosci. Biobehav. Rev. **21:** 207–217.
8. KRISTIAN, T. & B.K. SIESJÖ. 1998. Calcium in ischemic cell death. Stroke **29:** 705–718.
9. VORNOV, J.J., A.G. THOMAS & D. JO. 1996. Protective effects of extracellular acidosis and blockade of sodium/hydrogen ion exchange during recovery from metabolic inhibition in neuronal tissue culture. J. Neurochem. **67:** 2379–2389.
10. HALL, E.D. 1997. Brain attack: acute therapeutic interventions. Free radical scavengers and antioxidants. Neurosurg. Clin. North Am. **8:** 195–206.
11. IADECOLA, C. 1997. Bright and dark sides of nitric oxide in ischemic brain injury. Trends Neurosci. **20:** 132–139.
12. MASSA, S.M., R.A. SWANSON & F.R. SHARP. 1996. The stress gene response in brain. Cerebrovasc. Brain Metab. Rev. **8:** 95–158.
13. MACMANUS, J.P. & M.D. LINNIK. 1997. Gene expression induced by cerebral ischemia: an apoptotic perspective. J. Cereb. Blood Flow Metab. **17:** 815–832.
14. GINSBERG, M.D. 1993. Emerging strategies for the treatment of ischemic brain injury. *In* Molecular and Cellular Approaches to the Treatment of Neurological Diseases. S.G. Waxman, Ed.: 207–237. Raven Press, Ltd. New York.
15. GROTTA, J. 1994. The current status of neuronal protective therapy: why have all neuronal protective drugs worked in animals but none so far in stroke patients? Cerebrovasc. Dis. **4:** 115–120.

16. MUIR, K.W. & K.R. LEES. 1995. Clinical experience with excitatory amino acid antagonist drugs. Stroke **26:** 503–513.

17. BARINAGA, M. 1996. Finding new drugs to treat stroke. Science **272:** 664–666.

18. FISHER, M. 1997. Characterizing the target of acute stroke therapy. Stroke **28:** 866–872.

19. QUIÑONES-HINOJOSA, A., C.S. OGILVY & K.I. MAYNARD. 1998. Hypothermia during ischemia improves recovery of neuronal metabolism and function in the *in vitro* retina [abstract]. Soc. Neurosci. Abstr. **24:** 1506.

20. AMES III, A., K.I. MAYNARD, & S. KAPLAN. 1995. Protection against CNS ischemia by temporary interruption of function-related processes of neurons. J. Cereb. Blood Flow Metab. **15:** 433–439.

21. MAYNARD, K.I., T. KAWAMATA, C.S. OGILVY *et al.* 1998. Avoiding stroke during cerebral arterial occlusion by temporarily blocking neuronal functions in the rabbit. J. Stroke Cerebrovasc. Dis. **7:** 287–295.

22. MAYNARD, K.I., A. QUIÑONES & C.S. OGILVY. 1998. Magnesium plus mexiletine inhibit energy usage and protect retinas against ischemia. NeuroReport **9:** 4141–4144.

23. LAPTOOK, A.R., R.J. CORBETT, R. STERETT *et al.* 1995. Quantitative relationship between brain temperature and energy utilization: rate measured *in vivo* using ^{31}P and ^{1}H magnetic resonance spectroscopy. Pediatr. Res. **38:** 919–925.

24. WILLIAMS, G.D., B.J. DARDZINSKI, A.R. BUCKALEW *et al.* 1997. Modest hypothermia preserves cerebral energy metabolism during hypoxia-ischemia and correlates with brain damage: a ^{31}P nuclear magnetic resonance study in unanesthetized neonatal rats. Pediatr. Res. **42:** 700–708.

25. YAGER, J.Y. & J. ASSELIN. 1996. Effect of mild hypothermia on cerebral energy metabolism during the evolution of hypoxic-ischemic brain damage in the immature rat. Stroke **27:** 919–925.

26. ZAGER, E.L. & A. AMES III. 1988. Reduction of cellular energy requirements: screening for agents that may protect against CNS ischemia. J. Neurosurg. **69:** 568–579.

27. DONG, L.P., T.Y. WANG & L. ZHANG. 1992. Effect of mexiletine on energy metabolism of ischemic brain. Acta Pharmacol. Sin. **13:** 354–356.

28. BARONE, F.C., G.Z. FEUERSTEIN & R.F. WHITE. 1997. Brain cooling during transient focal ischemia provides complete neuroprotection Neurosci. Biobehav. Rev. **21:** 31–44.

29. KOCHS, E. & C. WERNER. 1995. Neuroprotection: fact or fantasy? Eur. J. Anaesthesiol. Suppl. **10:** 67–70.

30. COLBOURNE, F., G. SUTHERLAND & D. CORBETT. 1997. Postischemic hypothermia: a critical appraisal with implications for clinical treatment. Mol. Neurobiol. **14:** 171–201.

31. VACANTI, F.X. & A. AMES III. 1986. Mild hypothermia and Mg^{++} protect against irreversible damage during CNS ischemia. Stroke **15:** 695–698.

32. MARINOV, M.B., K.S. HARBAUGH, P.J. HOOPES *et al.* 1996. Neuroprotective effects of preischemia intraarterial magnesium sulfate in reversible focal cerebral ischemia. J. Neurosurg. **85:** 117–124.

33. ZHANG, X.S. & T.Y. WANG. 1993. Protection of mexiletine against hypoxic damage of synaptic function in hippocampal slices. Acta Pharmacol. Sin. **14:** 426–429.

34. STYS, P.K. & H. LESIUK. 1996. Correlation between electrophysiological effect of mexiletine and ischemic protection in central nervous system white matter. Neuroscience **71:** 27–36.

35. MAYNARD, K.I., D. CHEN, P.M. ARANGO *et al.* 1996. Nitro-L-arginine worsens and L-arginine improves functional recovery when added during ischemia in the *in vitro* rabbit retina. NeuroReport **8:** 81–85.

36. MAYNARD, K.I., P.M. ARANGO, D. CHEN *et al.* 1998. Acetylsalicylate administered during simulated ischemia impairs the recovery of neuronal function in the *in vitro* rabbit retina. Neurosci. Lett. **249:** 159–162.

37. MALEK, J.Y., A. QUIÑONES-HINOJOSA, C.S. OGILVY *et al.* 1998. An *in vitro* retina model to study neuronal function and metabolism following ischemia [abstract]. Soc. Neurosci. Abstr. **24:** 982.

38. AMES III, A. & R.H. MASLAND. 1990. The rabbit retina *in vitro*. *In* Preparation of Vertebrate Central Nervous System *In Vitro*. H. Jahnsen, Ed.: 183–202. John Wiley & Sons, Ltd. New York.

39. ASTRUP, J. 1982. Energy-requiring cell functions in the ischemia brain. Neurosurgery **56:** 482–497.

40. HOCHACHKA, P.W. 1986. Defence strategies against hypoxia and hypothermia. Science **231:** 234–241.

41. MICHENFELDER, J.D. & R.A. THEYE. 1973. The effects of anesthesia and hypothermia on canine cerebral ATP and lactate during anoxia produced by decapitation. Anesthesiology **33:** 430–439.

42. WRIGHT, R.L. & A. AMES III. 1964. Measurement of maximal permissible cerebral ischemia and a study of its pharmacologic prolongation. J. Neurosurg. **21:** 567–574.

43. LO, E.H. & G.K. STEINBERG. 1992. Effects of hypothermia on evoked potentials, magnetic resonance imaging, and blood flow in focal ischemia in rabbits. Stroke **23:** 889–893.

44. BUCHAN, A. & W.A. PULSINELLI. 1990. Hypothermia but not the N-methyl-D-aspartate antagonist, MK801, attenuates neuronal damage in gerbils subjected to transient global ischemia. J. Neurosci. **10:** 311–316.

45. BUSTO, R, W.D. DIETRICH, M. GLOBUS *et al.* 1987. Small differences in intraischemic brain temperature critically determine the extent of ischemic neuronal injury. J. Cereb. Blood Flow Metab. **7:** 729–738.

46. FIELD II, J., F.A. FUHRMAN & A.W. MARTIN. 1944. Effects of temperature on the oxygen consumption of brain tissue. J. Neurophysiol. **7:** 117–126.

47. LUST, W.D., A.B. WHEATON, G. FEUSSNER *et al.* 1989. Metabolism in the hamster brain during hibernation and arousal. Brain Res. **489:** 12–20.

48. RIDENOUR, T.R., D.S. WARNER, M.M. TODD *et al.* 1992. Mild hypothermia reduces infarct size resulting from temporary but not permanent focal ischemia in rats. Stroke **23:** 733–738.

49. XUE, D., Z.-G. HUANG, K.E. SMITH *et al.* 1992. Immediate or delayed mild hypothermia prevents focal cerebral infarction. Brain Res. **587:** 66–72.

50. ZEEVALK, G.D. & W.J. NICKLAS. 1996. Hypothermia and metabolic stress: narrowing the cellular site of early neuroprotection. J. Pharmacol. Exp. Ther. **279:** 332–339.

51. EDWARDS, A.D. & H. MEHMET. 1996. Apoptosis in perinatal hypoxic-ischaemic cerebral damage. Neuropathol. Appl. Neurobiol. **22:** 494–498.

52. SHIMIZU, H., L.H. CHANG, L. LITT *et al.* 1997. Effect of brain, body and magnet bore temperatures on energy metabolism during global cerebral ischemia and reperfusion monitored by magnetic resonance spectroscopy in rats. Magn. Reson. Med. **37:** 833–839.

53. BART, R.D., S. TAKAOKA, R.D. PEARLSTEIN *et al.* 1998. Interactions between hypothermia and the latency to ischemic depolarization: implications for neuroprotection. Anesthesiology **88:** 1266–1273.

54. NEHLS, D.G., M.M. TODD, R.F. SPETZLER *et al.* A comparison of the cerebral protective effects of isofluorane and barbiturates during temporary focal ischemia in primates. Anesthesiology **66:** 453–464.

55. THEYE, R.A. & J.D. MICHENFELDER. 1968. The effect of halothane on canine cerebral metabolism. Anesthesiology **29:** 1107–1112.

56. SANO, T., J.C. DRUMMOND, P.M. PATEL *et al.* 1992. A comparison of the cerebral protective effects of isoflurane and mild hypothermia in a model of incomplete forebrain ischemia in the rat. Anesthesiology **76:** 221–228.
57. ASTRUP, J., P. MOLLER, P. SORENSEN & H. RAHBEK SORENSEN. 1981. Inhibition of cerebral oxygen and glucose consumption in the dog by hypothermia, pentobarbital and lidocaine. Anesthesiology **55:** 263–268.
58. MICHENFELDER, J.D. 1973. Cerebral protection by thiopental during hypoxia. Anesthesiology **39:** 510–517.
59. NILLSON, L. & B.K. SIESJÖ. 1975. The effect of pentobarbitone anaesthesia on blood flow and oxygen consumption in the rat brain. Acta Anaesthesiol. Scand. Suppl. **57:** 18–24.
60. TODD, M.M. & D.S. WARNER. 1992. A comfortable hypothesis reevaluated: cerebral metabolic depression and brain protection during ischemia. Anesthesiology **76:** 161–164.
61. BRODERSEN, P. & E.O. JØRGENSEN. 1974. Cerebral blood flow and oxygen uptake, and cerebrospinal fluid biochemistry in severe coma. J. Neurol. Neurosurg. Psychiatry **37:** 384–391.
62. SCHWAB, S., M. SPRANGER, S. SCHWARTZ & W. HACKE. 1997. Barbiturate coma in severe hemispheric stroke: useful or obsolete? Neurology **48:** 1608–1613.
63. AMES III, A. 1992. Energy requirements of CNS cells as related to their function and to their vulnerability to ischemia: a commentary based on studies in retina. Can. J. Physiol. Pharmacol. **70:** S158–S164.
64. GORMAN, C. 1996. Damage control. Time **148:** 31–35.
65. LaMANNA, J.C. & W.D. LUST. 1997. Nutrient consumption and metabolic perturbations. Neurosurg. Clin. North Am. **8:** 145–163.
66. OBRENOVITCH, T.P. 1998. Neuroprotective strategies: voltage-gated Na-channel down-modulation. Rev. Neurosci. **9:** 203–211.
67. JONAS, S. 1995. Prophylactic pharmacologic neuroprotection against focal cerebral ischemia. Ann. N.Y. Acad. Sci. **765:** 21–25.

Questions and Answers

QUESTIONS FOR DR. ASCHNER

From Dr. Marchionni

Are these transient or stable transfections?

ANSWER: These are transient transfections.

QUESTION: Your current data do not support MT-I-mediated protection of astrocytes from MeHg toxicity. What about MT-2? Since this is expressed in astrocytes in addition to MT-I, perhaps MT-II is playing a role.

ANSWER: Your statement needs to be qualified, because as I have shown, the data support MT-I-mediated protection. The ^{51}Cr efflux measurements support the hypothesis that intracellular MT levels confer resistance to MeHg toxicity, but as I have said, MT-I-mediated protection attained statistical significance only in the 5-µM MeHg treatment group. The absence of a significant decrease in ^{51}Cr release in pGFAP-MT-I plasmid transfected astrocytoma at 10 µM MeHg was rather surprising, and it may represent the limited capacity of these cells to synthesize MT-I, such that the intracellular levels of MT-I do not attain a sufficiently high concentration to attenuate the effect of MeHg. We recognize that further work is required to optimize conditions that would allow for a greater increase of MT-I expression, and one way to approach this problem is obviously to study the astrocytes after stable transfections.

The possibility that MT-II may play a more important role in protection (compared to the MT-I isoform) is unlikely. Analysis of the regional distribution of MTs suggests that, in general, the relative abundance of MT mRNAs for all brain isoforms is quite identical, with MT-I and MT-II isoforms being constitutively expressed throughout the CNS. Please note that MT-III is also expressed in the CNS, but I have not discussed it today. It is well established that the distribution of MT-II mRNA mimics the distribution of MT-I mRNA, since their genes are coordinately expressed and respond in parallel to a variety of inducers.

QUESTIONS FOR DR. LOPACHIN

From Dr. Marchionni

Have you analyzed demyelinating lesions of MS patients or those seen in animal models such as experimental autoimmune encephalomyelitis (EAE)?

ANSWER: To date we have not had the opportunity to examine nervous tissue from "demyelinating" animal models or human disease states. We have analyzed peripheral nerve following induction of toxic neuropathies (e.g., acrylamide; 2,5-hexanedione) in rats where internodal thinning of the myelin sheath is observed. Corresponding data indicate axonal atrophy and a loss of axoplasmic K, Cl and water.[1,2]

From Dr. Jonas

What is the source of increased intraneuronal Ca^{2+}? Is it of extracellular origin only, or is there release of intercellular Ca^{2+}? Do you have studies done in Ca^{2+}-free medium that might clarify this?

ANSWER: Although ischemia is likely to promote subcellular redistribution of endogenous Ca^{2+}, we speculate that the major source of the observed Ca^{2+} rise is extraneuronal. As indicated in TABLE 1 of our paper, neuronal Ca^{2+} levels during control conditions are relatively low regardless of compartment considered and, therefore, release from these intracellular stores would contribute relatively little to the rather significant Ca^{2+} burden imposed by ischemia. In addition, our studies with glutamate receptor antagonists (FIGS. 4–6) show that during OGD/reperfusion compartmental Ca^{2+} levels remained normal. Presumably, Ca^{2+} release from internal stores would not be sensitive to membrane receptor blockage.[3,4]

From Dr. Narahashi

Have you done experiments similar to those of TTX and local anesthetics using calcium channel blockers and NMDA receptor blockers? Similar changes in Na, K, Ca and Mg to those caused by TTX and local anesthetics are expected to occur.

ANSWER: FIGURES 4–6 show that the P- and N-type Ca^{2+} channel blocker, ω-conotoxin, does not affect elemental derangement induced by OGD/reperfusion. To date, however, we have not used nifedipine or similar compounds to assess the role of L-type Ca^{2+} channels in experimental ischemia. As anticipated, NMDA receptor blockade with CPP afforded TTX-like protection against elemental disruption associated with OGD/reperfusion. Based on our pharmacologic data, we speculate that neuronal Ca^{2+} entry during ischemia is multifaceted and involves reverse operation of Na^{+}-Ca^{2+} exchange, ionophoric glutamate receptors and possibly Ca^{2+} channels.

From Dr. Faden

Where does the Mg^{2+} go if it disappears from intracellular and intramitochondrial spaces? Do the changes reflect chelating actions of, for example, lipid degradation products?

ANSWER: We think ischemic nerve cells lose Mg^{2+}, since all morphological compartments examined (cytoplasm, mitochondria, nucleus) exhibited nearly undetectable Mg levels following OGD (see Ref. 5 for details). EPMA measures total elemental concentrations irrespective of binding status. Therefore, Mg would have been detected by probe analysis regardless of lipid chelation or other nonspecific intraneuronal binding. The mechanism of Mg^{2+} efflux during OGD is not understood.

QUESTIONS FOR DR. MANEV

From Dr. Faden

You have presented intriguing date regarding 5-lipoxygenase pathways. What is known about the roles of 12- and 15-lipoxygenase pathways in neuronal injury? Is there evidence of shunting across these various lipoxygenase pathways?

ANSWER: We recently demonstrated a role for 5-lipoxygenase in aging-associated increased brain vulnerability.[6] *In vitro*, both 5-lipoxygenase[7] and 12-lipoxygenase[8] were shown to participate in neurodegeneration. Although 15-lipoxygenase could also participate in pathways of cell death, no clear evidence for its role in neurodegeneration has been reported. Whether these enzyme systems interact depends, probably, on the cell type and whether they are expressed in the same cells/neurons.

From Dr. Abbracchio

I have a question on the possible interaction between LO and COX-2. It has been reported that arachidonic acid metabolites may induce COX-2. Have you evaluated whether products of LO (i.e., leukotrienes) may mediate such an affect in your experimental model as well? You mentioned the fact that selective COX-2 inhibitors increase leukotriene production: may this reflect a compensatory mechanism consequent to enzymatic inhibition and aimed at increasing COX-2 expression?

ANSWER: It is currently believed that inhibition of one pathway of arachidonic acid metabolism may alter the rates of formation and quantities of products of other pathways. For example, inhibition of cyclooxygenase (COX) may elevate leukotriene production.[9] As yet, we have not investigated whether leukotrienes have any direct effect on COX-2 activity or expression, but we would like to explore this type of interaction in our future work.

From Dr. Youdim

Can you inform us whether you see the same changes in lipoxygenase in Parkinson's disease as those you showed so nicely in Alzheimer's disease brains?

ANSWER: Currently, of arachidonic acid metabolic pathways involved in neurodegeneration, the COX-2 pathway has attracted the most of attention. Our preliminary data indicate that 5-lipoxygenase is also upregulated during glutamate receptor-mediated excitotoxicity[10] and that it might participate in Alzheimer's pathology. Further research is needed to confirm this observation and to explore whether 5-lipoxygenase contributes to pathological changes in Parkinson's disease.

QUESTIONS FOR DR. COSI

From Dr. Abbracchio

If we consider PARP as a physiological means to eliminate cells with damaged DNA, when we rescue cells with PARP inhibitors, does this have any kind of long-term consequences on cell function? What I mean to say is, if a cell carries DNA damage and we rescue it from cell death, would DNA damage result in any future functional defects?

ANSWER: Poly(ADP-ribose) polymerase (PARP) is a multifunctional enzyme that utilizes NAD^+ as substrate and regulates the activity of proteins involved in DNA metabolism. Among its functions is DNA repair and the control of cell survival through the modulation of the NAD^+ pool. It has been hypothesized that when fully activated by damaged DNA, PARP can deplete cell energy stores in a matter of minutes and prime, in this way, the cell to death.

It is not known if inhibition of PARP by PARP inhibitors can lead to long-term consequences on cell functions if they are allowed to survive with a damaged DNA.

On the other hand, the extent of PARP inhibition seems to affect differently the survival of cells with free radical-damaged DNA. Shah and colleagues have reported that a complete inhibition of PARP by the potent PARP inhibitor 1,5-dihydroxyisoquinoline (DHIQ) potentiated oxidative damage and toxicity in C3H10T1/2 cells, while benzamide and 3-aminobenzamide were noted to promote survival of cells treated with oxidants.[11] They speculated that DHIQ, being a more potent PARP inhibitor than benzamide, does not permit any residual PARP activity which may be necessary for the cells to carry on the PARP-mediated excision-repair of DNA bases (i.e., a type of damage caused mostly by free radicals) which would allow the cell to recover.

Although the lack of a clear phenotype in PARP knocked-out mice might suggest that PARP is not critical for DNA repair in plasticity-related phenomena such as cell division and differentiation (see Dr. Vornov's comment below), it might still be important for repair in response to free radical-induced DNA damage; in this case a partial inhibition of PARP would be preferable to a complete inhibition, in order to prevent severe energy depletion and at the same time to allow DNA repair.

COMMENT (Dr. Vornov): PARP knockout mice have no clear phenotype, although this has been somewhat controversial. It may be dangerous to draw broad conclusions from knockout mice, since they have developed without the enzyme, but at least PARP is not critical to DNA repair.

From Dr. Slikker

PARP is involved in DNA repair. Does it respond to HIV therapeutic and other antivirals that block chain elongation by their incorporation into DNA?

ANSWER: It has been shown that inhibition of PARP activity by competitive PARP inhibitors, derivatives of benzamide, blocked retroviral infection of mammalian cells by inhibiting the integration of the provirus into the host cell DNA.[12]

From Dr. Ali

Did you observe any toxicity in mice at 640 ug/kg benzamide, and is there any change of body temperature at this dose?

ANSWER: At 640 mg/kg benzamide, no mortality was observed in the C57BL/6 strain of mice used in all our studies. Some transient sedation was apparent, and body temperature was lowered at this dose. However, this would not appear to explain the protective effect of the drug in our MPTP studies, since lowering of body temperature is not protective against and can even potentiate MPTP-induced nigrostriatal neurotoxicity in mice.[13,14] Also, we demonstrated previously that benzamide at 160 mg/kg can partially protect against methamphetamine-induced long-term striatal dopaminergic depletion in C57BL/6 mice, and that this neuroprotective dose did not affect body temperature.[15]

From Dr. Bowyer

Do PARP inhibitors block the long-term neurotoxicity (dopamine depletions and neuronal degeneration in the VTA and substrata nigra compacta)?

ANSWER: PARP inhibitors can block long term striatal dopamine and cortical noradrenaline depletions.[16] However, whether PARP inhibitors can affect the long-term depletions of dopamine and neuronal degeneration in the VTA and in substantia nigra zona compacta is not known yet and should be the subject for future studies. We did find that NAD^+ levels in the SN/VTA were reduced at 1 hour after a 4×20 mg/kg i.p. MPTP dose regimen, and that this NAD^+ loss could be prevented by co-treatments with benzamide (2×160 mg/kg i.p.).[17]

REFERENCES

1. LoPachin, R.M., C.M. Castiglia & A.J. Saubermann. 1992. Acrylamide disrupts elemental composition and water content of rat tibial nerve. I. Myelinated axons. Toxicol. Appl. Pharmacol. **115:** 21–23.
2. LoPachin, R.M., Jr., E.J. Lehning, E.C. Stack, S.J. Hussein & A.J. Saubermann. 1994. 2,5-Hexanedione alters elemental composition and water content of rat peripheral nerve myelinated axons. J. Neurochem. **63:** 2266–2278.
3. Lehning, E.J., R. Doshi, N. Isaksson, P.K. Stys & R.M. LoPachin, Jr. 1996. Mechanisms of injury-induced calcium entry into peripheral nerve myelinated axons: role of reverse sodium-calcium exchange. J. Neurochem. **66:** 493–500.
4. Stys, P.K. & R.M. LoPachin. 1998. Mechanisms of calcium and sodium fluxes in anoxic myelinated central nervous system axons. Neuroscience **82:** 21–32.
5. Taylor, C.P., M.L. Weber, C.L. Gaughan, E.J. Lehning & R.M. LoPachin. 1999. Oxygen/glucose deprivation in hippocampal slices: altered intraneuronal elemental composition predicts structural and functional damage. J. Neurosci. **19:** 619–629.
6. Uz, T., C. Pesold, P. Longone & H. Manev. 1998. Aging-associated up-regulation of neuronal 5-lipoxygenase expression: putative role in neuronal vulnerability. FASEB J. **12:** 439–449.
7. Maccarrone, M., M. Navarra, M.T. Corasaniti, G. Nisico & A. Finazzi Agro. 1998. Cytotoxic effect of HIV-1 coat glycoprotein gp120 on human neuroblastoma CHP100 cells involves activation of the arachidonate cascade. Biochem. J. **333:** 45–49.
8. Li, Y., P. Maher & D. Schubert. 1997. A role for 12-lipoxygenase in nerve cell death caused by glutathione depletion. Neuron **19:** 453–463.
9. Robinson, D.R., M. Skoskiewicz, K.J. Bloch et al. 1986. Cyclooxygenase blockade elevates leukotriene E4 production during acute anaphylaxis in sheep. J. Exp. Med. **163:** 1509–1517.
10. Manev, H., T. Uz & T. Qu. 1998. Early upregulation of hippocampal 5-lipoxygenase following systemic administration of kainate to rats. Restor. Neurol. Neurosci. **12:** 81–85.
11. Shah, M.G., D. Poirier, S. Desynoyers, S. Saint-Martin, J.-C. Hoflack, P. Rong, M. ApSimon, B.J. Kirkland & G.G. Poirier. 1996. Complete inhibition of poly(ADP-ribose)polymerase activity prevents the recovery of C3H10T1/2 cells from oxidative stress. Biochem. Biophys. Acta **1312:** 1–7.
12. Gaken, J.A., M. Tavassoli, S.U. Gan et al. 1996. Efficient retroviral infection of mammalian cells is blocked by inhibition of poly(ADP-ribose) polymerase activity. J. Virol. **70:** 3992–4000.
13. Freyaldenhoven, T.E., S.F. Ali & L.C. Schmued. 1997. Systemic administration of MPTP induces thalamic neuronal degeneration in mice. Brain Res. **759:** 9–17.

14. MOY, L.Y., D.S. ALBERS & P.K. SONSALLA. 1998. Lowering ambient or core body temperature elevates striatal MPP$^+$ levels and enhances toxicity to dopamine neurons in MPTP-treated mice. Brain Res. **790:** 264–269.
15. COSI, C., P. CHOPIN & M. MARIEN. 1996. Benzamide, an inhibitor of poly-(ADP-ribose) polymerase, attenuates methamphetamine-induced dopamine neurotoxicity in the C57B1/6N mouse. Brain Res. **735:** 343–348.
16. COSI, C., F. COLPAERT, W. KOEK, A. DEGRYSE & M. MARIEN. 1996. Poly(ADP-ribose) polymerase inhibitors protect against MPTP-induced depletions of striatal dopamine and cortical noradrenaline in C57B1/6 mice. Brain Res. **729:** 264–269.
17. COSI, C. & M. MARIEN. 1998. Decreases in mouse brain NAD$^+$ and ATP induced by 1-methyl-4-phenyl-1,2,3,6-tetrahydropyridine (MPTP): prevention by the poly(ADP-ribose) inhibitor, benzamide. Brain Res. **809:** 58–67.

Calpeptin and Methylprednisolone Inhibit Apoptosis in Rat Spinal Cord Injury

SWAPAN K. RAY, GLORIA G. WILFORD, DENISE C. MATZELLE, EDWARD L. HOGAN, AND NAREN L. BANIK[a]

Department of Neurology, Medical University of South Carolina, Charleston, South Carolina 29425, USA

ABSTRACT: Intracellular free Ca^{2+} and free radicals are increased following spinal cord injury (SCI). These can activate calpain to degrade cytoskeletal proteins leading to apoptotic and necrotic cell death. Primary injury triggers a cascade of secondary injury, which spreads to rostral and caudal areas. We tested calpain involvement in apoptosis in five 1-cm segments of rat spinal cord with injury (40 g-cm) induced at T12 by weight-drop. Animals were immediately treated with calpeptin (250 µg/kg) and methylprednisolone (165 mg/kg) and sacrificed at 48 hr. Untreated SCI rats manifested 68-kD neurofilament protein (NFP) degradation (indicating calpain activity), and internucleosomal DNA fragmentation (indicating apoptosis). Both calpain activity and apoptosis were highest in the lesion, and decreased with increasing distance from the lesion. Treatment decreased 68-kD NFP degradation with reduction in apoptosis in all five areas. Thus, calpeptin and methylprednisolone are found to be neuroprotective in SCI.

INTRODUCTION

The rat model of spinal cord injury (SCI) is useful to examine a role for calpain, the Ca^{2+}-dependent cysteine protease, in causing cytoskeletal protein degradation and programmed cell death (PCD) in the central nervous system (CNS). Apoptosis or PCD is mediated by activation of several cysteine proteases in response to a variety of factors including intracellular free Ca^{2+} and free radicals. The levels of these PCD-promoting factors are increased in SCI. One of the most important events in apoptosis is the activation of cysteine proteases.[1] Apoptotic death of neural cells, especially neurons and oligodendrocytes, in the spinal cord after trauma will disrupt and destroy the axon-myelin structural unit and, therefore, impair impulse conduction. Apoptosis has also been implicated in ischemia and in retinal ganglion cells after optic nerve axotomy.[2,3]

Since cytoskeletal and membrane proteins are degraded due to activation of calpain, many investigators have been interested in finding a role for calpain in apoptosis.[4] The level of intracellular free Ca^{2+} is increased during injury, causing activation of Ca^{2+}-dependent proteases and eventually apoptotic cell death.[5,6] It has

[a]Corresponding author: Naren L. Banik, Ph.D., Department of Neurology, Medical University of South Carolina, 171 Ashley Avenue, Charleston, SC 29425. Phone, 843/792-3946; fax, 843/792-8626.
e-mail, baniknl@musc.edu

been reported that intracellular free Ca^{2+} is greatly increased in experimental spinal cord trauma.[7] Intracellular free Ca^{2+} is absolutely required for activation of calpain, which may therefore be one of the cysteine proteases responsible for mediation of cell death in SCI. Cytoskeletal proteins, which maintain cellular integrity, are degraded by calpain activity during apoptosis.[8,9] A role for calpain in apoptosis of neurons has been reported.[10] Recently we have reported the involvement of calpain in mediation of apoptosis in glial cells.[11] Several enzymes including lipases and proteases are activated by Ca^{2+}. The activation of Ca^{2+}-dependent phospholipase A_2 (PLA$_2$) causes neurotoxicity by catalyzing release of arachidonic acid from membrane phospholipids followed by production of free radicals. Moreover, activated PLA$_2$ alters membranes facilitating influx of Ca^{2+} as well as release of Ca^{2+} from the internal stores.[12] Infiltration and activation of a variety of inflammatory cells in the CNS during the acute phase of SCI releases numerous inflammatory mediators and free radicals. Among proteases, calpain is activated in response to elevated intracellular free Ca^{2+} levels.[13,14] Activated calpain can induce proteolytic modifications in a number of proteins associated with multiple signaling cascades for mediating neural cell death.

Two major calpain isoforms are μcalpain and mcalpain, which are activated by μM and mM Ca^{2+} concentration, respectively. Each isoform consists of a 30-kD regulatory subunit and an 80-kD catalytic subunit.[15] The regulatory subunits are identical in both calpain isoforms, but the catalytic subunits are different. The regulatory subunit originates from one gene, and the catalytic subunits from different genes.[16] Calpastatin is an endogenous protein inhibitor, which regulates the activity of both calpain isoforms,[17] and the level and efficiency of calpastatin could play a critical role in preventing calpain-mediated proteolysis.[18] However, it should be noted that the level of calpastatin is decreased by calpain-mediated proteolysis.[19] It is also noteworthy that calpains exist in the cells as inactive proenzymes, which are activated by an increase in Ca^{2+} levels.

SOURCE OF CALPAIN IN SCI

The primary injury to the cord causes several changes, including disruption of blood vessels and alteration of membrane integrity, that play important roles in initiating the devastating secondary neuropathophysiological changes. Since degenerating of myelinated axons and degradation of proteins occur before infiltration of immune cells, it is likely that the early increase of calpain activity is derived from endogenous neural cells (neurons, oligodendrocytes, astrocytes, and microglia), while later there is a contribution from infiltrating inflammatory cells (lymphocytes and mononuclear phagocytes). Increased calpain levels have been found in macrophages, astrocytes, microglia, neurons and myelin in SCI.[20] Any increase in calpain expression and activity early in the injury is likely due to elevated levels of intracellular free Ca^{2+}, inflammatory cytokines, and arachidonic acid. Later, an increase in calpain activity in SCI may derive from reactive astrocytes and infiltrating immune cells. The current evidence indicates that arachidonic acid, its metabolites, and cytokines all accumulate in CNS injury.[21–23]

FREE Ca^{2+} AND FREE RADICALS IN SCI

It is now thought that Ca^{2+} influx in SCI results from cell damage in the lesion, and alteration in cell permeability in the penumbra.[7] An increase in intracellular free Ca^{2+} and free radicals causes cell death in CNS injury, ischemia, stroke, and glutamate neurotoxicity.[24] Free Ca^{2+} is also released from intracellular organelles such as mitochondria and microsomes.[25] Free radicals and other inflammatory mediators are generated during conversion of arachidonic acid to eicosanoids following activation of inflammatory cells,[26,27] which are infiltrated in the acute phase of SCI in animal models.[28–30] Lipid inflammatory mediators such as eicosanoids, prostaglandins, thromboxane, and leukotrienes accumulate following infiltration of inflammatory cells. Kininogen (the precursor of kinins) and kinins also progressively accumulate in SCI. Kinins activate phospholipases, which in turn release arachidonic acid and produce free radicals.[31] In addition to intracellular free Ca^{2+}, other factors including such kinins and free radicals can stimulate calpain activity in the mediation of cell death.

A ROLE FOR CALPAIN IN APOPTOSIS IN SCI

The primary injury to the cord causes cell membrane disruption, axon-myelin disintegration, and microvessel destruction.[32] The secondary injuries, initiated by a number of factors following primary injury, can cause cell death by necrosis or/and apoptosis. Necrosis is irreversible, and marked by damage to the plasma membrance and leakage of cell constituents in to extracellular space fluid. Apoptosis or PCD is preventable, as it is activated by a number of factors including Ca^{2+} and free radicals.[33] Cells undergoing apoptosis are cleared by proteolytic digestion.[34] There has been a long-held assumption that necrosis may be the mode of cell death in the SCI lesion,[28] and recent implication of excitotoxicity in the pathogenesis of SCI is consistent with this view.[35,36] Excitotoxicity is characterized by neuronal cell swelling, which is documented in the necrosis of cortical neurons in culture.[37] Although the death of neurons and glial cells in the lesion after SCI is likely to be necrotic, it may be largely apoptotic in the penumbra and adjacent areas. Apoptotic death is regulated by several factors initiating an intrinsic suicide program in the cells. The occurrence of apoptosis is an important part of secondary injuries in SCI, and has recently been reported by several laboratories besides ours.[38–40]

Since calpain expression and activity are increased in the SCI lesion,[41,42] calpain may be one of the proteases responsible for mediating apoptotic cell death after SCI. In response to increased intracellular Ca^{2+} levels, calpains are activated by autolytic cleavage of N-terminal peptides, and this limited autolysis is considered to be the key mechanistic step in the activation of calpains.[43] Structural proteins and other microtubular proteins have been shown to be partially degraded by calpain.[15,44] To this end, we have investigated the degradation of 68-kD neurofilament protein (NFP) in the lesion and adjacent areas of spinal cord in a rat model of SCI (FIG. 1). The loss of 68-kD NFP is found to be highest at the site of lesion, and decreases in neighboring regions in inverse relation to the distance from the lesion epicenter. The degradation of 68-kD NFP in SCI indicates the involvement of increased proteolytic

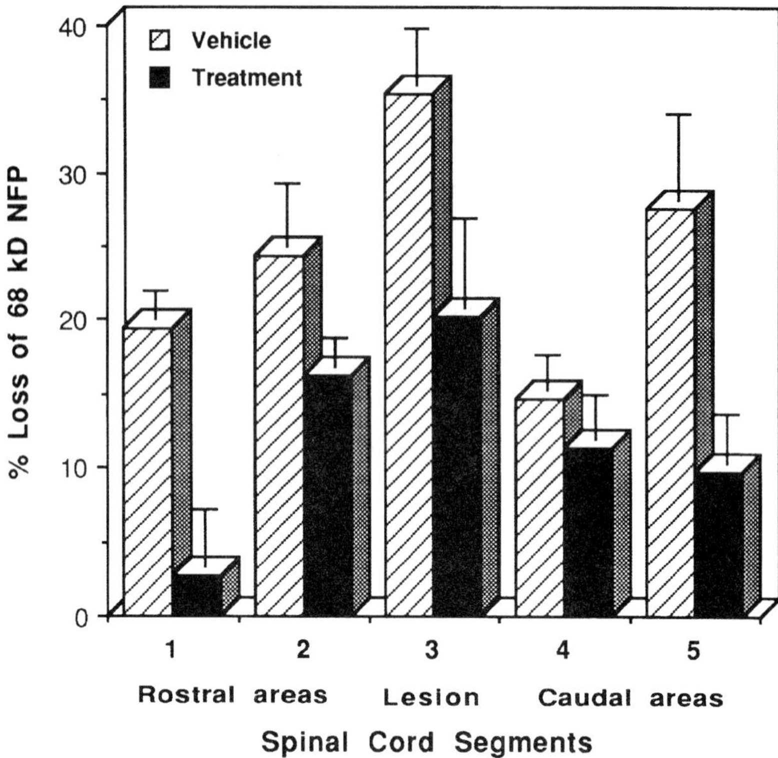

FIGURE 1. Extent of 68-kD NFP degradation in five different areas in SCI rat. Injury (40 g-cm) was induced on T12 by weight-drop. Calpain inhibitor CP (250 μg/kg) and anti-inflammatory agent MP (165 mg/kg) in 1.5% dimethyl sulfoxide (DMSO) as vehicle were administered intravenously within 30 min after injury. Following treatment, rats were sacrificed at 48 hr. A 5-cm section of spinal cord with lesion in the center was removed and divided into five 1-cm segments. Western analysis with proteins from SCI segments showed 68-kD NFP degradation in untreated (vehicle) SCI rats ($n = 7$), and prevention of 68-kD NFP degradation in drug-treated SCI rats ($n = 9$). Band intensities of 68-kD NFP were quantitated densitometrically using PDI Quantity One software. Percent loss of 68-kD NFP in SCI rats with or without treatment was calculated with respect to sham (uninjured) rats ($n = 4$). Data are presented as mean + SEM of separate expreiments.

activity of calpain. The treatment of SCI rats with calpeptin (CP) and methylpred-nisolone (MP) prevents degradation of 68-kD NFP. In untreated rats, neuronal cells with degraded 68-kD NFP and other cytoskeletal proteins are going to be structurally unstable and, therefore, prone to activate cellular machinery leading to apoptosis.

PREVENTION OF APOPTOSIS IN SCI

As calpain is involved in the patholphysiology of SCI, an intense research effort has been focused on examination of the effect of calpain inhibitors as therapeutic

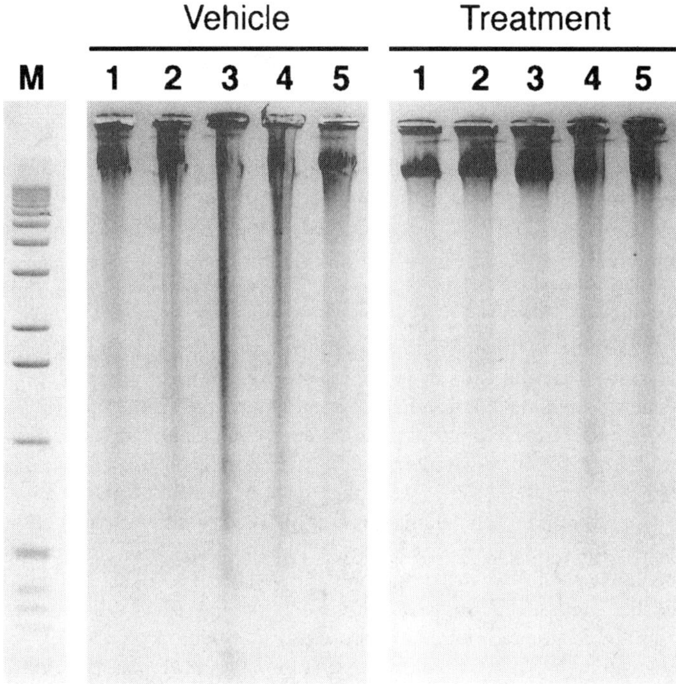

FIGURE 2. Extent of internucleosomal DNA fragmentation in five different areas in rat SCI. Induction of SCI, treatment of SCI rats, and collection of SCI segments are the same as described in FIGURE 1. Genomic DNA samples extracted from SCI segments were resolved on a 1.6% agarose gel by electrophoresis. *M*, marker (1 kb ladder); *vehicle*, DNA fragmentation occurred maximally in lesion (*lane 3*), and minimally in rostral areas (*lanes 1 and 2*) and caudal areas (*lanes 4 and 5*) of the spinal cord from untreated SCI rat; *treatment*, DNA fragmentation was prevented in all five segments of the spinal cord from drug-treated SCI rat. Results are representative of three separate experiments. There was no internucleosomal DNA fragmentation in these segments of the spinal cord from sham rat (data not shown).

agents in SCI. Calpastatin (110 kD), the natural inhibitor of calpain, is too large to be cell permeable. With an increased calpain:calpastatin ratio, calpastatin is degraded as a suicide substrate of calpain and, therefore, becomes ineffective. A cysteine residue (Cys108) at the catalytic site places calpains in the family of cysteine proteases. The thiol group (-SH) of Cys108 directly participates in covalent catalytic cleavage of peptide bond of the substrate. The inhibitors of calpain act by covalent interaction between the -SH of the active site Cys108 and an electrophilic center of the inhibitor. Calpeptin (CP), a dipeptide aldehyde, has been reported to inhibit proteolytic activity of calpain.[45] As CP is a small compound lacking charged groups, it is capable of penetrating the cell membrane by passive diffusion. Free radicals are generated by activation of inflammatory cells in SCI and, therefore, an antiinflammatory agent may ameliorate neural cell death in SCI. Glucocorticoids including methylprednisolone (MP) are antiinflammatory, and have been used in the treatment of SCI and inflammatory diseases such as multiple sclerosis. The exact mechanism of antiinflammatory action of glucocorticoids is not fully understood, but it is partly due to inhibition of PLA$_2$,[46] which catalyzes the release of arachidonic acid from membrane phospholipids with subsequent production of free radicals. The induction of inflammatory processes in SCI warranted the therapeutic use of a potent antiinflammatory agent such as MP, and its administration was neuroprotective in experimental and acute SCI.[47,48] Pharmacological studies suggest that MP is a neuroprotective agent.[49] Our recent *in vitro* study indicated a new mechanism of MP action with inhibition of calpain activity.[50] To a large extent, calpain and inflammatory mediators cause cell death and tissue destruction in SCI, and hence a therapeutic regimen containing a calpain inhibitor and an antiinflammatory agent may prevent apoptotic death of neural cells in SCI. Since many secondary destructive pathways are involved in tissue destruction in SCI, treatment with one therapeutic agent may not be highly effective. A combination therapy with calpain inhibitor CP and free radical inhibitor MP may have more synergistic neuroprotective effect than therapy with either one alone. We have investigated the efficacy of this combination therapy in SCI rats, and found that coadministration of CP (to inhibit calpain activity) and MP (to inhibit inflammatory process) in rat immediately after SCI reduced the extent of internucleosomal DNA fragmentation (apoptosis) in the lesion site and adjacent areas (FIG. 2). These results suggest that prevention of calpain-mediated protein degradation and inhibition of inflamatory process confer neuroprotection by prevention of apoptosis in rat SCI. The coadministration of CP and MP was more effective for inhibition of apoptosis than administration of CP or MP alone (data not presented).

CONCLUDING REMARKS

SCI initiates a complex neuropathological process stemming from a rapid increase in intracellular free Ca^{2+} and production of free radicals. These cause activation of Ca^{2+}-dependent proteases including calpain, and the progressive injury ultimately results in the loss of axon-myelin structural unit, degradation of cytoskeletal proteins, and massive apoptotic and also necrotic death of neural cells. Untreated SCI severely impairs motor function because of myelin loss, axonal degeneration, and neuronal cell death. The degradation of 68-kD NFP indicated the increased calpain activity in SCI lesion and adjacent areas, while the free radicals generated by inflammatory processes contribute to upregulation of intracellular free Ca^{2+} and several biochemical pathways to mediate cell death in the CNS. In an attempt to prevent apoptosis caused by calpain and free radicals in rat SCI, administration of CP and MP within 30 min of injury is found promising, and we think that inhibition of apoptosis by combination of CP and MP may help restore motor function in SCI.

ACKNOWLEDGMENTS

This investigation was supported in part by grants from the NIH-NINDS, the National MS Society, and the American Health Assistance Foundation.

REFERENCES

1. ZHIVOTOVSKY, B., D.H. BURGESS, D.M. VANAGS & S. ORRENIUS. 1987. Involvement of cellular machinery in apoptosis. Biochem. Biophys. Res. Commun. **230:** 481–488.
2. LINNEK, M.D., R.H. ZOBRIST & M.D. HATFIELD. 1993. Evidence supporting a role for programmed cell death in focal cerebral ischemia in rats. Stroke **24:** 2002–2028.
3. BERKELAAR, M., D.B. CLARKE, Y.C. WANG, G.M. BRAY & A.J. AGUAYO. 1994. Axotomy results in delayed death and apoptosis of retinal ganglion cells in adult rats. J. Neurosci. **14:** 4368–4374.
4. CARAFOLI, E. & M. MOLINARI. 1998. Calpain: a protease in search of a function? Biochem. Biophys. Res. Commun. **247:** 193–203.
5. TRUMP, B.F. & I.K. BEREZESKY. 1995. Calcium-mediated cell injury and cell death. FASEB J. **9:** 219–228.
6. NICOTERA, P. & S. ORRENIUS. 1998. The role of calcium in apoptosis. Cell Calcium **23:** 173–180.
7. HAPPEL, R.D., K.P. SMITH, N.L. BANIK, J.M. POWERS, E.L. HOGAN & J.D. BALENTINE. 1981. Ca^{2+}-accumulation in experimental spinal cord trauma. Brain Res. **211:** 476–479.
8. SAIDO, T.C., M. YOKOTA, S. NAGAO, I. YAMAURA, E. TANI, T. TSUCHIYA, K. SUZUKI & S. KAWASHIMA. 1993. Spatial resolution of fodrin proteolysis in postischemic brain. J. Biol. Chem. **268:** 25239–25243.
9. MARTIN, S.J., G.A. O'BRIEN, W.K. NISHIOKA, A.J. MCGAHON, A. MAHBOUBI, T.C. SAIDO & D.R. GREEN. 1995. Proteolysis of fodrin (non-erythroid spectrin) during apoptosis. J. Biol. Chem. **270:** 6425–6428.
10. JORDAN, J., M.F. GALINDO & R.J. MILLER. 1997. Role of calpain- and interleukin-1 β converting enzyme-like proteases in the β-amyloid-induced death of rat hippocampal neurons in culture. J. Neurochem. **68:** 1612–1621.
11. RAY, S.K., G.G. WILFORD, C.V. CROSBY, E.L. HOGAN & N.L. BANIK. 1999. Diverse stimuli induce calpain overexpression and apoptosis in C6 glioma cells. Brain Res. **829:** 18–27.
12. TRAYSTMAN, R.J., J.R. KIRSCH & R.C. KOEHLER. 1991. Oxygen radical mechanisms of brain injury following ischemia and reperfusion. J. Appl. Physiol. **71:** 1185–1195.
13. FOX, J.E., R.G. TAYLOR, M. TAFFAREL, J.K. BOYLES & D.E. GOLL. 1993. Evidence that activation of platelet calpain is induced as a consequence of binding of adhesive ligand to the integrin, glycoprotein IIb-IIIa. J. Cell Biol. **120:** 1501-1507.
14. INOMATA, M., M. HAYASHI, Y. OHNO-IWASHITA, S. TSUBUKI, T.C. SAIDO & S. KAWASHIMA. 1996. Involvement of calpain in integrin-mediated signal transduction. Arch. Biochem. Biophys. **328:** 129–134.
15. CROALL, D.E. & G.N. DEMARTINO. 1991. Calcium-activated neutral protease (calpain) system: structure, function, and regulation. Physiol. Rev. **71:** 813–847.
16. SUZUKI, K. 1987. Calcium activated neutral protease: domain structure and activity regulation. Trends Biochem. Sci. **12:** 103–105.
17. SUZUKI, K., S. IMAJOH, Y. EMORI, H. SAWASAKI, Y. MINAMI & S. OHNO. 1987. Calcium-acivated neutral protease and its endogenous inhibitor. Activation at the cell membrane and biological functions. FEBS Lett. **220:** 271–277.
18. PONTREMOLI, S., F. SALAMINO, B. SPARATORE, R. DE TULLIO, R. PONTREMOLI & E. MELLONI. 1988. Characterization of the calpastatin defect in erythrocytes from patients with essential hypertension. Biochem. Biophys. Res. Commun. **157:** 867–874.
19. PONTREMOLI, S., E. MELLONI, P.L. VIOTI, M. MICHETTI, F. SALAMINO & B.L. HORECKER. 1991. Identification of two calpastatin forms in rat skeletal muscle and their susceptibility to digestion by homologous calpains. Arch. Biochem. Biophys. **288:** 646–652.
20. LI, Z., E.L. HOGAN & N.L. BANIK. 1995. Role of calpain in spinal cord injury: increased mcalpain immunoreactivity in spinal cord after compression injury in the rat. Neurochem. Int. **27:** 425–432.

21. GIULAN, D. & L.B. LACHMAN. 1985. Interleukin-1 stimulation of astroglial proliferation after brain injury. Science **228:** 497–499.
22. OTT, L., C.J. MCCLAIN, M. GILLESPIE & B. YOUNG. 1994. Cytokines and metabolic dysfunction after severe head injury. J. Neurotrauma **11:** 447–472.
23. PERRY, V.H. 1994. Macrophage and microglia responses in CNS injury. *In* Macrophages and the Nervous System. V.H. Perry, Ed.: 62–86. R.G. Landes Company. Austin, TX.
24. LIPTON, S.A. & P. NICOTERA. 1998. Calcium, free radicals and excitotoxins in neuronal apoptosis. Cell Calcium **23:**165–171.
25. HOGAN, E.L., W. MCIVER, A. KRALL & N.L. BANIK. 1985. Subcellular distribution of calcium in spinal cord trauma. Trans. Am. Soc. Neurochem. **16:** 132.
26. GALLIN, J.I., I.M. GOLDSTEIN & R. SNYDERMAN. 1988. Inflammation: Basic Principles and Clinical Correlates. Raven Press. New York.
27. HSU, C.Y., P.V. HALUSHKA, E.L. HOGAN, N.L. BANIK, W.A. LEE & P.L. PEROT, JR. 1985. Alteration of thromboxane and prostacycline levels in experimental spinal cord injury. Neurology **35:** 1003–1009.
28. BALENTINE, J.D. 1978. Pathology of experimental spinal cord trauma. Lab. Invest. **39:** 254–266.
29. MEANS, E.D. & D.K. ANDERSON. 1983. Neuronophagia by leukocytes in experimental spinal cord injury. J. Neuropathol. Exp. Neurol. **42:** 707–719.
30. XU, J.A., C.Y. HSU, T.H. LIU, E.L. HOGAN, P.L. PEROT, JR. & H.H. TAI. 1990. Leukotriene B4 release and polymorphonuclear cell infiltration in spinal cord injury. J. Neurochem. **55:** 907–912.
31. KONTOS, H.A., E.P. WEI, J.T. POVLISHOCK & C.W. CHRISTMAN. 1984. Oxygen radicals mediate the cerebral arteriolar dilation from arachidonate and bradykinin in cats. Circ. Res. **55:** 295–303.
32. ANDERSON, D.K. & E.D. HALL. 1993. Pathophysiology of spinal cord trauma. Ann. Emerg. Med. **22:** 987–992.
33. ELLIS, R.E., J. YUAN & H.R. HORVITZ. 1991. Mechanisms and functions of cell death. Annu. Rev. Cell Biol. **7:** 663–698.
34. THOMPSON, C.B. 1995. Apoptosis in the pathogenesis and treatment of disease. Science **267:** 1456–1462.
35. FADEN, A.I. & R.P. SIMON. 1988. A potential role for excitotoxins in the pathophysiology of spinal cord injury. Ann. Neurol. **23:** 623–626.
36. PANTER, S.S., S.W. YUM & A.I. FADEN. 1990. Alteration in extracellular amino acids after traumatic spinal cord injury. Ann. Neurol. **27:** 96–99.
37. GWAG, B.J., J.Y. KOH, J.A. DEMARO, H.S. YING, M. JACQUIN & D.W. CHOI. 1997. Slowly triggered excitotoxicity occurs by necrosis in cortical cultures. Neuroscience **77:** 393–401.
38. CROWE, M.J., J.C. BRESNAHAN, S.L. SHUMAN, J.N. MASTERS & M.S. BEATTIE. 1997. Apoptosis and delayed degeneration after spinal cord injury in rats and monkeys. Nat. Med. **3:** 73–76.
39. LIU, X.Z., X.M. XU, R. HU, C. DU, S.X. ZHANG, J.W. MCDONALD, H.X. DONG, Y.J. WU, G.S. FAN, M.F. JACQUIN, C.Y. HSU & D.W. CHOI. 1997. Neuronal and glial apoptosis after traumatic spinal cord injury. J. Neurosci. **17:** 5395-5406.
40. RAY, S., D. DAVIS, D. SHIELDS, D. MATZELLE, G. WILFORD, E.L. HOGAN & N.L. BANIK. 1998. Increased calpain expression, cell death, and neuroprotection in rat spinal cord injury. J. Neurochem. **70**(Suppl. 1)**:** S63.
41. BANIK, N.L., D.L. MATZELLE, G. GANTT-WILFORD, A. OSBORNE & E.L. HOGAN. 1997. Increased calpain content and progressive degradation of neurofilament protein in spinal cord injury. Brain Res. **752:** 301–306.
42. RAY, S.K., D.C. SHIELDS, T.C. SAIDO, D.C. MATZELLE, G.G. WILFORD, E.L. HOGAN

& N.L. BANIK. 1999. Calpain activity and translational expression increased in spinal cord injury. Brain Res. **816:** 375–380.

43. BAKI, A., P. TOMPA, A. ALEXA, O. MOLNAR & P. FRIEDRICH. 1996. Autolysis parallels activation of μcalpain. Biochem. J. **318:** 897–901.

44. SAIDO, T.C., H. SORIMACHI & K. SUZUKI. 1994. Calpain: new perspectives in molecular diversity and physiological-pathological involvement. FASEB J. **8:** 814–822.

45. TSUJINAKA, T., Y. KAJIWARA, J. KAMBAYASHI, M. SAKON, N. HIGUCHI, T. TANAKA & T. MORI. 1988. Synthesis of a new cell penetrating calpain inhibitor (calpeptin). Biochem. Biophys. Res. Commun. **153:** 1201–1208.

46. HIRATA, F., E. SCHIFFMANN, K. VENKATASUBRAMANIAN, D. SALOMON & J. AXELROD. 1980. A phospholipase A_2 inhibitory protein in rabbit neutrophils induced by glucocorticoids. Proc. Natl. Acad. Sci. USA **77:** 2533–2536.

47. BRAUGHLER, J.M. & E.D. HALL. 1984. Effects of multidose methylprednisolone sodium succinate administration on injured cat spinal cord neurofilament degradation and energy metabolism. J. Neurosurg. **61:** 290–295.

48. BRACKEN, M.B. 1991. Treatment of acute spinal cord injury with methylprednisolone: results of a multicenter, randomized clinical trial. J. Neurotrauma **8**(Suppl. 1): S47–S52.

49. HALL, E.D. 1991. The neuroprotective pharmacology of methylprednisolone. J. Neurosurg. **76:** 13–22.

50. BANIK, N.L., D. MATZELLE, E. TERRY & E.L. HOGAN. 1997. A new mechanism of methylprednisolone and other corticosteroids action demonstrated *in vitro*: inhibition of a proteinase (calpain) prevents myelin and cytoskeletal protein degradation. Brain Res. **748:** 205–210.

Calpastatin Is Upregulated and Acts as a Suicide Substrate to Calpains in Neonatal Rat Hypoxia-Ischemia

KLAS BLOMGREN[a]

Perinatal Center, Department of Physiology, Göteborg University, SE-405 30 Göteborg, and Department of Pediatrics, Sahlgrenska University Hospital/Östra, SE-416 85 Göteborg, Sweden

The modified Levine preparation in 7-day-old rats[4] is the most widespread and well characterized model of hypoxia-ischemia (HI) in the immature brain. Transient cerebral HI is induced by unilateral occlusion of the common carotid artery plus 7.7% O_2 for 1 hr, producing widespread infarction and selective neuronal necrosis in the ipsilateral hemisphere, leaving the contralateral hemisphere undamaged. Long-term recovery is possible, and pups were followed for up to 14 days post HI.

In a previous study we found that calpains were equally translocated to cellular membranes in the ipsi- and contralateral hemispheres. This translocation, a prerequisite for protease activation, coincided with the appearance of fodrin (also called brain spectrin) breakdown product (FBDP) in the ipsilateral hemisphere, indicating calpain activation. No significant changes in FBDP were found in the contralateral, undamaged hemisphere. Calpastatin is an endogenous inhibitor protein specific for calpains, since no other protease tested so far is affected. We found an upregulation of calpastatin immunoreactivity in the contralateral hemisphere, both on Western blots and in tissue sections, after the insult, lasting for at least 24 hr, indicating that calpastatin may be the factor halting calpain activation in the contralateral hemisphere.

The upregulation in the contralateral hemisphere was concomitant with extensive degradation of calpastatin in the ipsilateral hemisphere (85% after 24 hr). This degradation was confined to the ipsilateral, damaged hemisphere, and it was discrete, since it produced a specific calpastatin breakdown product (CBDP) about half the size of the intact molecule. This CBDP seemed to be relatively resistant to further degradation, since it was accumulated in the P_2 fraction. The CBDP appeared to be membrane-bound, since it was not detected in the cytosolic fraction. Interestingly, it has been shown that calpastatin can be easily degraded by calpains *in vitro*[1,3] and in cultured cells, even more easily than other endogenous substrates, like fodrin.[2] Animals treated with CX295, a membrane-permeable calpain inhibitor, every 3 hr for 24 hr following the insult displayed significantly less degradation of calpastatin in the ipsilateral hemisphere (46% less degradation, $p = 0.003$). This is the first report

[a]Address for correspondence: Klas Blomgren, M.D., Ph.D., Perinatal Center, Department of Physiology, Göteborg University, P.O. Box 432, SE-405-30 Göteborg, Sweden. Phone, +46 31-773 33 76; fax, +46 31-773 35 12.

e-mail, klas.blomgren@fysiologi.gu.se

to our knowledge demonstrating degradation of calpastatin by calpains *in vivo*, indicating that calpastatin acts as a suicide substrate to calpain under hypoxia-ischemia.

REFERENCES

1. MELLGREN, R., M. MERICLE & R. LANE. 1986. Proteolysis of the calcium-dependent protease inhibitor by myocardial calcium-dependent protease. Arch. Biochem. Biophys. **246:** 233–239.
2. NAGAO, S., T. SAIDO, Y. AKITA, T. TSUCHIYA, K. SUZUKI & S. KAWASHIMA. 1994. Calpain-calpastatin interactions in epidermoid carcinoma KB cells. J. Biochem. **115:** 1178–1184.
3. NAKAMURA, M., M. INOMATA, S. IMAJOH, K. SUZUKI & S. KAWASHIMA. 1989. Fragmentation of an endogenous inhibitor upon complex formation with high- and low-Ca^{2+}-requiring forms of calcium-activated neutral proteases. Biochemistry **28:** 449–455.
4. RICE, J.E., R. VANNUCCI & J. BRIERLEY. 1981. The influence of immaturity on hypoxic-ischemic brain damage in the rat. Ann. Neurol **9:** 131–141.

Questions and Answers

QUESTION FOR DRS. BANIK AND BLOMGREN

From Dr. Palmer

Are there any calpain inhibitors available that can be administered orally or i.v.?
ANSWER (Dr. Blomgren): I am not aware of any calpain inhibitors that can be administered orally, but all the active site directed inhibitors can be given i.v.

QUESTION FOR DR. BLOMGREN

From Dr. Andrews

I enjoyed your excellent presentation, and only have a methodological comment regarding unilateral ischemia. In our swine model of unilateral brain retraction ischemia (which we talked about at the 3rd International Conference on Neuroprotective Agents), we found changes in evoked potentials and cerebral blood flow in the contralateral hemisphere during the ipsilateral retraction ischemia. These contralateral changes referred to baseline within 10 min of stopping retraction (retraction was for a maximum of 30 min). If we sectioned the corpus collosum, the contralateral changes were not seen—suggesting the inter- hemispheric connections were responsible (i.e., transcollsal or transhemispheric diaschisis).

It might be interesting to see if your contralateral effects would be present in a corpus callosum sectioned animal. Also, as a general comment it is probably not valid to use the contralateral hemisphere as a control.

ANSWER: The contralateral hemisphere is hypoxic, and the ipsilateral hemisphere is hypoxic-ischemic, so the contralateral hemisphere is never used as a control. We see great changes in the contralateral hemisphere, for example the upregulation of calpastatin I just described, compared with the real controls.

Thank you for your suggestion about sectioning of the corpus callosum, this is an interesting idea well worth trying.

High Extracellular Glutamate and Neuronal Death in Neurological Disorders

Cause, Contribution or Consequence?

TIHOMIR P. OBRENOVITCH[a]

Department of Pharmacology, School of Pharmacy, University of Bradford, Bradford, United Kingdom

ABSTRACT: In models of neurological disorders, increased extracellular glutamate and beneficial effects produced by glutamate-receptor antagonists are consistently taken as supporting evidence of excitotoxicity. This systematic interpretation is over-simplified and potentially misleading.

High extracellular glutamate is not a reliable indicator of *endogenous* excitotoxicity, i.e., the intrinsic, potential neurotoxicity of endogenous glutamate whenever it accumulates extracellularly. Firstly, because the extracellular levels of glutamate necessary to produce depolarization and death *in vivo*, are far above those measured in models of neurological disorders. Secondly, because changes in the concentration of glutamate in the synaptic cleft (i.e., the relevant compartment for endogenous excitotoxicity) are not reflected extracellularly.

Protection by glutamate-receptor antagonists does not necessarily imply inhibition of excitotoxic abnormalities. Indeed, neuronal death initiated by insults such as ischemia results from multifactorial processes that may be interrelated. Therefore, beneficial effects resulting from an interaction with glutamate-mediated transmission may actually render the cell more resistant to other deleterious mechanisms (e.g., mitochondrial injury, oxidative stress).

INTRODUCTION

The notion of excitotoxicity was introduced by Olney to describe the neurotoxicity associated with administration of very high concentrations of *exogenous* glutamate, or compounds acting as agonists onto glutamate receptors (FIG. 1a).[1,2] Exogenous excitotoxicity has been clearly demonstrated in laboratory animals, and exemplified by the severe, chronic neurological disorders affecting individuals who consumed mussels contaminated with domoic acid (i.e., a potent agonist of kainate receptors).[3,4]

In 1984, three discoveries in the field of cerebral ischemia have encouraged the extrapolation of exogenous excitotoxicity, to *endogenous* glutamate-mediated excitotoxicity, i.e., the intrinsic, potential neurotoxicity of glutamate whenever it accumulates in the extracellular space (FIG. 1b):

(*i*)   Extracellular levels of glutamate increase during ischemia;[5]

[a]Address for correspondence: Dr. T.P. Obrenovitch, Pharmacology, School of Pharmacy, University of Bradford, Bradford BD7 1DP, UK. Phone, +44 1274 233359; fax, +44 1274 233363. e-mail, t.obrenovitch@bradford.ac.uk

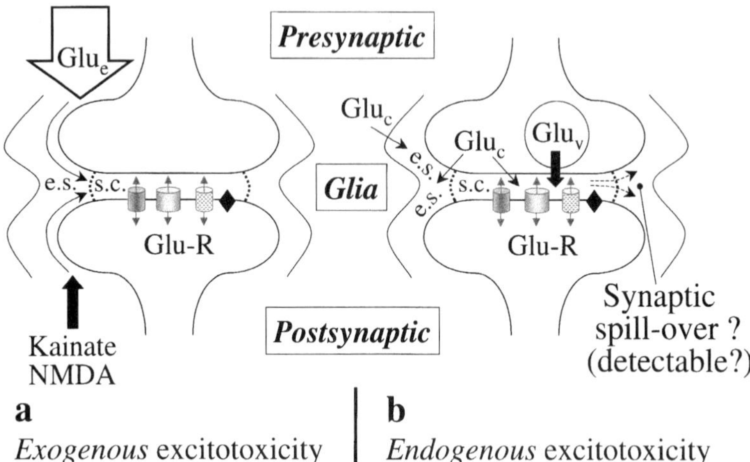

FIGURE 1. Diagram illustrating: **(a)** the initial concept of *exogenous* excitotoxicity, i.e., administration of very high concentration of exogenous glutamate, or glutamate receptor agonists (e.g., kainate, NMDA); and **(b)** its extrapolation to *endogenous* excitotoxicity, i.e., the intrinsic, potential neurotoxicity of endogenous glutamate (i.e., primarily of cytosolic origin) whenever it accumulates in the extracellular space. It has become clear that the concentrations of extracellular glutamate necessary to produce neuronal dysfunction and death *in vivo*, are far above those measured in models of neurological disorders (e.g., stroke and traumatic brain injury) (see text). The *dashed borders* between extracellular space (e.s.) and synaptic clefts (s.c.) indicate that "Changes in the concentration of glutamate in the synaptic cleft are NOT reflected at extracellular level," and the signs (?) adjacent to "Synaptic spill-over" and "(detectable)" reinforce this point. *Abbreviations*: e.s., extracellular space; Glu_c, cytosolic glutamate; Glu_e, very high extracellular glutamate of exogenous origin; Glu_v, vesicular glutamate releasable by exocytosis; GLU-R, postsynaptic receptor, ionotropic (*cylinder shape*) and metabotropic (*diamond shape*); s.c., synaptic cleft.

> *(ii)* blockade of glutamate receptors protects cultured neurons from both anoxia and the toxicity of exogenous glutamate and aspartate;[6]
>
> *(iii)* *N*-methyl-D-aspartate (NMDA)-receptor antagonists reduced ischemia-induced neuronal damage *in vivo*.[7]

Following these discoveries, increased extracellular concentrations of glutamate, and beneficial effects produced by glutamate receptor antagonists, have been consistently interpreted as indicative of endogenous excitotoxicity.

The main purpose of this article is to argue against these systematic interpretations, i.e., increased extracellular glutamate should not be taken as a reliable indicator of endogenous excitotoxicity, and protection against experimental or pathological events by glutamate receptor antagonists does not necessarily imply excitotoxic processes. More detailed and complementary arguments on this topic can be found in previous reviews.[8,9] Alternative mechanisms of endogenous excitotoxicity, such as accumulation of other endogenous ligands for glutamate receptors (e.g., quinolinate, aspartate, sulphur-containing excitatory amino acids) and postsynaptic abnormalities of glutamatergic transmission are beyond the scope of this article.

HIGH EXTRACELLULAR GLUTAMATE IS NOT A RELIABLE INDICATOR OF ENDOGENOUS EXCITOTOXICITY

In several experimental and clinical studies of focal ischemia or traumatic brain injury (TBI), the magnitude of increased extracellular glutamate correlated with neurological abnormalities and/or brain lesion volume, and this finding has been used to support the notion that glutamate efflux is a key determinant of the ultimate outcome.[10,11] However, correlation does not imply causality, and the widespread notion that high extracellular glutamate is a key contributor to neuronal death in neurological disorders conflicts with robust and important data.

The Extracellular Concentrations of Glutamate, Necessary to Produce Depolarization and Neuronal Death In Vivo, *Are Far above Those Measured following Cerebral Ischemia or TBI*

Early studies showed that very high amounts of glutamate must be applied to the brain in order to induce neuronal malfunction and death.[12–14] For example, repeated microinjections of a 1.8 M glutamate solution (0.5 µl, every 12 hours for 14 days) in the rat striatum or hippocampus caused neuronal degeneration only within 0.5 mm from the tip of the injection cannula, and continuous infusion of equivalent total daily doses did not produce any lesion.[13] As exogenous excitatory amino acids (e.g., kainate) were found to be much more potent excitotoxins,[15] these data were interpreted as suggesting that uptake systems for glutamate are very effective protective mechanisms, which can be only overcome by extremely high local concentration of glutamate.[13]

These findings were confirmed in our laboratory, by using microdialysis probes incorporating an electrode to apply glutamate-receptor agonists and measure the amplitude of the resulting depolarisation. When perfused through the probe at 1 µl/min, 10 to 100 mM glutamate (estimated EC_{50} = 42 mM) was necessary to produce marked deflection of the local direct current (DC) potential, and glutamate was 200- to 400-fold less potent than NMDA, α-amino-3-hydroxy-5-methyl-4-isoxazole-propionic acid (AMPA) or kainate in this preparation.[16] As did the authors of the previous studies outlined above, we hypothesized that the weak depolarizing potency of glutamate reflected its potent uptake mechanisms. However, subsequent studies with inhibitors of glutamate transports showed that extracellular concentrations of glutamate equivalent to those associated with ischemia or TBI are surprisingly well tolerated *in vivo.*

- Glutamate-induced depolarizations were not potentiated when a selective inhibitor of glutamate-uptake (L-*trans*-pyrrolidine-2,4-dicarboxylate, L-*trans*-PDC) was perfused together with glutamate through the probe;[17]

- Microdialysis perfusion of 10 mM L-*trans*-PDC for up to 10 min, which increased extracellular glutamate by >20-fold (i.e., a level comparable to that reached during spreading depression and 1–2 min after severe ischemia[18,19]) did not produce electrophysiological changes indicative of excessive excitation;[20]

- L-*trans*-PDC increased markedly extracellular glutamate in the hippocampus,

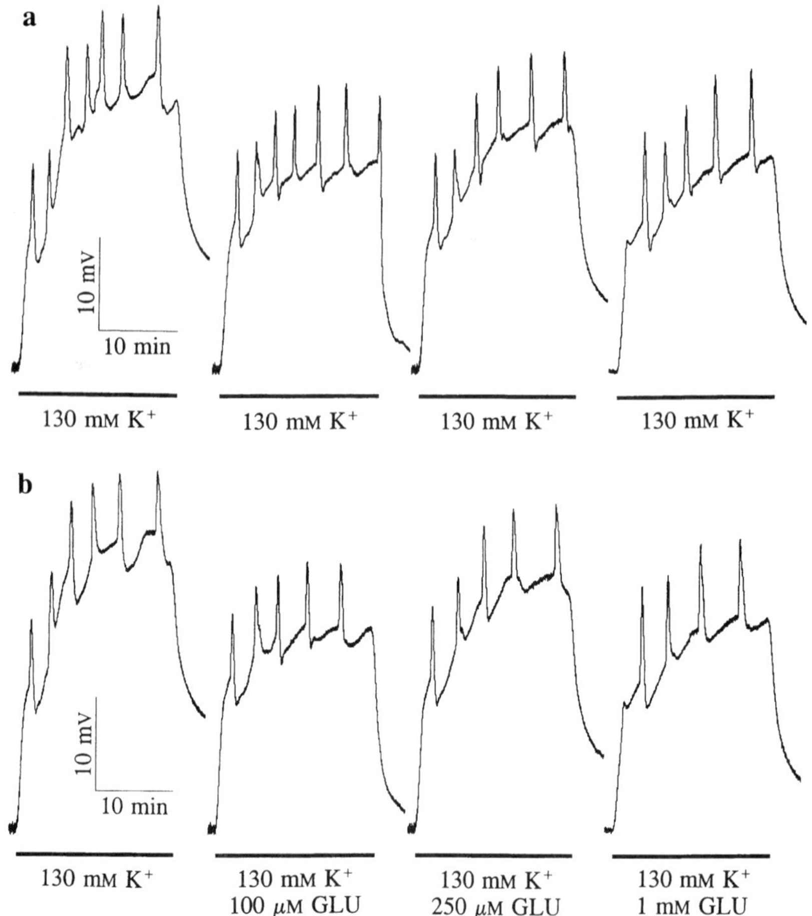

FIGURE 2. Effect of high extracellular glutamate on K^+-evoked spreading depression (SD). **(a)** Representative changes in the direct current (DC) potential produced by four repeated perfusion of 130 mM K^+ through a cortical microdialysis probe for 20 min (*horizontal bars*). **(b)** Representative changes in the DC potential, produced contra-laterally, by 130 mM K^+ onto which were superimposed increasing concentration of exogenous glutamate (0.1, 0.25 and 1 mM). These experiments were carried out in halothane-anesthetised rats. Changes in the DC potential were recorded with an electrode incorporated within the dialysis fiber. In each trace of (a) and (b), the sustained negative shifts of the DC potential correspond to persistent local depolarisation produced by the applied K^+, whereas each further transient depolarization reflects elicitation of an SD wave. Superimposition of glutamate on K^+ had no effect on SD elicitation, despite SD being exclusively sensitive to NMDA-receptor block. (From Obrenovitch *et al.*[23] Reprinted by permission from Lippincott Williams & Wilkins Publishers.)

striatum, and cortex of rats, but it produced a significant reduction of the latency for anoxic depolarization only in the cerebral cortex;[21]

- Increased extracellular glutamate did not promote the elicitation of spreading depression (SD).[22,23]

Emphasis needs to be placed on the last two points, i.e., tolerance to high extracellular glutamate early in ischemia and during SD. Indeed, one can argue that local, high extracellular concentrations of glutamate may be well tolerated in the intact brain (i.e., under physiological conditions), but not in situations where energy supply is limited (stroke and anoxia) or deficient (mitochondrial dysfunction), or when tissue integrity is altered (TBI). However, high extracellular glutamate precipitated neither anoxic depolarization nor SD. For example, the data in FIGURE 2 demonstrate that perfusion of up to 1 mM of glutamate through a microdialysis probe did not favour K^+-induced SD, despite the following features of SD: (i) remarkable sensitivity to NMDA-receptor block;[24,25] (ii) high energy demand;[26] (iii) reduced efficacy of glutamate uptake as extracellular K^+ increases;[27] and (iv) contribution to the progression of ischemic damage from the ischemic core to the periphery.[28,29]

Changes in the Concentration of Glutamate in the Synaptic Cleft Are NOT Reflected at Extracellular Level

The concentration of glutamate in the synaptic cleft is a critical determinant of *endogenous* excitotoxicity, because this is the compartment where glutamate interacts with postsynaptic receptors (FIG. 1b). Indeed, excitotoxic neuronal death is thought to be a consequence of intracellular Ca^{2+}-loading, resulting from excessive opening of NMDA-operated cation channels, superimposed on deficient Ca^{2+}-homeostasis as Na^+-influx associated with glutamatergic synaptic transmission increases and is not compensated for Na/K-ATPase overload or failure. Increased intracellular Ca^{2+} can promote cell death through activation of enzymes such as proteases, phospholipases, nitric oxide synthases and endonucleases.

Under normal physiological conditions, the concentration of glutamate within the synaptic cleft increases very briefly to 1–2 mM as it is released from presynaptic vesicles by exocytosis. Synaptic transmission is halted by the combination of glutamate re-uptake, its diffusion out of the synaptic cleft, and receptor di-sensitization.[30,31] Under experimental or pathological conditions, the exocytosis of glutamate may well be enhanced (e.g., epileptic seizures) and/or its re-uptake be reduced (FIG. 1b). Unfortunately, changes in extracellular concentrations of glutamate do not appear to reflect changes in the magnitude of synaptic spill-over.[32]

Reduction of Vesicular Neurotransmitter Release

In several studies, local inhibition of exocytosis by addition of the Na^+-channel blocker tetrodotoxin (TTX) to the microdialysis perfusion medium did not reduce the extracellular concentrations of glutamate (FIG. 3) (for review, see Timmerman & Westerink[32]). A similar discrepancy was found with regard to Ca^{2+}-dependency, another feature of transmitter output that can be assessed by omitting Ca^{2+} from the perfusion medium and/or infusing Ca^{2+}-channel blockers (e.g., Mg^{2+}).[33,34]

Enhanced Vesicular Neurotransmitter Release

The apparent lack of spill-over from glutamatergic synapses can be exemplified by data obtained with seizure activity and K^+-channel block. Enhanced glutamate-

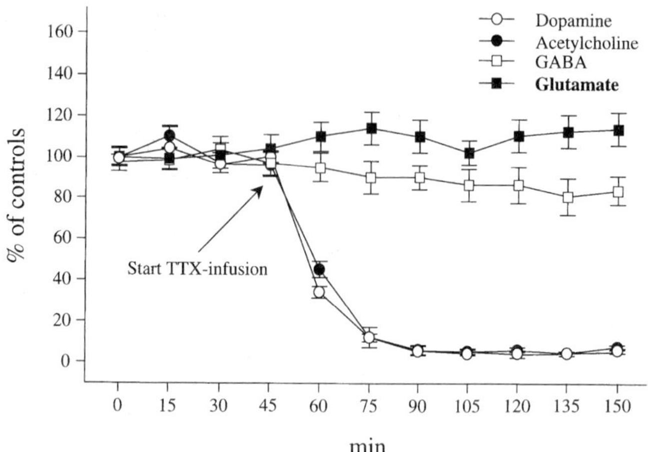

FIGURE 3. Effect of local inhibition of vesicular neurotransmitter release (exocytosis), by addition of the Na^+-channel blocker, tetrodotoxin (TTX, 1 µM) to the perfusion medium, on the extracellular levels of acetylcholine, dopamine, glutamate and GABA in the striatum of rats. Note the insensitivity of extracellular glutamate (■) to inhibition of exocytosis by TTX. (From Westerink.[35] Reprinted by permission from Elsevier Science B.V.)

mediated synaptic activity is clearly expected to be associated with seizure activity[36] but, in a number of studies, extracellular glutamate did not increase under this condition (for review, see Obrenovitch & Urenjak[8]). In two separate investigations, electrical activity and changes in extracellular glutamate were recorded at the same site of the dorsal hippocampus during drug-induced seizures in anesthetised rats.[20,37] No detectable change in dialysate levels of glutamate was associated with seizure activity, even when drugs were applied locally to inhibit glutamate uptake (i.e., dihydrokainate or L-*trans*-PDC), or when the K^+ concentration in the perfusion medium was increased slightly to compensate for a possible interference of microdialysis with the pathophysiology under study.[19]

The K^+-channel blocker 4-aminopyridine (4-AP) is considered to be one of the most suitable agents for "selective" induction of exocytosis, because unlike high K^+ and veratridine, it mimics enhanced, physiological presynaptic stimulation. 4-Aminopyridine induces the release of glutamate from synaptosomes in a Ca^{2+}-dependent manner.[38,39] In microdialysis experiments, this drug evoked the release of dopamine, and that of 5-hydroxytryptamine (5-HT) in some cases.[40,41] However, 4-AP (1, 5 and 10 mM) did not increase dialysate glutamate when it was perfused through probes implanted in the striatum of freely moving rats, either alone or in combination with an inhibitor of glutamate uptake.[42] In contrast, 4-AP decreased extracellular glutamine significantly,[42] which could reflect recycling of transmitter glutamate and γ-aminobutyric acid (GABA) via the glutamine synthesis pathway.[43,44]

In our laboratory, we have examined both the changes in extracellular glutamate and postsynaptic potentials evoked by stimulation of the perforant path, when 4-AP (1, 10 M) was perfused for 5 min through microdialysis probes implanted into the hippocampal dentate gyrus of anesthetised rats. 4-Aminopyridine markedly enhanced the amplitude of the evoked potentials recorded at the microdialysis sampling site, but the dialysate levels of glutamate remained unchanged.[45]

TTX Sensitivity of Stimuli-Induced Increase in Extracellular Glutamate: What Does It Mean?

In several studies, electrical stimulation of the prefrontal cortex increased extracellular glutamate in brain regions receiving projections from this area, and some of these changes have been linked to enhanced release of vesicular glutamate because they were inhibited by TTX.[46–48] However, when a compound has both transmitter

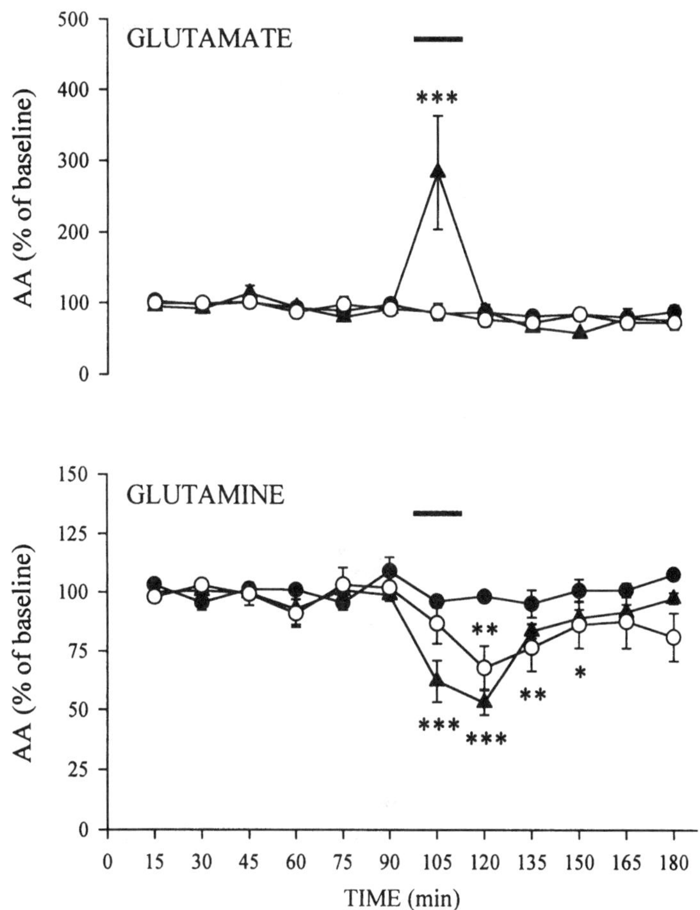

FIGURE 4. Effects of 4-aminopyridine (4-AP, 1 mM) and high K$^+$ (100 mM), added to the microdialysis perfusion medium, on extracellular glutamate and glutamine in the striatum of freely moving rats. Note that 4-AP did not increase the extracellular concentration of glutamate, but did reduce that of glutamine significantly. Values are mean ± SEM; (○–○), 4-AP 1 mM; (▲–▲), K$^+$ 100 mM; (●–●), control; $^*p < 0.05$; $^{**}p < 0.01$; $^{***}p < 0.001$. (From Segovia *et al.*[42] Reprinted by permission from Plenum Publishing Corporation.)

<u>and</u> metabolic functions (e.g., glutamate, adenosine, taurine), sensitivity of increased extracellular levels to TTX (and/or Ca^{2+}-dependency) does not necessarily imply that the change is a direct consequence of the compound being released by exocytosis. This point can be exemplified with lactate, which is devoid of neurotransmitter function. Enhanced synaptic activity produces an efflux of lactate in the extracellular space.[49] This change is certainly TTX and Ca^{2+} sensitive, because the brain energy demand, including anaerobic metabolism, is linked to synaptic activity.[50,51] But the origin of this change cannot be lactate exocytosis. The same rationale applies to cytosolic glutamate, i.e., efflux of cytosolic glutamate can be TTX sensitive or Ca^{2+} dependent because this change may be indirectly linked to synaptic activity.

Increased glutamate exocytosis may remain undetected extracellularly because of one or several of the following features: synapse ultrastructure;[52] relatively small contribution of synapses to the overall cell membrane area;[53] and efficient glutamate uptake mechanisms.[54] Alternatively, changes in extracellular glutamate of nonneuronal sources may mask those, much smaller, of synaptic origin (FIG. 1b).

Glutamate-receptor antagonists protect against traumatic brain injury (TBI)
⇨ *Excitotoxic mechanisms are involved in TBI* [55,56]

Mice with deficient neuronal nitric oxide synthase are more resistant to cerebral ischaemia
⇨ *Cerebral ischaemia may be associated with excessive formation of nitric oxide*[57,58]

Poly (ADP-ribose) polymerase (PARP) inhibitors are beneficial in models of cerebral ischaemia
⇨ *PARP activation may be involved in ischaemic neuronal damage*[59]

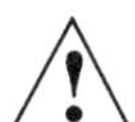 **Caution!** 

- Neuroprotection resulting from an interaction with a specific molecular target does not necessarily imply abnormal function of the target.

- The interaction may only render the cells more resistant to other deleterious mechanisms.

PROTECTION AGAINST EXPERIMENTAL OR PATHOLOGICAL EVENTS BY GLUTAMATE RECEPTOR ANTAGONISTS DOES NOT NECESSARILY IMPLY EXCITOTOXIC PROCESSES

A common experimental strategy in the field of neurodegeneration and neuroprotection is to interact with a specific molecular target, either pharmacologically or through specific mutations, and to examine whether this interaction modifies the sensitivity of a preparation to relevant stimuli. This is a pertinent approach, but the ensuing data are often interpreted in an oversimplified manner, i.e., any change subsequent to an interaction with a specific molecular target is taken as indicative of a

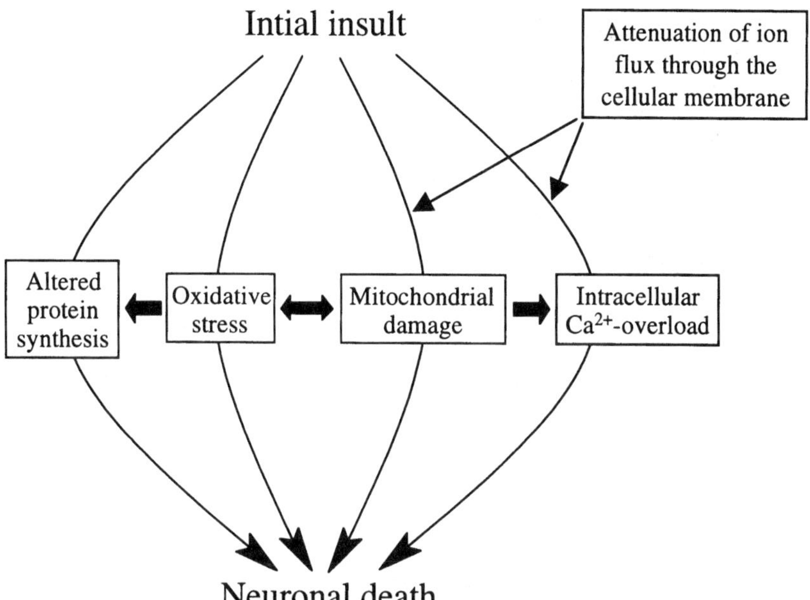

FIGURE 5. Diagram illustrating the multifactorial nature of the processes, triggered by an initial insult, which can lead to neuronal death. The four pathways represented here are only relevant examples. It is clear that a multitude of other malfunctions can promote neuronal death. With this degree of complexity, a specific treatment may actually increase the resistance of vulnerable cells to various deleterious mechanisms (see INSERT). For example, attenuation of ion flux through the cellular membrane, by administration of glutamate-receptor antagonists or Na^+-channel blockers, may be protective by helping brain cells to cope with intracellular Ca^{2+}-overload and/or mitochondrial injury.

direct involvement of the target in the pathology under study. This is not necessarily true (see INSERT). Neuronal death subsequent to ischemia, trauma and other insults is the consequence of multifactorial processes that may be inter-related (FIG. 5). Within such a complex picture, beneficial effects resulting from an interaction with a specific molecular target may actually render the cell more resistant to deleterious mechanisms that are not directly related to the target.

The above caution certainly applies to strategies based on reduction of cation flux through ligand-operated and/or voltage-gated channels (e.g., glutamate antagonists, Na^+-channel blockers),[60–62] designed to protect neurons when their energy demand cannot be matched by adequate supply or metabolism. Indeed, reduction of energy demand probably underlies neuroprotection with hypothermia, Na^+-channel blockers, and other strategies aiming to attenuate ion flux across the cellular membrane.[62–64] Therefore, reduction of ion flux across the cellular membrane can help cells to cope with mitochondrial damage or deficiency, as well as with intracellular Ca^{2+}-overload (FIG. 5), and this does not imply that the pathological conditions include excessive ion channel opening.

The following data illustrate that inhibition of cation influx into brain cells via one route can protect against enhancement of cation entry via a different route, as long as the latter challenge is not acute. Moderate glutamate toxicity in rat hippocampal neurons was attenuated by TTX.[65,66] Reciprocally, NMDA-receptor antagonists reduced the lethal effects of the Na^+-channel activator, veratridine, when 10–30 μM of the toxin was applied to brain neuronal cultures.[67,68] Several dihydropyridine Ca^{2+}-channel antagonists were found protective against excitotoxic conditions, both *in vivo* and *in vitro*.[69–71] It is pertinent to mention here that, in models of focal ischemia, the penumbra (i.e., where the severity of the insult is moderate) is the region that is often selectively rescued with protective treatments.[72]

The above caution (INSERT) also applies to oxidative stress because of the multiplicity of its potential origins: i.e., increased free radical formation from different sources (stimulation of NO synthesis, mitochondrial malfunction, lipid peroxidation, etc.); reduced efficacy of enzymatic free radical scavengers (superoxide dismutases, peroxidases, etc.); and reduced levels of endogenous antioxidants (ascorbic acid, tocopherol, etc.).[73]

CONCLUDING REMARKS

This analysis argues strongly against the oversimplified hypothesis that high extracellular glutamate is the key to excitotoxicity in neurological disorders. Accordingly, (i) application of exogenous glutamate agonists to nervous tissue is not a valid model of *endogenous* excitotoxicity; and (ii) the monitoring of brain extracellular glutamate in stroke and TBI patients is not a suitable aid for their therapeutic management.

Our data and rationale do not rule out the hypothesis that *endogenous* excitotoxic processes may contribute to neuronal death associated with some neurological disorders. Enhanced exocytosis of glutamate, and/or its deficient uptake, remain possible excitotoxic abnormalities, but only at synaptic level. In addition, a wide range of alternative abnormalities of glutamatergic transmission may occur (see Obrenovitch & Urenjak[8,9] for reviews), including increased permeability of AMPA-receptor-ionophore complexes to Ca^{2+},[74] and abnormal sensitivity and modulation of NMDA-receptors.[75]

ACKNOWLEDGMENTS

Financial support from the Thompson Fund and the Wellcome Trust (TG98/MEP/SRD/LR) is gratefully acknowledged.

REFERENCES

1. OLNEY, J.W. & O.L. HO. 1970. Brain damage in infant mice following oral intake of glutamate, aspartate or cysteine. Nature **227:** 609–611.
2. OLNEY, J.W. 1981. Kainic acid and other excitotoxins: a comparative analysis. Adv. Biochem. Psychopharmacol. **27:** 375–384.

3. TODD, E.C.D. 1993. Domoic acid and amnesic shellfish poisoning: a review. J. Food Prot. **56:** 69–83.

4. PENG, Y.G., T.B. TAYLOR, R.E. FINCH, R.C. SWITZER & J.S. RAMSDELL. 1994. Neuroexcitatory and neurotoxic actions of the amnesic shellfish poison, domoic acid. Neuroreport **5:** 981–985.

5. BENVENISTE, H., J. DREJER, A. SCHOUSBOE & N.H. DIEMER. 1984. Elevation of the extracellular concentrations of glutamate and aspartate in rat hippocampus during transient cerebral ischemia monitored by intracerebral microdialysis. J. Neurochem. **43:** 1369–1374.

6. ROTHMAN, S.M. 1984. Synaptic release of excitatory amino acid neurotransmitter mediates anoxic neuronal death. J. Neurosci. **4:** 1884–1891.

7. SIMON, R.P., J.H. SWAN, T. GRIFFITHS & B.S. MELDRUM. 1984. Blockade of *N*-methyl-D-aspartate receptors may protect against ischemic damage in the brain. Science **266:** 850–852.

8. OBRENOVITCH, T.P. & J. URENJAK. 1997. Altered glutamatergic transmission in neurological disorders: from high extracellular glutamate to excessive synaptic efficacy. Prog. Neurobiol. **51:** 39–87.

9. OBRENOVITCH, T.P. & J. URENJAK. 1997. Is high extracellular glutamate the key to excitotoxicity in traumatic brain injury? J. Neurotrauma **14:** 677–698.

10. SHIMIZU-SASAMATA, M., P. BOSQUE-HAMILTON, P.L. HUANG, M.A. MOSKOWITZ & E.H. LO. 1998. Attenuated neurotransmitter release and spreading depression-like depolarizations after focal ischemia in mutant mice with disrupted type I nitric oxide synthase gene. J. Neurosci. **18:** 9564–9571.

11. BULLOCK, R., A. ZAUNER, J.J. WOODWARD, J. MYSEROS, S.C. CHOI, J.D. WARD, A. MARMAROU & H.F. YOUNG. 1998. Factors affecting excitatory amino acid release following severe human head injury. J. Neurosurg. **89:** 507–518.

12. OLNEY, J.W. & T. DE GUBAREFF. 1978. Glutamate neurotoxicity and Huntington's chorea. Nature **271:** 557–559.

13. MANGANO, R.M. & R. SCHWARCZ. 1983. Chronic infusion of endogenous excitatory amino acids into rat striatum and hippocampus. Brain Res. Bull. **10:** 47–51.

14. TOTH, E. & A. LAJTHA. 1989. Motor effects of intracaudate injection of excitatory amino acids. Pharmacol. Biochem. Behav. **33:** 175–179.

15. SCHWARCZ, R., D. SCHOLZ & J.T. COYLE. 1978. Structure-activity relations for the neurotoxicity of kainic acid derivatives and glutamate analogues. Neuropharmacology **17:** 145–151.

16. OBRENOVITCH, T.P., J. URENJAK & E. ZILKHA. 1994. Intracerebral microdialysis combined with recording of extracellular field potential: a novel method for investigation of depolarizing drugs *in vivo*. Br. J. Pharmacol. **113:** 1295–1302.

17. OBRENOVITCH, T.P., J. URENJAK & E. ZILKHA. 1997. Effects of increased extracellular glutamate levels on the local field potential in the brain of anaesthetized rats. Br. J. Pharmacol. **122:** 372–378.

18. WAHL, F., T.P. OBRENOVITCH, A.M. HARDY, M. PLOTKINE, R. BOULU & L. SYMON. 1994. Extracellular glutamate during focal cerebral ischaemia in rats: time course and calcium-dependency. J. Neurochem. **63:** 1003–1011.

19. OBRENOVITCH, T.P., E. ZILKHA & J. URENJAK. 1995. Intracerebral microdialysis: electrophysiological evidence of a critical pitfall. J. Neurochem. **64:** 1884–1888.

20. OBRENOVITCH, T.P., J. URENJAK & E. ZILKHA. 1996. Evidence disputing the link between seizure activity and high extracellular glutamate. J. Neurochem. **66:** 2446–2454.

21. OBRENOVITCH, T.P., E. ZILKHA & J. URENJAK. 1998. Effect of pharmacological inhibition of glutamate-uptake on ischemia-induced glutamate efflux and anoxic depolarization latency. Naunyn-Schmiedeberg's Arch. Pharmacol. **357:** 225–231.

22. OBRENOVITCH, T.P. & E. ZILKHA. 1995. High extracellular potassium, and not extracellular glutamate, is required for the propagation of spreading depression. J. Neurophysiol. **73:** 2107–2114.

23. OBRENOVITCH, T.P., E. ZILKHA & J. URENJAK. 1996. Evidence against high extracellular glutamate promoting the elicitation of spreading depression by potassium. J. Cereb. Blood Flow Metab. **16:** 923–931.

24. MARRANNES, R., R. WILLEMS, E. DE PRINS & A. WAUQUIER. 1988. Evidence for a role of the N-methyl-D-aspartate (NMDA) receptor in cortical spreading depression in the rat. Brain Res. **457:** 226–240.

25. OBRENOVITCH, T.P. & E. ZILKHA. 1996. Inhibition of cortical spreading depression by L-701,324, a novel antagonist at the glycine site of the N-methyl-D-aspartate receptor complex. Br. J. Pharmacol. **117:** 931–937.

26. LAURITZEN, M. 1994. Pathophysiology of the migraine aura: the spreading depression theory. Brain **117:** 199–210.

27. KANNER, B.I. & A. BENDAHAN. 1982. Binding order of substrates to the sodium and potassium ion coupled L-glutamic acid transporter from rat brain. Biochemistry **21:** 6327–6300.

28. BACK, T., M.D. GINSBERG, W.D. DIETRICH & B.D. WATSON. 1996. Induction of spreading depression in the ischemic hemisphere following experimental middle cerebral artery occlusion: effect on infarct morphology. J. Cereb. Blood Flow Metab. **16:** 202–213.

29. BUSCH, E., M.L. GYNGEL, M. EIS, M. HOEHN-BERLAGE & K.A. HOSSMANN. 1996. Potassium-induced cortical spreading depressions during focal cerebral ischemia in rats: contribution to lesion growth assessed by diffusion-weighted NMR and biochemical imaging. J. Cereb. Blood Flow Metab. **16:** 1090–1099.

30. CLEMENTS, J.D., R.A. LESTER, G. TONG, C.E. JAHR & G.L. WESTBROOK. 1992. The time course of glutamate in the synaptic cleft. Science **258:** 1498–1501.

31. GLAVINOVIC, M.I. & H.R. RABIE. 1998. Monte Carlo simulation of spontaneous miniature excitatory postsynaptic currents in rat hippocampal synapse in the presence and absence of desensitization. Naunyn-Schmiedeberg's Arch. Pharmacol. **435:** 193–202.

32. TIMMERMAN, W. & B.H.C. WESTERINK. 1997. Brain microdialysis of GABA and glutamate: What does it signify? Synapse **27:** 242–261.

33. WESTERINK, B.H.C., H.M. HOFSTEEDE, G. DAMSMA & J.B. DE VRIES. 1988. The significance of extracellular calcium for the release of dopamine, acetylcholine and amino acids in conscious rats, evaluated by brain microdialysis. Naunyn-Schmiedeberg's Arch. Pharmacol. **337:** 373–378.

34. MIELE, M., M.G. BOUTELLE & M. FILLENZ. 1996. The source of physiologically stimulated glutamate efflux from the striatum of conscious rats. J. Physiol. (Lond.) **497:** 745–751.

35. WESTERINK, B.H.C. 1995. Brain microdialysis and its application for the study of animal behaviour. Behav. Brain Res. **70:** 103–124.

36. BRADFORD, H.F. 1995. Glutamate, GABA and epilepsy. Prog. Neurobiol. **47:** 656–659.

37. MILLAN, M.H., T.P. OBRENOVITCH, G.S. SARNA, S.-Y. LOK, L. SYMON & B.S. MELDRUM. 1991. Changes in rat brain extracellular glutamate concentration during seizures induced by systemic picrotoxin or focal bicuculline injection: an *in vivo* dialysis study with on-line enzymatic detection. Epilepsy Res. **9:** 86–91.

38. SANCHEZ-PRIETO, J., I. HERRERO, M.T. MIRAS-PORTUGA & F. MORA. 1994. Unchanged exocytotic release of glutamic acid in cortex and neostriatum of the rat during aging. Brain Res. Bull. **33:** 357–359.

39. TIBBS, G.R., J.O. DOLLY & D.G. NICHOLLS. 1996. Evidence for the induction of repetitive action potentials in synaptosomes by K^+-channel inhibitors: an analysis of plasma membrane ion fluxes. J. Neurochem. **67:** 389–397.

40. DAWSON, L.A. & C. ROUTLEDGE. 1995. Differential effects of potassium channel blockers on extracellular concentrations of dopamine and 5-HT in the striatum of conscious rats. Br. J. Pharmacol. **116:** 3260–3264.

41. PEI, Q., R.A. LESLIE, D.G. GRAHAM-SMITH & T.S.C. ZETTERSTRÖM. 1995. 5-HT efflux from rat hippocampus *in vivo* produced by 4-aminopyridine is increased by chronic lithium administration. Neuroreport **6:** 716–720.

42. SEGOVIA, G., A. PORRAS & F. MORA. 1997. Effects of 4-aminopyridine on extracellular concentrations of glutamate in striatum of the freely moving rat. Neurochem. Res. **22:** 1491–1497.

43. HERTZ, L. 1979. Functional interactions between neurons and astrocytes I. Turnover and metabolism of putative amino acid transmitters. Prog. Neurobiol. **13:** 277–323.

44. WESTERGAARD, N., U. SONNEWALD & A. SCHOUSBOE. 1995. Metabolic trafficking between neurons and astrocytes: the glutamate/glutamine cycle revisited. Dev. Neurosci. **17:** 203–211.

45. OBRENOVITCH, T.P. & J. URENJAK. 1998. The glutamate-excitotoxicity hypothesis: use and abuse. *In* Pharmacology of Cerebral Ischemia. J. Krieglstein, Ed. Medpharm. Stuttgart. In press.

46. LADA, M.W., T.W. VICKROY & R.T. KENNEDY. 1998. Evidence for neuronal origin and metabotropic receptor-mediated regulation of extracellular glutamate and aspartate in rat striatum *in vivo* following electrical stimulation of the prefrontal cortex. J. Neurochem. **70:** 617–625.

47. YOU, Z.-B., T.M. TZSCHENTKE, E. BRODIN & R.A. WISE. 1998. Electrical stimulation of the prefrontal cortex increases cholecystokinin, glutamate, and dopamine release in the nucleus accumbens: an *in vivo* microdialysis study in freely moving rats. J. Neurosci. **18:** 6492–6500.

48. ROSSETTI, Z.L., C. MARCANGIONE & R.A. WISE. 1998. Increase of extracellular glutamate and expression of Fos-like immunoreactivity in the ventral tegmental area in response to electrical stimulation of the prefrontal cortex. J. Neurochem. **70:** 1503–1512.

49. KORF, J. 1996. Intracerebral trafficking of lactate *in vivo* during stress, exercise, electroconvulsive shock and ischemia as studied with microdialysis. Dev. Neurosci. **18:** 405–414.

50. SOKOLOFF, L. 1993. Sites and mechanisms of function-related changes in energy metabolism in the nervous system. Dev. Neurosci. **15:** 194–206.

51. TAYLOR. D.L., D.A. RICHARDS, T.P. OBRENOVITCH & L. SYMON. 1994. Time course of changes in extracellular lactate evoked by transient K^+-induced depolarisation in the rat striatum. J. Neurochem. **62:** 2368–2374.

52. EDWARDS, F.A. 1995. Anatomy and electrophysiology of fast central synapses lead to a structural model for long-term potentiation. Physiol. Rev. **75:** 759–787.

53. RUSAKOV, D.A., E. HARRISON & M.G. STEWART. 1998. Synapses in hippocampus occupy only 1–2% of cell membranes and are spaced less than half-micron apart: a quantitative ultrastructure analysis with discussion of physiological implications. Neuropharmacology **37:** 513–521.

54. ELIASOF, S. & F. WERBLIN. 1993. Characterization of the glutamate transporter in retinal cones of the tiger salamander. J. Neurosci. **13:** 402–411.

55. IKONOMIDOU, C. & L. TURSKI. 1996. Prevention of trauma-induced neurodegeneration in infant and adult rat brain: glutamate antagonists. Metab. Brain Dis. **11:** 125–141.

56. OKIYAMA. K., D.H. SMITH, W.F. WHITE, K. RICHTER & T.K. MCINTOSH. 1997. Effects of the novel NMDA antagonists CP-98,113, CP-101,581 and CP-101,606 on cognitive function and regional cerebral edema following experimental brain injury in the rat. J. Neurotrauma **14:** 211–222.

57. HUANG, Z., P.L. HUANG, N. PANAHIAN, T. DALKARA, M.C. FISHMAN & M.A. MOSKOWITZ. 1994. Effects of cerebral ischemia in mice deficient in neuronal nitric oxide synthase. Science **265:** 1883–1885.

58. PANAHIAN, N., T. YOSHIDA, P.L. HUANG, E.T. HEDLEY-WHYTE, T. DALKARA, M.C. FISHMAN & M.A. MOSKOWITZ. 1996. Attenuated hippocampal damage after global cerebral ischemia in mice mutant in neuronal nitric oxide synthase. Neuroscience **72:** 343–354.

59. LO, E.H., P. BOSQUE-HAMILTON & W. MENG. 1998. Inhibition of poly(ADP-ribose) polymerase: reduction of ischemic injury and attenuation of N-methyl-D-aspartate-induced neurotransmitter dysregulation. Stroke **29:** 830–836.

60. AMES, A. III. 1992. Energy requirements of CNS cells as related to their function and to their vulnerability to ischemia: a commentary based on studies on retina. Can. J. Physiol. Pharmacol. **70**(Suppl.)**:** S158–S164.

61. AMES. A. III, K.I. MAYNARD & S. KAPLAN. 1995. Protection against CNS ischemia by temporary interruption of function-related processes of neurons. J. Cereb. Blood Flow Metab. **15:** 433–439.

62. URENJAK, J. & T.P. OBRENOVITCH. 1996. Pharmacological modulation of voltage-gated Na^+ channels: a rational and effective strategy against ischemic brain damage. Pharmacol. Rev. **48:** 21–67.

63. BACHER, A., J.Y. KWON & M.H. ZORNOW. 1998. Effects of temperature on cerebral tissue oxygen tension, carbon dioxide tension, and pH during transient global ischemia in rabbits. Anesthesiology **88:** 403–409.

64. HOFFMAN. W.E., F.T. CHARBEL, L. MUNOZ & J.I. AUSMAN. 1998. Comparison of brain tissue metabolic changes during ischemia at 35 degrees and 18 degrees C. Surg. Neurol. **49:** 85–88.

65. OGURA, A., M. MIYAMOTO & Y. KUDO. 1988. Neuronal death *in vitro*: parallelism between survivability of hippocampal neurones and sustained elevation of cytosolic Ca^{2+} after exposure to glutamate receptor agonist. Exp. Brain Res. **73:** 447–458.

66. YOON, K.W. 1995. Glutamate effect on synaptic transmission mediates neurotoxicity in dissociated rat hippocampal neurons. Brain Res. **669:** 320–324.

67. PAUWELS, P.J., H.P. VAN ASSOUW, J.E. LEYSEN & P.A. JANSSEN. 1989. Ca^{2+}-mediated neuronal death in rat brain neuronal cultures by veratridine: protection by flunarizine. Mol. Pharmacol. **36:** 525–531.

68. SCHRAMM, M., S. EIMERL & E. COSTA. 1990. Serum and depolarizing agents cause acute neurotoxicity in cultured cerebellar granule cells: role of the glutamate receptor responsive to N-methyl-D-aspartate. Proc. Natl. Acad. Sci. USA **87:** 1193–1197.

69. SUCHER, N.J., S.Z. LEI & S.A. LIPTON. 1991. Calcium-channel antagonists attenuate NMDA receptor-mediated neurotoxicity of retinal ganglion cells in culture. Brain Res. **551:** 297–302.

70. STUIVER, B.T., B.R.T. DOUMA, R. BAKKER, C. NYAKAS & P.G.M. LUITEN. 1996. *In vivo* protection against NMDA-induced neurodegeneration by MK-801 and nimodipine: combined therapy and temporal course of protection. Neurodegeneration **5:** 153–159.

71. KRIEGLSTEIN, J. 1997. Excitotoxicity and neuroprotection. Eur. J. Pharm. Sci. **5:** 181–187.

72. OBRENOVITCH, T.P. 1995. The ischaemic penumbra: twenty years on. Cerebrovasc. Brain Metab. Rev. **7:** 297–323.

73. WILSON, J.X. 1997. Antioxidant defence of the brain: a role for astrocytes. Can. J. Physiol. Pharmacol. **75:** 1149–1163.

74. PELLEGRINI-GIAMPIETRO, D.E., J.A. GORTER, M.V. BENNETT & R.S. ZUKIN. 1997. The GluR2 (GluR-B) hypothesis: Ca^{2+}-permeable AMPA receptors in neurological disorders. Trends Neurosci. **20:** 464–470.

75. DORIAT, J.F., A. CORTEY & J.L. DAVAL. 1998. Selective alterations in binding kinetic parameters and allosteric regulation of N-methyl-D-aspartate receptors after prolonged seizures in the developing rat brain. Pediatr. Res. **43:** 415–420.

Evidence Disputing the Importance of Excitotoxicity in Hippocampal Neuron Death after Experimental Traumatic Brain Injury

W. SHAWN CARBONELL AND M. SEAN GRADY[a]

Department of Neurological Surgery, University of Washington School of Medicine, Seattle, Washington, USA

ABSTRACT: The hippocampus is selectively vulnerable to experimental traumatic brain injury (TBI). Beneficial effects of glutamate receptor antagonists and increased extracellular levels of glutamate have suggested that glutamate-mediated excitotoxicity may be responsible for this selective damage. In order to clarify this important issue, we applied a severe parasagittal fluid percussion injury (FPI) to strains of mice shown to be susceptible and resistant to kainic acid (KA)-induced excitotoxic hippocampal damage. Dystrophic neurons were present by 10 min after FPI in the hippocampi of both strains. Damaged hippocampal neurons were absent at 4 days and 7 days. Additionally, there was no significant difference ($p = 1.00$) in CA3 neuron survival between KA-susceptible and -resistant mice at 4 days. In conclusion, excitotoxicity does not significantly contribute to hippocampal neuron loss after FPI and, in contrast to classic studies of excitotoxicity *in vivo*, the pattern of hippocampal cell death after TBI is extremely acute.

INTRODUCTION

Excitotoxicity has been proposed to play a role in hippocampal neuron death associated with traumatic brain injury (TBI) based on the findings in rats that (1) CA3 pyramidal neurons of the hippocampus are selectively lost after parasagittal fluid percusion injury (FPI), (2) extracellular (EC) glutamate levels are significantly elevated in CA3 after moderate and severe FPI, and (3) pharmacological blockade of glutamate receptors can improve neurological and behavioral outcome and, in some cases, attenuate CA3 neuron loss after experimental TBI.[8,12,16,18,35,34] Indeed, glutamate is the most abundant excitatory neurotransmitter in the brain, and the hippocampus has a particularly large endowment of glutamate receptors. However, although high levels of glutamate can cause death in *in vitro* preparations, the levels of EC glutamate necessary to produce neuronal dysfunction and death *in vivo* are far above those that may occur in models of stroke or TBI.[6,29] Further, N-methyl-D-aspartate (NMDA) and non-NMDA receptor agonists can improve outcome following FPI even when administered *after* the peak of EC glutamate.[29] Therefore, the ef-

[a]Corresponding author: M. Sean Grady, M.D., Chairman, Dept. of Neurosurgery, University of Pennsylvania, Hospital of the University of Pennsylvania, 3400 Spruce St., Philadelphia, PA 19104. Phone, 215/349-8325; fax, 215/349-5108.
e-mail, grady@mail.med.upenn.edu

ficacy of NMDA receptor antagonists does not necessarily imply the presence of excitotoxic processes.[30]

Several other lines of evidence suggest that the selective CA3 damage after FPI may not be due to excitotoxicity. For example, CA1 of the rat hippocampus has been shown to be preferentially damaged by high bath glutamate, kainate (KA), or NMDA compared to CA3 in the organotypic slice preparation.[37] In contrast, CA1 in rats is invulnerable to FPI, whereas CA3 is immediately damaged.[14,16,24] Further, in CA3 of rats, mice, and man, the predominant glutamate receptors are the high-affinity KA and α-amino-3-hydroxy-5-methylisoxazole-4-propionic acid (AMPA) type, whereas NMDA receptors are less concentrated.[9,15,28,38,39] Therefore, if there is excitotoxicity in CA3 after FPI, it would be preferentially mediated by KA and AMPA receptors rather than the NMDA class. However, non-NMDA-mediated excitotoxicity is slow-onset.[6] Even millimolar concentrations of either KA or AMPA will not kill neurons *in vitro* if exposed for less than 30 min and, *in vivo*, there are no pyknotic hippocampal neurons until at least 3 hr after systemic KA injection.[19,22] Additionally, maximal damage in the hippocampus due to KA is delayed with a peak seen several days after systemic injection.[31] In contrast, maximal hippocampal damage in both rats and mice is acute and present by *10 min* after parasagittal FPI.[3,16]

The aim of the present study was to characterize hippocampal damage in strains of mice, shown to be susceptible and resistant to KA-induced excitotoxic hippocampal damage, after parasagittal FPI of a severe magnitude. The post-TBI excitotoxicity hyposthesis would predict that if there is excitotoxicity after severe FPI, there will be (1) more overall hippocampal damage, (2) more delayed hippocampal neuron damage, and (3) more hippocampal neuron loss (especially in CA3) in the KA-susceptible mice compared to KA-resistant mice. In contrast, we found that both strains of mice displayed similarly *acute* patterns of hippocampal neuron damage with no evidence of delayed or spreading damage. Further, the KA-resistant mice had more neuron loss in CA1 than the KA-susceptible strain and, importantly, CA3 neuron survival was equivalent in both KA-susceptible and -resistant mouse strains.

MATERIALS AND METHODS

Animals

Adult male C57BL/6 (KA-resistant; B & K Universal, Inc, Kent, WA) and 129SvEMS (KA-susceptible; The Jackson Laboratory, Maine) were cared for in accordance with U.S. Public Health Service regulations under the supervision of the Department of Comparative Medicine, University of Washington.

Fluid Percussion Injury

Surgical preparation has been described in detail previously.[4] Briefly, mice were anesthetized with a xylazine (0.16 mg/kg)/ketamine (2.6 mg/kg) mixture and placed in a stereotaxic head holder for the neonatal rat (Stoelting Co., Wood Dale, IL). Lacrilube ointment was applied to the eyes. The scalp was reflected and the skull exposed through a midline incision. A 3.0-mm diameter, right-sided parasagittal craniectomy 0.5 mm lateral to the sagittal suture and centered between lambda and bregma was carefully created using a microdrill and scalpel. A single anchor screw was placed ipsilaterally approximately 3.0 mm rostral to bregma and 0.5 mm lateral to the sagittal suture. The 2.0-mm inner diameter rigid injury cannula (a modified Luer-Lok catheter hub 1.2 cm in height) was placed over the craniectomy site with stereotaxic assistance and secured with cyanoacrylate gel. All exposed cranial sutures were reinforced with the cyanoacrylate as well. After allowing time for the gel to dry, the anchor screw and injury cannula were encased with methyl methacrylate cement. Actifoam sponge (Coletica S.A., Lyons, France) was used to plug the injury cannula after the cement had hardened, and the animals were placed in a normothermic warming box until awake and alert.

After a 24-hr period to allow recovery from the effects of the general anesthesia, the mice were placed in a plexiglass chamber and administered halothane. The animals were then positioned on a normothermic heating pad and halothane (2% in 30% O_2) was continued via nose cone until the mice were unresponsive to a moderate paw pinch. The injury cannula was filled with isotonic saline and the animals were connected to the FPI device via high-pressure tubing.[4] For consistency, injuries were given within 5 sec of returning paw withdrawal reflex after discontinuation of halothane anesthesia. A severe injury magnitude of 3.5 atm was used. Sham-injured animals underwent identical procedures as the trauma group; however, no injury was delivered.

Acute Neurological Assessment

In order to assure equivalent injury response between strains, we examined acute neurological outcome. Immediately after injury, the animal was disconnected from the FPI device, the injury cannula fixture was removed, and the injury site was inspected for dural integrity, and then the animal was placed in a supine position for testing of righting reflex. We chose this test, because duration of unconsciousness has been shown to be predictive of histopathological outcome after TBI in rats.[27] We recorded the time it took for the animal to right three times consecutively. In order to maximize the equivalence and severity of FP injury across all time points, a minimum of righting time of 270 sec was selected as the cutoff for trauma animals for inclusion in this study. After testing, the animals were readministered halothane via nose cone, and the scalp was closed with 4-0 silk. Animals were inspected daily after injury.

Acute and Delayed Neuronal Injury

Animals were deeply anesthetized with pentobarbital sodium at 10 min ($n = 3$, each strain), 24 hr ($n = 3$, each strain), 4 days ($n = 4$, each strain), and 7 days ($n = 3$, each strain) after FPI and perfused transcardially with 10 ml saline and 75–100 ml of 4.0% paraformaldehyde in 0.1 M phosphate buffer solution (PBS; pH = 7.6). Sham animals ($n = 3$, each strain) were sacrificed at 24 hr and prepared in the same manner as above. Following perfusion, the brains were blocked to isolate the hippocampus, embedded in paraffin, and sectioned coronally at 6 μm. Selected sections were processed for standard acid fuchsin staining, and adjacent sections were stained with cresyl violet.[16] Damaged neurons were identified by intense acid fuchsin positivity combined with dystrophic morphology. Damage was confirmed with adjacent cresyl violet-stained sections.

Neuron Survival

Quantitative analysis of the hippocampus was made in areas selectively vulnerable to KA (CA1, CA3, and the dentate hilus) at 4 days post-FPI in both strains. Only neurons with a visible nucleus and apparent cell body were counted. For areas CA1 and CA3, nine representative sections of the entire hippocampus 240 μm apart were evaluated with a 100× oil immersion objective on a Leitz microscope. Six representative sections of the hilus (240 μm apart) at the mid-level of the hippocampus were evaluated in the same manner. The number of neurons per field were counted and averaged at all levels, and mean numbers were used for statistical analysis. Neuronal survival is expressed as a percent of sham mice.

Statistical Analysis

Righting times were compared with analysis of variance (ANOVA) followed by the Neuman-Keuls post hoc test for pairwise comparisons. Analysis of neuronal damage was qualitative in nature at the light microscopic level. Hippocampal neuron counts were subjected to Kruskal-Wallis ANOVA followed by post hoc pairwise comparisons with a t-test and the Bonferroni correction factor. A $p < 0.05$ was considered statistically significant.

RESULTS

During the course of the study there was one death (C57BL/6) immediately after injury. In addition, three mice of each strain were excluded from further study after injury cannula removal because the dura was broken (with severe cortical disruption) in these animals. Apneic episodes ranging from 5–30 sec occurred in all trauma animals immediately after injury. In addition, subdural hematoma could be visualized through the skull of all trauma animals most commonly over the posterior dorsolateral aspect of the ipsilateral hemisphere. Injury-induced pulmonary edema or acute convulsive episodes were not observed in any experimental animal immediately after injury.

All trauma animals demonstrated evidence of extensive cortical injury (FIG. 1) at all timepoints of the current study, which included damaged neurons, gliosis, subdural and intraparenchymal hemorrhage, and mild tissue loss consistent with a severe injury as described previously.[3]

Acute Neurological Outcome

Righting times between trauma and sham animals were significantly different for both strains (data not shown). FIGURE 2 plots righting times of trauma animals of each strain. The KA-susceptible mice righted after 470 ± 42 sec, and the KA-resistant mice righted after 413 ± 45 sec. This difference was not significant ($p = 0.32$), supporting equivalent response to severe FPI in both strains.

Hippocampal Neuron Damage

At 10 min both strains displayed extensive acid fuchsin-positive neurons in the hippocampus. At 24 hr this pattern was identical, if not reduced, with no evidence of

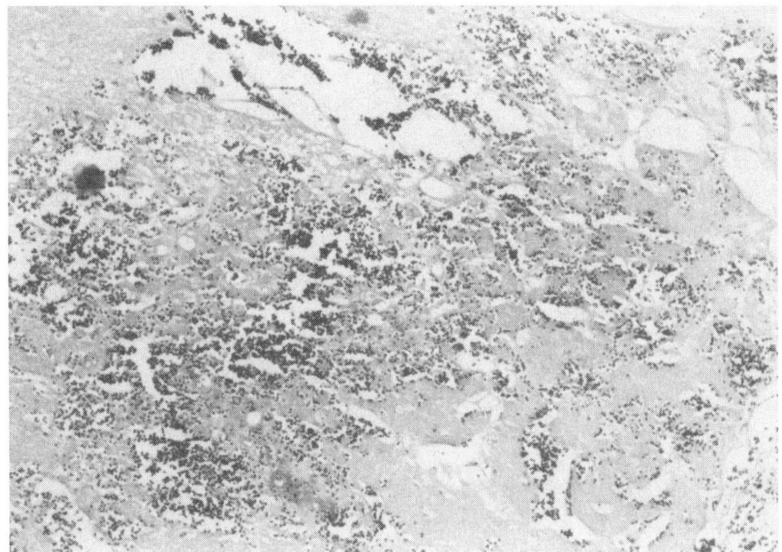

FIGURE 1. Acid fuchsin staining of the ipsilateral parietal cortex of a 129Sv/EMS mouse 4 days after severe FPI. Note the extensive blood and loss of neurons typical of this injury magnitude in both strains of mice (200×).

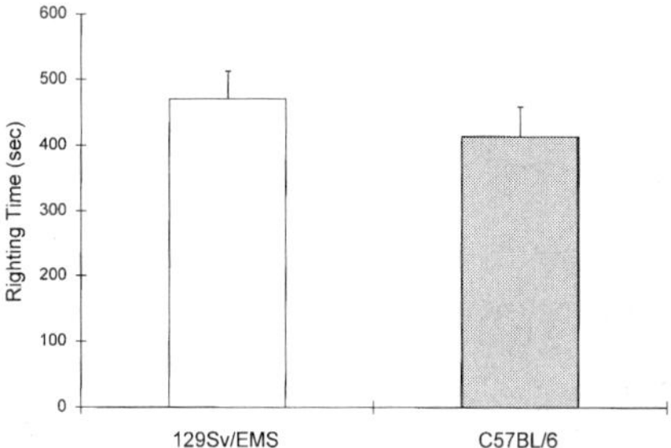

FIGURE 2. The righting time immediately after severe fluid percussion injury in KA-susceptible and -resistant mice. There is not significant difference in righting time between the two strains suggesting an equivalent response to injury ($p = 0.32$).

further damage recruitment. By 4 days there were rarely any acid fuchsin-labeled neurons in the hippocampi of either strain, demonstrating the acute nature of neuronal injury after FPI (FIG. 3A,B). In contrast to KA treatment in KA-susceptible mice, adjacent cresyl violet sections did not demonstrate any areas of overt frank pyramidal neuron loss at 4 days or 7 days in either mouse strain after severe FPI. Notably, several animals of both strains demonstrated visible loss of dentate granule cells in the dorsal blade of the dentate gyrus in 1–2 of the most medial brain sections at 4 days (data not shown). Hippocampi of both strains at 7 days appeared identical

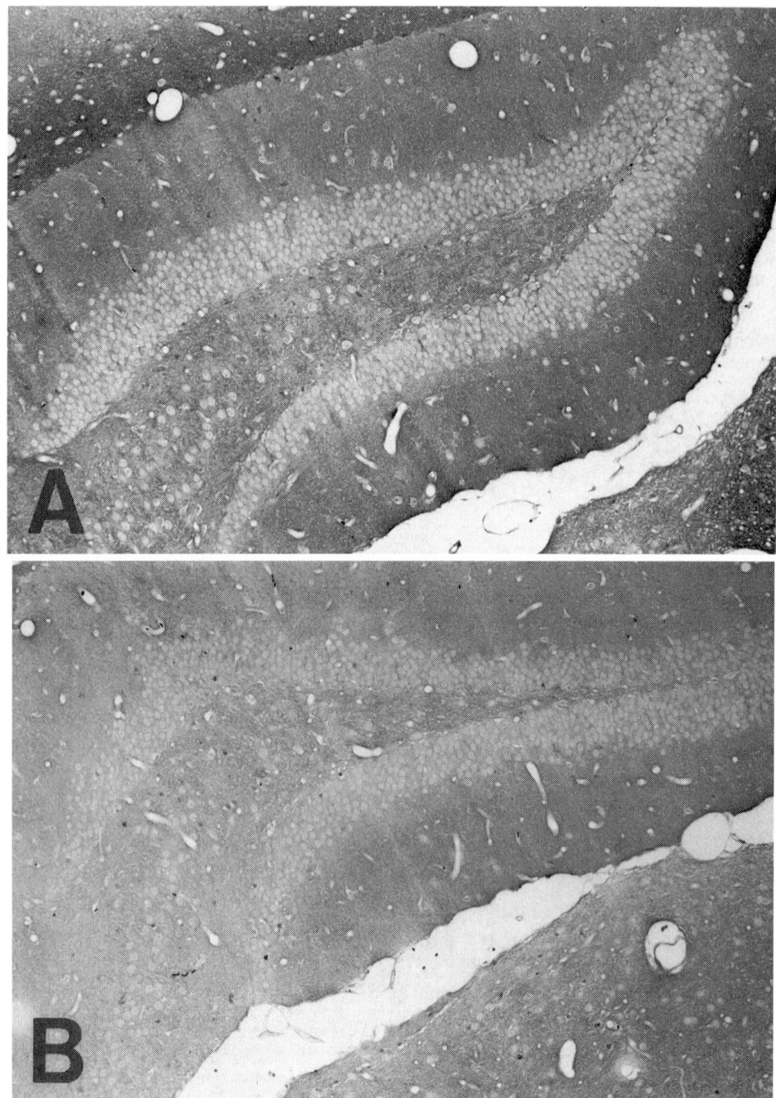

FIGURE 3. Acid fuchsin-stained sections of the hippocampus of KA-susceptible (**A**) and -resistant (**B**) mice 4 days following severe FPI. Note the large, intact cell bodies and the lack of acid fuchsin-positive, dystrophic neuronal profiles. Damage was uniformly absent by 4 days in both strains demonstrating the acute time course of hippocampal neuron damage and lack of delayed neuron damage following FPI (200×).

to those at 4 days, confirming the finding of acute hippocampal neuron injury and lack of delayed neuron damage after severe FPI.

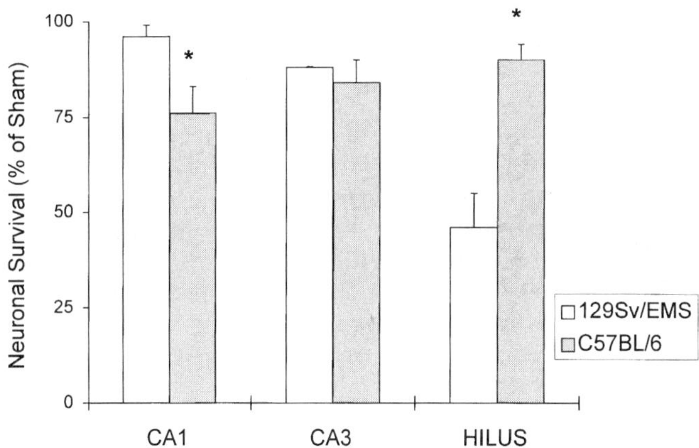

FIGURE 4. Regional patterns of hippocampal neuron loss following severe parasagittal FPI in KA-susceptible and -resistant mice. Contrary to what the post-TBI excitotoxicity hypothesis would predict, CA3 neuron survival was equivalent between KA-susceptible and -resistant mice ($p = 1.00$). Further, CA1 neuron loss was greater in the KA-resistant mice compared to the KA-susceptible mice (*$p < 0.05$). Hilar neuron loss was greater in the KA-susceptible mice compared to the KA-resistant mice (**$p < 0.005$); however, see Discussion).

Hippocampal Neuron Survival

FIGURE 4 compares hippocampal neuron survival between the KA-susceptible and -resistant strains 4 days after severe parasagittal FPI. The KA-resistant mice had significantly more neuron loss than the KA-susceptible mice in the CA1 pyramidal neuron layer ($p < 0.05$). Neuronal survival in area CA3 was equivalent between strains ($p = 1.00$). Lastly, KA-susceptible mice demonstrated significantly more hilar neuron loss than the KA-resistant mice ($p < 0.05$).

DISCUSSION

The current study tested the hypothesis that hippocampal damage after parasagittal FPI is mediated by an excitotoxic mechanism. We have demonstrated that this injury model causes an acute pattern of injury in the hippocampus of mice that are susceptible and resistant to KA-induced excitotoxic damage. Neuronal injury was detectable by 10 min, and there was no evidence for delayed damage in either strain. Further, we have shown that the patterns of neuron survival in CA1 and CA3 between these strains after FPI are not consistent with the post-FPI excitotoxicity hypothesis. Importantly, these findings suggest that excitoxicity may not contribute to hippocampal neuron loss after TBI, although we cannot yet completely rule out the role of other classes of glutamate receptors or voltage-sensitive ion channels.

We have shown in three separate studies that C57BL/6 mice have extremely acute patterns of hippocampal neuron injury after severe parasagittal FPI.[3,4] Similarly acute neuron damage was demonstrated in KA-susceptible 129Sv/EMS mice in the current study and in Sprague-Dawley rats after parasagittal FPI.[16] Such a rapid onset of damage is not consistent, temporally, with classic excitotoxicity, which is a delayed phenomenon.[6] Importantly, none of these studies found evidence for delayed hippocampal damage. It has, in fact, been demonstrated that the number of normal-appearing neurons in CA3 after parasagittal FPI in rats does not significantly decrease over time (from 10 min to 7 days post-FPI), arguing against the occurrence of delayed recruitment of neuron death.[16] Indeed, only in animal models combining TBI with a secondary insult such as transient hypoxia or ischemia is there apparent delayed damage and spread of damage to adjacent regions.[5,7,13] The extremely acute pattern of neuron damage after TBI has important implications for the design of pharmacological treatments. It is unclear whether TBI patients will benefit from therapies aimed at preventing cell death in the acute period or that such strategies are practical in the clinical setting given the small window of opportunity. Moreover, there is no consistent correlation between hippocampal neuronal sparing and improved outcome in experimental TBI.[1,13,25,26,35,41]

The patterns of hippocampal neuron survival in the present study are not consistent with the predictions of the post-TBI excitotoxicity hypothesis. This hypothesis would predict that neuronal loss in pyramidal regions of the hippocampus would be greater in KA-susceptible mice compared to KA-resistant mice after parasagittal FPI. This is especially true in CA3, which is selectively vulnerable after parasagittal FPI and is preferentially vulnerable to KA in mice.[31] In contrast, we have shown that mice susceptible and resistant to KA-induced excitotoxic hippocampal damage demonstrate equivalent neuron survival in CA3 after severe parasagittal FPI and, further, that KA-resistant mice have more CA1 neuronal loss than the KA-susceptible mice. Conversely, the hilus demonstrated a pattern of neuron loss that appeared to be consistent with the excitotoxicity hypothesis. However, this result is probably *not* due to excitotoxic processes, since it has been shown that hilar neurons are preferentially and instantaneously damaged by the mechanical insult resulting from FPI.[23,36] Consistent with this, as mentioned above, we found maximal hilar damage by 10 min post-FPI in both mouse strains. We are currently exploring the possibility that the difference in hilar neuron susceptibility to TBI lies in fundamental molecular cell damage/death mechanisms between the mouse strains.

Damage due to an insult as heterogeneous as TBI is likely dependent on similarly heterogeneous mechanisms. The selective hippocampal damage in rats and mice may be caused by a combination of (but not limited to) the following: mechanical injury; regionally selective glial impairment; spreading depression; and vascular events such as blood-brain barrier breakdown, hemorrhage, edema, and hypoperfusion.[10,11,20,32,36] Accordingly, Iijima *et al.* demonstrated selective loss of microtubule-associated protein 2 (MAP-2) staining in CA3 of the rat hippocampus with unilateral carotid artery occlusion combined with cortical spreading depression. Importantly, this selective damage was not present with either condition alone.[17]

The specific mechanisms by which certain strains of mice are more resistant to KA-induced excitotoxic damage are not currently known. However, it has recently been shown that the KA-resistant C57BL/6 mice have equal hippocampal affinity and binding of KA and AMPA when compared to DBA mice, a strain known to have a low threshold for behavioral seizures.[21] This supports the notion that differences in molecular responses to KA (rather than receptor property differences) may provide the neuroprotection from excitotoxic damage in the C57BL/6 strain. Several other studies have shown significant differences between mouse strains ranging from oral salt preference to susceptibility to brain damage from hypoxia-ischemia to neurovascular anatomy.[2,33,40] As in the present study, these differences may be easily exploited in order to investigate the molecular and genetic contributions to various biological processes. Wide commercial availability of these mice are a further advantage. However, these differences also suggest that one must be cautious when interpreting data from studies using transgenic and gene knockout mice that have been created in a hybrid background of two very different mouse strains.[31] Significantly, the majority of genetically altered mice available today are such hybrids. Indeed, our data suggest that knockout mice created from a background of C57BL/6 and 129Sv/EMS mice may not be appropriate for use in studies of TBI given their strikingly different patterns of hippocampal neuron survival after FPI.

In summary, severe parasagittal FPI applied to KA-susceptible and -resistant mice results in acute hippocampal neuronal damage without additional delayed recruitment. Further, the patterns of CA1 and CA3 pyramidal neuron loss between strains were not consistent with the predictions of the excitotoxicity hypothesis. Therefore, the hippocampal neuron damage and death seen after parasagittal FPI may not be mediated by an excitotoxic mechanism. These results suggest a reassessment is warranted of the treatment strategies for human TBI patients based on (1) the excitotoxic hypothesis and (2) the goal of preventing acute neuronal death.

ACKNOWLEDGMENTS

The authors gratefully thank Raimondo D'Ambrosio, Damir Janigro, and Philip Schwartzkroin (University of Washington) for helpful discussion and Tihomir Obrenovitch (Bradford University, UK), P. Elyse Schauwecker (University of Southern California), and Meredith Temple (University of Virginia) for the critical reading of the original manuscript. We also recognize Donald Maris, Paul Schwartz, and Janet Shukar for expert assistance with photography and Helen Marshall for technical assistance. This work was supported by NS30305, NS33107 (M.S.G.) and an NRSA Fellowship (W.S.C.).

REFERENCES

1. BAREYRE, F.M., K.E. SAATMAN, K. REESE & T.K. MCINTOSH. 1998. Magnesium deficiency exacerbates and treatment attenuates histological cell loss and cytoskeletal changes following brain injury in rats [abstract]. J. Neurotrauma **15:** 857.
2. BEAUCHAMP, G.K. & A.S. FISHER. 1993. Strain differences in consumption of saline solutions by mice. Physiol. Behav. **54:** 179–184.
3. CARBONELL, W.S. & M.S. GRADY. 1999. Regional and temporal characterization of neuronal, glial, and axonal response after traumatic brain injury in the mouse. Acta Neuropathol. **98:** 396–406.
4. CARBONELL, W.S., D.O. MARIS, T. MCCALL & M.S. GRADY. 1998. Adaptation of the fluid percussion injury model to the mouse. J. Neurotrauma **15:** 217–229.

5. CHERIAN, L., H.J. HANNAY, G. VAGNER, J.C. GOODMAN, C.F. CONTANT & C.S. ROBERTSON. 1998. Hyperglycemia increases neurological damage and behavioral deficits from posttraumatic secondary ischemic insults. J. Neurotrauma **15:** 307–321.

6. CHOI, D.W. 1992. Excitotoxic cell death. J. Neurobiol. **23:** 1261–1276.

7. CLARK, R.S., P.M. KOCHANEK, C.E. DIXON *et al.* 1997. Early neuropathologic effects of mild or moderate hypoxia after controlled cortical impact injury in rats. J. Neurotrauma **14:** 179–189.

8. CORTEZ, S.C., T.K. MCINTOSH & L.J. NOBLE. 1989. Experimental fluid percussion brain injury: vascular disruption and neuronal and glial alterations. Brain Res. **482:** 271–282.

9. COTMAN, C.W., D.T. MONAGHAN, O.P. OTTERSEN & J. STORM-MATHISEN. 1987. Anatomical organization of excitatory amino acid receptors and their pathways. Trends Neurosci. **10:** 273–280.

10. D'AMBROSIO, R., D.O. MARIS, M.S. GRADY & D. JANIGRO. 1998. Loss of glial potassium currents and impairment of potassium homeostasis, following fluid percussion injury [abstract]. J. Neurotrauma **15:** 864.

11. DIETRICH, W.D., O. ALONSO & M. HALLEY. 1994. Early microvascular and neuronal consequences of traumatic brain injury: a light and electron microscopic study in rats. J. Neurotrauma **11:** 289–301.

12. FADEN, A.I., P. DEMEDIUK, S.S. PANTER & R. VINK. 1989. The role of excitatory amino acids and NMDA receptors in traumatic brain injury. Science **244:** 798–800.

13. FORBES, M.L., R.S.B. CLARK, C.E. DIXON *et al.* 1998. Augmented neuronal death in CA3 hippocampus following hyperventilation early after controlled cortical impact. J. Neurosurg. **88:** 549–556.

14. GRADY, M.S., J.S. CHARLESTON & D.O. MARIS. 1996. Quantitation of rat hippocampal cells using the optical volume fractionator: a comparison of midline to lateral fluid percussion injury [abstract]. J. Neurotrauma **13:** 508.

15. GREENAMYRE, J.T., J.M. OLSON, J.B. PENNEY, JR. & A.B. YOUNG. 1985. Autoradiographic characterization of *N*-methyl-D-aspartate-, quisqualate-, and kainate-sensitive glutamate binding sites. J. Pharmacol. Exp. Ther. **233:** 254–263.

16. HICKS, R., H. SOARES, D. SMITH & T. MCINTOSH. 1995. Temporal and spatial characterization of neuronal injury following lateral fluid-percussion brain injury in the rat. Acta Neuropathol. **9:** 236–246.

17. IIJIMA, T., C. SHIMASE, H. SAWA & H. SANKAWA. 1998. Spreading depression induces depletion of MAP2 in area CA3 of the hippocampus in a rat unilateral carotid artery occlusion model. J. Neurotrauma **15:** 277–284.

18. IKONOMIDOU, C. & L. TURSKI. 1996. Prevention of trauma-induced neurodegeneration in infant and adult rat brain: glutamate antagonists. Metab. Brain Dis. **11:** 125–141.

19. KOH, J.-Y., M.P. GOLDBERG, D.M. HARTLEY & D.W. CHOI. 1990. Non-NMDA receptor-mediated neurotoxicity in cortical culture. J. Neurosci. **10:** 693–705.

20. KUBOTA, M., T. NAKAMURA, K. SUNAMI *et al.* 1989. Changes on local cerebral glucose utilization, DC potential and extracellular potassium in various degrees of experimental contusion. Brain Nerve (Japanese) **41:** 799–805.

21. KÜRSCHNER, V.C., R.L. PETRUZZI, G.T. GOLDEN, W.H. BERRETTINI & T.N. FERRARO. 1998. Kainate and AMPA receptor binding in seizure-prone and seizure-resistant inbred mouse strains. Brain Res. **780:** 1–8.

22. LASSMAN, H., H. BARAN, U. PETSCHE, K. KITZ, G. SPERK, O. HORNYKIEWICZ & F. SEITELBERGER. 1986. Ultrastructural analysis of rat brain tissue following systemic kainate administration. Adv. Exp. Med. Biol. **203:** 223–230.

23. LOWENSTEIN, D.H., M.J. THOMAS, D.H. SMITH & T.K. MCINTOSH. 1992. Selective vulnerability of dentate hilar neurons following traumatic brain injury: a potential

mechanistic link between head trauma and disorders of the hippocampus. J. Neurosci. **12:** 4846–4853.

24. LYETH, B.G., L.W. JENKINS, R.J. HAMM *et al.* 1992. Prolonged memory impairment in the absence of hippocampal cell death following traumatic brain injury in the rat. Brain Res. **452:** 39–48.

25. McDERMOTT, K.L., R. RAGHUPATHI, S.C. FERNANDEZ *et al.* 1997. Delayed administration of basic fibroblast growth factor (bFGF) attenuates cognitive dysfunction following parasagittal fluid percussion brain injury in the rat. J. Neurotrauma **14:** 191–200.

26. McINTOSH, T.K., D.H. SMITH, M. VODDI, B.R. PERRI & J.M. STUTZMANN. 1996. Riluzole, a novel neuroprotective agent, attenuates both neurologic motor and cognitive dysfunction following experimental brain injury in the rat. J. Neurotrauma **13:** 767–780.

27. MOREHEAD, M., R.T. BARTUS, R.L. DEAN *et al.* 1994. Histopathologic consequences of moderate concussion in an animal model: correlations with duration of unconsciousness. J. Neurotrauma **11:** 657–667.

28. PERRY, E.K., J.A. COURT, M. JOHNSON *et al.* 1993. Autoradiographic comparison of cholinergic and other transmitter receptors in the normal human hippocampus. Hippocampus **3:** 307–315.

29. OBRENOVITCH, T.P. & J. URENJAK. 1997. Altered glutamatergic transmission in neurological disorders: from high extracellular glutamate to excessive synaptic efficacy. Prog. Neurobiol. **51:** 39–87.

30. OBRENOVITCH, T.P. & J. URENJAK. 1998. The glutamate-excitotoxicity hypothesis: use and abuse. Pharmacol. Cereb. Ischemia. In press.

31. SCHAUWECKER, P.E. & O. STEWARD. 1997. Generic determinants of susceptibility to excitotoxic cell death: implications for gene targeting approaches. Proc. Natl. Acad. Sci. USA **94:** 4103–4108.

32. SCHMIDT, R.H. & M.S. GRADY. 1993. Regional patterns of blood-brain barrier breakdown following central and lateral fluid percussion injury in rodents. J. Neurotrauma **10:** 415–430.

33. SHELDON, R.A., C. SEDIK & D.M. FERRIERO. 1998. Strain-related brain injury in neonatal mice subjected to hypoxia-ischemia. Brain Res. **810:** 114–122.

34. SMITH, D.H., K. OKIYAMA, T.A. GENNARELLI & T.K. McINTOSH. 1993. Magnesium and ketamine attenuate cognitive dysfunction following experimental brain injury. Neurosci. Lett. **157:** 211–214.

35. SMITH, D.H., D.H. LOWENSTEIN, T.A. GENNARELLI & T.K. McINTOSH. 1994. Persistent memory dysfunction is associated with bilateral hippocampal damage following experimental brain injury. Neurosci. Lett. **168:** 151–154.

36. TOTH, Z., G.S. HOLLRIGEL, T. GORCS & I. SOLTESZ. 1997. Instantaneous perturbation of dentate interneuronal networks by a pressure wave-transient delivered to the neocortex. J. Neurosci. **17:** 8106–8117.

37. VORNOV, J.T., R.C. TASKER & J.T. COYLE. 1991. Direct observation of the agonist-specific regional vulnerability to glutamate, NMDA, and kainate neurotoxicity in organotypic hippocampal cultures. Exp. Neurol. **114:** 11–22.

38. WATANABE, M., M. FUKAYA, K. SAKIMURA, T. MANABE, M. MISHINA & Y. INOUE. 1998. Selective scarcity of NMDA receptor channel subunits in the stratum lucidum (mossy fibre-recipient layer) of the mouse hippocampal CA3 subfield. Eur. J. Neurosci. **10:** 478–487.

39. WERNER, P., M. VOIGT, K. KEINANEN, W. WISDEN & P.H. SEEBURG. 1991. Cloning of putative high-affinity kainate receptor expressed predominantly in hippocampal CA3 cells. Nature **351:** 742–744.

40. YANG, G., K. KITAGAWA, K. MATSUSHITA *et al.* 1998. C57BL/6 strain is most susceptible to cerebral ischemia following bilateral common carotid occlusion among

seven mouse strains: selective neuronal death in the murine transient forebrain ischemia. Brain Res. **752:** 209–218.

41. ZHANG, C., R. RAGHUPATHI, K.E. SAATMAN *et al.* 1998. Riluzole attenuates cortical lesion size, but not hippocampal neuronal loss, following traumatic brain injury in the rat. J. Neurosci. Res. **52:** 342–349.

Questions and Answers

QUESTION FOR DR. CARBONELL

From Dr. Manev

Did you verify in your experiments that C57BL mice are resistant to kainate? If there is no damage in this strain, do you know whether these mice are normal in terms of the expression of KA/AMPA receptors? For example, this particular mouse strain is known for having the mutation in the serotonin *N*-acetyl transferase gene and melatonin synthesis.

ANSWER: We performed positive control studies with both the C57BL/6 and 129Sv/EMS strains ($n = 2$, each strain) and were able to replicate the results seen by Schauwecker and Steward.[1] The 129Sv/EMS strain demonstrated frank neuronal loss in the hippocampus at 4 days, whereas the C57BL/6 strain did not. We did not attempt to quantify this neuron loss. Dr. Manev raises an important issue. Indeed, traits such as susceptibility to kainic acid (KA)-induced hippocampal neuron death may vary between different breeding colonies of the "same" mouse strain.[2] Further, one must be aware that there are striking *sub*strain differences in response to KA (O. Steward, personal communication).

We do not claim there is "no" damage in C57BL/6 mice after KA injection. Rather, they are more resistant to KA-induced hippocampal damage. If given a high enough dose (e.g., 40 mg/kg) C57BL/6 mice may show hippocampal neuron loss.[1] What is important to note is that 40 mg/kg is above the LD50 and is four times greater than doses commonly used to produce neuronal loss in rats. Receptor properties in these mice are currently under investigation by several laboratories. Importantly, Kurschner *et al.*[3] demonstrated that AMPA and KA binding and affinity in the hippocampus of C57BL/6 mice was not different than the seizure-prone DBA mouse strain.

QUESTIONS FOR DR. OBRENOVITCH

COMMENT (Dr. von Lubitz): Your lecture points at an extremely important distinction: extracellular space is *not* the same as the perisynaptic one. We saw the same problem with adenosine: despite a huge concentration of its A1 receptors in the hippocampus, there is not enough extracellular adenosine to stimulate them! Only due to T.V. Dumwiddie's work are we able to learn that in the perisynaptic compartment, the concentration of adenosine was more than sufficient to do the job. The problem of glutamate may be the same. Plus, it is unwise, a point you have made yourself, to believe glutamate is the "trigger." I agree with you—energy imbalance is. Neuronal death is simply the gross sum of all events, one of which is the excitotoxic cascade. Good work!!

COMMENT (Dr. Narahashi): I enjoyed your provocative talk, and agree with many points you raised. In particular, the traditional linear model does not necessarily explain the mechanism of cell death caused by ischemia, and there could be many

299

cascades of events, parallel and linear. I would like to point out that the glutamate concentration at the synaptic cleft momentarily becomes extraordinarily high, so it is not easy to compare the effect of externally applied glutamate with glutamate at the synaptic cleft. Another point is that glutamate cannot be directly compared with NMDA, kainate and AMPA in terms of their potencies, because only glutamate is a neurotransmitter.

From Dr. Jonas

With regard to the sequence of neuron-damaging events early in ischemia, particularly with regard to calcium ion-manipulating maneuvers: (1) If glutamate release is not a first step, is there a first step from which the others all follow? (2) What is your opinion of the use of glutamate to mimic the effects of early ischemia in a brain slice preparation in the laboratory?

ANSWER: (1) To the best of my understanding, the primary deleterious event in cerebral ischemia is: imbalance between energy supply (blood flow) and energy demand (intensity of synaptic activity). This justifies therapeutic strategies aiming at restoring or improving blood flow as soon as possible (e.g., thrombolysis, increase of perfusion pressure whenever possible and safe), or reducing energy demand (e.g., with hypothermia and/or modulators of voltage-gated Na channels such as riluzole). With regards to ischemia and calcium ions, opening of glutamate-operated ionophores may contribute to intracellular calcium loading (however, note that glutamate exocytosis is very rapidly inhibited in this condition as it is ATP dependent) but, more important contributors may be disruption of Ca homeostasis, opening of voltage-gated Ca channels, and release of calcium from intracellular stores. (2) Assuming that high extracellular glutamate mimics the effects of early ischemia, in any preparation, is fundamentally flawed.

COMMENT (Dr. Youdim): Your elegant studies have shown that there is not enough synaptic glutamate on excitosis of glutamate to induce nerve degeneration. I have to agree with you in that in Parkinson's disease brains or its animal models, MPTP or 6-hydroxydopamine, no direct evidence has been obtained to support the concept that glutamate excitotoxicity in Parkinson's disease. Furthermore, glutaminergic neurons innervate the substantia nigra pars reticulata and not the pars compacta where melanine-containing neurons degenerate.

REFERENCES

1. SCHAUWECKER, P.E. & O. STEWARD. 1997. Genetic determinants of susceptibility to excitotoxic cell death: implications for gene targeting approaches. Proc. Natl. Acad. Sci. USA **94:** 4103–4108.
2. LATHE, R. 1996. Mice, gene targeting and behavior: more than just genetic background. Trends Neurosci. **19:** 183–186.
3. KURSCHNER, V.C., R.L. PETRUZZI, G.T. GOLDEN, W.H. BERRETTINI & T.N. FERRARO. 1998. Kainate and AMPA receptor binding in seizure-prone and seizure-resistant inbred mouse strains. Brain Res. **730:** 1–8.

Neuroprotective Properties of Nitric Oxide

CHUANG C. CHIUEH[a]

Unit on Neurodegeneration and Neuroprotection, Laboratory of Clinical Science, National Institute of Mental Health, NIH Clinical Center, Bethesda, Maryland, USA

ABSTRACT: The discoveries of physiological roles of nitric oxide ($\cdot$NO) as the mediator of endothelium-derived relaxing factor (EDRF) action and the activator of guanylyl cyclase to increase cyclic guanosine monophosphate (cGMP), which lead to vasorelaxation in the cardiovascular system, have been awarded with the 1998 Nobel Prize of Medicine. The present review discusses putative beneficial effects of $\cdot$NO in the central nervous system (CNS). In addition to its prominent roles of the regulation of cerebral blood flow and the modulation of cell to cell communication in the brain, recent *in vitro* and *in vivo* results indicated that $\cdot$NO is a potent antioxidative agent. $\cdot$NO terminates oxidant stress in the brain by (i) suppressing iron-induced generation of hydroxyl radicals ($\cdot$OH) via the Fenton reaction, (ii) interrupting the chain reaction of lipid peroxidation, (iii) augmenting the antioxidative potency of reduced glutathione (GSH) and (iv) inhibiting cysteine proteases.

It is apparent that $\cdot$NO—a relative long half-life nitrogen-centered weak radical—scavenges those short-lived, highly reactive free radicals such as superoxide anion ($O_2^{\cdot-}$), $\cdot$OH, peroxyl lipid radicals (LOO$\cdot$) and thiyl radicals (i.e., GS$\cdot$), yielding reactive nitrogen species including nitrites, nitrates, *S*-nitrosoglutathione (GSNO) and peroxynitrite (ONOO$^-$). GSNO is 100-fold more potent than GSH; it completely inhibits the weak peroxidative effect of ONOO$^-$. Moreover, CO_2 and $\cdot$NO neutralize prooxidative effects of ONOO$^-$. CO_2 prevents protein oxidation but not 3-nitrotyrosine formation caused by ONOO$^-$. Finally, neuroprotective effects of GSNO and $\cdot$NO have been demonstrated in brain preparations *in vivo*.

These novel neuroprotective properties of $\cdot$NO and GSNO may have their physiological significance, since oxidative stress depletes GSH while increasing GS$\cdot$ and $\cdot$NO formation in astroglial and endothelial cells, resulting in the generation of a more potent antioxidant GSNO and providing additional neuroprotection at μM concentrations. This putative GSNO pathway (GSH $\rightarrow$ GS$\cdot$ $\rightarrow$ GSNO $\rightarrow$ $\cdot$NO + GSSG $\rightarrow$ GSH) may be an important part of endogenous antioxidative defense system, which could protect neurons and other brain cells against oxidative stress caused by oxidants, iron complexes, proteases and cytokines. In conclusion, $\cdot$NO is a potent antioxidant against oxidative damage caused by reactive oxygen species, which are generated by Fenton reaction or other mechanisms in the brain via redox cycling of iron complexes.

INTRODUCTION

Nitric oxide ($\cdot$NO) is generated *in vivo* in the endothelial cells, astroglias and a few neurons by three isoforms of nitric oxide synthase (NOS).[1,2] In the central ner-

[a]Address for correspondence: C.C. Chiueh, Ph.D.; LCS, NIMH; NIH, Bldg. 10, Rm. 3D-41; Bethesda, MD, 20892-1264. Phone, 301/496-3421; fax, 301/402-0188.
e-mail, chiueh@helix.nih.gov

vous system (CNS), through the activation of ·NO-sensitive guanylyl cyclase and the generation of cyclic guanosine monophosphate (cGMP),[3,4] ·NO modulates cell to cell modulation[5] and cerebral blood flow.[6–8] Based on the chemistry of ·NO—a nitrogen-centered free radical that scavenges reactive oxygen species—we investigated the putative beneficial effects of ·NO in the brain. Accumulated new data do not support a notion that ·NO mediates neurotoxicity in the CNS. Recent reports provide relevant *in vitro* and *in vivo* data to substantiate our working hypothesis[9] that ·NO and its congener *S*-nitrosoglutathione (GSNO) are potent antioxidants that protect brain dopamine neurons against oxidant stress and damage caused by reactive oxygen species.[10–13]

GENERATION OF REACTIVE OXYGEN SPECIES IN THE CNS

Free radicals are unavoidable side products of electron-transfer redox processes through either enzymatic or nonenzymatic reactions. Most of the redox enzymes generate hydrogen peroxide in the brain. The conversion of hydrogen peroxide to hydroxyl radical (·OH) is catalyzed by transition metals (i.e., iron and copper). Surprisingly, manganese, at neutral pH, does not convert hydrogen peroxide to hydroxyl radicals via the Fenton reaction.[14] It has been suggested that free radicals such as ·OH may mediate a common neurodegenerative pathway produced by ischemia/reperfusion injury, intracranial hemorrhage (e.g., hemoglobin), aggregated amyloid precursor protein and the dopaminergic toxin 1-methyl-4-phenyl-1,2,3,6-tetrahydropyridine (MPTP).[15] Inhibition of mitochondrial respiratory chain (complex I) could also lead to the accumulation of reactive oxygen species.[16] Owing to the ultrashort half-life of ·OH radicals, which may cause a site-specific oxidative stress and damage only at the site of generation (TABLE 1). For example, high concentrations of dopamine and oxygen plus an age-dependent accumulation of non-heme iron in the nigral neurons of human brain, resulting in the generation of ·OH and accumulation of dopamine neuromelanin, which is a free radical-mediated polymerization of oxidized metabolites of dopamine.[17,18] However, in the normal physiological situation, iron and oxygen are the cofactors for tyrosine hydroxylase, the rate-limit step for dopamine biosynthesis, which generate ·OH for the hydroxylation of L-tyrosine to L-DOPA.[19] This aromatic hydroxylation procedure has been successfully modified for the trapping of ·OH radicals by salicylate *in vivo*.[20]

NEUROBIOLOGY OF NITRIC OXIDE

As compared to highly neurotoxic ·OH radicals,[12,14,17,18] ·NO free radicals are several orders of magnitude less active than ·OH leading to opposite neurobiological actions, such as neuromodulation[4,5] and cytoprotection in the brain.[9–13] Most evidence confirms a prominent theory that ·NO activates guanylyl cyclase, which leads to an increase in cGMP and plays a role in neural modulation and vasodilation.[1–9] These and other biological actions of ·NO could be long lasting, and ·NO could act at a relatively long distance from its site of formation. ·NO thereby serves as a modulator in neurotransmission and neurogenic vasodilation.

TABLE 1. Free radicals-induced oxidative stress in the brain

I. The major source of ·OH generation

- Conversion of H_2O_2 to ·OH by Fe^{2+} and Cu^{2+} but not Mn^{2+}

- Redox cycling of small molecular weight iron complex: bidentate and tridentate iron citrate complexes

II. Chain reactions of brain lipid peroxidation

- Generation of free radicals (i.e., L·, LOO· and ·OH)

- Propagation by iron; termination by manganese

- Generation of toxic adducts of malondialdehyde and 4-hydroxy-2-nonenal

- Oxidative injury of cellular and subcellular membranes

III. Oxidation of enzymes and peptides

- Generation of carbonyl adducts

- Formation of active dimers of thiol containing peptides

- Free radical-induced polymerization and aggregation (i.e. , prion protein, amyloid, Lewy body and neuromelanin)

IV. Mutation and/or fragmentation of DNA and RNA

V. Neuronal death

- Necrotic and apoptotic cell death when oxidative stress overwhelms cellular defense and repair systems

·NO causes no increase in lipid peroxidation in the brain,[10–12] which is taken to be a cardinal sign of oxidant stress evoked by reactive oxygen species. This finding seems at odds with a prominent hypothesis that ·NO mediates oxidative damage and neurotoxicity in the brain. In fact, it suppresses brain lipid peroxidation induced by iron complexes (i.e., sodium nitroprusside and hemoglobin). Thus, previously proposed prooxidative effects of ·NO, based mostly on the results obtained from sodium nitroprusside (disodium nitroferricyanide) are debatable; unexpectedly, ·OH but not ·NO mediates sodium nitroprusside-induced neurotoxicity, since ·NO-exhausted, light-exposed nitroprusside is still neurotoxic.[21] Oxidative stress and damage are only observed following intracerebral administration of donors of ·OH but not ·NO *in vivo* (TABLE 2). Furthermore, our preliminary results indicate that ·NO may inactivate protease-induced apoptosis and neurotoxicity (Hawkins *et al.*, submitted). Based on results of *in vivo* brain preparations[10,11,13] and *in vitro* preparations[12,22–32] (i.e., brain, cardiac, endothelial, hepatic, retinal, gastric and bronchial cells), it is apparent that ·NO may act as a free radical scavenger *in vivo*.

ANTIOXIDATIVE AND NEUROPROTECTIVE PROPERTIES OF NITRIC OXIDE

Nitration or nitrosylation by ·NO of iron or thiol containing enzymes significantly alters their biological actions in the central nervous system. For example, ·NO binds to iron complexes[33,34] such as ferrous citrate, thiyl-iron and hemoglobin,

TABLE 2. *In vivo* neuroprotective versus neurotoxic effects of ·OH, ·NO and NOx

Agent	Dose (nmol)	Mechanisms	Toxicity	Protection*
·NO	2	$\downarrow$ ·OH $\downarrow$ LP	−	+
GSNO	16.8	$\downarrow$ ·OH $\downarrow$ LP	−	+
Iron	8.4	$\uparrow$ ·OH $\uparrow$ LP (+++)	+	−
SNP	16.8	$\uparrow$ ·OH $\uparrow$ LP (+)	+	−
ONOO⁻	33.6	$\uparrow$ ·OH $\uparrow$ LP (±)	−	−

NOTE: Based on the *in vivo* results of Rauhala *et al.*,[10,13,21] and Mohanakumar *et al.*,[11,36] solution containing ·NO or ·NO donors are intranigrally infused, and the chronic striatal dopamine depletion is used as the neurotoxicity marker. Photodegraded GSNO, which can no longer release ·NO, has no antioxidative effects.

ABBREVIATIONS: SNP, sodium nitroprusside either freshly prepared or ·NO exhausted; LP, nigral lipid peroxidation; NOx, ·NO-derived species such as *S*-nitrosoglutathione (GSNO) and peroxynitrite (ONOO⁻).

which in turn may reduce redox reactions, minimizing generation of reactive oxygen species and associated oxidative stress.[11,12] As mentioned above, *in vitro* results reveal that ·NO protects brain neurons and endothelial, hepatic, rectinal, gastric and cardiac cells from oxidant stress. We recently published several papers to answer the controversial question whether ·NO is a friend or foe in the brain[35] (TABLE 1). ·NO reverses exaggerated oxidative stress, dopamine turnover and related circling behavior evoked by intranigral infusion of small molecular weight iron complex—ferrous citrate.[10–14] Ferrous citrate generates ·OH directly from oxygen (not from hydrogen peroxide) through electron oscillation between bidentate and tridentate iron complexes.[36] Consistently, ·NO concentration-dependently suppresses the generation of ·OH stimulated by ferrous citrate.[11,13] Most of the ·NO donors, except sodium nitroprusside, completely suppressed ·OH generation and brain lipid peroxidation caused by ferrous citrate iron complex.[10,11,21] Interestingly, ascorbate inhibits ferrous citrate-induced ·OH generation while it augments sodium nitroprusside's action, since it contains unstable chelated iron complexes (i.e., $[(CN)_5\text{-Fe}]^{3-}$ and $[(CN)_4\text{-Fe}]^{2-}$), which can be reduced by ascorbate and thus increase ·OH generation, lipid peroxidation and nigral death.[21] Earlier studies, which may have misinterpreted the experimental results, obtained a stable ferricyanide $[(CN)_6\text{-Fe}]^{3-}$, which is not a proper sham control agent for nitroprusside, because it cannot undergo redox cycling in the presence of ascorbate. Pretreatment with deferoxamine, oxy-hemoglobin and ·NO decrease the prooxidative effects of sodium nitroprusside.

In addition, the less reactive ·NO scavenges highly reactive oxygen species (i.e., superoxide anion or $O_2^{\cdot-}$ and ·OH) and converts them into nonradicals such as nitrites and nitrate (TABLE 3). These acidic metabolites of ·NO are rapidly eliminated by brain anion transporters into circulation and thus minimized their cytotoxicity *in vivo*. However, the accumulation of nitrite and nitrates at mM concentrations in cell cultures is highly toxic. Furthermore, short-lived ·NO (e.g., min) can scavenge thiyl radicals such as GS· and CYS· converting to biological active *S*-nitrosothiols, which have much longer half-life *in vivo* (e.g., hr). In fact, GSNO—an endogenous *S*-nitrosylated reduced glutathione (GSH)—is approximately 100 times more potent than

TABLE 3. Reaction of unpaired electron: ·NO scavenges lipid, oxygen and thiyl radicals

(1)	$LOO· + ·NO \rightarrow LOONO$
(2)	$O_2^{·-} + ·NO \rightarrow [ONOO^-] \rightarrow NO_3^-$
(3)	$·OH + ·NO \rightarrow [HONO] \rightarrow NO_2^-$
(4)	$GS· + ·NO \rightarrow GSNO$
(5)	Peptide-CYS· + ·NO $\rightarrow$ peptide-CYSNO

the classic antioxidant GSH.[13] However, *S*-nitrosylation of cysteine moiety inactivates cysteine proteases[34] and HIV-1 proteases (Vivian Hawkins, Qian Shen, and C.C. Chiueh, Free Radical Research, in press). Therefore, ·NO is an atypical antioxidant terminating the lipid peroxidation chain reactions via scavenging highly reactive lipid peroxyl radicals not only in plasma low-density lipoprotein but also in brain polyunsaturated fatty acid. Finally, · NO inhibits brain lipid peroxidation in both *in vivo* and *in vitro* preparations[10–13] possibly through the scavenging or annihilation of lipid peroxyl radicals and also thiol-ferro radicals.

OPPOSITE ACTIONS OF TWO REACTIVE NITROGEN SPECIES: GSNO VERSUS ONOO⁻

·NO may interact with $O_2^{·-}$ [37] and GSH[38–42] generating biological active nitrogen species such as, ONOO⁻ and GSNO, respectively.[6–9] These ·NO-derived species may produce biological functions, either similar or opposite to that of ·NO. During and after oxidative stress, there are an immediate increase of oxidized GSH (i.e., GSSG and GS·) and a delayed increase of ·NO levels in the brain, which may scavenge toxic GS· and lead to the generation of a more potent antioxidant GSNO. GSNO has been identified in cells and tissues containing NOS and high mM concentrations of GSH.[38–42] Tissue levels of GSH are at mM concentrations in astroglial and endothelial cells, which are several orders of magnitude greater than $O_2^{·-}$ (<nM) and thus far more quantity of GSNO than ONOO⁻ can be generated in the brain (TABLE 4).

It has been proposed that GSNO may be an endogenous ·NO reservoir, which can release ·NO when it reacts with either Cu^+ or thioredoxin[43–46] (TABLE 4). Freshly prepared GSNO not only produces ·NO-like biological effects but also protects against oxidative stress in endothelium, myocardium and brain tissue.[10,13,46–48] GSNO is approximately 100-fold more potent than GSH in suppressing iron-induced generation of ·OH and the peroxidation of brain lipids; photodegraded and ·NO-exhausted old GSNO solution is devoid of such antioxidative properties.[13] Furthermore, these atypical antioxidant properties of freshly prepared GSNO, which have been demonstrated in the brain using either *in vitro* or *in vivo* preparations, seems to be mediated by the release of ·NO and GSH.

Contrary to antioxidative effects of GSNO, ONOO⁻ may cause oxidative stress and possibly neurotoxicity due to the possible generation of ·OH.[37] However, direct evidence of ONOO⁻ or ·NO in causing oxidative stress or injury in the brain could not be demonstrated *in vivo*,[13] since ONOO⁻ is easily detoxified by GSNO, CO_2 and

TABLE 4. The antioxidative, neuroprotective pathway of ·NO and GSH

I. Reactive oxygen species stimulate GSNO formation in the astroglial and endothelial cells, which contain GSH at mM concentrations

  (1) GSH → GS·

  (2) iNOS/eNOS: L-arginine → ·NO

  (3) LOO· + ·NO → LOONO

  (4) GS· + ·NO → GSNO

II. GSNO as a carrier of micromolar concentrations of GSH to brain neurons

  (1) $GSNO + Cu^+ \rightarrow GSSG + \cdot NO$

  (2) LOO· + ·NO → LOONO

  (3) Thioredoxin/GSSG redutase: GSSG → GSH

III. Suppression of oxidative stress induced by free radicals

  (1) Suppression of iron-induced ·OH generation

  (2) Termination of lipid peroxidation *in vitro;* GSNO is 100-fold more potent than GSH

  (3) Protection against iron-induced neurotoxicity (*in vivo*)

  (4) Suppression of proteolysis caused by cysteine proteases

IV. GSNO and ·NO: a part of the redox cycling of GSH and GSSG in the brain

·NO to nitrates,[13,25,49,50] which are readily excreted from the brain tissue. Interestingly, CO_2 inhibits protein oxidation but not tyrosine nitration caused by $ONOO^-$.[51] $ONOO^-$ is a weak prooxidative agent in the brain *in vitro* and *in vivo*,[13,25] since the saturated solution of $ONOO^-$ fails to evoke a significant oxidative stress in the brain. Furthermore, this rather weak prooxidative effect of $ONOO^-$ is completely blocked by GSNO, partially by GSH and ·NO.[13,25,30]

·NO AS A PART OF ANTIOXIDATIVE DEFENSE AGAINST CHAIN REACTIONS OF OXIDANT STRESS

Reactive oxygen species, such as the short-lived ·OH, trigger the oxidant stress chain reaction, which generates more cytotoxic free radicals. Reactive radicals of ·OH, lipid peroxyl radicals, thiyl or thiol-ferro radicals lead to (i) lipid peroxidation, (ii) protein oxidation and proteolysis, (iii) adenosine triphosphate (ATP) depletion and (iv) DNA fragmentation, all of which can be blocked by ·NO, which is known to protect endothelial cells from apoptosis evoked by cytokines.[32] The assay of fluorescent end products of lipid peroxidation and the detection carbonyl proteins are routinely used as the markers for oxidant stress even in *in vivo* studies.[12,20,36,51–55] Free radical-induced oxidative stress in cell and neuronal cultures is sometimes expressed as DNA fragmentation or apoptotic cell death, especially in differentiating neuronal cell lines. Due to effective endogenous DNA repair and antioxidative defense system, very limited mature brain neurons undergo apoptotic cell death, which is usually detected in the developing brain and differentiating neuronal cell lines.

Iron complexes elicited the following events in the nigrostriatal dopamine neurons.[11,36,55] Acutely, (i) it causes a brief generation of ·OH radicals for several hours. (ii) It exaggerated dopamine turnover for at least 24 hours. (iii) It is followed by a prolonged propagation of lipid peroxidation at the mid-brain substantia nigra area for seven days or longer. Finally, (iv) it produces a chronic and delayed oxidative damage reflected by nigral injury (i.e., decreases in nigral mRNA of tyrosine hydroxylase and terminal dopamine levels), which lasted for several weeks or even months. Most of the injured nigral neurons are eventually degenerated. Based on the intranigral dose of iron complexes, some of the partially injured dopamine neurons slowly recover from oxidant stress, since there are effective antioxidative enzymes in the brain. Significantly, iron-induced oxidant stress and damage to the midbrain dopamine neurons is blocked *in vivo* by atypical antioxidants such as manganese,[55] GSNO[13] and ·NO.[10,11]

Endogenous antioxidant enzymes, including superoxide dismutase (SOD), catalase, glutathione peroxidase and reductase, thiol specific antioxidant enzymes, thioredoxin, and protease inhibitors protect neurons against oxidative damage caused by cytotoxic ·OH, lipid peroxyl radicals and thiyl free radicals. This antioxidative cellular defense system is actively protecting brain cells and neurons from oxidant injury reflected by little peroxidation in normal control brain tissue. However, brain contains high levels of polyunsaturated fatty acids, which are easily peroxidized by reactive oxygen species, hemoglobin and ferrous citrate iron complexes. These neuroprotective effects of endogenous antioxidant enzymes and their products are supported by data obtained from cell cultures and transgenic experiment as well. SOD, glutathione peroxidase and other antioxidant enzymes can be increased by transgenic procedures. Transgenic SOD animals are less vulnerable than nontransgenic ones to oxidative damage caused by MPTP, methamphetamine, head trauma, and ischemia/reperfusion injury.[56] Clinically, defective enzyme as produced by mutated SOD_1 gene can increase free radical formation, cause a progressive degeneration of pyramidal motor neurons in familial amyotrophic lateral sclerosis.[57]

PROSPECTIVE: THE ANTIOXIDATIVE GSNO PATHWAY

Our results demonstrated that oxidative brain injury is protected by GSNO in low nanomole dosage *in vivo*. In addition, *S*-nitrosylated GSH or GSNO, at μM concentrations, produces greater antioxidative actions than GSH by approximately two orders of magnitude. Thus, GSNO/·NO may be the missing part of the antioxidative cellular defense system of GSH/GSSG,[58,59] since GSH is formed in the astroglias at mM concentrations, which cannot be transported to brain neurons. GSNO may serve as the carrier for GSH and provide GSH from astroglias to brain neurons. Elucidation of metabolic pathways involved in the proposed GSNO pathway (TABLE 4, GSH → GS· + ·NO → [GSNO] → GSSG + ·NO → GSH) in the CNS is necessary for understanding the biology of ·NO and its atypical antioxidative properties. Moreover, our unpublished observations indicate that GSNO also protects brain cells against oxidative stress caused by hemoglobin and proteases. This mechanism may also account for the fact that NOS containing neurons or nicotinamide-adenosine dinucleotide phosphate (NADPH) diaphorase positive neurons are less vulnerable to oxidative injury. Furthermore, this GSNO pathway may explain why the glial feeder layer is necessary for the long-term survival of primary neuronal cultures. This putative pathway of GSSG/·NO/GSNO/GSH provides new molecular insights of the redox cycling of GSH and GSSG.

Our recent results suggest that GSNO, but not GSH, at μM concentrations, inhibit iron-evoked ·OH generation and lipid peroxidation and protect brain dopamine neurons from oxidative damage.[13] These atypical antioxidative properties of GSNO are mediated by the release of ·NO instead of nitrosyl ions (NO^+). NO^+ may not terminate free radical chain reactions, since it does not scavenge LOO· radicals[13] to form inactive LOONO.[25] However, NO^+ may play an important role in transnitrosylation between thiol-containing amino acids.[60] Thus, this report on neuroprotective properties of GSNO and ·NO is somewhat at odds with a prominent hypothesis that ·NO causes neurotoxicity based on possible misinterpretation of experimental results of ·NO donors such as sodium nitroprusside.[21,61] Elucidation of these novel anitoxidative and neuroprotective mechanisms of ·NO and GSNO could stimulate the development of new neuroprotective agent for the treatment and/or prevention of oxidant-induced degenerative brain disorders in aging such as Parkinson's disease and Alzheimer's dementia, perhaps in stroke and head trauma as well.

REFERENCES

1. MONCADA, S., R.M.J. PALMER & E.A. HIGGS. 1991. Nitric oxide: physiology, pathophysiology, and pharmacology. Pharmacol. Rev. **43:** 109–142.
2. MURPHY, S., M.L. SIMMONS, L. AGULLO, A. GARCIA, D.L. FEINSTEIN, E. GALEA, D.J. REIS, D. MINC-GOLOMB & J.P. SCHWARTZ. 1993. Synthesis of nitric oxide in CNS glial cells. Trends Neurosci. **16:** 323–328.
3. MURAD, F., K. ISHII, U. FORSTERMANN, L. GORSKY, J.F. KERWIN, J. POLLOCK & M. HELLER. 1990. EDRF is an intracellular 2nd messenger and autacoid to regulate cyclic-GMP synthesis in many cells. Adv. Second Messenger Phosphoprotein Res. **24:** 441–448.
4. MIKI, N., Y. KAWABE & K. KURIYAMA. 1977. Activation of cerebral guanylate cyclase by nitric oxide. Biochem. Biophys. Res. Commun. **75:** 851–856.
5. GARTHWAITE, J. & C.L. BOULTON. 1995. Nitric oxide signalling in the central nervous system. Annu. Rev. Physiol. **57:** 683–706.
6. FURCHGOTT, R.F. 1996. The 1996 Albert Lasker Medical Research Awards: The discovery of endothelium-derived relaxing factor and its importance in the identification of nitric oxide. JAMA **276:** 1186–1188.
7. IGNARRO, L.J., G.M. BUGA, K.S. WOOD, R.E. BYRNS & G. CHAUDHURI. 1987. Endothelium-derived relaxing factor produced and released from artery and vein is nitric oxide. Proc. Natl. Acad. Sci. USA **84:** 9265–9269.
8. KOBARI, M., Y. FUKUUCHI, M. TOMITA, N. TANAHASHI & H. TAKEDA. 1994. Role of nitric oxide in regulation of cerebral microvascular tone and autoregulation of cerebral blood-flow in cat. Brain Res. **667:** 255–262.
9. CHIUEH, C.C. 1994. Neurobiology of ·NO and ·OH: basic research and clinical relevance. Ann. N.Y. Acad. Sci. **738:** 279–281.
10. RAUHALA, P., K.P. MOHANAKUMAR, I. SZIRAKI, A.M. LIN & C.C. CHIUEH. 1996. S-Nitrosothiols and nitric oxide, but not sodium nitroprusside, protect nigrostriatal dopamine neurons against iron-induced oxidative stress *in vivo*. Synapse **23:** 58–60.
11. MOHANAKUMAR, K.P., I. HANBAUER & C.C. CHIUEH. 1998. Neuroprotection by nitric oxide against hydroxyl radical-induced nigral neurotoxicity. J. Chem. Neuroanat. **14:** 195–205.

12. RAUHALA, P., I. SZIRAKI & C.C. CHIUEH. 1996. Peroxidation of brain lipids *in vitro*: nitric oxide versus hydroxyl radicals. Free Radical Biol. Med. **21:** 391–394.

13. RAUHALA, P., A.M.-Y. LIN & C.C. CHIUEH. 1998. Neuroprotection by *S*-nitrosoglutathione of brain dopamine neurons from oxidative stress. FASEB J. **12:** 165–173.

14. SZIRAKI, I., P. RAUHALA, K.K. KOH, P. VAN BERGEN & C.C. CHIUEH. 1999. Implication for atypical antioxidative properties of manganese in iron-induced brain lipid peroxidation and copper-dependent low density lipoprotein conjugation. Neurotoxicology. In press.

15. CHIUEH, C.C., D.L. GILBERT & C. COLTON, Eds. 1994. The Neurobiology of ·NO and ·OH. Ann. N.Y. Acad. Sci. **738:** 1–471.

16. YOSHINO, H., Y. NAKAGAWA-HATTORI, T. KONDO & Y. MIZUNO. 1992. Mitochondrial complex I and II activities of lymphocytes and platelets in Parkinson's disease. J. Neural Transm. Parkinson's Dis. Dement. Sect. **4:** 27–34.

17. CHIUEH, C.C., H. MIYAKE & M.T. PENG. 1993. Role of dopamine autoxidation, hydroxyl radical generation, and calcium overload in underlying mechanisms involved in MPTP-induced parkinsonism. Adv. Neurol. **60:** 251–258.

18. CHIUEH, C.C., D.L. MURPHY, H. MIYAKE, K. LANG, P.K. TULSI & S.J. HUANG. 1993. Hydroxyl free radicals (·OH) formation reflected by salicylate hydroxylation and neuromelanin: *in vivo* markers for oxidant injury of nigral neurons. Ann. N.Y. Acad. Sci. **679:** 370–375.

19. NAGATSU, T. & L. STJARNE. 1998. Catecholamine synthesis and release: an overview. Adv. Pharmacol. **42:** 1–14.

20. CHIUEH, C.C., G. KRISHNA, P. TULSI, T. OBATA, K. LANG, S.J. HUANG & D.L. MURPHY. 1992. Intracranial microdialysis of salicylic acid to detect hydroxyl radical generation though dopamine autooxidation in the caudate nucleus: effects of MPP$^+$. Free Radical Biol. Med. **13:** 581–583.

21. RAUHALA, P., A. KHALDI, K.P. MOHANAKUMAR & C.C. CHIUEH. 1997. Apparent role of hydroxyl radicals in oxidative brain injury induced by sodium nitroprusside. Free Radical Biol. Med. **24:** 1065–1073.

22. KANNER, J., S. HAREL & R. GRANIT. 1991. Nitric oxide as an antioxidant. Arch. Biochem. Biophys. **289:** 130–136.

23. IMAI, N., Y. TSUYAMA, K. MURAYAMA & E. ADACHI-USAMI. 1997. [Protective effect of nitric oxide on ischemic retina.] Nippon Ganka Gakkai Zasshi **101:** 639–643.

24. HOGG, N., B. KALYANARAMAN, J. JOSEPH, A. STRUCK & S. PARTHASARATHY. 1993. Inhibition of low-density lipoprotein oxidation by nitric oxide: Potential role in atherogenesis. FEBS Lett. **334:** 170–174.

25. RUBBO, H., R. RADI, M. TRUJILLO, R. TELLERI, B. KALYANARAMAN, S. BARNES, M. KIRK & B.A. FREEMAN. 1994. Nitric oxide regulation of superoxide and peroxynitrite-dependent lipid peroxidation: formation of novel nitrogen-containing oxidized lipid derivatives. J. Biol. Chem. **269:** 26066–26075.

26. WINK, D.A., I. HANBAUER, M.C. KRISHNA, W. DEGRAFF, J. GAMSON & J.B. MITCHELL. 1993. Nitric oxide protects against cellular damage and cytotoxicity from reactive oxygen species. Proc. Natl. Acad. Sci. USA **90:** 9813–9817.

27. CHANG, J., N.V. RAO, B.A. MARKEWITZ, J.R. HOIDAL & J.R. MICHAEL. 1996. Nitric oxide donor prevents hydrogen peroxide-mediated endothelial cell injury. Am. J. Physiol. **270:** L931–L940.

28. SERGENT, O., B. GRIFFON, I. MOREL, M. CHEVANNE, M.P. DUBOS, P. CILLARD & J. CILLARD. 1997. Effect of nitric oxide on iron-mediated oxidative stress in primary rat hepatocyte culture. Hepatology **25:** 122–127.

29. CASINI, A., E. CENI, R. SALZANO, P. BIONDI, M. PAROLA, A. GALLI, M. FOSCHI, A. CALIGIURI, M. PINZANI & C. SURRENTI. 1997. Neutrophil-derived superoxide anion induces lipid peroxidation and stimulates collagen synthesis in human hepatic stellate cells: role of nitric oxide. Hepatology **25:** 361–367.

30. GUTIERREZ, H.H., B. NIEVES, P. CHUMLEY, A. RIVERA & B.A. FREEMAN. 1996. Nitric oxide regulation of superoxide-dependent lung injury: oxidant-protective actions of endogenously produced and exogenously administered nitric oxide. Free Radical Biol. Med. **21:** 43–52.

31. BRUCKDORFER, K.R., G. DEE, M. JACOBS & C.A. RICE-EVANS. 1989. The protective action of nitric oxide against membrane damage induced by myoglobin radicals. Biochem. Soc. Trans. **18:** 285–286.

32. CENEVIVA, G.D., E. TZENG, D.G. HOYT, E. YEE, A. GALLAGHER, J.F. ENGELHARDT, Y.M. KIM, T.R. BILLIAR, S.A. WATKINS & B.R. PITT. 1998. Nitric oxide inhibits lipopolysaccharide-induced apoptosis in pulmonary artery endothelial cells. Am. J. Physiol. **19:** L717–L728.

33. DRAPIER, J.C. 1997. Interplay between NO and [Fe-S] clusters: relevance to biological systems. Methods **11:** 319–329.

34. LI, J.R., T.R. BILLIAR, R.V. TALANIAN & Y.M. KIM. 1997. Nitric oxide reversibly inhibits seven members of the caspase family via *S*-nitrosylation. Biochem. Biophys. Res. Commun. **240:** 419–424.

35. CHOI, D.W. 1993. Nitric oxide: Foe or friend to injured brain? Proc. Natl. Acad. Sci. USA **90:** 9741–9743.

36. MOHANAKUMAR, K.P., A. DE BARTOLOMEIS, R.M. WU, K.J. YEH, L.M. STERNBERGER, S.Y. PENG, D.L. MURPHY & C.C. CHIUEH. 1994. Ferrous-citrate complex and nigral degeneration: evidence for free-radical formation and lipid peroxidation. Ann. N.Y. Acad. Sci. **738:** 392–399.

37. BECKMAN, J.S., T.W. BECKMAN, J. CHEN, P.A. MARSHALL & B.A. FREEMAN. 1990. Apparent hydroxyl radical production by peroxynitrite: implications for endothelial injury from nitric oxide and superoxide. Proc. Natl. Acad. Sci. USA **87:** 1620–1624.

38. WINK, D.A., R.W. NIMS, J.F. DARBYSHIRE, D. CHISTODOULOU, I. HANBAUER, G.W. COX, F. LAVAL, J. LAVAL, J.A. COOK, M.C. KRISHNA, W. DEGRAFF & J.B. MITCHELL. 1994. Reaction kinetics for nitrosation of cysteine and glutathione in aerobic nitric oxide solutions at neutral pH. Insights into the fate and physiological effects of intermediates generated in the NO/O_2 reaction. Chem. Res. Toxicol. **7:** 519–525.

39. DO, K.Q., B. BENZ, G. GRIMA, U. GUTTECK-AMSLER, I. KLUGE & T.E. SALT. 1996. Nitric oxide precursor arginine and *S*-nitrosoglutathione in synaptic and glial function. Neurochem. Int. **29:** 213–224.

40. GOW, A.J., D.G. BUERK & H. ISCHIROPOULOS. 1997. A novel reaction mechanism for the formation of *S*-nitrosothiol *in vivo*. J. Biol. Chem. **272:** 2841–2845.

41. CLANCY, R.M., D. LEVARTOVSKY, J. LESZCZYNSKA-PIZIAK, J. YEGUDIN & S.B. ABRAMSON. 1994. Nitric oxide reacts with intracellular glutathione and activates the hexose monophosphate shunt in human neutrophils: evidence for *S*-nitrosoglutathione as a bioactive intermediary. Proc. Natl. Acad. Sci. USA **91:** 3680–3684.

42. GASTON, B., J. REILLY, J.M. DRAZEN, J. FACKLER, P. RAMDEV, D. ARNELLE, M.E. MULLINS, D.J. SUGARBAKER, C. CHEE, D.J. SINGEL, J. LOSCALZO & J.S. STAMBLER. 1993. Endogenous nitrogen oxides and bronchodilator *S*-nitrosothiols in human airways. Proc. Natl. Acad. Sci. USA **90:** 10957–10961.

43. SINGH, R.J., N. HOGG, J. JOSEPH & B. KALYANARAMAN. 1996. Mechanism of nitric oxide release from *S*-nitrosothiols. J. Biol. Chem. **271:** 18596–18603.

44. NIKITOVIC, D. & A. HOLMGREN. 1996. *S*-Nitrosoglutathione is cleaved by the thioredoxin system with liberation of glutathione and redox regulating nitric oxide. J. Biol. Chem. **271:** 19180–19185.

45. GORREN, A.C., A. SCHAMMEL, K. SCHMIDT & B. MAYER. 1996. Decomposition of *S*-nitrosoglutathione in the presence of copper ions and glutathione. Arch. Biochem. Biophys. **330:** 219–228.

46. RADOMSKI, M.W., D.D. REES, A. DUTRA & S. MONCADA. 1992. *S*-Nitrosoglutathione inhibits platelet activation *in vitro* and *in vivo*. Br. J. Pharmacol. **107:** 745–749.

47. KONOREV, E.A., M.M. TARPEY, J. JOSEPH, J.E. BAKER & B. KALYANARAMAN. 1995. *S*-Nitrosoglutathione improves functional recovery in thc isolated rat heart after cardioplegic ischemic arrest-evidence for a cardioprotective effect of nitric oxide. J. Pharmacol. Exp. Ther. **274:** 200–206.

48. KONOREV, E.A., J. JOSEPH, M.M. TARPEY & B. KALYANARAMAN. 1996. The mechanism of cardioprotection by *S*-nitrosoglutathione monoethyl ester in rat isolated heart during cardioplegic ischaemic arrest. Br. J. Pharmacol. **119:** 511–518.

49. PLUM, R.C. & J.O. EDWARDS. 1994. The chemistry of peroxynitrites. Prog. Inorg. Chem. **41:** 599–635.

50. SQUADRITO, G.L. & W.A. PRYOR. 1998. Oxidative chemistry of nitric oxide: the roles of superoxide, peroxynitrite, and carbon dioxide. Free Radical Biol. Med. **25:** 392–403.

51. BERLETT, B.S., R.L. LEVINE & E.R. STADTMAN. 1998. Carbon dioxide stimulates peroxynitrite-mediated nitration of tyrosine residues and inhibits oxidation of methionine residues of glutamine synthetase: both modifications mimic effects of adenylylation. Proc. Natl. Acad. Sci. USA **95:** 2784–2789.

52. DILLARD, C.J. & A.L. TAPPEL. 1973. Fluorescent products from reaction of peroxidizing polyunsaturated fatty acids with phosphatidyl ethanolamine and phenylalanine. Lipids **8:** 183–189.

53. KIKUGAWA, K., T. KATO, M. BEBBU & A. HAYASAKA. 1989. A fluorescent and cross-linked proteins formed by free radicals and aldehyde specifics generated during lipid peroxidation. Adv. Exp. Med. Biol. **266:** 345–356.

54. SMITH, M.A., L.M. SAYRE, V.E. ANDERSON, P.L. HARRIS, M.F. BEAL, N. KOWALL & G. PERRY. 1998. Cytochemical demonstration of oxidative damage in Alzheimer's disease by immunochemical enhancement of the carbonyl reaction with 2,4-dinitrophenylhydrazine. J. Histochem. Cytochem. **46:** 731–735.

55. SZIRAKI, I., K.P. MOHANAKUMAR, P. RAUHALA, H.G. KIM, K.J. YEH & C.C. CHIUEH. 1998. Manganese: a transition metal protects nigrostriatal neurons from oxidative stress in the iron-induced animal model of parkinsonism. Neuroscience **85:** 1011–1111.

56. CHAN, P.H., C.J. EPSTEIN, Y. LI, T.T. HUANG, E. CARLSON, H. KINOUCHI, G. YANG, H. KAMII, S. MIKAWA, T. KONDO *et al.* 1995. Transgenic mice and knockout mutants in the study of oxidative stress in brain injury. J. Neurotrauma **12:** 815–824

57. BROWN, R.H., Jr. 1998. SOD_1 aggregates in ALS: cause, correlate or consequence? Nature Med. **4:** 1362–1364.

58. DENEKE, S.M. & B.L. FABURG. 1989. Regulation of cellular glutathione. Am. J. Physiol. **257:** L-163–L-173.

59. MEISTER, A. 1995. Glutathione metabolism. Methods Enzymol. **251:** 3–7.

60. ARNELLE, D.R. & J.S. STAMBLER. 1995. NO^+, NO, and NO^- donation by *S*-nitrosothiols: implications for regulation of physiological functions by *S*-nitrosylation and acceleration of disulfite formation. Arch. Biochem. Biophys. **318:** 279–285.

61. FEELISCH, M. 1998. The use of nitric oxide donors in pharmacological studies. Naunyn Schmiedebergs Arch. Pharmacol. **358:** 113–122.

Neuroprotective Strategies for HIV-1-Associated Neurologic Disease

HARRIS A. GELBARD[a]

Division of Child Neurology, Department of Neurobiology, University of Rochester, Rochester, New York, USA

It is widely accepted that HIV-1 infection of the central nervous system (CNS) may result in productive infection of brain-resident macrophages and microglia and restricted infection (i.e., regulatory gene products expressed without production of progeny virus) of astrocytes, without direct cytolytic infection of neurons. Based on these findings, the most plausible hypothesis to explain neurologic disease in patients with HIV-1 infection is that HIV-1-infected macrophages and microglia initiate production of HIV-1 gene products and cellular metabolites that act as toxicants to vulnerable neurons, as well as impair normal astrocyte homeostatic functions.

Death of vulnerable neurons in pediatric patients with HIV-1-associated neurologic disease is due to apoptosis[1] by a mechanism that does not involve overexpression of the pro-apoptotic gene product Bax.[2] We have recently extended these findings to demonstrate that marked upregulation of the pro-apoptotic gene product caspase 3 occurs in neurons in pediatric patients with HIV-1-associated neurologic disease.[3] Because HIV-1 infection of the CNS results in apoptosis of vulnerable neurons, we have used *in vitro* models to identify novel relationships between several HIV-1 neurotoxins that may be critical to inducing disruption of normal neuronal functions and ultimately causing neuronal apoptosis. We initially investigated the role of the pro-inflammatory cytokine tumor necrosis factor alpha (TNFα), produced by HIV-1-infected macrophages and microglia, and antigenically stimulated, uninfected macrophages and microglia, because levels of TNFα in vulnerable brain regions correlate with neurologic disease in HIV-1-infected patients. We demonstrated that TNFα induces neuronal apoptosis by a mechanism that involves oxidative stress, but is independent of nuclear factor kappa B (NFκB) activation,[4] and in part involves excitotoxic activation of the α-amino-3-hydroxy-5-methylisoxazole-4-propionic acid (AMPA) subtype of glutamate receptors[5] and downregulation of high-affinity glutamate uptake sites in astrocytes.[6] We extended these findings to demonstrate that the HIV-1 regulatory gene product Tat increases release of TNFα, and also results in activation of AMPA receptors to induce neuronal apoptosis by a NFκB-independent mechanism.[7] We identified another neurotoxin, the pro-inflammatory phospholipid mediator platelet-activating factor (PAF), which is produced by HIV-1-infected, antigenically stimulated macrophages, and activates the *N*-methyl-D-aspartate (NMDA) subtype of glutamate receptors to induce neuronal apoptosis, and is positively correlated with dementia and immunosuppression in HIV-1-infect-

[a]Address for correspondence: Harris A. Gelbard, M.D., Ph.D., Division of Child Neurology, Box 631, Department of Neurobiology, University of Rochester, Rochester, NY 14642-8677. Phone, 716/275-4784; fax, 716/275-3683.

e-mail, hgelbard@neurology.rochester.edu

ed patients.[8] We have demonstrated that TNFα induces PAF release from macrophages, and that the majority of neuronal apoptosis that occurs after exposure to neurotoxins secreted by antigenically stimulated, HIV-1-infected macrophages can be blocked by catabolism of PAF, suggesting that PAF may be a key initiator step for HIV-1 neuropathogenesis.[9]

Thus agents that reduce oxidative stress mediated by TNFα, antagonize PAF receptor activation, catabolize PAF or related oxidized phospholipids, or antagonize NMDA and non-NMDA receptor subtypes can markedly ameliorate neuronal death from these HIV-1 neurotoxins. The available data suggest that combination chemotherapy with these agents is likely to ameliorate neurologic disease associated with HIV-1 infection of the CNS by reducing inflammation that results in excitotoxicity.

ACKNOWLEDGMENTS

This work was supported in part by NIH grants PO1 MH57556 and RO1 MH56838.

REFERENCES

1. GELBARD *et al.* 1995.
2. KRAJEWSKI *et al.* 1997.
3. JAMES *et al.* Submitted.
4. TALLEY *et al.* 1995.
5. GELBARD *et al.* 1993.
6. FINE *et al.* 1996.
7. NEW *et al.* 1998.
8. GELBARD *et al.* 1994
9. PERRY *et al.* 1998.

Changes in mRNA Levels for Heat-Shock/ Stress Proteins (Hsp) and a Secretory Vesicle Associated Cysteine-String Protein (Csp1) after Amphetamine (AMPH) Exposure

JOHN F. BOWYER[a,c] AND DAVID L. DAVIES[b]

[a]*Division of Neurotoxicology, National Center for Toxicological Research/FDA, Jefferson, Arkansas 72079-9502, USA*

[b]*Department of Anatomy, University of Arkansas for Medical Sciences, Little Rock, Arkansas 72205-7199, USA*

ABSTRACT: Damage to nerve terminals, reactive gliosis and somatic degeneration can result when pronounced hyperthermia occurs during amphetamine (AMPH) exposure. The effects of AMPH-induced hyperthermia and damage on the relative mRNA levels for several heat shock/stress proteins (Hsp27, Hsp60, Hsp70 and Hsc70), as well as secretory vesicle associated cysteine-string protein (Csp1) were determined in both the striatum and substantia nigra using reverse transcriptase polymerase chain reaction (RT-PCR). These changes were compared to changes in Hsp mRNA levels seen in primary rat cerebral astrocyte cultures after heat shock/stress. Striatal Hsp70 mRNA increased about 2-fold over control levels at 16 hr after AMPH-induced hyperthermia, and was the only Hsp species to significantly increase in response to AMPH. Hsp70 mRNA levels returned to control within 14 days after AMPH. Two-fold increases in Hsp70 mRNA were also seen in primary cultures of rat cerebrum 24 hr after heat shock. In primary cultures and brain tissue, the increased Hsp70 mRNA levels were still more than 500-fold less than constitutive Hsc70 mRNA and 50-fold less than Hsp60 levels. Hsp27 mRNA was not present in the striatum, nigra and primary cell cultures. Thus, the expression of Hsp species mRNA measured was very similar in brain tissue and primary cell cultures. Because only a modest induction of Hsp 70 mRNA occurred, the Hsp species evaluated may only play a minor role in AMPH neurotoxicity. However, further studies are necessary to determine whether large increases in Hsp 70 are occurring in selected neurons or glia in the striatum. RT-PCR products for Csp1 were produced in total RNA obtained from brain but not from cultured astrocytes, suggesting that the Csp1 mRNA measured by RT-PCR is of neuronal origin. Csp1 mRNA levels were acutely downregulated in neurons in the substantia nigra, possibly in response to damage, but not the striatum after AMPH exposure. A slight long-term upregulation at 4 months of Csp1 mRNA may occur in the striatum but not in nigra.

[c]Corresponding author: John Bowyer, Ph.D., Division of Neurotoxicology, National Center for Toxicological Research/FDA, 3900 NCTR Road, Jefferson, AR 72079-9502. Phone, 870/543-7194; fax, 870/543-7745.

e-mail, Jbowyer@nctr.fda.gov

"

INTRODUCTION

The hyperthermia produced by amphetamine (AMPH) and methamphetamine (METH) is well document to play an important role in their lethality.[1,11,36,25] As well, hyperthermia greatly potentiates the dopamine depletion, nerve terminal damage and expression of reactive gliosis in the striatum of rat and mouse after exposure to AMPH and METH.[7,2,25] In addition, significant hyperthermia and seizures are important components in the neurodegeneration of the cortex, limbic system and thalamus that occurs after either AMPH or METH exposure.[6,14,17] Thus, it follows that psychoactive drugs such as lysergic acid diethylamide (LSD) and AMPH, which induce hyperthermia, also induce Hsp70 mRNA in the brain, and in particular the hippocampus.[15,24,18,30] It has been postulated that the expression of Hsp 70 in the hippocampus affects the development of neurotoxicity as well as being a biomarker for its occurrence.

However, less is known about how neurotoxic doses of AMPH and METH affect mRNA and protein for Hsp at sites of dopamine terminal degeneration in the striatum and the cell bodies of these terminals. A significant increase in Hsp70 has been observed in the striatum of mice given a single dose of 20 mg/kg METH at time points up to 39 hr. However, there was no mention of Hsp70 changes in the substantia nigra where the dopaminergic cell bodies for the terminals in the striatum.[20] In addition, single-dose paradigms of AMPH or METH do not consistently produce long-term dopamine depletions.[5] This study was designed to look at the relative changes in mRNA for Hsp70, Hsc70, Hsp60 and Hsp27 after multiple doses of either AMPH or saline. Also, the relative changes in mRNA for secretory vesicle associated cysteine-string protein (Csp1), a DnaJ-Hsp40-related protein, which has previously been called Hsp34, were determined.[37,23,22]

The substantia nigra and striata used for isolating the total RNA in these studies were obtained from 15-month-old rats in which consistent long-term reductions in striatal dopamine and tyrosine hydroxylase were produced.[3] Older rats were used, because they are more sensitive to the neurotoxic effects of amphetamines. The relative mRNA levels for HSP in the substantia nigra and striatum were determined using reverse transcriptase polymerase chain reaction (RT-PCR). Total RNA was isolated from striatum and substantia nigra after AMPH at 1 day (24 hr after the start of dosing but only 14–16 hr after the end of hyperthermia above 40.0°C) up to 4 months after AMPH. Changes in brain Hsp and Csp1 mRNA after AMPH were compared to changes in Hsp and Csp1 mRNA levels *in vitro* using primary adult rat cerebral cultures subjected to heat shock/stress. These primary cultures consisted predominantly of vimentin positive epithelioid astrocytes and a small subpopulation of processes bearing astrocytes positive for glial fibrillary acidic protein (GFAP); neurofilament positive neurons were absent. Therefore, the Hsp profile of these primary cultures is primarily glial in nature.

METHODS

The aliquots of total RNA used to determine the relative changes in Hsp and Csp1 mRNA levels in the substantia nigra and striatum used in this paper have been previously tested for changes in tyrosine hydroxylase mRNA after AMPH.[3] The description of some of the methods used (such as: dosing and sacrifice, total RNA isolation, and phosphorimaging) have been abbreviated here but can be found in more detail in Bowyer *et al.*[3]

Drug Administration

Animals used in these experiments were 15-month-old male Sprague-Dawley rats from the National Center for Toxicological Research (NCTR) colony. The rats were administered 4 injections intraperitoneally (i.p.) once every 2 hr of 3 mg/kg *d*-amphetamine at an environmental temperature of 24°C. Rats were euthanized at 1, 3, or 14 days or 4 months postamphetamine treatment. Brains were rapidly removed, and the striata and substantia nigra were dissected as described and stored at –70°C until total RNA isolation.[3]

Measurement of Hsp, Csp1 and Glyceraldehyde-3-phosphate Dehydrogenase (GAPDH) mRNA Using RT-PCR

Total cellular RNA was isolated essentially by the procedure of Chomczynski[12] and stored at 70°C. Ten µl of the 70-µl RNA sample from each striatum and nigra were used to measure total RNA concentration, and 10–20 µl was used to measure Hsp, Csp1 and glyceraldehyde-3-phosphate dehydrogenase (GAPDH) mRNA using the quantitative RT-PCR assay. RNA concentration was estimated as previously described.[3] For relative quantification of Hsp, Csp1 and GAPDH mRNA using RT-PCR, aliquots of 0.4 µg total cellular RNA were subjected to RT using either oligodeoxythymidine (oligo dT) primers or random hexamers. Aliquots of the resulting singlestranded cDNA product were used along with the appropriate primers (see below) in the PCR to incorporate ^{32}PdATP into doublestranded products encoding for 433 bp Hsp27 cDNA, 441 bp Hsp60 cDNA, 332 bp Hsp70, 303 bp Hsc70, 374 bp Csp1 (Hsp34) or 626 bp GAPDH cDNA. This enabled the radiolabeled Hsp and Csp1 cDNA PCR products to be compared to the GAPDH products as well as to the µg of total cellular RNA used in the RT step.

Reverse Transcription (RT)

At least two separate reverse transcription (RT) reactions, using 8 ul of either 0.6 µg/µl oligo(dT)1218 (Sigma, St. Louis) or 8 µl of 0.4 µg/µl random hexamers and 2 µl of 0.2 µg/µl total RNA, were performed in a thin-walled PCR reaction tube (Gene AmpR). The reactions were first heated to 70°C for 5 min and then cooled to 5°C for annealing the oligo dT or random hexamer primers to mRNA. Subsequently, 10 ul of reaction buffer was added to the reaction mixtures (final volume = 20 µl). Final concentrations of reactants were as follows: 50 mM Tris (pH 8.3), 75 mM KCl, 3 mM MgCl$_2$, 10 mM dithiothreitol, 0.5 mM dNTPs, 0.5 units/µl RNase inhibitor and 50 units reverse transcriptase. The reaction mixtures were warmed to 42°C for 15 min, heated to 99°C for 5 min and then cooled to 5°C. MMLV reverse transcriptase or Superscript RNase H reverse transcriptase (Gibco/BRL) were used for these reactions. The RT reaction produced enough product for at least 8 separate PCR amplifications.

PCR Reaction Mixture and Buffers

The PCR amplification of Hsp, Csp1 or GAPDH mRNAs from RT product were performed, in separate reaction tubes for optimization of each PCR product, using a 2-µl aliquot of the 20-µl RT reaction solution of the first strand template for the PCR amplification. The PCRs were performed in a 50 µl reaction volume containing (final concentrations): 10 mM TrisHCl (pH 9.0), 50 mM KCl, 3 mM $MgCl_2$, 200 µM dNTPs, 1.5 units Taq DNA polymerase (GIBCO/BRL), 0.2 µM of both 5′ and 3′ primers and 5 µCi (3000 Ci/mmol) of alpha ^{32}PdATP (DuPont NEN). The primers for the PCR (NBI; Plymouth, MN) amplification of Hsp, Csp1 or GAPDH mRNAs were selected using the cDNA sequences for these mRNAs in GenBank (NCI/ Frederick Biomedical Supercomputing Center) and the program Oligo® (NBI/ Genovus Inc., Plymouth, MN).

PCR Primers

The 5′ GAPDH sense primer encoded cDNA sequences 298 to 318 (5′-gct gag tat gtc gtg gag tct), and the 3′ antisense primer was complementary to GAPDH cDNA sequences 903 to 923 (5′-cca gcc cca gca tca aag gtg-3′). The 5′ Csp1 (also known as Hsp34; GeneBank accession, Gb S81917) sense primer encoded cDNA sequences 154 to 174 (5′-ctg aca aga acc ctg ata acc-3′) and the 3′ antisense primer was complementary to Csp1 cDNA sequences 507 to 527 (5′-gtc tgt agc ctc cct ctc atc-3′). The 5′ Hsp27 sense primer encoded sequences 156 to 176 (5′-ggt ttc ccg atg agt ggt ctc-3′) and the 3′ antisense primer was complementary to Hsp27 cDNA sequences 569 to 589 (5′-ctc cgc tga ttg tgt gac tgc-3′). The 5′ Hsp60 sense primer encoded cDNA sequences 346 to 366 (5′-aga ggt gtg atg ttg gct gtt-3′) and the 3′ antisense primer was complementary to Hsp60 cDNA sequences 766 to 786 (5′-caa aac cag tgt gct aag agc-3′). The 5′ Hsp70 sense primer encoded cDNA sequences 842 to 862 (5′-acc gtg gag ccc gtg gag aag-3′) and the antisense primer was complementary to Hsp70 cDNA sequences 1153 to 1173 (5′-ttg gtg ggg atg gtg gag ttg-3′). The 5′ Hsc70 sense primer encoded cDNA sequences 176 to 196 (5′-ttg ctt tca ccg aca cag aac-3′) and the antisense primer was complementary to the Hsc70 cDNA sequences 458 to 478 (5′-cgg cat tgg taa cag tct ttc-3′).

PCR Cycling Conditions

All PCR reaction mixtures were kept at 5°C and the Taq polymerase was added seconds prior to the start of PCR. To optimize fidelity, the PCR tubes, with reactants, were transferred directly to the PCR machine, which was already at 94°C (denaturing temperature). Each PCR cycle, with the exception of the first cycle, which had a longer denaturing period at 94°C for 2 min, and the final cycle, which had an extension period of 7 min, consisted of 3 steps: 1 min at 94°C (denaturing); 1 min at 51–70°C (annealing, depended on which mRNA was to be amplified by RT-PCR); and 1 min at 72°C (primer extension) for amplification of RT product. The annealing temperatures for the various amplifications are: Hsp27, 61°C; Hsp60, 64°C; Hsp70, 70°C; Hsc70, 65°C; Csp1, 62°C; GAPDH, 57°C. The number of cycles used for PCR varied for each cDNA bp species from 19 (GAPDH) to 34 (Hsp27 and Hsp70). Following the last PCR cycle the reactions were cooled to 5°C.

After PCR amplification 10 µl of 6× loading buffer (0.25% xylene cyanol FF, 0.25% bromophenol blue and 15% Ficoll) was added to each 50 ul PCR reaction to prepare it for electrophoresis on a 6% nondenaturing polyacrylamide gel. Twelve ul of the RT-PCR products were loaded per lane for isolation of radioactive bands. Each gel was run for 3 hr at 25 mamps, such that the PCR products traveled at least 6 cm from the origin, and then the gel was dried down onto Whatman 1MM paper (Schleicher & Schuell). The levels of ^{32}P-labeled RT-PCR products separated on the gels were quantified using the PhosphorImager system from Molecular Dynamics (Sunnyvale, CA) after exposure to the phosphor screens for 2 to 6 hr. The ImageQuant™ software (Molecular Dynamics) methods of volume integration were used to quantify the intensity of the RT-PCR bands. In some instances, 2% agarose gels were used to separate RT-PCR products for ethidium bromide visualization.

Tissue Culture Techniques

Primary cultures were prepared from the cerebra of 3-month-old CD rats using procedures similar to those described previously for neonatal cerebra.[16] Using sterile procedures, the cortical grey matter was isolated and minced into 1–2-mm^3 fragments and incubated in phosphate buffered saline (PBS) containing 0.2% trypsin for 20 min at 37°C. Tissue fragments were then dissociated by trituration, the cell suspension was mixed with Dulbecco's modified Eagle's medium (DMEM) containing 10% fetal bovine serum (HyClone) and allowed to settle for 5 min. The supernatant containing suspended cells was saved, and 4 ml of fresh DMEM was used to tritiate the pellet. This procedure was repeated 2 times to maximize recovery of harvested cells.[19] The pooled supernatants were centrifuged at $200 \times g$ for 5 min, and the pellet was resuspended in fresh medium. The suspended cells were then filtered through a 70-µm nylon sieve (Falcon #2350). The cells were plated in DMEM containing 10% fetal bovine serum, 2 mM glutamine, 100 U/ml penicillin and 100 µg/ml streptomycin into 25-cm^2 flasks. Cultures were incubated in a 5% CO_2 humidified atmosphere at 37°C. The culture medium was changed at 2-day intervals.

Confluent cultures at 21 days were subjected to stress by placing them into an incubator set at 42°C for 1 hr, and then harvested 16–18 hr later. The medium was decanted, and each culture was carefully rinsed with 6 ml of PBS. The cells were then immediately frozen on dry ice and transferred to −70°C until total RNA isolation.

Immunohistochemistry

The cellular composition of the cultures was characterized after 22 days. Sister cultures to those tested for Hsp were rinsed with PBS, and then fixed for 10 min in a 4% paraformaldehyde in 0.12 Sorensen's buffer. Cells were washed several times with PBS after fixation, and then incubated in PBS containing 0.2% Triton-X 100 and primary antibodies (1:500) overnight at 4°C. After primary antibody exposure a modification of the unlabeled peroxidase-antiperoxidase method similar to that of Sternberger et al.[29] was used for localization of GFAP, vimentin and neurofilament. All immunological reagents were obtained from Dako Corp. (Carpinteria, CA) with 3,3′-diaminobenzidene as an enzyme substrate. The cultures were primarily vimentin positive epitheliod astrocytes, and also contained a subpopulation (about 5%) of process-bearing astrocytes, which were GFAP positive. Cells positive for neurofilament were not found.

RESULTS

The time course of the changes in striatal levels of dopamine as well as the protein and mRNA levels for tyrosine hydroxylase for the striatum and substantia nigra of animals used in this study have already been reported elsewhere.[3] The RT-PCR prod-

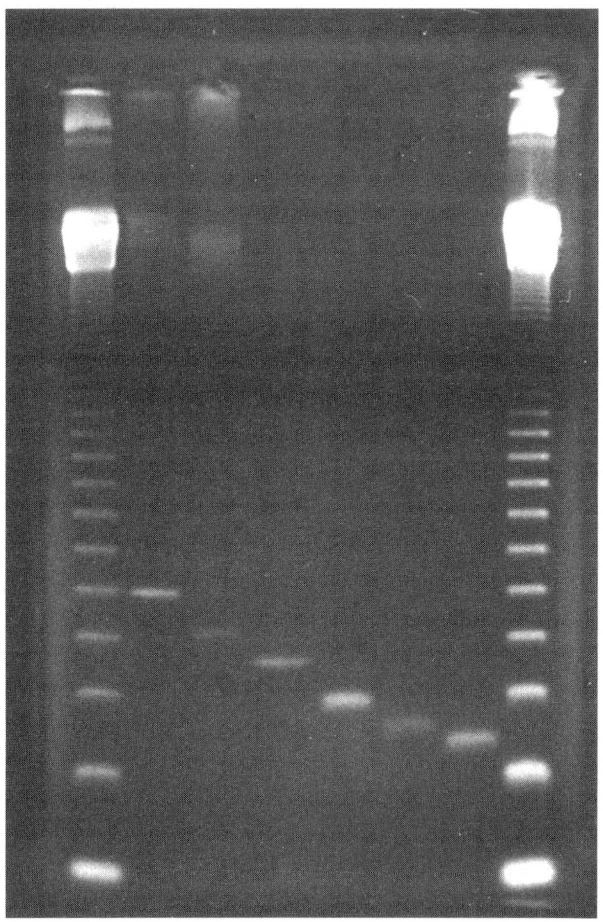

FIGURE 1. Ethidium bromide-labeled RT-PCR products from substantia nigra total RNA. Ethidium bromide stain of RT-PCR products (RT used oligo dT_{12-18} primers) from 0.4 µg total RNA from substantia nigra separated on a nondenaturing 2% agarose gel. From *left* to *right* are: 2 µg 123 bp standards, 626 bp GAPDH (21 PCR cycles), 519 bp TH (23 PCR cycles), 441 bp Hsp60 (25 PCR cycles), 374 bp Csp1 (30 PCR cycles), 332 bp Hsp70 (34 PCR cycles), 303 bp Hsc70 (23 PCR cycles) and 4 µg 123 bp standards. Twelve µl of the total 50 µl of PCR reaction mixture were loaded in *lanes 2–7*. Sizes of the PCR products correspond to what would be predicted by mRNA sequences of the respective proteins.

TABLE 1. Summary of the relative[a] mRNA changes (as determined by RT-PCR) in substantia nigra and striatum after amphetamine

PT-PCR Product	1 Day Post Amphetamine ($n = 6$)		3 Days Post Amphetamine ($n = 6$)		14 Days Post Amphetamine ($n = 6$)		120 Days Post Amphetamine ($n = 10$)	
	S.N.	Striatum	S.N.	Striatum	S.N.	Striatum	S.N.	Striatum
GAPDH	$80 \pm 8\%$	$105 \pm 4\%$	$74 \pm 9\%$	$92 \pm 4\%$	$85 \pm 8\%$	N.D.	$87 \pm 15\%$	$96 \pm 5\%$
TH	$77 \pm 17\%^{b}$	N.D.	$87 \pm 14\%^{b}$	N.D.	$75 \pm 5\%^{b}$	N.D.	$99 \pm 15\%^{b}$	$250\%^{b}$
Csp1	$59 \pm 15\%$	$89 \pm 5\%$	$83 \pm 7\%$	$97 \pm 4\%$	$86 \pm 18\%$	N.D.	$90 \pm 10\%$	$125 \pm 6\%$
Hsp70b	$107 \pm 19\%$	$184 \pm 13\%$	$118 \pm 9\%$	$118 \pm 18\%$	N.D.	N.D.	98 ± 11	$91 \pm 5\%$
Hsp70c	$108 \pm 8\%$	$83 \pm 6\%$	$103 \pm 7\%$	N.D.	N.D.	N.D.	$100 \pm 4\%$	N.D.
Hsp60	$90 \pm 3\%$	N.D.	$88 \pm 9\%$	N.D.	N.D.	N.D.	$102 \pm 9\%$	N.D.

[a]Levels for mRNA RT-PCR products are shown as a percentage of control values (N.D. = not determined).

[b]Data on tyrosine hydroxylase (TH) were previously reported by Bowyer *et al.*[3]

ucts for the Hsp, Csp1 and GAPDH generated from 0.4 ug of control substantia nigra total RNA are shown separated on a gel stained with ethidium bromide (FIG. 1). From left to right are 123 bp standards, 626 bp GAPDH, 519 bp tyrosine hydroxylase, 374 bp Csp1, 341 bp Hsp60, 322 bp Hsp70b, 303 bp Hsc 70c and 123 bp standard. Sizes of the RT-PCR products correspond to what would be predicted by mRNA/cDNA sequences of the respective proteins. Note that a wide variation in the number of PCR cycles was necessary to generate the bands because of the many orders of magnitude differences in the levels of these mRNA species. PCR product for Hsp27 could be not detected from nigra or striatum at up to 34 cycles in either control or AMPH-treated rats, and only a weak signal could be generated at 34 cycles for Hsp70. The number of PCR cycles chosen for relative quantitation of each mRNA RT-PCR product was set so that linearity in the ^{32}P-radiolabeled PCR product occurred at 3 cycles fewer and 3 cycles greater than the number chosen.

GAPDH mRNA RT-PCR product levels were relatively stable only dipping slightly 1 and 3 days post AMPH in substantia nigra, and GAPDH levels in the striatum were not significantly reduced at any time point (TABLE 1, note that levels are shown as a percent of the saline controls). In the substantia nigra, Hsp70 mRNA RT-PCR product levels were not affected at 16 hr after the end of AMPH-induced hyperthermia but were increased 2-fold in the striatum (TABLE 1, FIG. 2). Levels of Hsp70 mRNA were increased only slightly at 3 days after AMPH in the nigra and striatum. The relative levels of Hsp70, as determined by RT-PCR, were also increased 2-fold in primary cultures of adult rat cerebrum 24 hr after heat shock/stress (FIGS. 2B and 4A). In comparison, level of induction was orders of magnitude less than for cell lines, such as the 9Lvar.SF cell line, sensitive to Hsp70 induction by heat shock/stress (FIG. 2B). Interestingly, the 9Lvar.SF cell line barely had detectable levels of the constitutive Hsc70 or Hsp60 mRNA even when heat-stressed (FIG. 2B).

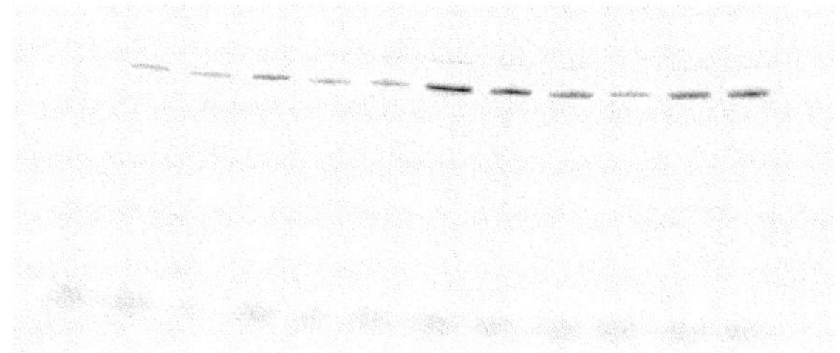

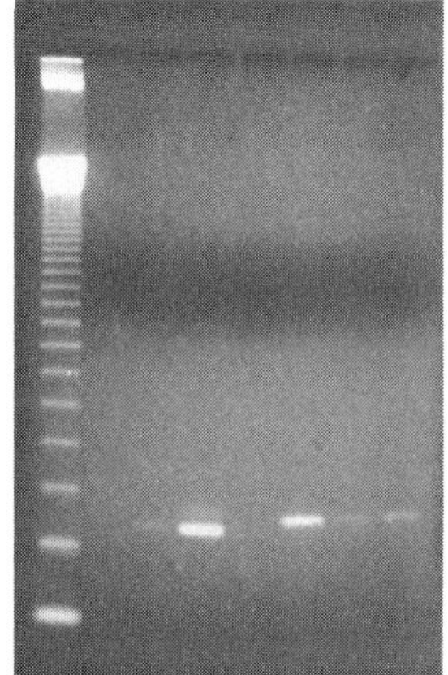

FIGURE 2. RT-PCR amplification of Hsp70 and Hsc70 mRNA. **(A)** Phosphorimage of 12 µl of 50 µl RT-PCR product from total RNA using Hsp70 primers was separated on a nondenaturing 5% acrylamide gel. Blank control (no total RNA in the RT step, 30 cycles), *L1*; total RNA from striatum at 18 hr post 4 × saline (30 cycles), *L2–L6*; total RNA from striatum at 16 hr after the end of AMPH-induced hyperthermia (30 cycles), *L7–L12*. Each lane contains the RT-PCR products derived from the total RNA of different rats. **(B)** Ethidium bromide-labeled RT-PCR products in 12 µl of 50 µl RT-PCR reaction using either Hsp70 or Hsc70 primers from total RNA derived from striatum, primary glial cultures or the mRNA from 9Lvar.SF rat cell line containing Hsp70 inducible by heat-shock (from Stress Gen) were separated on a nondenaturing 2% agarose gel. Two µg of 123 kb ladder standards, *L1*; 303 bp Hsc70 product (23 PCR cycles, no product visible) from control 9Lvar.SF cells, *L2*; Hsc70 product (23 PCR cycles, faint band) from heat-stressed cells 9Lvar.SF cells, *L3*; Hsc70 product (23 PCR cycles, bright band) from control primary cortical glial cultures, *L4*; 332 bp Hsp70 product (30 PCR cycles, no product visible) from control cells 9Lvar.SF cells, *L5*; Hsp70 product (30 PCR cycles, bright band) from heat-stressed cells 9Lvar.SF cells, *L6*; Hsp70 product (30 PCR cycles, faint band) from control primary cortical glial cultures, *L7*; Hsp70 product (30 PCR cycles, faint band) from heat stressed primary cortical glial cultures, *L8*.

However, the relative levels of constitutive Hsc70 and Hsp60 mRNA were very high in both the substantia nigra and striatum of control rats with levels of over 500 and 100 times, respectively, that of Hsp70 mRNA but were not significantly affected by AMPH exposure in either brain region (FIG. 3). This same profile of Hsc70 and Hsp60 was also observed in primary cultures of cerebrum (data not shown). Hsp27 mRNA [32]P- labeled RT-PCR products were not detected in substantia nigra or striatum in control or AMPH-treated rats after 32 PCR cycles (data not shown). Also, RT-PCR products for Hsp27 were not produced from total RNA derived from primary cerebral cultures (FIG. 4). In contrast, RNA from a HeLa cell line expressed a prominent band for the RT-PCR product for Hsp27 mRNA after 30 PCR cycles.

A

120 Days Post | 3 Days Post

Control | AMPH | Control | AMPH

L1 L2 L3 L4 L5 L6 L7 L8 L9 L10 L11 L12 L13 L14 L15

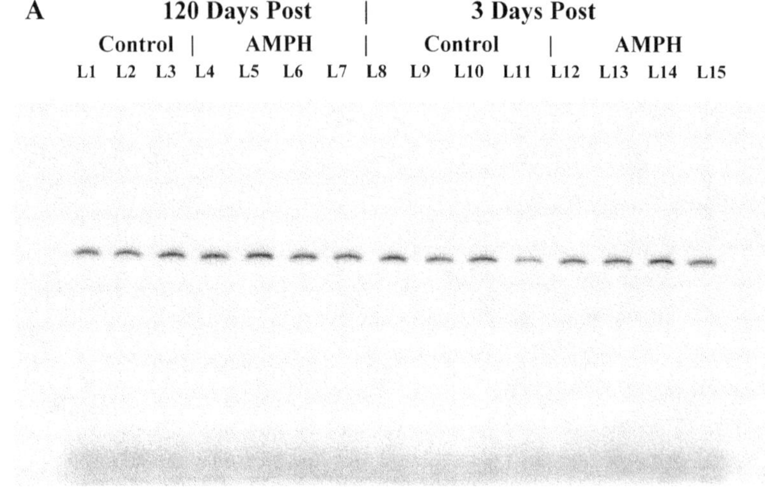

B

120 Days Post | 3 Days Post

Control | AMPH | Control | AMPH

L1 L2 L3 | L4 L5 L6 | L7 L8 L9 L10 | L11 L12 L13 L14

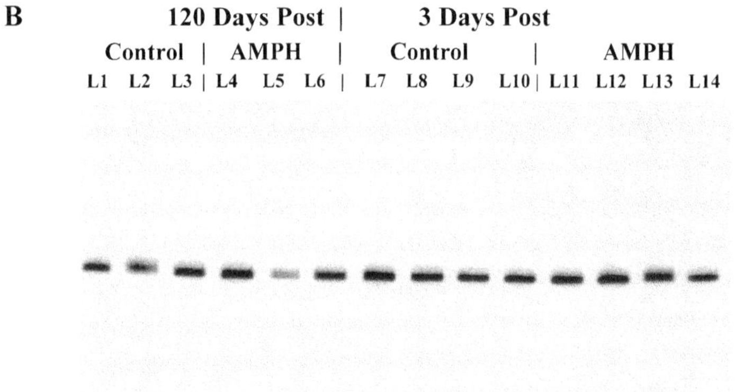

FIGURE 3. RT-PCR amplification of Hsc70 and Hsp60 mRNA in substantia nigra total RNA. **(A)** Phosphorimage of 12 µl of 50 µl RT-PCR product using Hsc70 primers and 21 PCR cycles obtained from total RNA from substantia nigra is shown. Total RNA was obtained at either 120 (control, *L1–L3*; AMPH, *L4–L7*) or 3 days (control, *L8–L11*; AMPH, *L12–L15*), and PCR products were separated on a nondenaturing 5% acrylamide gel. Each lane contains the RT-PCR products derived from the total RNA of different rats. **(B)** Phosphorimage of 12 µl of 50 µl RT-PCR product using Hsp60 primers and 23 PCR cycles obtained from total RNA from substantia nigra is shown. Total RNA was obtained at either 120 (control, *L1–L3*; AMPH, *L4–L6*) or 3 days (control, *L7–L10*; AMPH, *L11–L15*), and PCR products were separated on a non-denaturing 5% acrylamide gel. Each lane contains the RT-PCR products derived from the total RNA of different rats.

The phosphorimages of RT-PCR products of Csp1 mRNA are shown in FIGURE 5. The products were not produced with total RNA from primary cultures of cerebrum but were from total RNA from both substantia nigra and striatum. Up to 60% de-

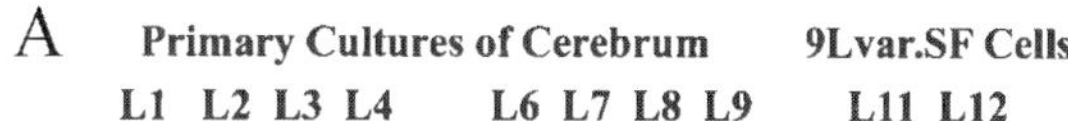

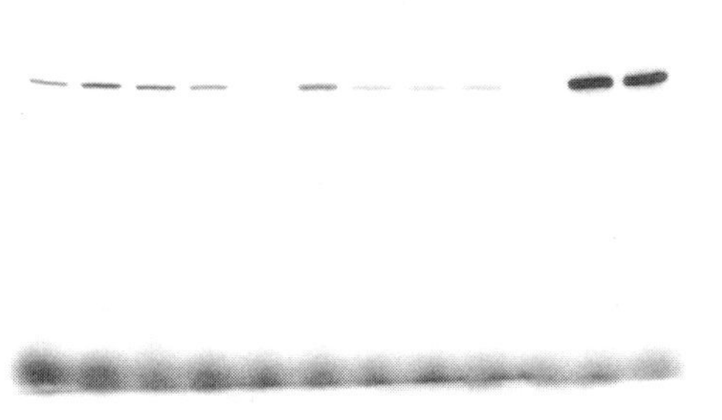

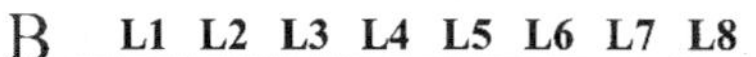

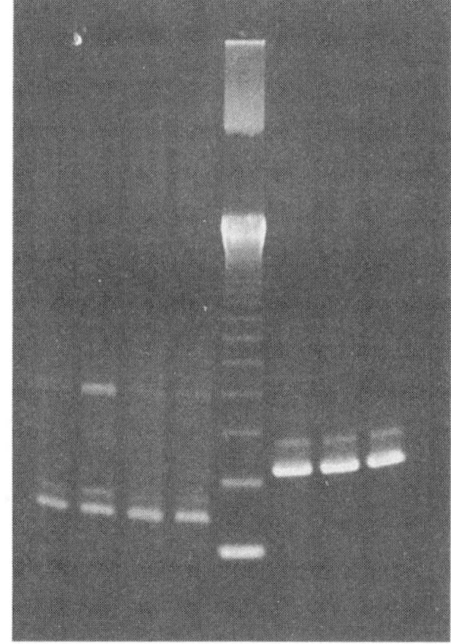

FIGURE 4. RT-PCR amplification of Hsp70 and Hsp27 mRNA in total RNA from cultured cells. **(A)** Phosphorimage of 12 µl of 50 µl RT-PCR products from Hsp70 primers and total RNA isolated from primary cortical cultures at 16–18 hr after exposure to 42°C. The RT-PCR products (*L1*, control; *L2–L4*, heat-stressed; *L5*, blank; *L6*, heat-stressed; *L7*, control; *L8* & *L9*, heat-stressed & interleukin-1β (IL-1β); *L10*, blank; *L11* & *L12*, heat-stressed 9Lvar.SF cells) were separated on a nondenaturing 5% acrylamide gel. **(B)** Ethidium bromide-labeled RT-PCR products in 12 µl of 50 µl RT-PCR products from Hsp27 primers and RNA isolated from control primary cortical cultures (*L1–L2*) primary cortical cultures at 16–18 hr after exposure to 42°C (*L3–L4*) or Hela cells after heat-stress (*L6–L8*). RT-PCR products were separated on a 2% agarose gel (*L5* contains 2 µg of 123 bp standards).

creases in the RT-PCR products for Csp1 were seen in the substantia nigra of individual rats at 16 hr and 3 days after the end of AMPH-induced hyperthermia but not 14 or 120 days post AMPH (FIG. 5, TABLE 1). Although changes in Csp1 mRNA were not seen in the striatum at the 2 early time points, at 4 months the apparent levels for Csp1 mRNA were slightly increased (TABLE 1).

CONCLUSIONS

The modest increases in Hsp70 mRNA in the rat striatum at 16 hr and 3 days after hyperthermia produced by 4 × 3 mg/kg AMPH reported herein are generally in agreement with Hsp70 protein increases in mouse striatum after a single dose of

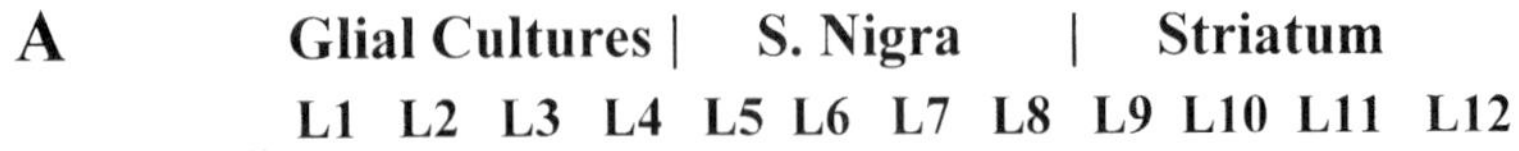

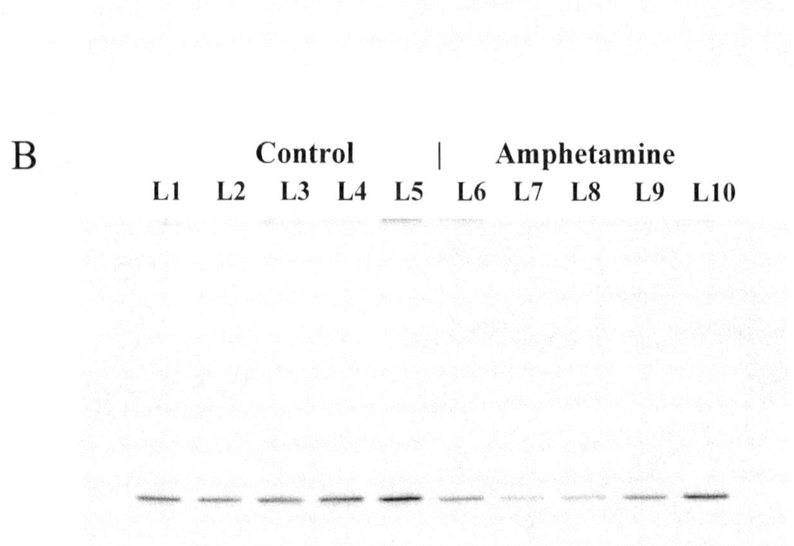

FIGURE 5. RT-PCR amplification for secretory vesicle associated cysteine-string protein (Csp1) mRNA. (**A**) Phosphorimage of 12 µl of 50 µl RT-PCR product from total RNA and Csp1 primers. RT-PCR products were separated on a nondenaturing 5% acrylamide gel. RT-PCR products from total RNA isolated from cortical primary glial cultures (*L1* & *L3*, 25 PCR cycles; *L2* & *L4*, 35 PCR cycles), substantia nigra 4 months post AMPH (25 cycles; *L5* & *L6*, control; *L7* & *L8*, AMPH), or striatum 4 months post AMPH (25 cycles; *L9* & *L10*, control; *L11* & *L12*, AMPH) are shown. (**B**) Phosphorimage of 12 µl of 50 µl RT-PCR product from Csp1 primers and total RNA isolated from substantia nigra at 1 day post either saline (*L1–L5*) or AMPH (*L6–L10*) were separated on a nondenaturing 5% acrylamide gel. Each lane contains the RT-PCR products derived from the total RNA of different rats.

20 mg/kg METH.[20] AMPH and METH would be expected to produce similar changes in Hsp, since the dose necessary to produce neurotoxicity and the neurotoxic profile of AMPH and METH to dopaminergic neurons is nearly the same in both rat and mouse.[5,6,2,13,25,21,27] Kuperman *et al.*[20] reported wide fluctuations in Hsp70 protein levels over 6-hr intervals from 12 to 48 hr after dosing. However, large fluctuations in neurotoxicity are seen after a single high dose of either AMPH or METH. The duration of hyperthermia above 40.0°C from a single high dose of either AMPH or METH is usually less than 2 hr, and is often insufficient to produce long-term dopamine depletions.[7,2,13] Consistent and pronounced long-term depletions in dopamine and tyrosine hydroxylase in the striatum were seen in the rats used in our studies. Thus, the changes in the mRNA species reported herein are truly reflective of what can occur after a exposure to neurotoxic doses of AMPH.

A minimal increase in Hsp70 mRNA was only observed at 3 days in the substantia nigra, and not 16 hr post AMPH. These changes are less than that observed in the striatum, and much less than the Hsp70 mRNA and protein increases seen in the hippocampus in mouse after high doses of METH.[18] However, although there is clear evidence for neurotoxicity occurring in the striatum, there does not appear to be significant damage to the substantia nigra compacta via the dosing regimen, age and species of rodent used in our studies.[6,3] Irrespective of the dosing paradigm, the substantia nigra does not show signs of neurodegeneration after AMPH or METH exposure.[5,28] There are two likely explanations for the discrepancy in Hsp70 increases between the substantia nigra compared to the striatum and hippocampus. Either there are fewer of the types of cells that express Hsp70 in the nigra after hyperthermia or the expression of Hsp70 is more dependent on neuronal damage than hyperthermia.

Why would a single dose of METH produce a much larger increase in Hsp70 in the hippocampus compared to the striatum when multiple dosing paradigms produce larger increases in GFAP in the striatum than in the hipporcampus?[25,20] One plausible explanation, other than that the hippocampus contains cell type(s) more susceptible to Hsp70 induction, is that a single high dose of either METH or AMPH produces seizure activity, thus, more damage to the hippocampus. This possibility is supported by the findings that more extensive damage to hippocampal and septal cells, possibly astrocytes and microglia, occur after exposure to multiple doses of either AMPH or METH that are sufficient, 4 × 15 mg/kg, to induce seizures.[6,27] Further studies are necessary to determine what type(s) of neurons or glia increase Hsp70 expression after neurotoxic doses of AMPH or METH. Also, the dosing paradigms tested should range from those that damage primarily the striatum and parietal cortex, lower doses, to higher doses that damage the hippocampus and thalamus. Our studies in rat indicate that the profiles of Hsp60, Hsc70 and Hsp70 mRNA in the striatum or substantia nigra in control and after AMPH exposure are very similar to the profile of these Hsp seen in primary cultures of rat cerebrum. These cultures contain primarily astrocytic, with few, if any, neurons present. It is possible that the increases for Hsp60, Hsc70 and Hsp70 mRNA in striatum and substantia nigra after amphetamine exposure are primarily from astrocyte mRNA. The best way to be certain which cells contribute to the Hsp70 signal would be with future studies using *in situ* hybridization techniques with cDNA probes to detect Hsp mRNA species.

Csp1 mRNA changes after AMPH exposure were also determined, since Csp1 was also known as Hsp34 and is similar to the classic type of Hsp40 and can interact with Hsp70.[8,9] Csp1 is also involved in vesicular neurotransmitter release,[37,32,23] and its effects are regulated by environmental temperature.[33,38] Therefore, changes in nigral and striatal Csp1 may even be very relevant to neurotoxicity resulting from AMPH exposure. The Csp1 described in *Drosophila* contains a series of cysteine amino acids adjacent to the Dnaj site in its protein sequence.[22,8] Csp1 deletion/dysfunction mutation blocks impulse-mediated neurotransmitter release at elevated environmental temperatures, and plays a role in the coupling of Ca^{2+} influx to vesicular release of neurotransmitter in invertebrates.[31,9,10] Because its sequence is so closely conserved between species, and the protein is concentrated in presynaptic nerve terminals,[37,8] it is likely that it also interacts with vesicular release in rat and other mammals as it does in *Drosophila*.

Two likely causes for the transient decrease in Csp1 mRNA in the substantia nigra after AMPH exposure are 1) a response to damage and/or 2) a downregulation in reaction to AMPH exposure. There were no "classic" signs of neurotoxicity in substantia nigra at any time point, and Hsp70 levels were minimally increased at 3 days after AMPH exposure. Therefore, Csp1 changes may not be a direct effect of damage. However, the Csp1 decreases could be an indirect result of the damage that occurs in the striatum. There are regulatory changes that occur after AMPH or METH exposure that lead to the behavioral phenomenon of AMPH "sensitization,"[34] and it is possible that downregulation of Csp1 may be due to a similar type of phenomenon. A significant release of vesicular stores of dopamine may occur during exposure to neurotoxic doses of AMPH and METH, although much of the dopamine released during METH and AMPH exposure may be of nonvesicular origin.[4] Therefore, downregulation of Csp1 would be a response that could decrease dopamine release at elevated environmental temperatures, and thus be a neuroprotective adaptation. It is not known why or how a slight long-term increase in Csp1 mRNA in the striatum occurs after 4 months. Long-term increases in the catecholamine synthesizing enzyme tyrosine hydroxylase also occur 4 months after AMPH.[3] It is possible that these changes are in response to the damage produced in dopaminergic terminals by AMPH.

In summary, only 2-fold changes in inducible Hsp70 mRNA were only seen in the striatum and not in the substantia nigra after AMPH, while changes in Hsp60 and Hsc70 mRNA levels did not occur. The moderate increase in Hsp70 may reflect that the striatum, but not the substantia nigra, most often shows histological evidence for neuronal damage.[28] However, the overall increase in Hsp70 mRNA would not appear to be sufficient to protect against, or be involved in the generation of, AMPH and METH toxicity unless the increase was due to a large increase in selected neurons or glia. The profile of Hsp27, Hsp60, Hsc70 and Hsp70 in the striatum is very similar to that of primary cultures of adult cerebrum (primarily consisting of astrocytes) under control and heat-stressed conditions. Thus whole tissue levels of Hsp mRNA could primarily reflect glia and not neuronal levels. The changes seen in Csp1 mRNA levels after AMPH exposure may indicate either a response to damage or a neuroregulatory response.

REFERENCES

1. ASKEW, B.M. 1962. Hyperpyrexia as a contributory factor in the toxicity of amphetamine to aggregated mice. Br. J. Pharmacol. **19:** 245–257.

2. BOWYER, J.F., D.L. DAVIES, L. SCHMUED, H.W. BROENING, G.D. NEWPORT, W. SLIKKER & R.R. HOLSON. 1994. Further studies of the role of hyperthermia in methamphetamine neurotoxicity. J. Pharmacol. Exp. Ther. **268:** 1571–1580.

3. BOWYER, J.F., L.T. FRAME, P. CLAUSING, K. NAGAMOTO-COMBS, C.A. OSTERHOUT, C. STERLING & A.W. TANK. 1998. Long-term effects of amphetamine neurotoxicity on tyrosine hydroxylase mRNA and protein in aged rats. J. Pharmacol. Exp. Ther. **286:** 1074–1085.

4. BOWYER, J.F., B. GOUGH, H.W. BROENING, G.D. NEWPORT & L. SCHMUED. 1993. Fluoro-gold and pentamidine inhibit the *in vitro* and *in vivo* release of dopamine in the striatum of rat. J. Pharmacol. Exp. Ther. **266:** 1066–1074.

5. BOWYER, J.F. & R.R. HOLSON. 1995. Methamphetamine and amphetamine neurotoxicity. *In* Handbook of Neurotoxicology. L.W. Chang & R.S. Dyer, Eds.: 845–870. Marcel Dekker. New York.

6. BOWYER, J.F., S.J. PETERSON, R.L. ROUNTREE, J. TOR-AGBIDYE & G.J. WANG. 1998. Neuronal degeneration in rat forebrain resulting from *d*-amphetamine-induced convulsions is dependent on seizure severity and age. Brain Res. **809:** 77–90.

7. BOWYER, J.F., A.W. TANK, G.D. NEWPORT, W. SLIKKER, JR., S.F. ALI & R.R. HOLSON. 1992. The influence of environmental temperature on the transient effects of methamphetamine on dopamine levels and dopamine release in rat striatum. J. Pharmacol. Exp. Ther. **260:** 817–824.

8. BRAUN, J.E. & R.H. SCHELLER. 1995. Cystein string protein, a DnaJ family member, is present on diverse secretory vesicles. Neuropharmacology **34:** 1361–1369.

9. CHAMBERLAIN, L.H. & R.D. BURGOYNE. 1997. Activation of the ATPase activity of heat-shock proteins Hsc70/Hsp70 by cysteine-string protein. Biochem. J. **322:** 853–858.

10. CHAMBERLAIN, L.H. & R.D. BURGOYNE. 1998. Cysteine string protein functions directly in regulated exocytosis. Mol. Biol. Cell **9:** 2259–2267.

11. CHANCE, M.R.A. 1947. Factors influencing the toxicity of sympathomimetic amines in solitary mice. JPET **89:** 289–296.

12. CHOMCZYNSKI, P. 1993. A reagent for the single-step simultaneous isolation of RNA, DNA and proteins from cell and tissue samples. Biotechnology **15:** 532–537.

13. CLAUSING, P., B. GOUGH, R.R. HOLSON, W. SLIKKER, JR., & J.F. BOWYER. 1995. Amphetamine levels in brain microdialysate, caudate putamen, substantia nigra and plasma after dosage that produces either behavioral or neurotoxic effects. J. Pharmacol. Exp. Ther. **274:** 614–621.

14. COMMINS, D.L. & L.S. SEIDEN. 1986. Alpha-methyltyrosine blocks methylamphetamine-induced degeneration in the rat somatosensory cortex. Brain Res. **365:** 15–20.

15. COSGROVE, J.W. & I.R. BROWN. 1983. Heat shock protein in mammalian brain and other organs after a physiologically relevant increase in body temperature induced by D-lysergic acid diethylamide. Proc. Natl. Acad. Sci. USA **80:** 569–573.

16. DAVIES, D.L. & W.E. COX. 1991. Delayed growth and maturation of astrocytic cultures following exposure to ethanol: electron microscopic observations. Brain Res. **546:** 53–61.

17. EISCH, A.J. & J.F. MARSHALL. 1998. Methamphetamine neurotoxicity: dissociation of striatal dopamine terminal damage from parietal cortical cell body injury. Synapse **30:** 433–445.

18. GOTO, S., K. KOREMATSU, T. OYAMA, K. YAMADA, J. HAMADA, N. INOUE, S. NAGAHIRO & Y. USHIO. 1993. Neuronal induction of 72-kDa heat shock protein following methamphetamine-induced hyperthermia in the mouse hippocampus. Brain Res. **626:** 351–356.

19. KNUSEL, B. & F. HEFTI. 1988. Development of cholinergic pedunculopontine neurons *in vitro*: comparison with cholinergic septal cells and response to nerve

growth factor, cilliary neurotrophic factor and retinoic acid. J. Neurosci. Res. **21:** 365–375.

20. KUPERMAN, D.I., T.E. FREYALDENHOVEN, L.C. SCHMUED & S.F. ALI. 1997. Methamphetamine-induced hyperthermia in mice: examination of dopamine depletions and heat-shock protein induction. Brain Res. **771:** 221–227.

21. MELEGA, W.P., A.E. WILLIAMS, D.A. SCHMITZ, E.W. DISTEFANO & A.K. CHO. 1995. Pharmacokinetic and pharmacodynamic analysis of the actions of *d*-amphetamine and *d*-methamphetamine on the dopamine terminal. J. Pharmacol. Exp. Ther. **274:** 90–96.

22. MOSTROGIACOMO, A. & C.B. GUNDERSEN. 1995. The nucleotide and deduced amino acid sequence of a rat cysteine string protein. Mol. Brain Res. **28:** 12–18.

23. MOSTROGIACOMO, A., S.M. PARSONS, G.A. ZAMPIGHI, D.J. JENDEN, J.A. UMBACH & C.B. GUNDERSEN. 1994. Cysteine string proteins: a potential link between synaptic vesicles and presynaptic Ca^{2+} channels. Science **263:** 981–982.

24. NOWAK, T.S. 1988. Effects of amphetamine on protein synthesis and energy metabolism in mouse brain: role of drug-induced hyperthermia. J. Neurochem. **50:** 285–294.

25. O'CALLAGHAN, J.P. & D.B. MILLER. 1994. Neurotoxicity profiles of substituted amphetamines in the C57BL/6J mouse. J. Pharmacol. Exp. Ther. **270:** 741–751.

26. RANJAN, R., P. BRONK & K.E. ZINSMAIER. 1998. Cysteine string protein is required for calcium secretion coupling of evoked neurotransmission in *Drosophila* but not for vesicle recycling. J. Neurosci. **18:** 956–964.

27. SCHMUED, L.C. & J.F. BOWYER. 1997. Methamphetamine exposure can produce neuronal degeneration in mouse hippocampal remnants. Brain Res. **759:** 135–140.

28. SEIDEN, L.S. & K.E. SABOL. 1995. Neurotoxicity of methamphetamine-related drugs and cocaine. *In* Handbook of Neurotoxicology. L.W. Chang & R.S. Dyer, Eds. Vol. 2: 824–844. Marcel Dekker, Inc. New York, Basel, Hong Kong.

29. STERNBERGER, L.A., P.H. HARDY, J.J. CUCULIS & H.G. MEYER. 1970. The unlabeled antibody-enzyme method of immunohistochemistry: preparation and properties of soluble antigen-antibody complex (horseradish peroxidase-anti-horseradish peroxidase) and its use in the identification of spirochetes. J. Histochem. Cytochem. **18:** 315–333.

30. TYTELL, M., M.F. BARBE & I.R. BROWN. 1993. Stress (heat shock) protein accumulation in the central nervous system: its relationship to cell stress and damage. Adv. Neurol. **59:** 293–303.

31. UMBACH, J.A. & C.B. GUNDERSON. 1997. Evidence that cyteine string proteins regulate an early step in the Ca^{2+}-dependent secretion of neurotransmitter at *Drosophila* neuromuscular junctions. J. Neurosci. **17:** 7203–7209.

32. UMBACH, J.A., K.E. ZINSMAIER, K.K. EBERLE, E. BUCHNER, S. BENZER & C.B. GUNDERSON. 1994. Presynaptic dysfunction in *Drosophila* csp mutants. Neuron **13:** 899–908.

33. VAN DE GOOR, J., M. RAMASWAMI & R. KELLY. 1995. Redistribution of synaptic vesicles and their proteins in temperature-sensitive shibire (ts1) mutant *Drosophila*. Proc. Natl. Acad. Sci. USA **92:** 5739–5743.

34. WOLF, M.E. 1998. The role of excitatory amino acids in behavioral sensitization to psychomotor stimulants. Prog. Neurobiol. **54:** 679–720.

35. ZALIS, E.G., G.D. LUNDBERG & R.A. KNUTSON. 1967. The pathophysiology of acute amphetamine poisoning with pathologic correlation. J. Phrrmacol. Exp. Ther. **158:** 115–127.

36. ZALIS, E.G. & L. F. PARMLEY, JR. 1963. Fatal amphetamine poisoning. Arch. Int. Med. **112:** 822–826.

37. ZINSMAIER, K.E., A. HOFBAUER, G.O. HEINBECK, G.O. PFLUGFELDER, S. BUCHNER & E. BUCHNER. 1990. A cysteine-string protein is expressed in retina and brain of *Drosophila*. J. Neurogenet. **7:** 15–19.
38. ZINSMAIER, K.E., K.K. EBERLE, E. BUCHNER, N. WALTER & S. BENZER. 1994. Paralysis and early death in cysteine string protein mutants of *Drosophila*. Science **263:** 997–980.

Benzamide, a Poly(ADP-Ribose) Polymerase Inhibitor, Is Neuroprotective against Soman-Induced Seizure-Related Brain Damage[a]

H.L. MEIER,[b,d] G.P.H. BALLOUGH,[c] J.S. FORSTER,[b] AND M.G. FILBERT[b]

[b]*Pharmacology Division, US Army Medical Research Institute of Chemical Defense, Aberdeen Proving Ground, Maryland 21010-5400, USA*

[c]*La Salle University, Department of Biology, Philadelphia, Pennsylvania 19141-1199, USA*

INTRODUCTION

Soman is an organophosphorous nerve agent that irreversibly inhibits acetylcholinesterase, causing a rapid rise in acetylcholine levels. This high elevation of acetylcholine over a 5–20-min period leads to limbic seizures and seizure-related brain damage (SRBD).[1] There is considerable evidence that soman-induced SRBD stems from glutamate excitotoxicity,[2] which, in turn, generates DNA-damaging free radicals. This hypothesis is supported by the exacerbation in excitotoxicity of glutamate due to a decrease in adenosine triphosphate (ATP).[3,4] The linkage of DNA damage, metabolic impairment, and cell death was first formulated by Berger.[5] He formulated an energy-dependent hypothesis to explain the cytotoxic action of DNA alkylating agents. He proposed that alkylation of DNA causes activation of the nuclear enzyme poly(ADP-ribose) polymerase (EC 2.4.2.30, PARP) and results in depletion of ATP. This hypothesis appears to be relevant to any cytotoxic event in which DNA damage causes depletion of cellular ATP. Bis-(2-chloroethyl) sulfide (SM), a potent DNA alkylating agent, was used to study and validate Berger's hypothesis. The mechanism of SM cytotoxicity in human lymphocytes was shown to result in necrotic cell death,[6] which is a consequence of decreasing ATP.[7] SM also causes disruption of the nuclear and plasma membranes[8] as well as other biochemical and morphologic changes in the lymphocytes consistent with necrotic cell death.[9] Inhibitors of PARP (PARPI) were effective at altering or blocking the SM-dependent changes.[6,7,9] PARPI converts the SM-initiated necrotic pattern of cell death to what appears to be non-inflammatory apoptotic changes.[6] Since both soman and SM have been shown to cause energy-dependent necrotic cell death, it was decided to examine whether PARPI would be as effective at blocking the cellular damage of SRBD as the PARPI were in reducing SM-induced cellular injury. This decision was supported by the findings that the prevention of ATP depletion by administration of PARPI provides considerable neuroprotection in various excitotoxic models.[11,12]

[a]In conducting the research described in this report, the investigators adhered to the Guide for the Care and Use of Laboratory Animals, published by the Institute of Laboratory Animal Resources, National Research Council.

[d]Address for correspondence: Commander, USAMIRCD, Attn.: MCMR-UV-PB (Dr. Meier), 3100 Ricketts Pt. Rd., APG, MD 21010-5400. Fax, 410/436-1960.

e-mail, Henry.Meier@AMEDD.Army.Mil

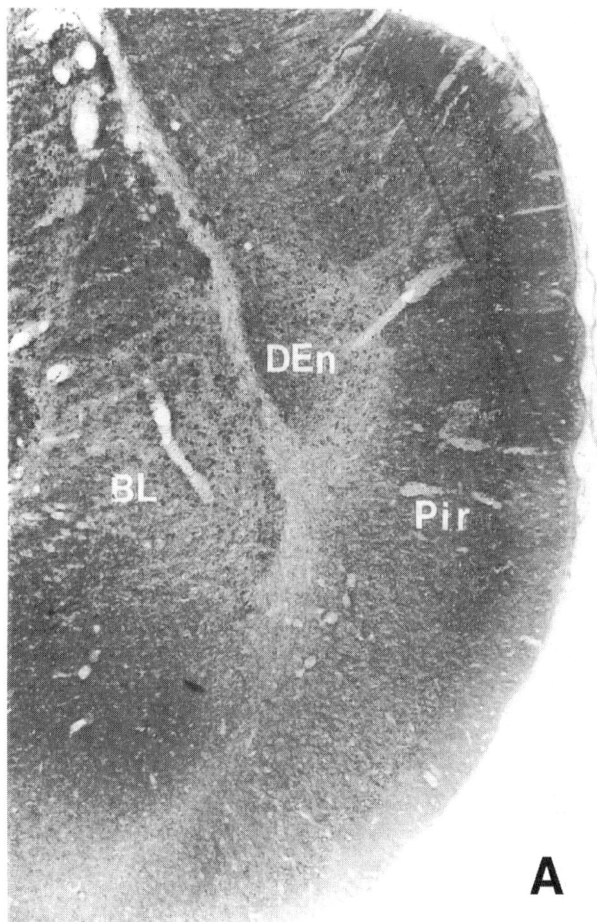

FIGURE 1. MAP-2 immunohistochemical staining of rat temporal lobe shows lesions produced by soman and neuroprotection by benzamide therapy at 40 min and 120 min after onset of seizures. This figure contains pictures of similar rat brain sections exposed to control (**A**), soman alone (**B**), and soman with the PARP inhibitor added at 40/120 min post-soman initiated seizure onset (**C**). The sections are labeled to identify the dorsal endopiriform nucleus (Den), basolateral amygdala (BL), and the piriform cortex (Pir) for orientation. The brown staining is the presence of the MAP-2 protein in the viable neurons. The staining of the piriform cortex is greatly decreased in the brains from soman-treated animals (**B**). There is a protection of the axons in the piriform cortex in the rats given benzamide.

METHODS

Male Sprague-Dawley rats were challenged with 180 μg/kg, s.c. soman (i.e., 1.6 LD_{50}). HI-6 (125 mg/kg, i.p.) and atropine methylnitrite (2 mg/kg, i.m.) were administered to protect against the peripheral effects of soman. Animals were subsequently

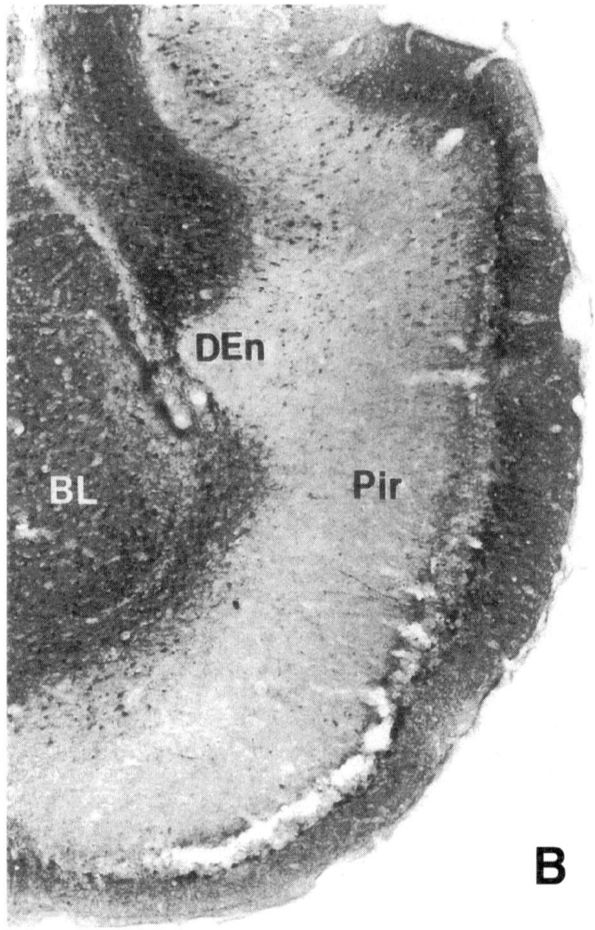

FIGURE 1B

given two intraperitoneal injections of either saline or 320 mg/kg benzamide in saline 5 and 40 min post-seizure onset. Rats were observed for convulsions during the 5-hr post-soman injection period. They were also assessed for convulsions at 29 hr after soman administration just before they were euthanized.[10] Their brains were longitudinally divided into left and right hemispheres, and alternate hemispheres were processed for microtubule-associated protein 2 (MAP-2) immunohistochemical staining.[10] Macroscopic temporal lobe necrosis was assessed using morphometric image analysis of MAP-2-negative immunostaining. The above paradigm yielded five treatment groups: (1) soman positive controls, $n = 18$; (2) non-soman negative controls, $n = 6$; (3) benzamide controls, $n = 2$; (4) soman and benzamide, 5/40-min regimen, $n = 7$; (5) soman and benzamide, 40/120-min regimen, $n = 5$. Lesion volumes were determined by summing cross-sectional areas of temporal lobe necrosis

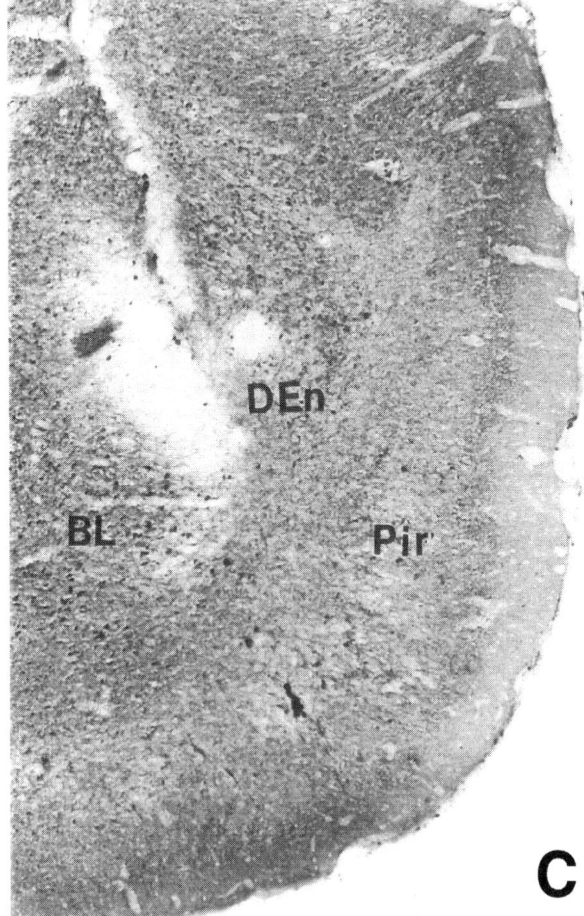

FIGURE 1C

in coronal brain sections, along the anterior posterior axis. Median lesion volumes
were compared between groups using Kruskal-Wallis and Mann-Whitney nonparametric analysis of variance by ranks.

RESULTS

Soman initiated convulsions and seizures in rats within 5–12 min post-exposure
appeared to result in SRBD.[10] Rats not treated with benzamide convulsed throughout the 5-hr observation period after soman administration and still had evidence of
convulsions until they were euthanized. Animals experiencing unabated soman-induced convulsions exhibited profound SRBD. Soman-induced SRBD was evident
when the brain sections from a control rat (FIG. 1A) were compared with brain sections from a soman-treated rat (FIG. 1B). The latter exhibited temporal lobe necrosis

involving the piriform cortex and contiguous brain regions. In the temporal lobe, SRBD appeared white, a result of the loss of MAP-2 immunostaining that correlates to neuronal necrosis. The median lesion volume in the soman-treated animals was 10.8 mm^3. No lesions were detected in the control animals.

When soman-treated rats were given benzamide, their convulsions stopped within 5 min of the initial injection. The cessation of convulsions in the rats was independent of the time course of the injection of benzamide. The continuous occurrence of convulsions did not resume during the experimental period. These animals, like the control benzamide rats, were nonambulatory for less than an hour after the injection of benzamide. When the brains from the benzamide-treated rats were assessed for lesion size (FIG. 1C), there was a marked decrease in the median volume of temporal lobe necrosis. A 67% reduction in the median lesion volume was seen in rats receiving the 5/40-min regimen (FIG. 2). However, if the administration of the benzamide regimen was delayed for a longer period of time (i.e., 40/120-min regimen) the amount of protection (i.e., decrease in lesion volume) increased to 87% (FIG. 2). Rats given benzamide in the 40/120-min regimen demonstrated a similar recovery to those receiving the 5/40-min regimen.

DISCUSSION

Berger's hypothesis concerning the activation of PARP as an integral part of the cytotoxicity mechanism of alkylating agents[5] appears to center around energy deple-

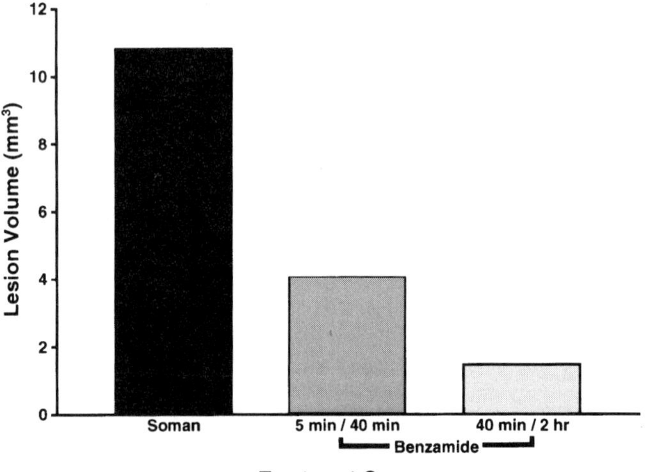

FIGURE 2. Histogram of the median volume of lesion size in the piriform cortex of soman-challenged rats. Three groups of rats were studied: Group A received soman alone, Group B received soman and then at 5 min and 40 min after seizure onset they were injected i.p. with benzamide, and Group C received soman and then at 40 min and 120 min after seizure onset they were injected i.p. with benzamide. Group C demonstrated an 87% decrease in the median volume of the soman-induced SRBD. The volumes of SRBD were calculated by measuring the lesion of many slices of each brain using image analysis.

tion resulting in necrotic cell death. However, based on the investigation of other cytotoxic agents, it appears that the energy depletion due to DNA damage may contribute to many other toxic events not involving alkylating agents. In many of these models, the ability of PARPI to alter the cytotoxic responses of broad classes of toxic events[7,11,13] suggests that the activation of PARP may play a pivotal role in the mechanism of cell death due to these events. To explore this hypothesis, benzamide, a potent PARPI that had already been shown, *in vitro*, to alter the cytotoxicity of alkylating agents,[8] was studied to determine whether it could offer neuroprotection against soman-induced SRBD in rats. Benzamide produced a reverse time-dependent neuroprotection against the loss of MAP-2. The increase in protection seen in the 40/120-min benzamide regimen suggests that there may be a delay in the generation of SRBD and that benzamide, perhaps due to a short half-life in the brain, needs to be added later when the damage is occurring. This delay in SRBD could result from a delay in DNA damage produced by free radicals. The increase in protection seen in the 40/120 regimen might result from increased benzamide availability coincident with the initiation of DNA damage. Many questions, such as why benzamide appears to better protect the 40/120 group, still need to be addressed. However, based on our results it appears that Berger's hypothesis[5] is relevant to the mechanism by which soman initiates SRBD.

REFERENCES

1. TAYLOR, P. 1985. Anticholinesterase agents. *In* The Pharmacological Basis of Therapeutics. 6th edit. A.G. Gilman, L.S. Goodman, T.W. Rall & F. Musad, Eds.: 110–129. Macmillan. New York.
2. GREENE, J.O. & J.T. GREENAMYRE. 1996. Prog. Neurobiol. **48:** 613–634.
3. ZEEVALK, G.D. L. BERNARD, C. SINHA, J. EHRHART & W. NICKLAS. 1998. Dev. Neurosci. **20:** 444–453.
4. HOYT, K.R., I.J. REYNOLDS & T.G. HASTINGS. 1997. Exp. Neurol. **143:** 269–281.
5. BERGER, N.A., G.W. SIKORSKI, S.J. PETZOLD & K.K. KUROHARA. 1979. J. Clin. Invest. **63:** 1164–1171.
6. MEIER, H.L. & C.B. MILLARD. 1998. Biochim. Biophys. Acta **1404:** 367–376.
7. MEIER, H.L., E.T. CLAYSON, S.A. KELLY & C.M. CORUN. 1996. *In Vitro* Toxicol. **9:** 135–139.
8. MILLARD, C.B., H.L. MEIER & C.A. BROOMFIELD. 1994. Biochim. Biophys. Acta **1224:** 389–394.
9. CLAYSON, E.T., S.A. KELLY & H.L. MEIER. 1993. Cell Biol. & Toxicol. **9:** 165–175.
10. BALLOUGH, G.P.H., L.J. MARTIN, G.J. CANN, J.S. GRAHAM, C.D. SMITH, C.E. KLING, J.S. FORSTER, S. PHANN & M.G. GILBERT. 1995. J. Neurosci. Methods **61:** 23–32.
11. COSI, C., H. SUZUKI, S.D. SKAPER, D. MILANI, L. FACCI, M. MENEGAZZI, G. VANTINI, Y. KANAI, A. DEGRYSE, F. COLPAERT, W. KOEK & M.R. MARIEN. 1997. Ann. N.Y. Acad. Sci. **825:** 366–379.
12. HIVERT, B. 1998. Neuroreport **9:** 1835–1838.
13. SZABO, C., L.H. LIM, S. CUZZOCREA, S.J. GETTING, B. ZINGARELLI, R.J. FLOWER, A.L. SALZMAN & M. PERRETTI. 1997. J. Exp. Med. **186:** 1041–1049.

Central Noradrenergic Neurotoxicity of DSP4 in Mice

Studies on the Neuroprotective Potential of the Poly(ADP-Ribose) Polymerase Inhibitor, Benzamide

MARC MARIEN[a] AND CRISTINA COSI

Divisions of Neurobiology I and II, Centre de Recherche Pierre Fabre, Castres, France

Poly(ADP-ribose) polymerase (PARP) is a DNA binding enzyme that uses nicotinamide adenine nucleotide (NAD^+) as a substrate in the poly(ADP-ribosyl)ation of nuclear proteins (including histones, topoisomerases, DNA and RNA polymerases, DNA ligases and endonucleases) that are involved in DNA plasticity-related phenomena. PARP is activated by nicks in the DNA molecule induced by different damaging agents, including free radicals. When fully activated, PARP can deplete NAD^+ and consequently adenosine triphosphate (ATP) energy stores within a matter of minutes, and to an extent that would conceivably lead to severe cellular dysfunction and death.[1] Inhibitors of PARP, including benzamide (BNZ), have been shown to protect against brain catecholamine depletions induced by 1-methyl-4-phenyl-1,2,3,6-tetrahydropyridine (MPTP)[2] and methamphetamine[3] in the C57BL/6 mouse, suggesting a role for PARP in these models of neurotoxicity where free radicals are thought to play a causative role. In addition, the ability of BNZ to prevent MPTP-induced decreases in striatal and midbrain levels of ATP and NAD^+ have suggested an involvement of PARP in the control of brain energy metabolism during this type of neurotoxic insult (Ref. 4, and this meeting). To extend these studies to another model of central catecholamine neurotoxicity, but one which is induced by a different mechanism of action, BNZ was tested against the cortical noradrenergic terminal degeneration, i.e., the long-lasting depletion of cortical noradrenaline (NA), produced in the C57BL/6 mouse by DSP4 (*N*-2-chloroethyl-2-bromobenzylamine), a neurotoxin whose action involves hydrolysis to a quaternary aziridium ion (a highly reactive alkylating species) and whose selectivity for NA terminals is dependent on a functional NA transporter (i.e., desipramine-sensitive).[5]

Male C57BL/6 mice were injected intraperitoneally (i.p.) with drugs as indicated in the TABLE legends, and killed by head-focused microwave irradiation.[4] Monoamines and metabolites, adenine nucleotides and NAD^+ levels were quantified in perchloric acid extracts of frontoparietal cortical tissue by high-performance liquid chromatography (HPLC).[4] In an acute time-course study (TABLE 1), DSP4 produced an initial transient increase (at 0.5–2 hr) and a later decrease (at 6 and 24 hr) in normetanephrine levels (index of NA release[6]), and a rapid and progressive deple-

[a]Corresponding author: Marc Marien, Ph.D., Division de Neurobiologie I, Centre de Recherche Pierre Fabre, 17 ave. Jean Moulin, 81106 Castres, France. Phone, +33-5-63-71-42-86; fax, +33-5-63-71-43-63.

e-mail, marc.marien@pierre-fabre.com

TABLE 1. Acute time-course effects of DSP4 (single injection of 40 mg/kg, i.p.) on frontocortical levels of noradrenaline, normetanephrine, adenosine triphosphate (ATP) and nicotinamide adenine nucleotide (NAD^+)

Treatment	Time (hr) after treatment	Normetanephrine fmol/mg Tissue		Noradrenaline fmol/mg Tissue		ATP pmol/mg Tissue		NAD+ pmol/mg Tisssue	
Vehicle	0.5	38.3 ± 2.6		2696 ± 41		2523 ± 44		533 ± 11	
DSP4	0.5	77.2 ± 1.9**	*+102%*	2320 ± 42**	*−14%*	2075 ± 65**	*−18%*	449 ± 14**	*−16%*
DSP4	1	76.1 ± 5.8**	*+99%*	1895 ± 35**	*−30%*	2077 ± 40**	*−18%*	458 ± 6**	*−14%*
DSP4	1.5	58.0 ± 2.9**	*+51%*	1738 ± 87**	*−36%*	2022 ± 133**	*−20%*	458 ± 20**	*−14%*
DSP4	2	65.4 ± 2.1**	*+71%*	1420 ± 38**	*−47%*	2041 ± 74**	*−19%*	452 ± 7**	*−15%*
DSP4	3	38.7 ± 4.0		1075 ± 44**	*−60%*	2115 ± 22**	*−16%*	453 ± 6**	*−15%*
DSP4	4	39.7 ± 1.7		945 ± 18**	*−65%*	2185 ± 47**	*−13%*	454 ± 10**	*−15%*
DSP4	6	23.2 ± 4.3*	*−39%*	690 ± 81**	*−74%*	2215 ± 42**	*−12%*	459 ± 6**	*−14%*
Vehicle	24	34.0 ± 1.7		2651 ± 29		2461 ± 45		526 ± 11	
DSP4	24	15.8 ± 3.0††	*−53%*	547 ± 83††	*−79%*	2209 ± 40††	*−10%*	463 ± 11††	*−12%*

NOTE: Each analyte was measured in the same tissue sample. Values are means ± SEM, 6–7 mice per group. Values in italics are % change vs corresponding vehicle control. $*p < 0.05$, $**p < 0.01$ vs levels in vehicle-treated group at 30 min; $††p < 0.01$ vs vehicle group at 24 hr (Kruskal-Wallis ANOVA + Mann-Whitney U-test).

TABLE 2. Acute effects of benzamide (BNZ) on DSP4-induced decreases in frontocortical noradrenaline and NAD$^+$ levels, and ATP/ADP ratios

Treatment	Noradrenaline pmol/mg Tissue		NAD$^+$ pmol/mg Tissue		ATP/ADP	
Veh + veh	2850 ± 74		490 ± 9		2.771 ± 0.080	
Veh + DSP4	812 ± 68 **	*−72%*	448 ± 20*	*−9%*	2.558 ± 0.085*	*−8%*
BNZ + DSP4	1169 ± 104**†	*−59%*	460 ± 12		2.622 ± 0.089	
BNZ + veh	2579 ± 139		472 ± 15		2.875 ± 0.091	

NOTE: Each measure was made in the same tissue sample of mice killed 6 hr after DSP4 (40 mg/kg, i.p.). BNZ (160 mg/kg, i.p.) or its vehicle (veh) was injected at 0.5 hr before and 3.5 hr after DSP4 or its vehicle. Values are means ± SEM, 13–14 mice per group. Values in *italics* are % change vs corresponding vehicle control. *$p < 0.05$, **$p < 0.01$ vs veh + veh group. †$p < 0.01$ vs veh + DSP4 group (Kruskal-Wallis ANOVA + Mann-Whitney U-test).

TABLE 3. Frontocortical noradrenaline levels in mice 7 days after DSP4 (40 mg/kg, i.p.)

Treatment Group	Noradrenaline fmol/mg Tissue	% Change vs. Veh + Veh Group
veh + veh	3017 ± 28	
veh + DSP4	1034 ± 218**	−66%
DMI 20 + DSP4	1909 ± 61** ††	−37%
DMI 40 + DSP4	2524 ± 107** ††	−16%
DMI 20 + veh	2879 ± 72	−5%
DMI 40 + veh	2903 ± 61	−4%
BNZ 160 + DSP4	1140 ± 66**	−62%
BNZ 640 + DSP4	1438 ± 85** †	−52%
BNZ 160 + veh	3019 ± 78	0%
BNZ 640 + veh	2902 ± 43	−4%

NOTE: Effects of cotreatments with benzamide (BNZ; 160 mg/kg or 640 mg/kg, i.p., 0.5 hr before and 3.5 hr after DSP4) or desipramine (DMI; 20 mg/kg or 40 mg/kg, i.p., 0.5 hr before DSP4). Values are means ± SEM, 13–14 mice per group. *$p < 0.05$, **$p < 0.01$ vs veh + veh group. †$p < 0.05$, ††$p < 0.01$ vs veh + DSP4 group (Kruskal-Wallis ANOVA + Mann-Whitney U-test).

tion of NA (but not dopamine or serotonin; not shown) which was maximal (74–79% reduction) at 6 and 24 hr post-injection. A novel finding was the rapid (at 0.5 hr) and persistent (at 1, 2, 3, 4, 6 and 24 hr) decreases (by 10–20%) in the cortical levels of ATP and NAD$^+$ (TABLE 1). In a second study (TABLE 2), cortical levels of NA and NAD$^+$ and the ATP/ADP ratio were decreased by 72%, 9% and 8%, respectively, at 6 hr after DSP4; cotreatment with BNZ (2×160 mg/kg, i.p.) did not significantly affect the changes in the ATP/ADP ratio or NAD$^+$ levels, and only slightly reduced the NA loss. In a third study (TABLE 3), at 7 days after DSP4, cortical NA was depleted by 66%; cotreatment with the NA transport blocker desipramine largely reduced the DSP4-induced depletion of NA, while BNZ, in dose regimens that completely prevented MPTP-induced depletions of cortical NA,[2] had little or no effect. These studies indicate that acute DSP4 toxicity (rapid cortical NA depletion within 24 hr) is associated with an early and sustained deficit in cortical ATP and

NAD[+], and show that BNZ, when coadministered with DSP4, does not exert a marked protective (i.e., desipramine-like) effect against the cortical NA loss measured at 7 days. While the results indicate little or no effect of BNZ on the early disruption of cortical NA terminals in this model, a possible influence on the delayed progressive loss of NA cell bodies in the locus coeruleus occurring at much later times after DSP4 intoxication[5] remains to be examined.

REFERENCES

1. GAAL, J.C., K.R. SMITH & C.K. PEARSON. 1987. Cellular euthanasia mediated by a nuclear enzyme: a central role for nuclear ADP-ribosylation in cellular metabolism. Trends Biochem. Sci. **12:** 128–129.
2. COSI, C., F. COLPAERT, W. KOEK, A.-D. DEGRYSE & M. MARIEN. 1996. Poly(ADP-ribose)polymerase inhibitors protect against MPTP-induced depletions of striatal dopamine and cortical noradrenaline in C57Bl/6 mice. Brain Res. **729:** 264–269.
3. COSI, C., P. CHOPIN & M. MARIEN. 1996. Benzamide, an inhibitor of poly(ADP-ribose) polymerase, attenuates methamphetamine-induced dopamine neurotoxicity in the C57Bl/6N mouse. Brain Res. **735:** 343–348.
4. COSI, C. & M. MARIEN. 1998. Decreases in mouse brain NAD[+] and ATP induced by 1-methyl-4-phenyl-1,2,3,6-tetrahydropyridine (MPTP): prevention by the poly(ADP-ribose) polymerase inhibitor, benzamide. Brain Res. **809:** 58–67.
5. JAIM-ETCHEVERRY, G. 1998. 2-Chloroethylamines (DSP4 and xylamine). *In* Highly Selective Neurotoxins: Basic and Clinical Applications. R.M. Kostrzewa, Ed.: 131–140. Humana Press. Totowa, NJ.
6. WOOD, P.L., H.S. KIM & C.A. ALTAR. 1987. *In vivo* assessment of dopamine and norepinephrine release in rat neocortex: gas chromatography–mass spectrometry measurement of 3-methoxytyramine and normetanephrine. J. Neurochem. **48:** 574–579.

The Antioxidative Effect of Carboxyfullerenes (C3/D3) on Iron-Induced Oxidative Injury in CNS

ANYA M.Y. LIN,[a,b,d] T.-Y. LUH,[c] C.K. CHOU,[a] AND L.T. HO[a,d]

[a]*Department of Medical Research and Education, Veterans General Hospital-Taipei, Taipei, Taiwan*

[b]*Department of Physiology, National Yang-Ming University, Taiwan*

[c]*Department of Chemistry, National Taiwan University, Taipei, Taiwan*

ABSTRACT: Carboxyfullerenes, including two regioisomers C3 and D3, were investigated as antioxidants against iron-induced oxidative stress *in vivo* and *in vitro*. Both C3 and D3 dose-dependently inhibited autoxidation and iron-elevated lipid peroxidation in cortical homogenates. The antioxidative property of C3 was compared to Trolox (a water-soluble analogue of vitamin E) and glutathione. C3 was more effective than glutathione but was less effective than Trolox in inhibiting iron-induced elevation in lipid peroxidation. In urethane-anesthetized rats, intranigral infusion of iron degenerated the nigrostriatal dopaminergic system, including as elevation in lipid peroxidation in the infused substantia nigra (SN) and reductions in K^+-evoked dopamine overflow and dopamine content in the ipsilateral striatum 7 days after the infusion. Local application of iron with C3 or D3 prevented iron-induced oxidative injuries. Our data suggest that carboxyfullerenes have a neuroprotective effect in preventing iron-induced oxidative injury in CNS.

INTRODUCTION

In the 1980's, fullerenes, as cage molecules, were first deduced, successfully synthesized and well characterized.[1,2] Due to their low water solubility, the investigation of the biological activity of fullerenes was hindered. Recently, two water-soluble derivatives of fullerenes have been developed, including carboxyfullerenes (carboxylic derivatives of fullerenes) and polyhydroxylated fullerenes (fullerenol-1). Since then, more biological studies have been performed on these molecules, and the action of fullerenes has become a focus of interest in the field of antioxidative research. For example, carboxyfullerenes reportedly prevented neurotoxicity evoked by *N*-methyl-D-aspartate (NMDA), by serum deprivation or exposure to the Alzheimer's disease amyloid peptide ($A\beta_{1-42}$) in cortical cell cultures.[3,4] Fullerenol-1 has been found to attenuate exsanguination-induced bronchoconstriction, which is mediated via an increase in free radicals.[5] Moreover, an electrophysiological study

[d]Corresponding authors: Drs. Anya M.Y. Lin and L.T. Ho, Department of Medical Research and Education, Veterans General Hospital-Taipei, Taipei, Taiwan. Phone, +886-2-28712121, ext.2688; fax, +886-2-28751562.

e-mail, myalin@vghtpe.gov.tw

demonstrated that inhibition by hydrogen peroxide of population spikes was prevented by fullerenol-1 in the rat hippocampal slice preparation.[6] So far, few *in vivo* studies have been reported. One animal study by Dugan and her colleagues demonstrated that chronic infusion of carboxyfullerenes by implanting miniosmotic pumps delayed both functional deterioration and death of rats carrying the human mutant superoxide dismutase gene responsible for familial amyotrophic lateral sclerosis.[3]

Due to its antioxidative property, carboxyfullerenes may be employed to suppress iron-induced oxidative stress in biological organisms. Iron, a transitional metal, is known to produce hydroxyl radicals via Fenton's reaction *in situ*.[7] In addition to the attenuated antioxidative enzyme systems,[8–11] excess iron is observed in substantia nigra in Parkinson's patients.[12,13] Accordingly, accumulated oxidative stress is suggested to be responsible for the deterioration of nigrostriatal dopaminergic system.[14–18] To prevent the oxidative injury, supplementation of iron chelators, antioxidants and upregulation of antioxidative defense enzyme systems may become therapeutic for Parkinsonism.[19] The purpose of the present study was to study the antioxidative effect of carboxyfullerenes, including two regioisomers, C3 and D3, on iron-induced oxidative stress in rat brain. First, the antioxidative property of carboxyfullerenes in inhibiting autoxidation and iron-elevated lipid peroxidation was evaluated in cortical homogenates. The antioxidative property of carboxyfullerenes was compared to other well-known antioxidants, including vitamin E and glutathione *in vitro*. In addition, the antioxidative activity of C3 and D3 was tested *in vivo* using a Parkinson's animal model, in which iron was infused in substantia nigra to induce neurodegeneration in nigrostriatal dopaminergic system of rat brain.[20–25]

METHODS

Lipid Peroxidation of Cortical Homogenates

Rats were decapitated, and cortical samples were dissected and homogenized in ice-cold Ringer's solution using a homogenizer. Cortical homogenates (50 mg/ml) were used for autoxidation and iron-induced lipid peroxidation as follows. Autoxidation: the homogenates (320 µl/tube) were incubated at 37°C for 4 hr with or without C3 or D3 (10–500 µM). Iron-induced lipid peroxidation: the homogenates were incubated at 37°C for 4 hr following an addition of ferrous citrate (iron, 1 µM) ± C3 or D3 (10–500 µM). At the end of incubation, an aliquot sample (300 µl) was transferred to a tube containing 100 µl methanol and 300 µl chloroform. The slurry was mixed and kept in ice for 15 min. After centrifugation at 8000 g for 5 min, 400 µl of chloroform extract (lower layer) was transferred to another tube containing 100 µl methanol. Lipid peroxidation was determined by measuring the levels of malondialdehyde and its dihydropyridine polymers, which emit fluorescence at 426 nm when activated by UVa at 356 nm using a spectrofluorometer (Aminco Bowman-2, USA). Statistical comparisons were made using one-way ANOVA followed by post hoc analyses.

In Vivo *Electrochemical Detection*

Adult, male Sprague-Dawley (SD) rats, weighing 250–350 g, were used. These animals were maintained according to the guidelines established in Guide for the

Care and Use of Laboratory Animals prepared by the Committee on Care and Use of Laboratory Animals of the Institute of Laboratory Animal Resources Commission on Life Sciences, National Research Council, USA (1985).

Rats were anesthetized with chloral hydrate (450 mg/kg, intraperitoneally (i.p.), Sigma, St. Louis, MO, USA) and placed in a stereotaxic instrument (David Kopf Instruments, Palo Alto, CA, USA). Rectal temperature was maintained at $37 \pm 1°C$ by a homeothermic blanket (Harvard Instruments, Southnatick, MA, USA). After skin incision and exposure of the parietal bone, holes were drilled above the cortical surface for intranigral infusion of drugs. To induce oxidative stress in the nigrostriatal dopaminergic system, iron (4.2 nmol/µl Ringer's solution) $\pm$ C3 (4.5 mM) or D3 (4.5 mM) was infused stereotaxically into substantia nigra of each hemisphere using the following coordinates: 3.2 mm anterior and 2 mm above the interaural zero; 2.1 mm lateral to the midline; 3.5 mm below the mouth bar.[26] Drug solutions were infused at a rate of 0.2 µl/min through a 30-gauge stainless steel needle for 5 min. The injection needle was held in place for an additional 5 min following drug infusion. After the surgery, rats recovered from anesthesia and were placed in home cages for 7 days.

The iron-induced oxidative effect on K^+-evoked dopamine releases in the nigrostriatal system was studied using the technique of *in vivo* electrochemical detection 7 days after intranigral infusion of drugs. Urethane-anesthetized rats (1.25 g/kg, i.p.) were placed in a stereotaxic instrument with rectal temperature maintained at $37 \pm 1°C$ as aforementioned. Regions of the skull overlaying the anterior cortex were removed bilaterally and holes were drilled above the cortical surface for implantation of electrochemical Ag/AgCl reference electrodes in the brain regions remote from the recording sites. These electrodes were cemented by dental acrylic. Chrono-amperometric measurements were recorded at 5 Hz, averaged and expressed at 1 Hz, by a computer-controlled electrochemical instrument (IVEC-10, Medical System Corporation, Greenvale, NY, USA) as previously described.[27] The working electrodes consisted of three 30-µm diameter carbon fibers, which were sealed with epoxylite in a glass pipette and then coated with nafion (5% solution; Aldrich Chemical Co., Milwaukee, WI, USA) to increase sensitivity and selectivity of electrodes for dopamine.[28] Calibration of the recording electrode was performed at room temperature using 0.1 M phosphate buffered saline solution (pH = 7.4). The linearity obtained from 4 accumulating dopamine concentrations (2–8 µM) exceeded 0.997 (i.e., correlation coefficient). The selectivity for dopamine against ascorbic acid (250 µM) was greater than 500:1. Detection limits for the measurement of extracellular dopamine was averaged 30–100 nM with a signal-to-noise ratio of 3 for recording sensors. Square-wave pulses (5 Hz) of 0V to + 0.55 V with respect to the reference were applied to the working electrode. The resulting oxidation and reduction currents were digitally integrated during the final 80% of the recording period. The ratios of peak reduction current-to-peak oxidation current (redox ratio) were used to identify the primary monoamines generating the electrochemical signals. The redox ratio of dopamine is 0.4–0.6.[29]

Drug barrels made of single glass pipettes (1.00 mm o.d; 0.58 mm i.d., World Precision Instruments Sarasota, FL, USA) were attached to the working electrode by sticky wax at a distance of 260–320 µM as an electrochemical recording assembly.[27] The solution used to evoke dopamine releases containing 110 mM KCl, 30 mM

NaCl, 2.5 mM $CaCl_2$ in micropipettes was ejected using a pneumatic pump (BH-2, Medical System Corporation, Greenvale, NY, USA) with pressure of 2.5–40 psi and duration of 5–10 sec. The amount of K^+ solution ejected was determined by measuring the changes in the fluid meniscus then calculating the volume of fluid ejected (70 nl per mm segment of the pipette). The effective tissue concentration of drugs achieved by pressure ejection is generally 3–10-fold lower than that of the drugs in the barrel.[30] The electrochemical recording assembly was lowered into the striatum with a micromanipulator (MO-10, Narishige, Japan) using the following stereotaxic coordinates: 2.0–0 mm anterior to bregma; 2.0–3.5 mm lateral to the midline and 3.0–6.0 mm in 1.0-mm steps from the surface of cortex.[26] Once a stable baseline signal was achieved, K^+-evoked dopamine releases were measured. The amplitude as concentration (μM) of neurotransmitter of an electrochemical signal was analyzed. Statistical comparisons were made using an unpaired Student *t*-test or one-way ANOVA followed by post hoc analyses.

Fluorescence Assay of Lipid Peroxidation in Substantia Nigra

At the end of each *in vivo* experiment, rats were sacrificed by decapitation. Brains were removed and substantia nigra was dissected from both hemispheres. A fluorescence assay procedure was modified to measure lipid peroxidation in substantia nigra.[31,32] The dissected tissue was homogenized in chilled 400 μl chloroform and 200 μl methanol. After centrifugation, an aliquot of the chloroform and methanol layer was scanned. The relative fluorescent intensities of samples in a cuvette were measured as relative fluorescent units (RFU) using a spectrofluorometer as aforementioned.

High-Performance Liguid Chromotography with Electrochemical Detection (HPLC-EC) Analysis of Striatal Dopamine Content

Rats were decapitated and regional dissections were performed and striata were immediately frozen in liquid nitrogen and stored at −70°C until analysis. A high-performance liquid chromotography with electrochemical detection (HPLC-EC) procedure was used to quantify dopamine content in striatum.[32]

RESULTS AND DISCUSSION

Effects of Carboxyfullerenes on Lipid Peroxidation of Brain Homogenates

The discovery of fullerenes has shed illumination on the field of the antioxidative research. In the present study, the antioxidative properties of C3 and D3 against iron-induced oxidative stress were compared using an autoxidation study that was induced by endogenous iron and an iron-induced lipid peroxidation study. Brain homogenates were incubated at 37°C for 4 hr, and the formation of peroxidized lipids was increased compared to those incubated at 0°C. Coincubation of C3 or D3 dose-dependently suppressed autoxidation (FIG. 1). C3 was more potent than D3 (FIG. 1). Addition of iron (1 μM) further enhanced lipid peroxidation in brain homogenates following a 4-hr incubation at 37°C. Coincubation with C3 or D3 (10–500 μM) pre-

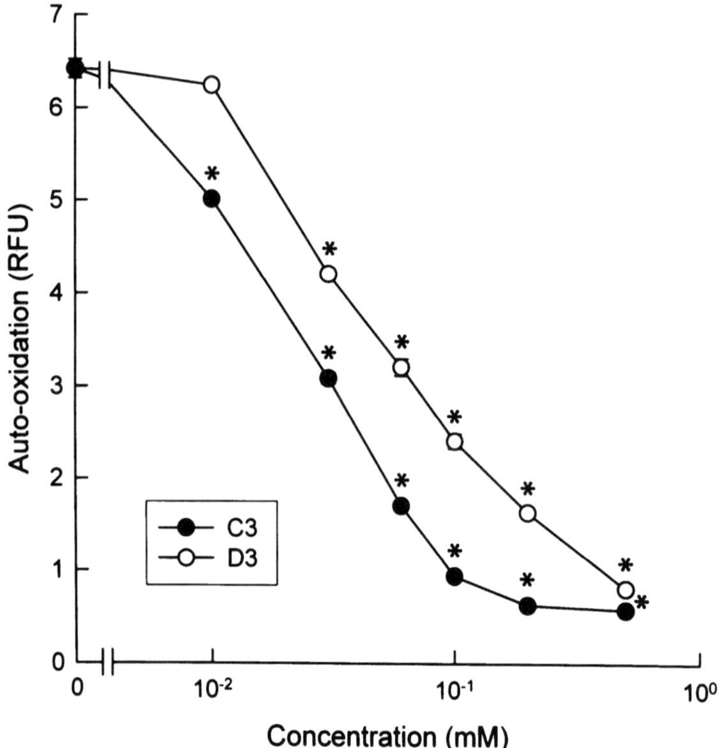

FIGURE 1. Effects of C3 and D3 on autoxidation in cortical homogenates. The brain lipid peroxidation (LP) was reported as relative fluorescence units (RFU). Values are the mean $\pm$ SEM ($n = 4$–5) from a representative experiment that was replicated with similar results. *$p < 0.05$ in C3 ($\bullet$) group or D3 ($\circ$) group compared to the control group by one-way ANOVA followed by post hoc analyses.

vented iron-induced increase in lipid peroxidation in a concentration-dependent manner (FIG. 2). C3 were more efficacious than D3 in inhibiting iron-induced lipid peroxidation (FIG. 2). In addition to our data, which demonstrated discrepancies between these two regioisomers in suppressing iron-oxidative stress, other studies have reported that C3 was more effective than D3 in preventing NMDA- and in α-amino-3-hydroxy-5-methylisoxazole-4-propionic acid (AMPA)-induced neurotoxicity.[4] The mechanisms underlying different potencies of the regioisomers, C3 and D3 require more investigation.

Furthermore, the antioxidative potency of C3 was compared to other well-known antioxidants. Our data showed that C3 was less effective than Trolox (a water-soluble analogue of vitamin E) in inhibiting lipid peroxidation in cortical homogenates (FIG. 3). However, C3 was much more potent than glutathione and melatonin,[25] which has been proposed as a potent antioxidant.[33]

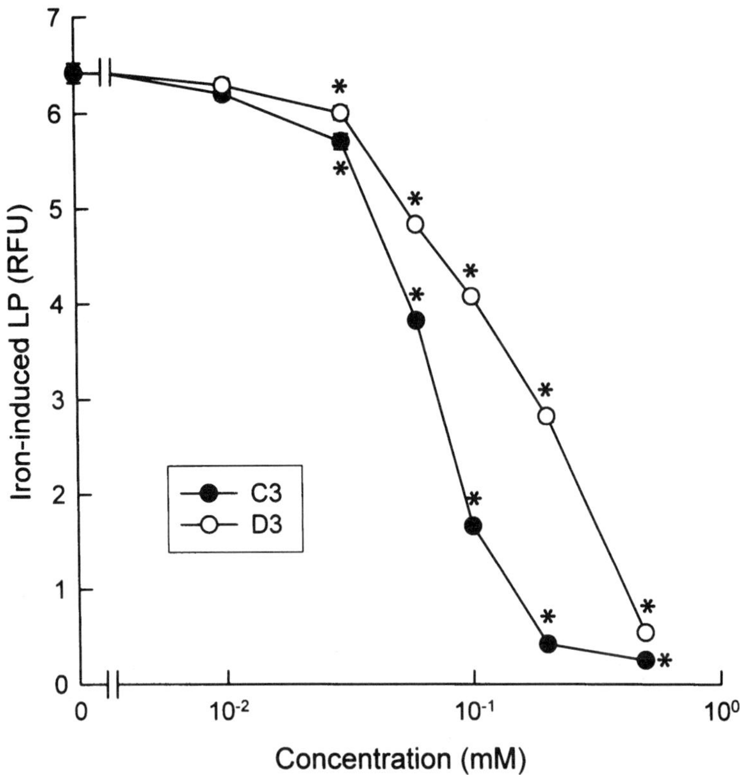

FIGURE 2. Effects of C3 and D3 on iron-induced lipid peroxidation (LP) in cortical homogenates. The brain LP was reported as relative fluorescence units (RFU). Values are the mean ± SEM (n = 4–5) from a representative experiment that was replicated with similar results. *p < 0.05 in C3 group (●) or in D3 (○) group compared to the control group by one-way ANOVA followed by post hoc analyses.

Chronic Effect of Intranigral Infusion of C3 in Rat Brain

Although the discovery of fullerenes has generated much interest in the field of antioxidative research, there is much controversy about whether fullerenes are antioxidants and/or prooxidants. For example, several studies have shown fullerene-induced production of free radicals.[34–36] Antioxidants, such as β-carotene reportedly scavenged single oxygens generated by fullerenes.[36] Furthermore, fullerenes were found to antagonize nitric oxide-induced vasodilatation through formation of superoxide radicals.[37] Both *in vitro* and *in vivo* studies have shown that fullerenes, via reactive oxygen species, abnormally controlled the cell differentiation of mouse embryos.[38] Several lines of evidence have even suggested that fullerenes may cause damage to biological tissues, including nephrotoxicity[39] and mutagenesis.[40] Nevertheless, our data showed that carboxyfullerenes may not be harmful to the nigrostriatal dopaminergic system, since intranigral infusion of C3 did not increase the lipid

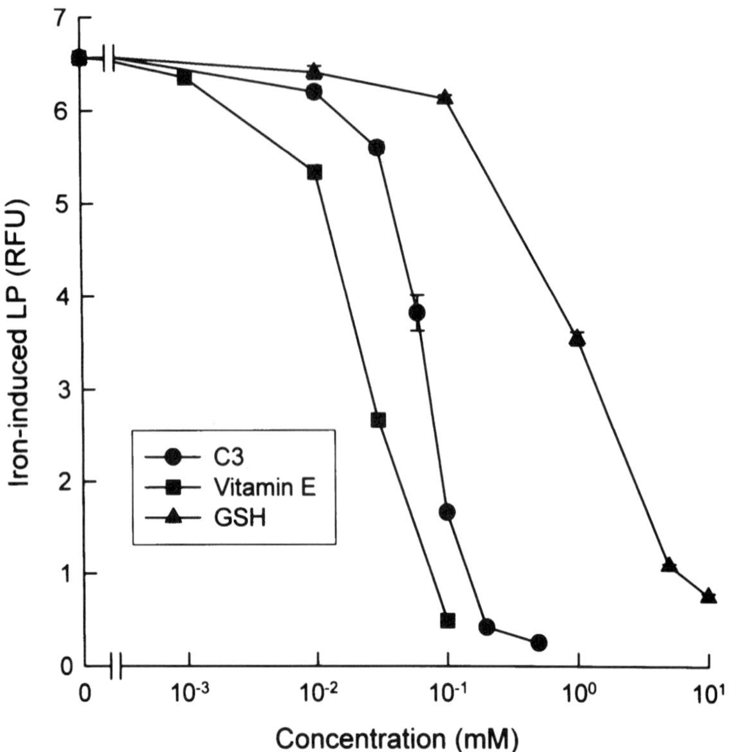

FIGURE 3. Dose-response curves for C3, Trolox (a water-soluble analogue of vitamin E) and glutathione (GSH) on iron-induced elevation of lipid peroxidation (LP) of cortical homogenates. The brain LP was reported as relative fluorescence units (RFU). Values are the mean ± SEM (n = 4) from a representative experiment that was replicated with similar results.

peroxidation in infused substantia nigra, did not deplete striatal dopamine content and did not reduce K^+-evoked dopamine release in striatum ipsilateral to the infused substantia nigra.[25]

Effects of C3 or D3 on Iron-Induced Degeneration of the Nigrostriatal System

Our previous studies and those of others have shown that infusion of iron in substantia nigra degenerates the nigrostriatal dopamine system. An elevated lipid peroxidation in lesioned substantia nigra was used to confirm an oxidative injury *in situ*.[22–24] Functional alterations include decreases in K^+-evoked dopamine release and tyrosine hydroxylase mRNA, a depletion of striatal dopamine content, and a neuronal loss in the striatum ipsilateral to lesioned substantia nigra.[20–24] In our study, *in vivo* electrochemical detection was employed to measure the dynamics of dopamine transmission, while the HPLC-EC measurements of dopamine content[20–23] is time limited in relaying spatial and temporal information about the dopamine system. In

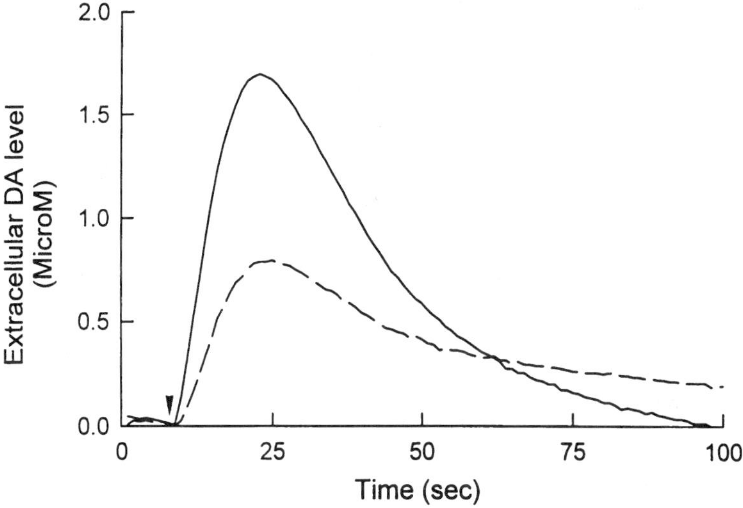

FIGURE 4. Chronoamperometric measurement of K⁺-evoked dopamine (DA) release from the DA-containing nerve terminals in rat striatum. *Solid tracing* represents oxidation current recording and the *dashed tracing* represents reduction current recording. The electrochemical signals, expressed as dopamine concentration (μM), are evoked by applications of K⁺ at the *arrow* above the tracings.

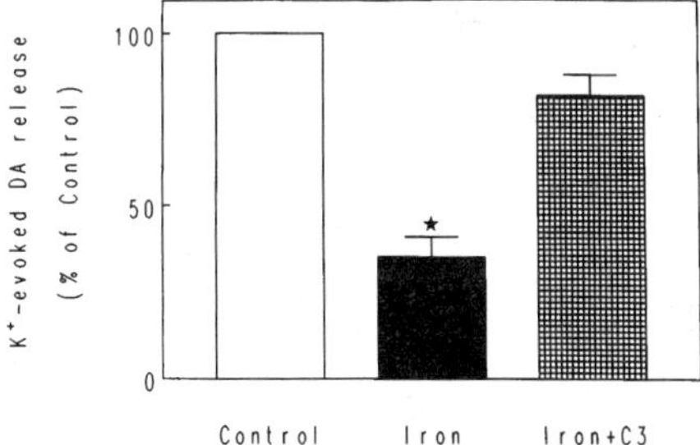

FIGURE 5. Effects of C3 on iron-attenuated K⁺-evoked dopamine release 7 days after an intranigral infusion of iron. Evoked dopamine release was determined using *in vivo* electrochemical detection. Values are the mean $\pm$ SEM (n = 26–30). *$p < 0.05$ in the iron group compared to intact controls and the iron + C3 group by one-way ANOVA followed by post hoc analyses. (Modified from Lin *et al.*[25])

the present study, iron $\pm$ carboxyfullerenes was infused unilaterally in substantia nigra of anesthetized rat. The contralateral striatum of the same rat brain served as a control group. Moreover, the data sets for each rat were obtained using the same electrochemical assembly and thus reduced the variabilities in the construction of the working assembly. *In vivo* electrochemical detection, coupled with microejection of K⁺, which simulates the physiological dopamine release by depolarization, dynamically records the evoked dopamine release in striatum. Seven days after iron infusion, local application of K⁺ (10 nmol) was pressure-ejected to induce dopamine release from the dopamine-containing nerve terminals in the striatal extracellular space. A representative electrochemical signal of K⁺-evoked dopamine release, expressed as the changes in dopamine concentration (μM), is shown in FIGURE 4. Averaged dopamine release in striatal cortex with iron-lesioned substantia nigra was

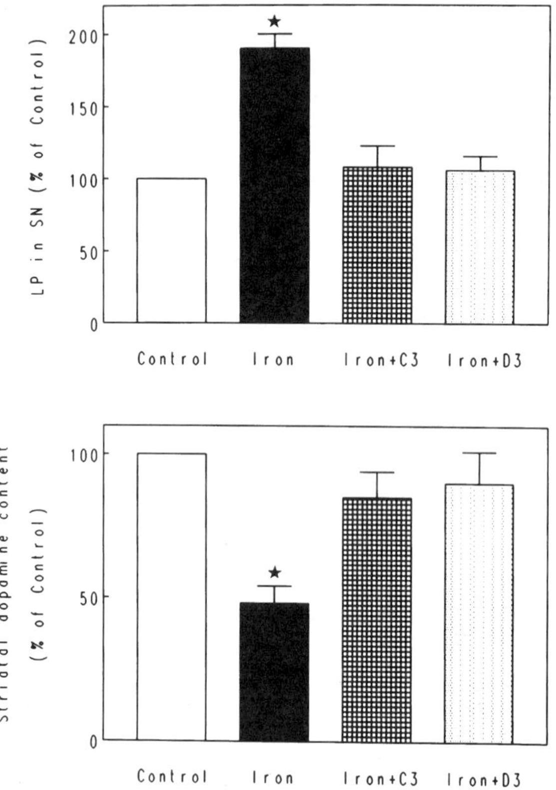

FIGURE 6. Effects of C3 and D3 on iron-attenuated oxidative injury in the nigrostriatal dopaminergic system. Seven days after an intranigral infusion of iron, striatal dopamine
content and lipid peroxidation in substantia nigra were determined. Values are the mean
$\pm$ SEM (n = 4–12). *$p < 0.05$ in the iron group compared to the intact controls, and the
iron + C3, and iron + D3 groups by one-way ANOVA followed by post hoc analyses.

decreased compared to that evoked by an equal amount of K^+ in the corresponding
areas in striatum with intact substantia nigra (FIG. 5). Furthermore, lipid peroxidation of the lesioned substantia nigra was elevated, and striatal dopamine content was
depleted (FIG. 6). Concomitant infusion of C3 prevented the iron-induced attenuation in K^+-evoked dopamine release (FIG. 5). C3 was equally potent as D3 in inhibiting iron-induced depletion of dopamine content in striatum and iron-elevated lipid
peroxidation in substantia nigra (FIG. 6). It is possible that the doses of C3 and D3
were in the high-dose range compared to those used in the *in vitro* study.

SUMMARY AND CONCLUSION

Antioxidants have increasingly become the focus of research in preventing central nervous system (CNS) degenerative diseases.[19] Several strategies, including

supplementation with antioxidants as well as upregulation of endogenous antioxidative defense systems by neurotrophic factors have been proposed.[41,42] Carboxyfullerenes, with their unusual structure possessing a very large electronegative center, have been suggested to be antioxidative as free radical scavengers.[3,6] Our results demonstrate that C3 and D3 carboxyfullerenes prevent iron-induced oxidative stress in biological organisms in several ways. In cortical homogenates, both C3 and D3 inhibited both autoxidation and iron-elevated lipid peroxidation. Furthermore, the antioxidative property of C3 was compared to Trolox and glutathione, and the following rank order was observed: Trolox > C3 > glutathione $\approx$ melatonin. Moreover, our *in vivo* study demonstrates that both C3 and D3 are capable of preventing iron-elevated lipid peroxidation in substantia nigra and iron-reduced dopamine content and evoked dopamine releases in striatum. These results strongly suggest that carboxyfullerenes have a neuroprotective effect in preventing iron-induced oxidative injury in the nigrostriatal dopaminergic system. While more investigation, including that of toxic side effects, are required to evaluate the utilization of carboxyfullerenes for therapeutic treatment, the results presented here clearly indicate that these compounds can reverse oxidative damaged biological systems thought to be involved in Parkinson's disease as well as the normal aging process.

ACKNOWLEDGMENTS

The authors express their gratitude to Dr. Chai C.Y. at the Institute of Biomedical Sciences, Academia Sinica, for his encouragement and support. Special thanks are due to Dr. R.K. Freund at the Health Sciences Center, University of Colorado at Denver, CO., USA, in editing this paper. This study was supported by NSC88-2413-B-075-009-M35 and VGH89-438, Taipei, Taiwan.

REFERENCES

1. KROTO, H.W., S. HEATH, S.C. O'BRIEN, R.F. CURL & R.E. SMALLEY. 1985. C_{60}: Buckminsterfullerene. Nature **318:** 162–163.
2. KRATSCHMER, W., L.D. LAMB, K. FOSTIROPOULOS & D.R. HUFFMAN. 1990. Solid C_{60}: a new form of carbon. Nature **347:** 354–358.
3. DUGAN, L.L., J.K. GABRIELESEN, S.P. YU, T.S. LIN & D.W. CHOI. 1996. Buckminsterfullerenol free radical scavengers reduce excitotoxic and apoptotic death of cultured cortical neurons. Neurobiol. Dis. **3:** 129–135.
4. DUGAN, L.L., D.M. TURETSKY, C. DU, D. LOBNER, M. WHEELER, C.R. ALMLI, C.K. SHEN, T.Y. LUH, D.W. CHOI & T.S. LIN. 1997. Carboxyfullerenes as neuroprotective agents. Proc. Natl. Acad. Sci. USA **94:** 9434–9439.
5. LAI, Y.L. & L.Y. CHIANG. 1997. Water-soluble fullerene derivatives attenuate exsanguination-induced bronchoconstriction of guinea-pigs. J. Auton. Pharmacol. **17:** 229–235.
6. TSAI, M.C., Y.H. CHEN & L.Y. CHIANG. 1997. Polyhydroxylated C_{60}, fullerenol, a novel free radical trapper, prevented hydrogen peroxide- and cumene hydroperoxide-elicited changes in rat hippocampus *in vitro*. J. Pharm. Pharmacol. **49:** 438–445.
7. HALLIWELL, B. & J.M. GUTTERIDGE. 1984. Oxygen toxicity, oxygen radicals, transition metals and diseases. Biochem. J. **219:** 1–14.
8. PERRY, T.L., D.V. GODIN & A. HANSEN. 1982. Parkinson's disease: a disorder due to nigral glutathione deficiency. Neurosci. Lett. **33:** 305–310.

9. SOFIC, E., K.W. LANGE, K. JELLINGER & P. RIEDERER. 1992. Reduced and oxidized glutathione in the substantia nigra of patients with Parkinson's disease. Neurosci. Lett. **142:** 128–130.

10. YOUDIM, M.B., D. BEN-SHACHAR, G. ESHEL, J.P.M. FINBERG & P. RIEDERER. 1993. The neurotoxicity of iron and nitric oxide relevance to the etiology of Parkinson's disease. *In* Advances in Neurology. H. Narabyashi, T. Nagatsu, N. Yanagisawa & Y. Mizuno, Eds.: 259–266. Raven Press. New York.

11. DE LA TORRE, M.R., A. CASADO, M.E. LOPEZ-FERNANDEZ, D. CARRASCOSA, M.C. CASADO, D. VENARUCCI & V. VENARUCCI. 1996. Human aging brain disorders: role of antioxidant enzymes. Neurochem. Res. **21:** 885–888.

12. SOFIC, E., W. PAULUS, K. JELLINGER, P. RIEDERER & M.B.H. YOUDIM. 1991. Selective increase of iron in substantia nigra zona compacta of Parkinsonian brains. J. Neurochem. **56:** 978–982.

13. DEXTER, D.T., F.R. WELLS, A.J. LEES, F. AGID, Y. AGID, P. JENNER & C.D. MARSDEN. 1989. Increased nigral iron content and alteration in other metal ions occurring in brain in Parkinson's disease. J. Neurochem. **52:** 1830–1836.

14. HALLIWELL, B. 1992. Reactive oxygen species and the central nervous system. J. Neurochem. **59:** 1609–1623.

15. AMES, B.N., M.K. SHIGENAGA & T.M. HAGEN. 1993. Oxidants, antioxidants and the degenerative disease of aging. Proc. Natl. Acad. Sci. USA **90:** 7915–7922.

16. COHEN, G. & P. WERNER. 1994. Free radicals, oxidative stress and neurodegeneration. *In* Neurodegenerative Diseases. D.B. Calne, Ed.: 139–162. W.B. Saunders. Philadelphia.

17. JENNER, P. & C.W. OLANOW. 1996. Oxidative stress and the pathogenesis of Parkinson's disease. Neurology **47:** S161–S170.

18. HIRSCH, E.C. 1993. Does oxidative stress participate in nerve cell death in Parkinson's disease. Eur. Neurol. **33** (Suppl. 1): 52–59.

19. EBADI, M., S.K. SRINIVASAN & M.D. BAXI. 1996. Oxidative stress and antioxidant therapy in Parkinson's disease. Prog. Neurobiol. **48:**1–19.

20. BEN-SHACHAR, D. & M.B.H. YOUDIM. 1991. Intranigral iron injection induced behavioral and biochemical "Parkinsonism" in rats. J. Neurochem. **57:** 2133–2135.

21. SENGSTOCK, G.J., C.W. OLANOW, A.J. DUNN, S. BARONE, JR. & G.W. ARENDASH. 1994. Progressive changes in striatal dopaminergic markers, nigral volume, and rotational behavior following iron infusion into the rat substantia nigra. J. Exp. Neurol. **130:** 82–94.

22. RAUHALA, P., K.P. MOHANAKUMAR, I. SZIRAKI, A.M.Y. LIN & C.C. CHIUEH. 1996. *S*-Nitrosothiols and nitric oxide, but not sodium nitroprusside protect nigrostriatal dopamine neurons against iron-induced oxidative stress *in vivo*. Synapse **23:** 58–60.

23. RAUHALA, P., A.M.Y. LIN & C.C. CHIUEH. 1998. Neuroprotection by *S*-nitroso glutathione of brain dopamine neurons from oxidative stress. FASEB J. **12:** 165–173.

24. LIN, A.M.Y., C.H. YANG & C.Y. CHAI. 1998. Striatal dopamine dynamics are altered following an intranigral infusion of iron in SD rat. Free Radical Biol. Med. **24:** 988–993.

25. LIN, A.M.Y., B.Y. CHYI, S.D. WANG, H.-H. YU, P.P. KANAKAMMA, T.-Y. LUH, C.K. CHOU & L.T. HO. 1999. Carboxyfullerene prevents iron-induced oxidative stress in rat brain. J. Neurochem. **72:** 1634–1640.

26. PAXINOS, G. & C. WATSON. 1986. The Rat Brain in Stereotaxic Coordinates. Academic Press. New York.

27. FRIEDEMANN, M.N. 1992. *In vivo* electrochemical studies of dopamine diffusion and clearance in the striatum of young and aged F344 rats. Age **15:** 23–28.

28. GERHARDT, G.A., A.F. OKE, G. NAGY, B. MOGHADDAM & R.N. ADAMS. 1984. Nafion-coated electrodes with high selectivity for CNS electrochemistry. Brain Res. **290:** 390–395.

29. Su, M.T., T.V. Dunwiddie, M. Mynlieff & G.A. Gerhardt. 1990. Electrochemical characterization of stimulated norepinephrine overflow in locus coeruleus-hippocampus double brain grafts grown in oculo. Neurosci. Lett. **110:** 186–192.

30. Gerhardt, G.A. & M. Palmer. 1987. Characterization of the techniques of pressure ejection and microiontophoresis using *in vivo* electrochemistry. J. Neurosci. Methods **22:** 147–159.

31. Kikugawa, K., T. Kato, M. Beppu & A. Haysaaka. 1989. Fluorescent and crosslinked protein formed by free radical and aldehyde species generated during lipid peroxidation. Adv. Exp. Med. Biol. **266:** 345–356.

32. Mokanakumar, K.P., A. DeBartolomeis, R.M. Wu, K.J. Yeh, L.M. Sternberger, S. Peng, D.L. Murphy & C.C. Chiueh. 1994. Ferrous citrate complex and nigral degeneration: evidence for free radical formation and lipid peroxidation. Ann. N.Y. Acad. Sci. **738:** 392–399.

33. Reiter, R., L. Tang, J.J. Garcia & A. Munoz-Hoyos. 1997. Pharmacological actions of melatonin in oxygen radical pathophysiology. Life Sci. **60:** 2255–2271.

34. Hung, R.R. & J.J. Grabowski. 1991. A precise determination of the triplet energy of C_{60} by photoacoustic calorimetry. J. Phys. Chem. **95:** 6073–6075.

35. Krasnovsky, Jr., A.A. & C.S. Foote. 1993. Time-resolved measurements of singlet oxygen dimol-sensitized luminescence. J. Am. Chem. Soc. **115:** 6013–6016.

36. Nagano, T., K. Arakane, A. Ryu, T. Masunaga, K. Shinmoto, S. Mashiko & M. Hirobe. 1994. Comparison of singlet oxygen production efficiency of C_{60} with other photosensitizer, based on 1268 nm emission. Chem. Pharm. Bull. **42:** 2291–2294.

37. Satoh, M., K. Matsuo, H. Kiriya, T. Mashino, T. Nagano, M. Hirobe & I. Takayanagi. 1997. Inhibitory effects of fullerene derivative, dimalonic acid C_{60}, on nitric-oxide-induced relaxation of rabbit aorta. Eur. J. Pharmacol. **327:** 175–181.

38. Tsuchiya, T., I. Oguri, Y.N. Yamakoshi & N. Miyata. 1996. Novel harmful effects of [60] fullerene on mouse embryos *in vitro* and *in vivo*. FEBS Lett. **393:** 139–145.

39. Chen, H.H, C. Yu, T.H. Ueng, S. Chen, B.J. Chen, K.J. Huang & L.Y. Chiang. 1998. Acute and subacute toxicity study of water-soluble polyalkylsulfonated C_{60} in rats. Toxicol. Pathol. **26:** 143–151.

40. Sera, N., H. Tokiwa & N. Miyata. 1996. Mutagenicity of the fullerene C_{60}-generated singlet oxygen dependent formation of lipid peroxides. Carcinogensis **17:** 2163–2169.

41. Hou, J.G., G. Cohen & C. Mytilineou. 1997. Basic fibroblast growth factor stimulation of glial cells protects dopamine neurons from 6-OHDA toxicity: involvement of the glutathione system. J. Neurochem. **69:** 76–83.

42. Furukawa, K., S. Estus, W. Fu, R.J. Mark & M.P. Mattson. 1997. Neuroprotective action of cycloheximide involves induction of bcl-2 and antioxidant pathways. J. Cell Biol. **136:** 1137–1149.

Questions and Answers

QUESTIONS FOR DR. CHIUEH

From Dr. Banik

Do you think HIV-1 protease has some similarities to calpain?

ANSWER: Calpain is a calcium-activated protease, whereas calcium ions do not mediate the cytotoxicity evoked by the HIV-1 protease. Our recent data indicate that ferrous ions may form a reactive cysteinyl thioferrous complex with Cys 67 and 95 of the HIV-1 protease to promote oxidative stress, apoptosis and neurotoxicity. These neurotoxic effects of HIV-1 protease are prevented by either double mutation of the cysteine residues or the chelation of iron.[1] Interestingly, *S*-nitrosylation of cysteine residues by GSNO inactivates both caspase-3 and HIV-1 protease. Therefore, we propose that there is a common mechanism underlying the neurotoxicity induced by caspase-3 and HIV-1 protease.[2] HIV-1 protease may act like a caspase (cysteinyl aspartate-specific proteinase) rather than calpain.

COMMENT (Dr. Youdim): I have to mention that we do not agree with Dr. Chiueh's finding that NO is neuroprotective. In cell culture studies where L-arginine is introduced in microglia-mesencephalic dopamine neurons, the neurons die. The iron chelator disferrioxamine is neuroprotective. We believe the mechanism of NO toxicity is not only peroxynitrite formation but that NO is capable of releasing iron from ferretin similar to what we and others have shown with other neurotoxins such as 6-hydroxy dopamine, MPP^+ and kainate.

ANSWER: This controversial notion that nitric oxide (NO) releases iron from ferritin may be due to a misinterpretation of the experimental results using an iron-containing NO donor of sodium nitroprusside (SNP or disodium nitroferricyanide, $Na_2[NO\text{-}Fe\,(CN)_5]$). These experimental results[3,4] have never been replicated using non-iron-containing NO donors. Moreover, earlier studies employed a stable potassium ferricyanide, $K_3Fe(CN)_6$, instead of the proper sham control of NO-depleted old SNP solution that contains redox iron complexes such as $Fe(CN)_5$ and $Fe(CN)_4$. Due to redox cycling of these SNP-derived iron complexes, NO-depleted SNP is more toxic than the freshly prepared SNP that releases NO. In fact, hydroxyl radicals (OH•) generated by these reactive iron complexes[5] mediate SNP-induced dopamine injury. SNP-induced oxidative stress (such as OH• generation and lipid peroxidation) is blocked by not only iron chelating agent deferoxamine but also NO. In fact, these antioxidative, neuroprotective effects of NO have been replicated *in vivo*.[6]

From Dr. Maynard

Have you or anyone looked at the effect of L-arginine on iron-induced lipid peroxidation? My reason for asking is that although exogenous NO introduced by NO donors may be helpful, one may address more directly the effect of endogenously generated NO by providing the NOS precursor L-arginine.

ANSWER: We have not investigated this interesting question. The mid-brain dopaminergic nigral neurons do not contain NOS in our animal models. We propose that GSNO/NO but not GSH synthesized in endothelial and astroglial cells can reach neighboring neurons to provide antioxidative protection.[2] However, other studies have shown that NOS (NADPH diaphorase positive) containing neurons/cells are not sensitive to oxidative brain injury. For example, gerbils are more sensitive than rats to reperfusion brain injury, because little NO is generated in the gerbil brain following the ischemia-reperfusion procedure. Oxidative stress increases NOS in rat brain; NO is increased slowly and profoundly after the ischemia-reperfusion procedure resulting in lesser neurodegeneration in rats.

NOTE: Our newly obtained results indicate that induction of human nNOS leads to neuroprotection rather than neurotoxicity (Andoh, T., S.Y. Lee & C.C. Chiueh, in preparation).

QUESTIONS FOR DR. GELBARD

From Dr. Obrenovitch

Could you comment on the possible role of quinolinic acid (i.e., potent endogenous NMDA-receptor agonist) associated with brain inflammation?

ANSWER: Quinolinate levels in SIV models of lentiviral-induced neurologic disease have been extensively studied by Dr. Heyes and his colleagues. In general, quinolinate levels in the CSF correlate very well with neurologic impairment in this model. However, using exogenously infected (with a neurovirulent, monocytotropic stain of HIV-1) human monocyte-derived macrophages that are antigenically stimulated to produce a number of potent HIV-1 associated neurotoxins, Dr. Gendelman and Drs. Flanagan and Reinhard reported in the *Journal of Neurovirology* in 1996 that quinolinate levels measured in the culture medium were quite low, well below a neurotoxic dose range.[7]

From Dr. Youdim

You have mentioned that Tat induced apoptosis is NFκB independent. Is the same true for TNF, and is NFκB activated in the microglia and macrophages? If you have these brains you should stain them for iron and ferritin. I would bet that these are increased.

ANSWER: In 1995 we reported that TNFinduced apoptosis in a human neuronal cell line was independent of NFκB activation. We are still not certain of all the signal transduction pathways involved in apoptosis of neurons vulnerable to HIV-1-associated neurotoxins in the CNS. It is a very complicated story that involves dysregulation of multiple homeostatic mechanisms involving microglia and astrocytes as well. We have not stained the brains with HIV-1 encephalitis for iron and ferritin, but will plan to do so shortly. It is an excellent suggestion.

From Dr. Banik

Do you find activated T-lymphocytes expressing interferon gamma (IFNγ) in AIDS brains, since these cells do secrete detrimental factors that could also cause neuronal apoptosis?

ANSWER: We have not looked for activated T-lymphocytes expressing IFNγ in either our *in vitro* or *in vivo* models, but again, that is an excellent suggestion and we will follow up on it.

REFERENCES

1. HAWKINS, V., Q. SHEN & C.C. CHIUEH. 1999. Kynostatin and 17β-estradiol prevent the apoptotic death of human neuroblastoma cells exposed to HIV-1 protease. J. Biomed. Sci. **6:** 433–438.
2. CHIUEH, C.C. & P. RAUHALA. 1999. The redox pathway of *S*-nitrosoglutathione, glutathione and nitric oxide in cell to neuron communications. Free Radical Res. **31:** 641–650.
3. REIF, D.W. & R.D. SIMMONS. 1990. Nitric oxide mediates iron release from ferritin. Arch. Biochem. Biophys. **283:** 537–541.
4. YOUDIM, M.B., D. BEN-SHACHAR, G. ESHEL, J.P. FINBERG & P. RIEDERER. 1993. The neurotoxicity of iron and nitric oxide: relevance to the etiology of Parkinson's disease. Adv. Neurol. **60:** 259–266.
5. RAUHALA, P., A. KHALDI, K.P. MOHANAKUMAR & C.C. CHIUEH. 1998. Apparent role of hydroxyl radicals in oxidative brain injury induced by sodium nitroprusside. Free Radical Biol. Med. **24:** 1065–1073.
6. MOHANAKUMAR, K.P., I. HANBAUER & C.C. CHIUEH. 1998. Neuroprotection by nitric oxide against hydroxyl radical-induced nigral neurotoxicity. J. Chem. Neuroanat. **14:** 195–205.
7. NOTTET, H.S., E.M. FLANAGAN, C.R. FLANAGAN, H.A. GELBARD, H.E. GENDELMAN & J.F. REINHARD, JR. 1996. The regulation of quinolinic acid in human immunodeficiency virus-infected monocytes. J. Neurovirol. **2:** 111–117.

Neuregulin Signaling in Brain Injury and in Animal Models of Ischemia

MARK A. MARCHIONNI,[a,c] MARC A. SORIANO,[b] IAN MURDOCH,[b]
ELIZEBETH McCRACKEN,[b] DEBORAH DEWAR,[b] AND JAMES McCULLOCH[b]

[a]*Cambridge NeuroScience, Inc., Cambridge, Massachusetts 02139, USA*

[b]*Wellcome Surgical Institute, University of Glasgow, Glasgow G61 1QH, UK*

Neuregulin signaling is involved in the survival, proliferation, differentiation and migration of cells throughout the peripheral and central nervous systems. Many aspects of neuron/glial interactions necessary for neural development have been shown to be mediated via the neuregulin peptide growth factors and the erbB receptor tyrosine kinases. In adult peripheral nerve, the expression of neuregulin signaling components appears to be upregulated following injury. Further, parenteral administration of recombinant neuregulin proteins, such as recombinant human glial growth factor 2 (rhGGF2) appears to be neuroprotective, and led to improved recovery in animal models of peripheral nerve damage or peripheral neuropathy. Thus the induced expression of neuregulin signaling in models of disease or injury might suggest potential indications for treatment using rhGGF2. Hence we have investigated the expression of neuregulin immunoreactivity following focal ischemia in rat and in human head injury. After permanent and transient middle cerebral artery occlusion (MCAO), we observed a substantial increase in neuregulin immunoreactivity in shrunken neurons, astrocytes and oligodendrocytes in the ischemic tissue. Interestingly, increased expression also was remarkable in the grey matter from the cingulate gyrus of head-injured patients compared to controls, but was unaltered in white matter.

[c]Corresponding author: Mark Marchionni, Ph.D., Cambridge NeuroScience, One Kendall Square, Building 700, Cambridge, MA 02139. Phone, 617/225-0600, ext. 140; fax, 617/225-2741.

e-mail, Mark_Marchionni@cambneuro.com

Protective and Rescuing Abilities of IGF-I and Some Putative Free Radical Scavengers against β-Amyloid-Inducing Toxicity in Neurons

SYLVAIN DORÉ, STÉPHANE BASTIANETTO, SATYABRATA KAR,
AND RÉMI QUIRION[a]

Douglas Hospital Research Center, McGill University, Montreal, Quebec, Canada

ABSTRACT: β-Amyloid (Aβ) peptides are most likely involved in the neurodegenerative process occurring in Alzheimer's Disease (AD) and are enriched in senile plaques. The mechanisms of Aβ toxicity are not clear but likely involve free radicals and apoptosis. Much interest is currently aiming at developing effective approaches to block Aβ toxicity in order to slow down disease progression. In that context, we are particularly interested in studying the role of insulin-like growth factors, particularly IGF-I and purported free radical scavengers including a Gingko biloba extract (EGb761) as blocker of Aβ toxicity in a simple *in vitro* model of hippocampal primary cultures. We observed that both IGF-I and EGb761 are unique in that they are able not only to protect but even to rescue neurons against Aβ toxicity. These results are summarized here and possible mechanisms of action are discussed to explain the protective properties of these two classes of agents.

IGF ACTIONS IN THE NERVOUS SYSTEM

Insulin-like growth factors (IGF-I and IGF-II) play an important role in the normal development and maintenance of the cellular integrity of the organism, including the central nervous system (CNS).[1] Both trophic factors are selectively localized in the brain and their specific receptors are uniquely distributed in various neuroanatomical regions, being especially concentrated in the hippocampal formation.[2] The IGF-I receptor is composed of two α-chains where the ligand binds and two β-chains possessing a tyrosine kinase domain.[3] In contrast, the IGF-II receptor is made of a single transmembrane segment containing a binding site for IGF-II and another for mannose-6-phosphate residues. Both receptors bind specifically to their cognate ligands but can also recognize the other with lower affinity. We have recently shown that cultured hippocampal neurons are highly enriched with IGF-I and IGF-II receptors each being differentially internalized,[4] and serving distinct functions.[5]

Among various biological effects, it was shown that IGF-I can promote the survival, proliferation and maturation of cultured neurons,[6] reduce neuronal loss in adult rat brain following hypoxic-ischemic injury,[7] induce the differentiation of oligodendrocytes,[8] stimulate DNA synthesis[9] and neurite outgrowth,[10] and direct the

[a]Corresponding author: Rémi Quirion, Ph.D., Douglas Hospital Research Center, McGill University, 6875, LaSalle Blvd., Montreal, Quebec, Canada, H4H 1R3. Phone, 514/762-3048; fax, 514/762-3034.
e-mail, mcou@musica.mcgill.ca

sprouting of spared afferents into a deafferented hippocampus.[11] More recently, we have shown that IGFs can modulate hippocampal acetylcholine release.[5]

Considering the broad actions of IGFs on the maintenance of normal cellular functions and the presence of high levels of IGF receptors in the hippocampus, the region that is severely affected in Alzheimer's disease brain, we investigated here the potential neuroprotective effects of IGF-I and some free radical scavengers against β-amyloid-induced toxicity in rat hippocampal neurons.

PRIMARY HIPPOCAMPAL CELL CULTURES

It is now rather well established that various Aβ derivatives, especially in their aggregated forms, are toxic to neurons.[12–14] The main amyloidogenic components of the neuritic plaques are the $A\beta_{1-42}$ and $A\beta_{1-40}$ fragments.[15,16] The $A\beta_{25-35}$ peptide, which contains the active toxic domain, is highly toxic to rat primary hippocampal neurons.

Aβ peptide ($A\beta_{25-35}$) was purchased from Bachem (Torrance, CA) was used in the present study. hIGF-I was obtained from Genentech Canada Inc. (Burlington, Ontario, Canada). The Ginkgo biloba extract (EGb761) was obtained from IPSEN Laboratories (France). Materials used for cell culture were obtained from Gibco BRL (Burlington, Ontario, Canada). Unless stated otherwise, all other chemicals were purchased from Sigma Chemical Co. (St. Louis, MO).

Primary rat hippocampal neuronal cultures were prepared as described earlier.[17] Experiments were performed after 6 days in culture. Aβ peptides were dissolved in dimethyl sulfoxide (DMSO) and used immediately by directly diluting to the indicated concentrations in the chemically defined experimental culture medium. Sister cultures were treated with appropriate vehicle control. Following treatments, neurons were maintained for an additional period of 6 days and their survival was assessed by phase-contrast microscopy and quantified using the thiazoyl blue (MTT) colorimetric assay, an indicator of mitochondrial activity. The neuroprotective effect of the different agents was evaluated by treating the cells simultaneously with them and different Aβ peptides, while the neurorescuing action was determined by treating the cells for different hours or days following initial exposure to Aβ peptides. All experiments were repeated at least with three separate batches of cultures and the means were analyzed and represented as the mean ± SEM with p <0.01 being considered significant.

NEUROPROTECTIVE ACTIONS OF THE IGF-I

Exposure of rat primary hippocampal neurons to $A\beta_{25-35}$ (25–30 μM) produced marked toxicity (TABLES 1 and 2), while similar concentrations of Aβ scrambled sequence ($A\beta_{25-35}$) failed to exhibit any significant effect on neuronal survival. IGF-I (30–100 nM) significantly protected hippocampal neurons against neurotoxicity induced by Aβ derivatives (TABLE 1). Most interestingly, IGF-I (100 nM) was even

TABLE 1. Neuroprotective effect of IGF-I against toxicity induced by $A\beta_{25-35}$ in rat hippocampal neuronal cultures

Treatment	Neuron Survival (% MTT Values)	
IGF-I (nM)	$A\beta_{25-35}$ (30 µM) + IGF-I	Control + IGF-I
0	45 ± 2	100 ± 7
0.3	46 ± 2	93 ± 2
1.0	38 ± 2	102 ± 6
3.0	37 ± 3	103 ± 2
10.0	40 ± 1	99 ± 3
30.0	$70 \pm 2^*$	109 ± 2
100.0	$94 \pm 5^*$	109 ± 2
300.0	$111 \pm 8^*$	114 ± 3
Number of Days after $A\beta$ Treatment	$A\beta_{25-35}$ (30 µM) + IGF-I (100 nM)	Control + IGF-I (100 nM)
No IGF-I	36 ± 1	100 ± 2
0	$75 \pm 1^*$	110 ± 1
1	$73 \pm 2^*$	109 ± 1
2	$71 \pm 2^*$	108 ± 1
3	$61 \pm 2^*$	108 ± 1
4	$55 \pm 3^*$	106 ± 3
5	$44 \pm 2^*$	107 ± 2

NOTE: Values are the mean $\pm$ SEM of three separate batches of cultures with $^*p$ <0.01 as $A\beta$-treated neurons.

able to rescue neurons preexposed (up to 5 days) to amyloidogenic peptide (TABLE 1). Similar neuroprotective and neurorescueing effects of IGF-I were observed against AB_{1-42} (5 µM).[17]

MECHANISMS OF IGF ACTIONS

The mechanism of action involved in the neuroprotective and especially neurorescuing properties of IGF-I against $A\beta$-induced toxicity remains to be clarified. The activation of the IGF-I tyrosine kinase receptor induces protein phosphorylation followed by a cascade of intracellular events, which include the activation of insulin receptor substrates (IRS-1 and IRS-2), and phosphoinositide 3-kinase, phosphotyrosine phosphatases, S6 kinase, Ras-MAP kinase and transcription factors leading to alterations in Ca^{2+} storage and mobilization, and mitochondrial respiration.[18,19] The toxic properties of $A\beta$-derivatives could also relate to their abilities to stimulate apoptotic genes/cellular events.[20–22] Accordingly, IGF-I could interfere at different stages of the necrotic or apoptotic pathway to block and even rescue neurons against $A\beta$-induced cell death. IGF-I is known to block programmed cell death in various models.[23–27] IGF-I has also been shown to prevent apoptosis associated with K^+-

deprivation in cerebellar granule neurons, while other trophic factors tested such as acidic fibroblast growth factor (aFGF), basic fibroblast growth factor (bFGF), platet-derived growth factor (PDGF) and neurotrophin-3 (NT-3) were found to be inactive.[26] Similar protective effects were observed in a hybrid dopaminergic cell line against oxidation and hypoglycemia-induced cell death, IGF-I being more potent than bFGF, epidermal growth factor (EGF) and nerve growth factor (NGF). It was also demonstrated that IGF-I can activate the phosphoinositide 3-kinase and the serine-threonine protein kinase Akt and promote the survival of rat primary cerebellar neurons after induction of apoptosis by serum deprivation.[27] A similar activation by IGF-I is likely to occur in our Aβ toxicity model. Hence, IGF-I by acting on necrotic and/or apoptotic cellular events could protect and more importantly rescue neurons against Aβ-induced toxicity.

IMPORTANCE OF DEVELOPING IGF MIMETICS
FOR ALZHEIMER'S DISEASE

In addition to their neuroprotective actions, IGF-I is critically involved in maintenance of body homeostasis. Aging is associated with changes in basic functions including altereation in glucose metabolism in the nervous system. In aged rats and humans, poor cognitive performances have been correlated with impaired glucose regulation.[28] In sporadic AD cases, significant reductions in glucose utilization have been reported.[29] Moreover, IGF-I receptor binding levels are apparently increased in affected areas of the AD brain,[30] maybe as an attempt to counteract energy metabolism deficits and cell losses. Interestingly, IGF-I is also known to be neuroprotective against toxicity induced by glucose deprivation,[29,31] and it has been shown that exposure to subthreshold doses of Aβ derivatives render neurons more susceptible to glucose deprivation.[32] The unique capacity of IGF-I to protect and rescue neurons against Aβ-induced toxicity, in parallel to its homeostatic potential to insure adequate glucose/energy metabolism exemplified even further the critical relevance of this trophic factor in normal and pathological brain functioning.

Hyperphosphorylated tau is the major component of paired helical filaments in neurofibrillary lesions associated with AD. Hyperphosphorylation reduces the affinity of tau for microtubules and is thought to be a critical event in the pathogenesis of this disease. Interestingly, it was recently demonstrated that insulin and IGF-I reduce tau phosphorylation and promote tau binding to microtubules in cultured human neuronal NT2N cells.[33] Hence IGF-I could also decrease tau phosphorylation in addition to diminishing Aβ toxicity—two key events in AD pathogenesis.

It is well established that IGF-I does not penetrate well the blood-brain barrier. In addition, it is relatively unstable chemically and is highly sensitive to enzymatic degradation. Accordingly, the use of an IGF-I-based therapy in AD depends on the development of small mimetics preferably of nonpeptidic nature that are chemically stable and could easily penetrate the brain. Alternatively, small molecules having neuroprotective properties similar to IGF-I could be another strategy. In that regard, we have recently obtained promising results with a gingko biloba extract (see below).

TABLE 2. Effects of the Ginkgo biloba extract (EGb761), the neurosteroid DHEA and its sulfated form (DHEAS) against toxicity induced by $A\beta_{25-35}$ in rat hippocampal cellular cultures

Treatment	Cell Survival (% MTT Values)
Control	100 ± 2
$A\beta_{25-35}$ (25 μM)	64 ± 6
+ EGb761 (100 μg/ml)	$95 \pm 3^*$
+ DHEA 10^{-7}M	66 ± 5
+ DHEA 10^{-6}M	68 ± 6
+ DHEA 10^{-5}M	70 ± 7
+ DHEAS 10^{-7}M	66 ± 6
+ DHEAS 10^{-6}M	66 ± 6
+ DHEAS 10^{-5}M	67 ± 8

NOTE: Values are the mean $\pm$ SEM of three separate batches of cultures with $^*p$ <0.01 as $A\beta$-treated cells.

PUTATIVE FREE RADICAL SCAVENGERS AGAINST $A\beta$ TOXICITY

Other trophic factors have been reported to protect neurons against various types of insults. For example, NGF,[34] bFGF,[35] tumor necrosis factor-α (TNFα) and TNFβ[36] have been shown to protect cultured hippocampal neurons against $A\beta$-induced toxicity. However, none of these trophic factors was effective post-$A\beta$ treatment hence lacking neurorescuing properties. Interestingly, TGFβ1 and TGFβ2, but not TGFβ3, were apparently able to have a slight protective effect in neurons preexposed to $A\beta_{25-35}$ for 24 hours, while such effect was not observed with TNF, NGF, aFGF or bFGF.[37] The rescuing ability of TGFβ1 and TGFβ2 was not as pronounced as the one observed with IGF-I and was not as effective against longer exposures to $A\beta_{25-35}$. Experiments testing melatonin (10^{-10}–10^{-6} M), different steroids (dehydroepiandrosterone (DHEA), sulfated form of DHEA (DHEAS), 10^{-7}–10^{-5} M) (TABLE 2) and progesterone, pregnenolone, and estradiol (10^{-10}–10^{-5} M) failed to reveal clear neurorescuing abilities against $A\beta$ toxicity.

Interestingly, similar neuroprotective properties to those of IGF-I were observed with the Ginkgo biloba extract (EGb761, "Tanakan," IPSEN laboratories, France) (TABLE 2), a well-defined and complex product containing 24% flavonoids and 6% terpenoids.[38] These protective effects could be partly attributable to the purported antioxidant properties of EGb761[39] and may depend upon the polyvalent action of its active constituents including flavonoids.[40] These results support its therapeutic usefulness in treating mild cognitive impairments in elderly patients[41] and neurodegenerative diseases of multifactorial origin such as AD and vascular dementia.[42,43]

While various neurotrophins and neurotrophic factors[44] have been shown to block the toxic effects of $A\beta$ derivatives *in vitro* and *in vivo*, the rescuing actions of IGF-I and Ginkgo biloba extract are rather unique. The multiple properties of these compounds suggest that the development of related mimetics could be a promising strategy toward the treatment of various neurodegenerative disorders.

CONCLUSIONS

An effective therapeutic approach in the treatment of neurodegenerative diseases would most likely be one that has a variety of beneficial properties Optimally, it should also be effective at various stages of the disease process. In that regard, IGF-I (or its mimetic) is certainly worth considering. It is well known that one of the first steps triggering neuronal death is the lack of adequate energy supply in the form of glucose. Recently, Sapolski and colleagues have shown that the transfection of glucose transporters into neurons protected them against a variety of toxic insults.[45,46] Interestingly, one of the classical actions of IGF-I is its ability to facilitate glucose uptake by neurons.[47,48] Additionally, IGF-I, apart from inhibiting apoptosis,[27] has been shown to promote outgrowth and facilitate proper connectivity, two key features to be considered for an effective therapeutic intervention. In parallel, a Gingko extract is known to properly scavenge toxic free radical species[39,49] and to limit apoptosis[50] and inflammatory insults via its anti-platelet-activating factor (PAF) activity.[51,52] Hence, the combination of an IGF-I mimetic with a gingko extract could prove most useful in the treatment of neurodegenerative diseases because of their multifaceted, complementary actions.

REFERENCES

1. DE PABLO, F. & E.J. DE LA ROSA. 1995. The developing CNS: a scenario for the action of proinsulin, insulin and insulin-like growth factors. Trends Neurosci. **18:** 143–150.
2. DORÉ, S., S. KAR, W. ROWE & R. QUIRION. 1997. Distribution and levels of [^{125}I]IGF-I, [^{125}I]IGF-II and [^{125}I]insulin receptor binding sites in the hippocampus of aged memory-unimpaired and -impaired rats. Neuroscience **80:** 1033–1040.
3. LeROITH, D., H. WERNER, D. BEITNER-JOHNSON & C.T. ROBERTS, JR. 1995. Molecular and cellular aspects of the insulin-like growth factor I receptor. Endocr. Rev. **16:** 143–163.
4. DORÉ, S., S. KAR & R. QUIRION. 1997. Presence and differential internalization of two distinct insulin-like growth factor receptors in rat hippocampal neurons. Neuroscience **78:** 373–383.
5. KAR, S., D. SETO, S. DORÉ, U. HANISCH & R. QUIRION. 1997. Insulin-like growth factors-I and -II differentially regulate endogenous acetylcholine release from the rat hippocampal formation. Proc. Natl. Acad. Sci. USA **94:** 14054–14059.
6. DiCICCO-BLOOM, E. & I.B. BLACK. 1988. Insulin growth factors regulate the mitotic cycle in cultured rat sympathetic neuroblasts. Proc. Natl. Acad. Sci. USA **85:** 4066–4070.
7. GUAN, J., C. WILLIAMS, M. GUNNING, C. MALLARD & P. GLUCKMAN. 1993. The effects of IGF-1 treatment after hypoxic-ischemic brain injury in adult rats. J. Cereb. Blood Flow Metab. **13:** 609–616.
8. McMORRIS, F.A., R.L. MOZELL, M.J. CARSON, Y. SHINAR, R.D. MEYER *et al.* 1993. Regulation of oligodendrocyte development and central nervous system myelination by insulin-like growth factors. Ann. N.Y. Acad. Sci. **692:** 321–334.
9. LENOIR, D. & P. HONEGGER. 1983. Insulin-like growth factor I (IGF I) stimulates DNA synthesis in fetal rat brain cell cultures. Brain Res. **283:** 205–213.
10. RUIZ, P., J.A. PULIDO, C. MARTINEZ, J.M. CARRASCOSA, J. SATRUSTEGUI *et al.* 1992. Effect of aging on the kinetic characteristics of the insulin receptor autophosphorylation in rat adipocytes. Arch. Biochem. Biophys. **296:** 231–238.
11. GUTHRIE, K.M., T. NGUYEN & C.M. GALL. 1995. Insulin-like growth factor-1 mRNA is increased in deafferented hippocampus: spatiotemporal correspondence of a trophic event with axon sprouting. J. Comp. Neurol. **352:** 147–160.

12. MAURICE, T., B.P. LOCKHART & A. PRIVAT. 1996. Amnesia induced in mice by centrally administered beta-amyloid peptides involves cholinergic dysfunction. Brain Res. **706:** 181–193.

13. HAASS, C. 1996. The molecular significance of amyloid beta-peptide for Alzheimer's disease. Eur. Arch. Psychiatry Clin. Neurosci. **246:** 118–123.

14. IVERSEN, L.L., R.J. MORTISHIRE-SMITH, S.J. POLLACK & M.S. SHEARMAN. 1995. The toxicity *in vitro* of beta-amyloid protein. Biochem. J. **311:** 1–16.

15. ROHER, A.E., J.D. LOWENSON, S. CLARKE, A.S. WOODS, R.J. COTTER *et al.* 1993. Beta-amyloid-(1–42) is a major component of cerebrovascular amyloid deposits: implications for the pathology of Alzheimer disease. Proc. Natl. Acad. Sci. USA **90:** 10836–10840.

16. SELKOE, D.J. 1994. Normal and abnormal biology of the beta-amyloid precursor protein. Annu. Rev. Neurosci. **17:** 489–517.

17. DORÉ, S., S. KAR & R. QUIRION. 1997. Insulin-like growth factor I protects and rescues hippocampal neurons against beta-amyloid- and human amylin-induced toxicity. Proc. Natl. Acad. Sci. USA **94:** 4772–4777.

18. LIENHARD, G.E. 1994. Insulin. Life without the IRS. Nature **372:** 128–129.

19. WATERS, S.B., D. CHEN, A.W. KAO, S. OKADA, K.H. HOLT *et al.* 1996. Insulin and epidermal growth factor receptors regulate distinct pools of Grb2-SOS in the control of Ras activation. J. Biol. Chem. **271:** 18224–18230.

20. LOO, D.T., A. COPANI, C.J. PIKE, E.R. WHITTEMORE, A.J. WALENCEWICZ *et al.* 1993. Apoptosis is induced by beta-amyloid in cultured central nervous system neurons. Proc. Natl. Acad. Sci. USA **90:** 7951–7955.

21. FORLONI, G., R. CHIESA, S. SMIROLDO, L. VERGA, M. SALMONA *et al.* 1993. Apoptosis mediated neurotoxicity induced by chronic application of beta amyloid fragment 25–35. Neuroreport **4:** 523–526.

22. GSCHWIND, M. & G. HUBER. 1995. Apoptotic cell death induced by beta-amyloid 1–42 peptide is cell type dependent. J. Neurochem. **65:** 292–300.

23. SELL, C., R. BASERGA & R. RUBIN. 1995. Insulin-like growth factor I (IGF-I) and the IGF-I receptor prevent etoposide-induced apoptosis. Cancer Res. **55:** 303–306.

24. RODRIGUEZ-TARDUCHY, G., M.K. COLLINS, I. GARCIA & A. LOPEZ-RIVAS. 1992. Insulin-like growth factor-I inhibits apoptosis in IL-3-dependent hemopoietic cells. J. Immunol. **149:** 535–540.

25. HARRINGTON, E.A., M.R. BENNETT, A. FANIDI & G.I. EVAN. 1994. c-Myc-induced apoptosis in fibroblasts is inhibited by specific cytokines. EMBO J. **13:** 3286–3295.

26. D'MELLO, S.R., C. GALLI, T. CIOTTI &. P. CALISSANO. 1993. Induction of apoptosis in cerebellar granule neurons by low potassium: inhibition of death by insulin-like growth factor I and cAMP. Proc. Natl. Acad. Sci. USA **90:** 10989–10993.

27. DUDEK, H., S.R. DATTA, T.F. FRANKE, M.J. BIRNBAUM, R. YAO *et al.* 1997. Regulation of neuronal survival by the serine-threonine protein kinase Akt. Science **275:** 661–665.

28. LONG, J.M., B.J. DAVIS, P. GAROFALO, E.L. SPANGLER & D.K. INGRAM. 1992. Complex maze performance in young and aged rats: response to glucose treatment and relationship to blood insulin and glucose. Physiol. Behav. **51:** 411–418.

29. HOYER, S. 1994. Neurodegeneration, Alzheimer's disease, and beta-amyloid toxicity. Life Sci. **55:** 1977–1983.

30. CREWS, F.T., R. MCELHANEY, G. FREUND, W.E. BALLINGER, JR. & M.K. RAIZADA. 1992. Insulin-like growth factor I receptor binding in brains of Alzheimer's and alcoholic patients. J. Neurochem. **58:** 1205–1210.

31. CHENG, B. & M.P. MATTSON. 1994. NT-3 and BDNF protect CNS neurons against metabolic/excitotoxic insults. Brain Res. **640:** 56–67.

32. COPANI, A., J.Y. KOH & C.W. COTMAN. 1991. Beta-amyloid increases neuronal susceptibility to injury by glucose deprivation. Neuroreport **2:** 763–765.

33. HONG, M. & V.M. LEE. 1997. Insulin and insulin-like growth factor-1 regulate tau phosphorylation in cultured human neurons. J. Biol. Chem. **272:** 19547–19553.

34. RABIZADEH, S., C.M. BITLER, L.L. BUTCHER & D.E. BREDESEN. 1994. Expression of the low-affinity nerve growth factor receptor enhances beta-amyloid peptide toxicity. Proc. Natl. Acad. Sci. USA **91:** 10703–10706.

35. MATTSON, M.P., S.W. BARGER, B. CHENG, I. LIEBERBURG, V.L. SMITH-SWINTOSKY *et al.* 1993. Beta-amyloid precursor protein metabolites and loss of neuronal Ca^{2+} homeostasis in Alzheimer's disease. Trends Neurosci. **16:** 409–414.

36. BARGER, S.W., D. HORSTER, K. FURUKAWA, Y. GOODMAN, J. KRIEGLSTEIN *et al.* 1995. Tumor necrosis factors alpha and beta protect neurons against amyloid beta-peptide toxicity: evidence for involvement of a kappa B-binding factor and attenuation of peroxide and Ca^{2+} accumulation. Proc. Natl. Acad. Sci USA **92:** 9328–9332.

37. REN, R.F. & K.C. FLANDERS. 1996. Transforming growth factors-beta protect primary rat hippocampal neuronal cultures from degeneration induced by beta-amyloid peptide. Brain Res. **732:** 16–24.

38. OYAMA, Y., L. CHIKAHISA, T. UEHA, K. KANEMARU & K. NODA. 1996. Ginkgo biloba extract protects brain neurons against oxidative stress induced by hydrogen peroxide. Brain Res. **712:** 349–352.

39. MARCOCCI, L., L. PACKER, M.T. DROY-LEFAIX, A. SEKAKI & M. GARDES-ALBERT. 1994. Antioxidant action of Ginkgo biloba extract EGb 761. Methods Enzymol. **234:** 462–475.

40. BASTIANETTO, S., C. RAMASSAMY, S. DORÉ, J. POIRIER & R. QUIRION. 1996. Neurosteroids and ginkgo biloba extract prevent cell death induced by hydrogen peroxide in hippocampal neuronal cell cultures. Soc. Neurosci. Abstr. **22:** 1119.

41. RAI, G.S., C. SHOVLIN & K.A. WESNES. 1991. A double-blind, placebo controlled study of Ginkgo biloba extract ('Tanakan') in elderly outpatients with mild to moderate memory impairment. Curr. Med. Res. Opin. **12:** 350–355.

42. LE BARS, P.L., M.M. KATZ, N. BERMAN, T.M. ITIL, A.M. FREEDMAN *et al.* 1997. A placebo-controlled, double-blind, randomized trial of an extract of Ginkgo biloba for dementia. North American EGb Study Group. JAMA **278:** 1327–1332.

43. MAURER, K., R. IHL, T. DIERKS & L. FROLICH. 1997. Clinical efficacy of Ginkgo biloba special extract EGb 761 in dementia of the Alzheimer type. J. Psychiatr. Res. **31:** 645–655.

44. YANKNER, B.A., A. CACERES & L.K. DUFFY. 1990. Nerve growth factor potentiates the neurotoxicity of beta amyloid. Proc. Natl. Acad. Sci. USA **87:** 9020–9023.

45. LAWRENCE, M.S., G.H. SUN, D.M. KUNIS, T.C. SAYDAM, R. DASH *et al.* 1996. Overexpression of the glucose transporter gene with a herpes simplex viral vector protects striatal neurons against stroke. J. Cereb. Blood Flow Metab. **16:** 181–185.

46. HO, D.Y., T.C. SAYDAM, S.L. FINK, M.S. LAWRENCE & R.M. SAPOLSKY. 1995. Defective herpes simplex virus vectors expressing the rat brain glucose transporter protect cultured neurons from necrotic insults. J. Neurochem. **65:** 842–850.

47. CHENG, B. & M.P. MATTSON. 1992. IGF-I and IGF-II protect cultured hippocampal and septal neurons against calcium-mediated hypoglycemic damage. J. Neurosci. **12:** 1558–1566.

48. WERNER, H., M.K. RAIZADA, L.M. MUDD, H.L. FOYT, I.A. SIMPSON *et al.* 1989. Regulation of rat brain/HepG2 glucose transporter gene expression by insulin and insulin-like growth factor-I in primary cultures of neuronal and glial cells. Endocrinology **125:** 314–320.

49. DROY-LEFAIX, M.T., J. CLUZEL, J.M. MENERATH, B. BONHOMME & M. DOLY. 1995. Antioxidant effect of a Ginkgo biloba extract (EGb 761) on the retina. Int. J. Tissue React. **17:** 93–100.

50. NI, Y., B. ZHAO, J. HOU & W. XIN. 1996. Preventive effect of Ginkgo biloba extract

on apoptosis in rat cerebellar neuronal cells induced by hydroxyl radicals. Neurosci. Lett. **214:** 115–118.

51. AKISU, M., N. KULTURSAY, I. COKER & A. HUSEYINOV. 1998. Platelet-activating factor is an important mediator in hypoxic ischemic brain injury in the newborn rat. Flunarizine and Ginkgo biloba extract reduce PAF concentration in the brain. Biol. Neonat. **74:** 439–444.

52. SMITH, P.F., K. MACLENNAN & C.L. DARLINGTON. 1996. The neuroprotective properties of the Ginkgo biloba leaf: a review of the possible relationship to platelet-activating factor (PAF). J. Ethnopharmacol. **50:** 131–139.

Questions and Answers

QUESTION FOR DR. MARCHIONNI

From Dr. Banik

Have you looked at whether neuregulin is upregulated in MS or EAE brain, or is expressed more in particular cell types?

ANSWER: Clearly this is an important experiment, and it will receive a high priority for our work in the coming year. In particular, analyzing tissues from MS patients can help to underscore the relevance of our recent finding that GGF2 significantly reduced relapses in the chronic phase of EAE in mice and produced a substantial increase in remyelination.

QUESTION FOR DR. QUIRION

From Dr. Abbracchio

Is it possible that IGF-1-induced protection is anyhow related to a better utilization of glucose by cells? In this respect, is β-amyloid altering fructose metabolism, which would result in hyperglycemia? We heard yesterday how toxic hyperglycemia can be cells, through generation of radicals; along the same line, were any other antioxidants (e.g., acetylcysteine or other GSH-preserving agents) protective as well?

ANSWER: Very little information and hard data are currently available on the effect of β-amyloid on fructose metabolism. It would certainly be most pertinent to investigate. As to the second part of your question, various antioxidants can be protective against amyloid toxicity, but it is not at all clear that it relates directly to a better utilization of glucose by cells (of course, it would have an impact at some point likely not direct). Other neuroprotective/neurorescuing agents include *Gingko biloba* extracts as summarized here.

The Unique Histopathological Responses of the Injured Spinal Cord

Implications for Neuroprotective Therapy

LLOYD GUTH,[a,b,c] ZIYIN ZHANG,[a] AND OSWALD STEWARD[a,d]

[a]*Department of Neuroscience, University of Virginia School of Medicine, Charlottesville, Virginia 22908, USA*

[b]*Department of Biology, College of William and Mary, Williamsburg, Virginia 23187, USA*

ABSTRACT: Tissue destruction at the primary site of a spinal cord injury leads to persistent necrosis that progressively enlarges the lesion. Steroids attenuate this necrotizing process and promote tissue repair even though such anti-inflammatory drugs interfere with wound healing in non-CNS organs. To address this paradox, the spinal cord of rats and mice was crushed extradurally and the effects of the following anti-inflammatory agents studied by light microscopical image analysis: allopurinol, aminoguanidine, indomethacin, a bacterial lipopolysaccharide, naproxen, and pregnenolone. The contribution of Wallerian degeneration to progressive necrosis was studied in a mutant mouse strain (Wld^S) that is characterized by delayed Wallerian degeneration.

In rats, the anti-inflammatory agents *selectively* attenuated progressive necrosis and encouraged wound healing. In mice, considerable tissue repair occurred without pharmacological intervention; this wound-healing process was delayed in the mutant Wld^S strain. Since spinal cord injury results in concomitant tissue necrosis and wound healing, a goal of neuroprotective therapy is to regulate the dynamic balance between these destructive and reparative processes.

RELATION OF INFLAMMATORY PROCESSES TO THE HISTOPATHOLOGY OF SPINAL CORD INJURY

Overview of the Inflammatory Response

Anti-inflammatory agents are among the most useful neuroprotective agents for treating spinal cord trauma. It is puzzling why this should be so, since steroidal and non-steroidal anti-inflammatory agents generally inhibit tissue repair. In order to explain the paradoxical neuroprotective effects of anti-inflammatory agents, we begin with a review of the mechanisms by which inflammation leads to tissue repair.

[c]Corresponding author: Dr. Lloyd Guth, 111 Gullane, Williamsburg, VA 23188-7438. Phone, 757/258-3705.

e-mail, lloydguth@erols.com

[d]Present address: Department of Anatomy and Neurobiology, College of Medicine, University of California at Irvine, Irvine, CA 92697-4292, USA.

Inflammation is set in motion when tissue is injured, be it from microorganisms, allergens, chemicals, or physical trauma. By a sequential and coordinated series of biochemical responses of specific cells, injurious agents are neutralized, damaged tissues removed, ingrowth of parenchymal and stromal cells facilitated, and wound healing initiated. The endothelial cell is the first to be affected by injury; its metabolic responses attract neutrophils and expedite their entry into the injured region. The neutrophils destroy infectious agents, initiate the degradation of necrotic cellular debris, synthesize vasoactive lipids that loosen the extracellular matrix,[1] and secrete chemotactic substances that attract the ingrowth of monocytes. Upon entering the inflamed region, the monocytes differentiate into macrophages which phagocytose cell debris and secrete cytokines and growth factors[2–5] that promote the ingrowth of parenchymal cells. In this way, the inflammatory response corrects the cellular and intercellular disarray, reestablishes the tissue fabric, restores normal structure and function and, in short, regulates every aspect of the wound-healing process.

Initiation of the Inflammatory Response

The rapidity with which edema develops after injury is an indication that vascular alterations initiate the inflammatory response; but only after the discovery of "reperfusion injury" did the biochemical explanation for this phenomenon become clear. Reperfusion injury is the mechanism by which tissue ischemia leads to necrosis. The extraordinary finding is that the tissue damage does not occur during the ischemic episode, but subsequently when blood flow is resumed.[6] Reperfusion injury has been observed in virtually every organ of the body, but studies on lung tissue have provided definitive evidence that oxygen is the critical ingredient responsible for reperfusion injury.[7] In these experiments, the lung was rendered ischemic by clamping its blood supply while the organ was ventilated with either nitrogen or air. Pulmonary infarction occurred if the ischemic lung was ventilated with air, and not if it was ventilated with nitrogen (anoxic-ischemia). However, pulmonary infarction developed rapidly when the lung that had been subjected to anoxic-ischemia was reperfused with oxygenated blood. The finding that ischemia produced damage only in oxygenated tissues raised the important question of the mechanism by which the presence of oxygen leads to tissue destruction.

Endothelial cells are ubiquitous in all organs and are the very first cells exposed to oxygen upon reperfusion. Therefore, it is not altogether surprising that reperfusion injury reflects ischemia-induced metabolic changes in these cells. Under normal conditions, the endothelial cell's xanthine dehydrogenase enzyme oxidizes hypoxanthine and xanthine to uric acid by transferring electrons to nicotinamide adenine dinucleotide (NAD). However, during ischemia this enzyme undergoes limited proteolysis. The resulting modified enzyme (now designated xanthine oxidase) can only transfer the electron to molecular oxygen, and not to NAD),[6] a reaction that produces cytotoxic superoxide and hydroxyl radicals.[8,9] Consequently, the precipitous reintroduction of oxygen during reperfusion initiates the enzymatic reaction that gives rise to reactive oxygen species[10] that are cytotoxic to the endothelial cell and thereby damaging to the blood vessels. Neutrophils aggregate in regions of vascular damage where they secrete superoxide and other reactive oxygen species by a nicotinamide adenine dinucleotide phosphate (NADPH) oxidase reaction unrelated to xanthine oxidase.[6] This cytotoxic activity further damages the vascular integrity and facilitates migration of neutrophils across the vessel wall.[6] Thus begins the neutrophil-dominated phase of the acute inflammatory reaction.

Tissue necrosis resulting from reperfusion injury can be attenuated by various anti-inflammatory agents such as allopurinol (an inhibitor of xanthine oxidase) and superoxide dismutase (a scavenger of free radicals). However, as would be expected, such agents are protective only if administered within minutes after the onset of reperfusion.[6,11–13]

The Phenomenon of Progressive Necrosis after Spinal Cord Injury

In the following experiments the spinal cord with overlying dura intact was exposed by laminectomy and crushed extradurally between the blades of a fine (#5) jeweler's forceps.[14] FIGURE 1 illustrates characteristic histological changes during the first 8 postoperative weeks: In FIGURE 1A,B,C, the epicenter of the primary lesion (i.e., the site of necrosis caused by mechanical trauma) is indicated by *e*. The secondary dorsal column lesion, whose extent is demarcated by arrowheads, will be described and discussed later. At 6 hr after injury, the primary lesion is bounded rostrally and caudally by an edematous area or penumbra (FIG. 1A). By 1 wk (FIG. 1B) the tissues of the penumbra undergo necrosis and thereby enlarge the primary lesion. During succeeding weeks, the tissue at the margin of the lesion gradually undergoes further necrosis such that by 8 wk (FIG. 1C) the primary lesion is characterized by the presence of large cavities that are partially walled off by astroglial scar tissue.[15] Thus, the necrotizing process destroys nerve pathways that had been initially spared from damage, replaces the normal spinal tissue fabric with fibroglial scars and fluid-filled cavities, and creates an environment that precludes any possibility of meaningful tissue repair and functional recovery.[16]

The extent to which the primary lesion expands varies with the severity of the injury. Spinal transection injuries produce a lesion that may extend for several centimeters;[16] while severe crush lesions extend only for several millimeters.[17] FIGURE 2 illustrates the growth of the primary lesion after a severe crush injury.

ROLE OF INFLAMMATORY REACTIONS IN THE PATHOGENESIS OF PRIMARY AND SECONDARY SPINAL CORD LESIONS

Pathogenesis of the Primary Lesion

During the first 6–12 hr after injury, neutrophils appear in the postcapillary venules at or near the primary lesion (FIG. 3A,B), and by 24 hr they migrate into the tissue parenchyma (FIG. 3C). Between 24 and 48 hr vascular damage has resulted in the extravasation of erythrocytes as well (FIG. 3D). By 48 hr, the neutrophils have been largely replaced by mononuclear cells (FIG. 3E). By 72 hr these cells have already differentiated into macrophages and are now engorged with phagocytosed debris (FIG. 3F). The macrophages do not seem to leave the inflamed region; rather they remain and degenerate, perhaps thereby prolonging the inflammatory response. The presence of large numbers of degenerated macrophages within and around

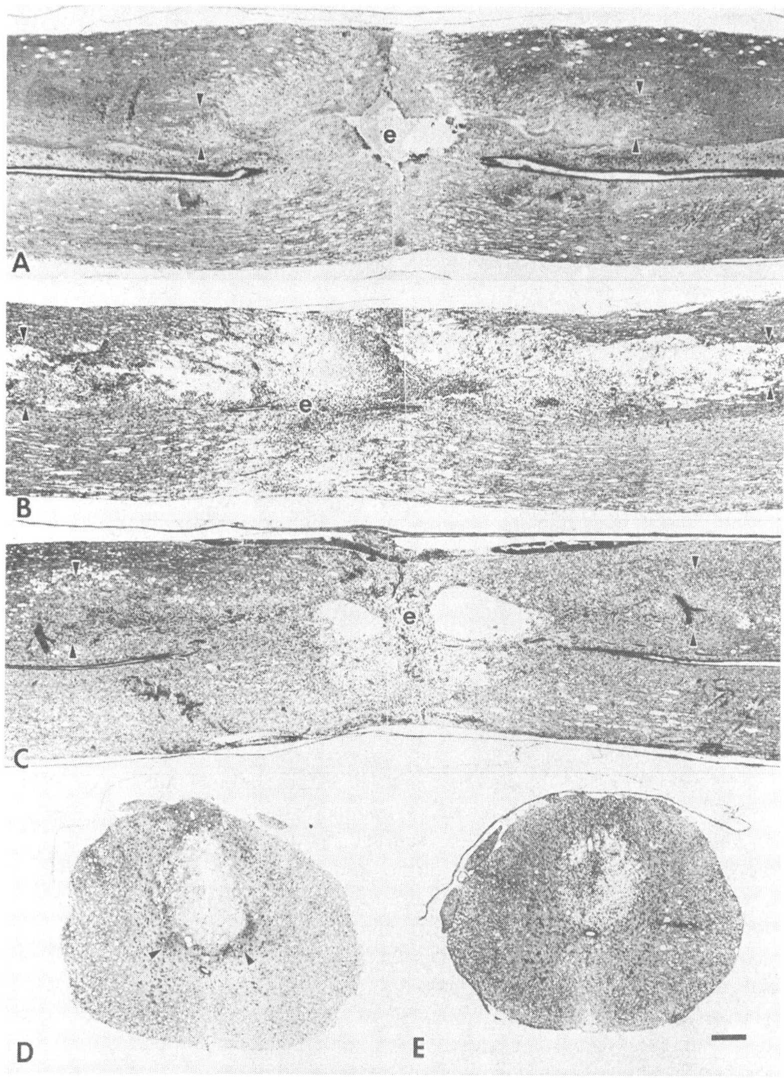

FIGURE 1. Midsagittal (**A,B,C**) and transverse (**D, E**) sections of spinal cord subjected to crush injury. In (A,B,C) the epicenter of the primary lesion is designated by *e*, and the extent of the dorsal column lesion by *arrow heads*. (H&E, scale bar = 480 μm). (A) 6 hr postoperative. (B) 1 wk postoperative. (C) 8 wk postoperative. (D,E) Transverse sections 1 mm caudal from the margin of the primary lesion. (D) At 3 d postoperative a region of hemorrhage (*arrow heads*) partially surrounds the lesion. (E) By 7 d postoperative the lesion is more cellular.

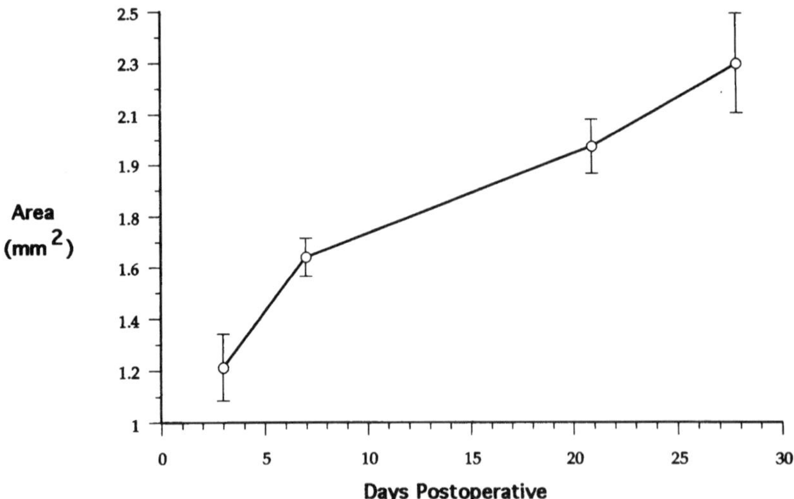

FIGURE 2. Progressive enlargement of the primary lesion after a crush lesion of the rat spinal cord. Analysis of variance showed that the lesion increased significantly in size from 3 to 28 d postoperative (p <0.01), and regression analysis revealed a statistically significant linear trend (p <0.001) during this 4-wk period.

cavities[17] suggests that degeneration of these cells contributes to the development of cavitation during progressive spinal cord necrosis.

Pathogenesis of the Secondary Dorsal Column Lesion

A second feature shown in FIGURE 1 is the development of a secondary lesion, which is located in the dorsal column. By 6 hr after spinal crush injury (FIG. 1A), an edematous (pale-staining) region extends rostrocaudally from the primary lesion within the ventral part of the dorsal column. Its extent is demarcated by arrowheads. At 1 wk (FIG. 1B) after injury the dorsal column lesion is so greatly enlarged as to extend beyond the margins of the photograph. At this time, tissue necrosis has resulted in loss of cellularity and cavitation within dorsal column lesions. By 8 wk, however (FIG. 1C), the dorsal column lesion is significantly shorter, shows less cavitation, and has regained much of its original cellularity and vascularity. In transverse section (FIG. 1D,E) the lesion is seen to occupy the ventralmost portion of the dorsal column which, in rodents, is the site of the main corticospinal tract.[18–21] Quantitative measurements of the dorsal column lesion (FIG. 4) showed evidence of wound healing not seen in the primary lesion. Between 1 and 8 wk the dorsal column lesion decreased significantly in overall size and in amount of cavitation, whereas in the primary lesion these measures remained unchanged.

As early as 6 hr after injury, the tissues of the dorsal column are in disarray (compare FIGS. 5A and 5B); the nuclei of the oligodendroglial cells have become pyknotic, and the myelin is dispersed and pale-staining. At this very time, inflammatory responses are also evident; neutrophils begin to accumulate in the venules of the white matter (top of FIG. 5C) and, by 12 hr, they have begun to migrate from the venules (middle of FIG. 5D) into the tissue parenchyma. The dorsal column lesion elongates

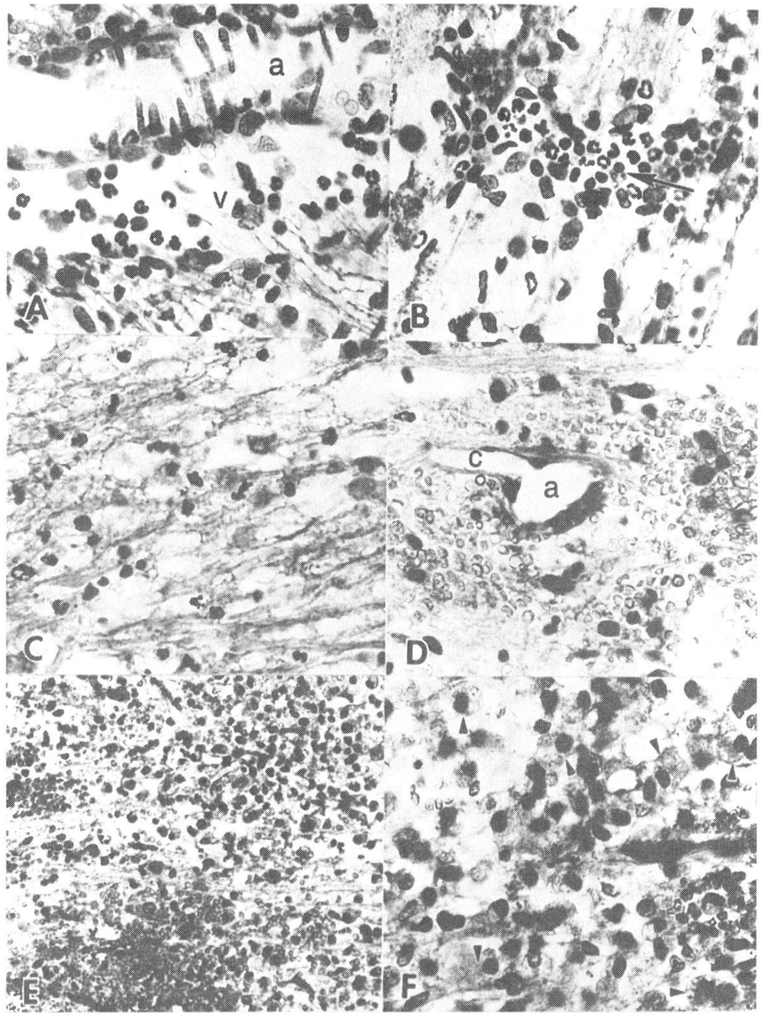

FIGURE 3. High-power photomicrographs of sections from the spinal cord of vehicle-treated control rats. H&E; ×620 (**A,B,C,D,F**); ×310 (**E**). (A) 6 hr postoperative, ventral aspect of the cord, 0.3 mm from the epicenter (a, arteriole; v, venule). (B) 12 hr postoperative, ventral cord, 0.4 mm from epicenter (*arrow* points to neutrophils). (C) 24 hr postoperative, dorsal column, 1 mm from the epicenter (a, arteriole; c, capillary). (D) 48 hr postoperative, central gray matter, 1 mm from epicenter. (E) 48 hr postoperative, interface of dorsal column and subjacent gray matter, 1 mm from the epicenter. (F) 72 hr postoperative, central gray matter, 1.5 mm from epicenter (*arrowheads* point to macrophages).

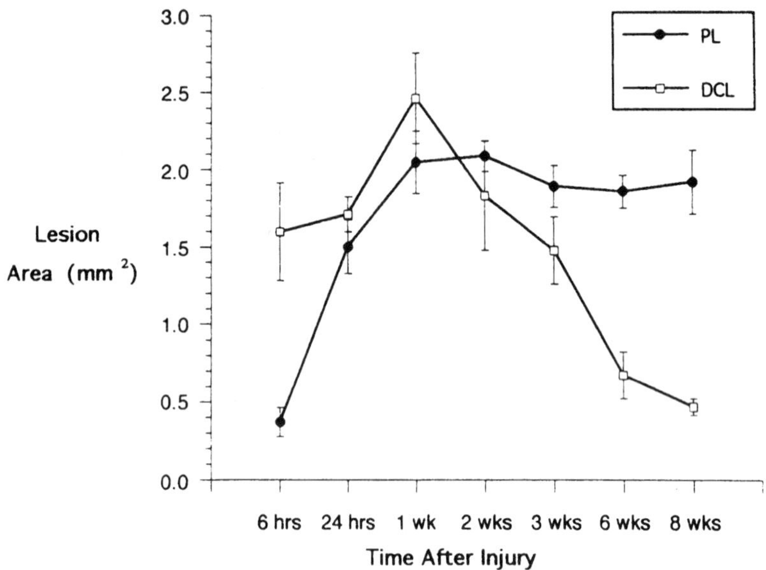

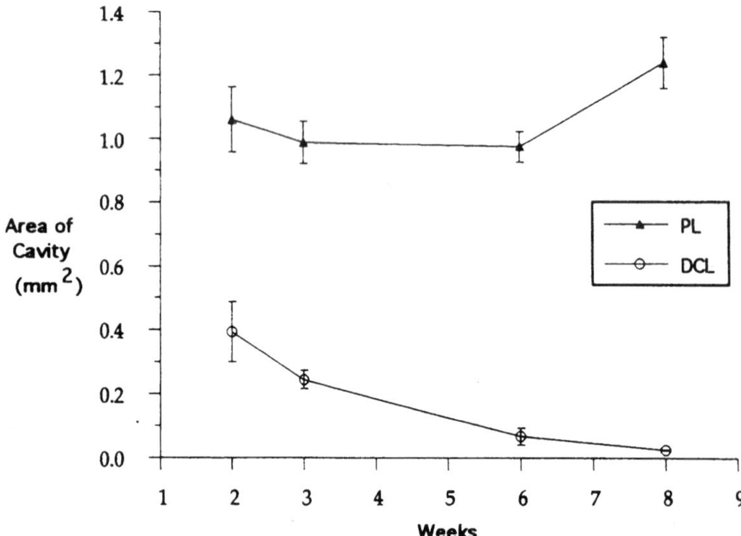

FIGURE 4. Comparison of changes in dorsal column and the primary lesions as a function of weeks postoperative. *Top.* The size of the dorsal column lesion diminished significantly between 1 and 8 weeks ($p < 0.01$), whereas that of the primary lesion remained unchanged. *Bottom.* The amount of cavitation in the dorsal column lesion declined significantly from 2 to 8 weeks ($p < 0.01$), while that of the primary lesion remained unchanged.

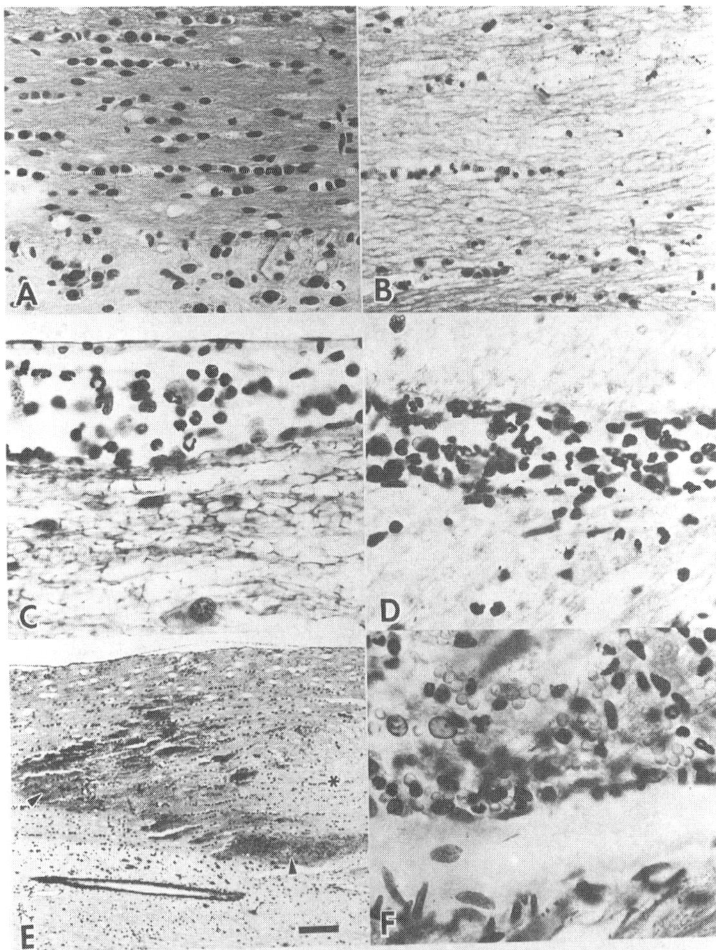

FIGURE 5. Midsagittal sections of the normal dorsal column (**A**) and of the dorsal column lesion (**B–F**) stained with H&E. Scale bar: 60 μm (A,B), 30 μm (C,D,F), and 300 μm (E). (A) Distribution of glial cells (presumably oligodendrocytes) of myelinated fiber tracts in the dorsal column of the normal spinal cord. (B) Six hr postoperative showing myelin and glial disarray. (C) Six hr postoperative showing accumulation of neutrophils in venules (*top* of figure). (D) Twelve hr postoperative showing neutrophils emerging from a venule (*center* of figure) and infiltrating the tissue parenchyma. (E) From 6 hr (illustrated) to 3 d after injury, a characteristic cap-like area of hemorrhage (*arrowheads*) was consistently found at the rostral termination (*asterisk*) and the caudal termination (not shown) of the dorsal column lesion. (F) Higher magnification of the margin of the dorsal column lesion at 48 hr illustrates the extravasated red blood cells among the neutrophils.

rostrocaudally from 6 hr to 3 d, and at every stage of this process a characteristic region of hemorrhage caps the rostral and caudal terminations of the lesion (FIG. 5E,F).

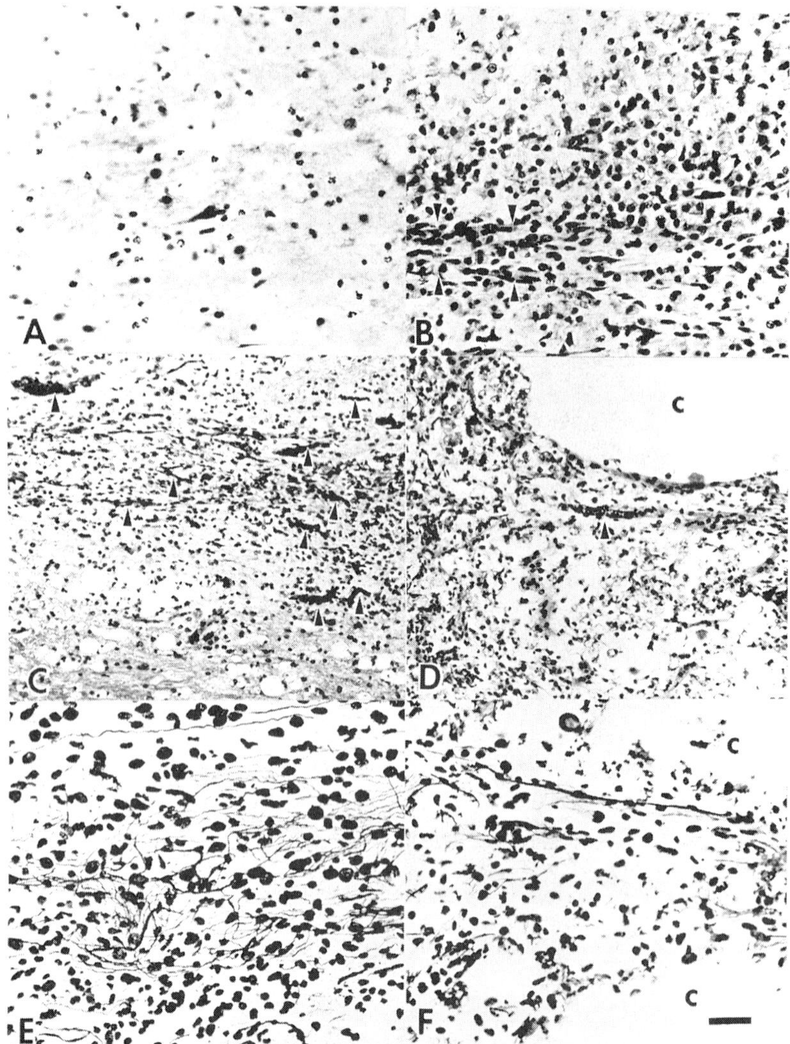

FIGURE 6. Midsagittal sections of the dorsal column lesion **(A,B,C,E)** and the primary lesion **(E,F)**. Scale bar = 60 μm (A,B,E,F), 120 μm (C,D). (A) H&E stain, 24 hr postoperative. (B) H&E stain, 1 wk postoperative. *Arrowheads* indicate spindle-shaped glial cells. (C) H&E stain, 8 wk postoperative. *Arrowheads* indicate longitudinally oriented blood vessels. (D) H&E stain, primary lesion site, 8 wk postoperative. A large cavity is indicated by *c* and a blood vessel by an *arrowhead*. (E) Protargol impregnation, dorsal column lesion, 8 wk postoperative. (F) Protargol, primary lesion, 8 wk postoperative.

The subsequent inflammatory processes in the dorsal column lesion are quite different from those of the primary lesion. By 24 hr, the tissue of the dorsal column is heavily infiltrated by neutrophils (FIG. 6A), but within 1 wk, these cells disappear and are replaced by large, foamy-appearing, macrophages (FIG. 6B) and by spindle-shaped glial cells (arrowheads) which begin to grow into the lesion. The macrophages do not persist as they do at the primary lesion site; they disappear, and their place is increasingly taken by glial cells. By 8 wk postoperative, few macrophages are found, cysts remain only at the margin of the lesion, the glial cells provide a densely cellular environment, and there is extensive ingrowth of longitudinally-oriented blood vessels (FIG. 6C). Numerous regenerating nerve fibers are now seen in the dorsal column lesion (FIG. 6E). By contrast, the primary lesion shows extensive cavitation and cystic degeneration, persisting macrophages, and little ingrowth of blood vessels or nerve fibers (FIG. 6D,F). These differences are seen to advantage by comparing FIGURES 6C vs 6D and 6E vs 6F.

In summary, spinal cord injury is followed by progressively increasing damage at the primary lesion and by wound healing at the secondary dorsal column lesion. The fact that these two distinctive histopathological reactions occur within the same animal raises the possibility that wound healing of the primary lesion might also be achieved if necrotizing processes were attenuated by administration of specific anti-inflammatory "neuroprotective" agents. The following experiments bear on this issue.

MODULATION OF PROGRESSIVE NECROSIS BY ANTI-INFLAMMATORY AGENTS

The Primary Lesion: Immunomodulatory Agents

Two macrophage-activating (immunomodulatory) agents were tested; lipopolysaccharide (LPS, a preparation from the cell walls of *Salmonella enteritidis*) and Imuvert (a preparation that does not contain LPS and that derives from cytosolic membranes of *Serratia marcescens*). These agents were chosen because they activate the secretion of cytokines by various cell types including macrophages, neuroglia and microglia;[4,5,22–24] they were administered for 28 d after crushing the spinal cord of rats. As summarized in TABLE 1, neither agent affected the size of the primary lesion, but both significantly reduced the amount of cavitation within the lesion. Of particular importance was the finding that indomethacin—which inhibits the synthesis of prostaglandins thought to be detrimental to healing of spinal cord injuries[25]—had no effect by itself but significantly potentiated the ability of LPS to reduce the amount of cavitation ($p < 0.01$). This finding indicates that agents that selectively modulate different inflammatory processes should be evaluated both separately and in combination.

The Primary Lesion: Effect of Steroids, Indomethacin and LPS

Because the combination of LPS and indomethacin significantly attenuated histological damage, and because steroids are effective neuroprotective agents in animal models and human injuries,[25–28] a comprehensive experiment was done to compare the efficacy of these three classes of drugs both individually and in combination.[29] We selected pregnenolone and dehydroepiandrosterone (DHEA), because they are natural rather than synthetic, they are progenitors of the glucocorticoids,

TABLE 1. Area of lesion (mm^2) and area of cavitation (mm^2) 28 days after crush injury of the rat spinal cord

	N	Area of Lesion Mean ± SEM	p	Area of Cavitation Mean ± SEM	p
Control	6	1.62 ± 0.113	ns	0.93 ± 0.102	—
LPS	7	1.64 ± 0.043	ns	0.49 ± 0.099	<0.001
Imuvert	7	1.53 ± 0.108	ns	0.29 ± 0.043	<0.001
Indomethacin	5	1.61 ± 0.109	ns	1.05 ± 0.128	ns
LPS+indomethacin	7	1.23 ± 0.140	ns	0.11 ± 0.040	<0.001

DOSAGE: LPS, 1 μg/gm daily, i.p.; indomethacin, 1 μg/gm daily, i.p.; Imuvert, 0.5 μg/gm biweekly, i.p. Statistical analysis (vehicle controls vs experimental treatments) by analysis of variance and Student-Newman-Keuls multiple comparison test.

TABLE 2. Effect of anti-inflammatory drug treatments on lesion size and cavitation 21 days after spinal cord crush injury in the rat

Treatment	N	Area of Lesion (mm^2) Mean ± SEM	p	Area of Cavitation (mm^2) Mean ± SEM	p
Control	6	1.62 ± 0.11	—	0.94 ± 0.11	ns
Indomethacin (IM)	6	1.63 ± 0.14	ns	1.05 ± 0.13	ns
LPS	4	1.64 ± 0.08	ns	0.63 ± 0.09	ns
Pregnenolone (Preg)	6	1.84 ± 0.10	ns	1.00 ± 0.11	ns
LPS+IM	4	1.63 ± 0.13	ns	0.49 ± 0.11	<0.05
Preg+LPS+IM	6	1.14 ± 0.14	<0.01	0.30 ± 0.04	<0.01
DHEA	6	1.68 ± 0.12	ns	0.94 ± 0.10	ns
DHEA+LPS+IM	8	1.12 ± 0.08	<0.01	0.33 ± 0.03	<0.01

DOSAGE: LPS, 1 μg/gm daily, i.p.; indomethacin, 1 μg/gm daily, i.p.; PREG+DHEA, 2.4 mg daily via a 50-mg, 21-day, timed-release, subcutaneously implanted pellet (Innovative Research of America, Inc.). Statistical analysis (vehicle controls vs experimental treatments) by analysis of variance and Student-Newman-Keuls multiple comparison test.

mineral corticoids and sex steroids, and they have neuroexcitatory properties by virtue of their actions on γ-aminobutyric acid (GABA) and glutamate receptors.[30,31]

As seen in TABLE 2, both the size of the primary lesion and the amount of its cavitation were significantly reduced when LPS, indomethacin and pregnenolone or DHEA were administered in combination. This effect seemed so remarkable that the experiment was performed again on a larger number of subjects per group; the results (TABLE 3) verify that combination treatment with pregnenolone, LPS, and indomethacin significantly attenuated progressive necrosis and that the inclusion of indomethacin was essential for this effect. In addition, this treatment significantly improved recovery of locomotor function.[29,32]

TABLE 3. Effect of treatment with pregnenolone, LPS and indomethacin on lesion size and cavitation 21 days after spinal cord injury

Treatmen	N	Area of Lesion (mm^2) Mean ± SEM	p	Area of Cavitation (mm^2) Mean ± SEM	p
Vehicle	9	1.89 ± 0.12	—	0.99 ± 0.09	
Preg+LPS	10	1.77 ± 0.14	ns	0.94 ± 0.12	ns
Preg+LPS+IM	9	1.33 ± 0.14	<0.05	0.49 ± 0.08	<0.01

Dosage as per TABLE 2. Statistical analysis (vehicle controls vs experimental treatments) by analysis of variance and Student-Newman-Keuls multiple comparison test.

The Primary Lesion:
Early Intervention with Anti-inflammatory Agents

Since progressive expansion of a spinal cord lesion begins soon after spinal cord injury, the question arose whether specific neuroprotective treatments might attenuate or retard early steps in the process of progressive necrosis. In the first experiment, we compared the effects of two anti-inflammatory treatments on the size of the lesion at 3 d postoperative. One treatment was the combination of pregnenolone, LPS, and indomethacin (PLI), and the other was aminoguanidine, an inhibitor of inducible nitric oxide synthase (i-NOS)[33,34] that reduces the release of nitric oxide by activated neutrophils and macrophages. Nitric oxide is cytotoxic at early stages of inflammation.[35] The results (TABLE 4) show that PLI treatment, which markedly reduced the size of the lesion at 21–28 d, had no significant effect at 3 d, whereas aminoguanidine significantly reduced the size of the lesion at 3 d. Combining the aminoguanidine with indomethacin or naproxen conferred no additional benefit.[32] We conclude that inhibition of the release of nitric oxide is neuroprotective during the acute period after spinal cord injury, while the combined pregnenolone, LPS, and indomethacin treatment is beneficial only after 21–28 d of treatment.

The Secondary Dorsal Column Lesion:
Selective Effects of Anti-inflammatory Drugs

The unique location and extent of the dorsal column lesion raised the possibility that this secondary degeneration might be related to Wallerian degeneration of its long propriospinal and corticospinal tracts. If so, the inflammatogenic nature of axonal and myelin fragments would be responsible for the occurrence of hemorrhage, leukocytic infiltration, and tissue necrosis far from the site of primary injury. Since the dorsal column lesion is transient, we studied the effect of allopurinol and aminoguanidine, two agents that act at early stages of the inflammatory process. Allopurinol, a competitive inhibitor of xanthine oxidase, attenuates the endothelial cell damage caused by reperfusion injury.[6,10] Aminoguanidine, an inhibitor of i-NOS,[33,34] attenuates early damage at the primary lesion site (TABLE 4). The results (TABLE 5) permit three conclusions: (a) Both allopurinol and aminoguanidine reduced the size of the primary lesion at 3 d postoperative, but the effect of aminoguanidine was significantly greater than that of allopurinol. (b) Allopurinol significantly reduced the size of the dorsal column lesion, while aminoguanidine did not. (c) The distinctive effects of inhibitors of i-NOS and xanthine oxidase are consistent with the

TABLE 4. Effect of anti-inflammatory drugs on the response to spinal cord injury at 3 days postoperative

Treatment	N	Area of Lesion Mean ± SEM	p
Vehicle control	5	1.38 ± 0.110	—
Pregnenolone+LPS+indomethacin	5	1.22 ± 0.081	ns
Naproxen+aminoguanidine	5	0.96 ± 0.086	<0.01
Aminoguanidine	5	0.99 ± 0.049	<0.05

Statistical analysis (vehicle controls vs experimental treatments) by analysis of variance and Student-Newman-Keuls multiple comparison test.

TABLE 5. Effect of allopurinol or aminoguanidine treatment on size of the primary and dorsal column lesions 3 days after spinal cord injury

Treatment	N	Primary Lesion Area (mm^2) Mean	SEM	Secondary Dorsal Column Lesion (mm^2) Mean	SEM
Vehicle control	6	1.53	0.044	2.11	0.149
Aminoguanidine	10	1.17	0.045	1.95	0.116
Allopurinol	7	1.31	0.057	1.53	0.069
Statistical Comparisons[a]					
Vehicle vs aminoguanidine			<0.001		>0.05 (ns)
Vehicle vs allopurinol			<0.01		<0.05
Aminoguanidine vs allopurinol			<0.05		<0.05

[a]Statistical analysis by analysis of variance and Student-Newman-Keuls multiple comparison test.

hypothesis that multiple inflammatory processes contribute to the pathogenesis of progressive necrosis.

DEGENERATION AND REPAIR
AFTER SPINAL CORD INJURY IN THE MOUSE

Introduction

Many issues in neurotrauma research can best be addressed by use of genetic approaches; for this purpose, the mouse is an especially appropriate species.[36] We have studied *Wld^s* mice, a naturally-occurring mutant strain in which the process of Wallerian degeneration is substantially delayed. Indeed, axonal structure is preserved for 1 wk or more after nerve transection and the distal stump remains capable of conducting action potentials during this time.[37,38] Although the mutation also delays the onset of myelin breakdown degeneration and the activation of macrophages,[39] several lines of evidence indicate that the mutation regulates the nerve degeneration process directly rather than via an effect on macrophage function.[38,40] The *Wld^s*

TABLE 6. Area of primary and dorsal column lesions after spinal cord injury in C57BL/6J and *Wld^S* mice

Primary Lesion

| Weeks | Area of Lesion (mm^2) | | | | Statistical Analysis[a] | | | |
| | C57BL | | *Wld^S* | | By Strain | | By Weeks | |
Postop.	Mean ± SEM	(n)	Mean ± SEM	(n)	C57 vs *Wld^S*	Weeks	C57BL	*Wld^S*
1	1.03 ± 0.014	(5)	1.03 ± 0.121	(4)	ns	1 vs 2	<0.001	ns
2	0.84 ± 0.032	(6)	0.95 ± 0.071	(4)	ns	2 vs 3	<0.001	ns
3	0.32 ± 0.031	(6)	0.89 ± 0.063	(7)	<0.001	3 vs 4	<0.05	<0.001
4	0.24 ± 0.012	(7)	0.36 ± 0.030	(6)	<0.01	4 vs 8	ns	ns
8	0.22 ± 0.020	(5)	0.38 ± 0.044	(6)	<0.01			

Secondary Dorsal Column Lesion

| Weeks | Area of Lesion (mm^2) | | | | Statistical Analysis[a] | | | |
| | C57BL | | *Wld^S* | | By Strain | | By Weeks | |
Postop.	Mean ± SEM	(n)	Mean ± SEM	(n)	C57 vs *Wld^S*	Weeks	C57BL	*Wld^S*
1	0.87 ± 0.043	(5)	0.48 ± 0.008	(4)	<0.001	1 vs 2	<.001	ns
2	0.61 ± 0.048	(6)	0.60 ± 0.100	(4)	ns	2 vs 3	<0.001	ns
3	0.12 ± 0.045	(6)	0.44 ± 0.088	(7)	<0.001	3 vs 4	<0.05	<0.01
4	0.02 ± 0.031	(7)	0.22 ± 0.095	(6)	<0.01	4 vs 8	ns	ns
8	0.03 ± 0.036	(5)	0.11 ± 0.070	(6)	<0.05			

[a]Statistical analysis by analysis of variance and Student-Newman-Keuls multiple comparison test.

mutation in our mice was on a C57BL/6J background genotype, and the non-mutant C57BL/6J mice were therefore used for comparison.

Histopathology of the Primary Lesion in C57BL/6J and Wld^S *Mice*

The sequelae of crush injury in mice are significantly different from those in rats. As illustrated in FIGURE 7, at 1 wk postoperatively, mice show far less destruction and cavitation (FIG. 7A) than rats (FIG. 7B). At 8 wk, the tissue damage and cavitation in mice has decreased, and healing is evidenced by the near-approximation of the re-forming central canal (FIG. 7C). At 8 wk in rats, on the other hand, the primary lesion consists of several huge cavities (FIG. 7D). Healing of the primary lesion in mice is similar to wound healing in other organs. The tissue at the site of injury is a variety of loosely arranged connective tissue, in which macrophages are the predominant cell type and collagenous connective tissue the predominant fibrous component. In time, this connective tissue becomes increasingly dense as the wound contracts, diminishes in size, and becomes encapsulated by hypertrophied astrocytic processes.[39,4]

We observed no qualitative differences in the primary or secondary dorsal column lesions of C57BL/6J and *Wld^S* mice, but quantitative differences were demonstrable by image analysis (TABLE 6). At 1 wk after injury, the size of the primary lesion was the same in *Wld^S* as in C57BL/6J mice. The lesion diminished in size thereafter, and by 8 wk was very small in both strains. However, at every postoperative interval, after week 2, the lesion was significantly larger in the *Wld^S* than in the C57BL/6J strain (TABLE 6, top). We therefore conclude that healing of the primary spinal cord lesion is slower in *Wld^S* than in C57BL/6J mice.

Secondary Dorsal Column Lesion (TABLE 6, Bottom)

At 1 wk, the secondary dorsal column lesion was smaller in *Wld^S* than in C57BL/6J mice. Thereafter, the size of the dorsal column lesion diminished in both strains, but the change was slower and less complete in the *Wld^S* strain. For many weeks after injury, the dorsal column lesion in the *Wld^S* mouse could be distinguished from that in the C57BL/6J by greater macrophage infiltration and a denser fibrotic reaction.[39,41] The following conclusions are consistent with hypothesis that Wallerian degeneration contributes to the formation of the dorsal column lesion: the dorsal column lesion develops after the primary lesion, the onset and healing of the dorsal column lesion is delayed in *Wld^S* mice, and the cellular inflammatory response is delayed and prolonged in *Wld^S* mice.

Thus, Wallerian degeneration in the dorsal column triggers histopathological changes that produce an inflammatory response by which the damaged tissues are removed and the wound repaired. As was noted by Dusart and Schwab,[42] the dorsal column lesion cannot result from cytotoxic secretions of macrophages, because the lesion develops prior to macrophage infiltration. Presumably the temporally prolonged and spatially widespread process of Wallerian degeneration produces necrotizing changes in regions of the dorsal column far from the initial site of trauma and thereby initiates an inflammatory response that leads to repair of the damage.

DYNAMIC ASPECTS OF TISSUE REPAIR
AFTER SPINAL CORD INJURY

Beginning with the seminal experiments of David and Aguayo,[43] the results of numerous animal studies have attested to the regenerative capacity of the injured mammalian spinal cord. However, the expression of this growth potential has been demonstrable only under highly controlled laboratory conditions. We do not know precisely why this so, but insights can be inferred from these histopathological observations: In rats, the primary lesion does not heal; it progressively enlarges as it undergoes additional necrosis and cavitation. However, in the secondary dorsal column lesion of rats, wound-healing processes restore tissue architecture to a considerable degree. In mice, on the other hand, necrosis and cavitation are milder than in the rat, and both primary and secondary lesions gradually diminish in size as they undergo wound healing (FIG. 7). Even though tissue repair and nerve regeneration are not brought to completion in traumatic (primary) spinal cord lesions of rats, certain cellular responses are indicative of incipient wound-healing processes. These re-

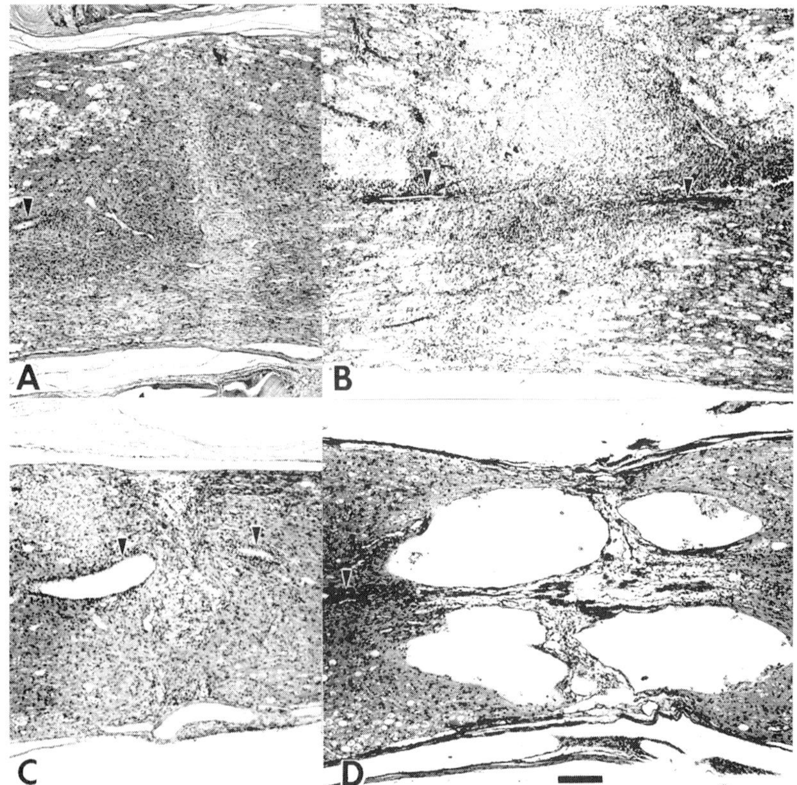

FIGURE 7. Midsagittal sections through the primary spinal cord lesion in mice and rats. (**A**) H&E, 1 wk postoperative, mouse (C57BL/6J). (**B**) H&E, 1 wk postoperative, rat. (**C**) H&E, 8 wk postoperative, mouse (C57BL/6J). (**D**) H&E, 8 wk postoperative, rat.

sponses include proliferation and migration of endothelial, ependymal, and glial cells, and the abortive growth of nerve fibers.[14,42,44,45]

These observations imply that wound-healing processes are initiated after spinal cord injury in rats but are subsequently thwarted by destructive events. Consequently, the outcome of progressive necrosis vs tissue repair depends on the dynamics of the balance between these reparative and destructive processes.[17,26,27,29] For this reason, the fundamental goal of neuroprotective therapy is to redress the imbalance between the destructive and reparative physiological cascades and, thereby, to allow the intrinsic physiological healing mechanisms to be expressed. It follows that neuroprotective agents should not be chosen solely for their ability to interfere with destructive reactions; indeed, seemingly "destructive processes" may actually promote tissue repair (e.g., by removing obstructive debris and loosening extracellular matrix so that cells can move more freely through the site of injury) . The goal of neuroprotective therapy is to restore the dynamics of wound healing in order to facilitate the coordinated integration of cellular activities that will lead to structural and functional reconstitution of the injured spinal cord.

REFERENCES

1. GOETZL, E.J., R.A. LEWIS & M. ROLA-PLESZCZYNSKI, Eds. 1994. Cellular Generation, Transport, and Effects of Eiconosoids. Ann. N.Y. Acad. Sci. **744:** 1–340.
2. HUNT, T.K., D.R. KNIGHTON, K.K. THAKRAL *et al.* 1984. Studies on inflammation and wound healing: angiogenesis and collagen synthesis stimulated *in vivo* by resident and activated wound macrophages. Surgery **96:** 48–54.
3. NATHAN, C.F. 1987. Secretory products of macrophages. J. Clin. Invest. **79:** 319–326.
4. RAPPOLEE, D.A., D. MARK, M.J. BANDA *et al.* 1988. Wound macrophages express TGF-α and other growth factors *in vivo*. Analysis by mRNA phenotyping. Science **241:** 708–712.
5. SPORN, M.B. & A.B. ROBERTS, Eds. 1990. Peptide Growth Factors and Their Receptors. Springer-Verlag. Berlin.
6. SUSSMAN, M.S. & G.B. BULKLEY. 1990. Oxygen-derived free radicals in reperfusion injury. *In* Methods in Enzymology: Oxygen Radicals in Biological Systems. Vol. 186, Part B. L. Packer & A.N.Glazer, Eds.: 711–723. Academic Press. San Diego.
7. FISHER, A.B., C. DODIA, I. AYENE *et al.* 1994. Ischemia-reperfusion injury to the lung. Ann. N.Y. Acad. Sci. **723:** 197–207.
8. COHEN, G. 1994. Enzymatic/nonenzymatic sources of oxyradicals and regulation of antioxidant defenses. Ann. N.Y. Acad. Sci. **738:** 8–14.
9. CHIUEH, C.C., D.L. GILBERT & C.A. COLTON, Eds. 1994. The Neurobiology of NO and OH. Ann. N.Y. Acad. Sci. **738:** 1–467.
10. KUROSE, I. & D.N. GRANGER. 1994. Evidence implicating xanthine oxidase and neutrophils in reperfusion-induced microvascular dysfunction. Ann. N.Y. Acad. Sci. **723:** 158–179.
11. HOSHINO, T., W.R. MALEY, G.B. BULKLEY *et al.* 1988. Ablation of free radical-mediated reperfusion injury for the salvage of kidneys taken from non-heart-beating donors. A quantitative evaluation of the proportion of injury caused by reperfusion following periods of warm, cold and combined warm and cold ischemia. Transplantation **45:** 284–289.
12. PARK, P.O., U. HAGLUND, G.B. BULKLEY *et al.* 1990. The sequence of development of intestinal tissue injury after strangulation ischemia and reperfusion. Surgery **107:** 574–580.
13. HAGLUND, U., G.B. BULKLEY & D.N. GRANGER. 1987. On the pathophysiology of intestinal ischemic injury. Acta Chir. Scand. **153:** 321–324.
14. GUTH, L., C.P. BARRETT, E.J. DONATI *et al.* 1985. Essentiality of a specific cellular terrain for growth of axons into a spinal cord lesion. Exp. Neurol. **88:** 1–12.
15. BALENTINE, J.D. 1978. Pathology of experimental spinal cord trauma. I. The necrotic lesion as a function of vascular injury. Lab. Invest. **39:** 236–253.
16. GUTH, L., E.X. ALBUQUERQUE, S.S. DESHPANDE *et al.* 1980. Ineffectiveness of enzyme therapy on regeneration in the transected spinal cord of the rat. J. Neurosurg. **52:** 73–86.
17. GUTH, L., Z. ZHANG, N.A. DIPROSPERO *et al.* 1994. Spinal cord injury in the rat: treatment with bacterial lipopolysaccharide and indomethacin enhances cellular repair and locomotor function. Exp. Neurol. **126:** 76–87.
18. LINOWIECKI, A.J. 1914. The comparative anatomy of the pyramidal tract. J. Comp. Neurol. **24:** 509–530.
19. TERASHIMA, T., T. OCHIISHI & T. YAMAUCHI. 1994. Immunohistochemical detection of calcium/calmodulin-dependent protein kinase II in the spinal cord of the rat and monkey with special reference to the corticospinal tract. J. Comp. Neurol. **340:** 469–479.
20. JOOSTEN, E.A., R.L.SCHUITMAN, M.E. VERMELIS *et al.* 1992. Postnatal development of the ipsilateral corticospinal component in rat spinal cord: a light and electron microscopic anterograde HRP study. J. Comp. Neurol. **326:** 133–146.

21. PIPPENGER, M.A., T. SIMS & S.A. GILMORE. 1990. Development of the rat corticospinal tract through an altered glial environment. Brain Res. **55:** 43–50.
22. JOHNSON, W. & C.P. SUNG. 1987. Rat macrophage treatment with lipopolysaccharide with leads to a reduction in respiratory burst product secretion and a decrease in NADPH oxidase affinity. Cell. Immunol. **108:** 109–119.
23. KOCH, A.E., P.J. POLVERINI & S.J. LEIBOVICH. 1986. Induction of neovascularization by activated human monocytes. J. Leukocyte Biol. **39:** 233–238.
24. STRASSMAN, G., T.A. SPRINGER, S.J. HASKILL *et al.* 1985. Antigens associated with the activation of murine mononuclear macrophages *in vivo*: differential expression of lymphocyte function-associated antigen in the several stages of development. Cell. Immunol. **94:** 265–275.
25. HALL, E.D., D.L. WOLF & J.M. BRAUGHLER. 1985. Pathophysiology, consequences and pharmacological prevention of posttraumatic CNS ischemia. *In* Processes of Recovery from Neural Trauma. G. Gilad, Ed.: 63–73. Springer-Verlag. Berlin.
26. BEHRMANN, D.L., J.C. BRESNAHAN & M.S. BEATTIE. 1994. Modeling of acute spinal cord injury in the rat: neuroprotection and enhanced recovery with methylprednisolone, U-74006F and YM-14673. Exp. Neurol. **126:** 61–75.
27. BARTHOLDI, D. & M.E. SCHWAB. 1995. Methylprednisolone inhibits early inflammatory processes but not ischemic cell death after experimental spinal cord lesion in the rat. Brain Res. **672:** 177–186.
28. BRACKEN, M.B., M. J. SHEPARD, W.F. COLLINS *et al.* 1990. A randomized, controlled trial of methylprednisolone or naloxone in the treatment of acute spinal cord injury. N. Engl. J. Med. **322:** 1405–1411.
29. GUTH, L., Z. ZHANG & E. ROBERTS. 1994. Key role for pregnenolone in combination therapy that promotes recovery after spinal cord injury. Proc. Natl. Acad. Sci. USA **91:** 12308–12312.
30. MAJEWSKA, M.D. 1992. Endogenous bimodal modulators of the GABA receptor: mechanism of action and physiological significance. Prog. Neurobiol. **38:** 379–395.
31. WU, F.S., T.T. GIBBS & D.H. FARB. 1991. Pregnenolone sulfate: a positive allosteric modulator at the NMDA receptor. Mol. Pharmacol. **40:** 333–336.
32. ZHANG, Z., C.J. KREBS & L. GUTH. 1997. Experimental analysis of progressive necrosis after spinal cord trauma in the rat: etiological role of the inflammatory response. Exp. Neurol. **143:** 141–152.
33. GRIFFITHS, M.J.D., M. MESSENT, R.J. MACALLISTER *et al.* 1994. Aminoguanidine selectively inhibits inducible nitric oxide synthase. Br. J. Pharmacol. **110:** 963–968.
34. MISKO, T.P., W.M. MOORE, T.P. KASTEN *et al.* 1993. Selective inhibition of the inducible nitic oxide synthase by aminoguanidine. Eur. J. Pharmacol. **233:** 119–125.
35. LIPTON, W.A., Y.B. CHOI, Z.H. PAN *et al.* 1993. A redox-based mechanism for the neuroprotective and neurodestructive effects of nitric oxide and related nitroso-compounds. Nature **364:** 626–632.
36. STEWARD, O., P.E. SCHAUWECKER, L. GUTH *et al.* 1999. Genetic approaches to neurotrauma research: opportunities and potential pitfalls of murine models. Exp. Neurol. **157:** 19–42.
37. PERRY, V.H., E.R. LUNN, M.C. BROWN *et al.* 1990. Evidence that the rate of Wallerian degeneration is controlled by a single autosomal dominant gene. Eur. J. Neurosci. **2:** 408–413.
38. PERRY, V.H., M.C. BROWN, E.R. LUNN *et al.* 1990. Evidence that very slow Wallerian degeneration in C57BL/Ola mice is an intrinsic property of the peripheral nerve. Eur. J. Neurosci. **2:** 802–808.

39. FUJIKI, M., Z. ZHANG, L. GUTH & O. STEWARD. 1996. Genetic influences on cellular reactions to spinal cord injury: activation of macrophages/microglia and astrocytes is delayed in mice carrying a mutation (Wld^s) that causes delayed Wallerian degeneration. J. Comp. Neurol. **371:** 469–484.

40. GLASS, J.D., T.M. BRUSHART, E.B. GEORGE *et al.* 1993. Prolonged survival of transected nerve fibers in C57BL/Ola mice is an intrinsic characteristic of the axon. J. Neurocytol. **22:** 311–321.

41. ZHANG, Z., M. FUJIKI, L. GUTH & O. STEWARD. 1996. Genetic influences on cellular reactions to spinal cord injury: a wound-healing response present in normal mice is impaired in mice carrying a mutation (Wld^s) that causes delayed Wallerian degeneration. J. Comp. Neurol. **371:** 485–495.

42. DUSART, I. & M.E. SCHWAB. 1994. Secondary cell death and the inflammatory reaction after dorsal hemisection of the rat spinal cord. Eur. J. Neurosci. **6:** 712–724.

43. DAVID, S. & A.J. AGUAYO. 1981. Axonal elongation into peripheral nervous system "bridges" after central nervous system injury in adult rats. Science **214:** 931–933.

44. CURTIS, R., D. GREEN, R.M. LINDSAY *et al.* 1993. Up-regulation of GAP-43 and growth of axons in rat spinal cord after compression injury. J. Neurocytol. **2:** 51–64.

45. WINDLE, W.F. 1956. Regeneration of axons in the vertebrate central nervous system. Physiol. Rev. **36:** 427–440.

Ion Channel Modulation as the Basis for Neuroprotective Action of MS-153

HIROAKI UENISHI, CHAO-SHENG HUANG, JIN-HO SONG,
WILLIAM MARSZALEC, AND TOSHIO NARAHASHI[a]

*Department of Molecular Pharmacology and Biological Chemistry, Northwestern
University Medical School, Chicago, Illinois, USA*

ABSTRACT: MS-153, (*R*)-(−)-5-methyl-1-nicotinoyl-2-pyrazoline, is a new neuroprotective drug. Recent data in the literature suggest that it inhibits glutamate accumulation occurring during ischemia and the translocation of protein kinase C gamma (PKCγ). The present study was undertaken to prove the hypothesis that MS-153 blocks neuroreceptors and ion channels involved in glutamate accumulation. Neurons isolated from rat dorsal root ganglia and frontal cortex were used for recording channel currents by the whole-cell patch clamp technique. The effects of bath-applied MS-153 were examined on tetrodotoxin-sensitive and tetrodotoxin-resistant sodium channels and high voltage-gated calcium channels of dorsal root ganglion neurons, and channels activated by glutamate, *N*-methyl-D-aspartate (NMDA), kainate, α-amino-3-hydroxy-5-methyl-4-isoxarole propionic acid (AMPA), γ-aminobutyric acid (GABA) and acetylcholine (ACh) in cortical neurons.

MS-153 at a concentration of 300 μM had no effect on either tetrodotoxin-sensitive or tetrodotoxin-resistant sodium channels. High voltage-gated calcium channels were either suppressed or not affected by 1–300 μM MS-153. The variable blocking effect of MS-153 was due to the variable activity of intracellular components in individual neurons, especially that of PKC, whose translocation is known to be inhibited by MS-153. When 100 nM phorbol 12-myristate-13-acetate (PMA) was applied to neurons, MS-153 suppressed the calcium channel current more frequently. Calphostin C (0.5 μM), a specific PKC inhibitor, applied intracellularly via recording patch pipette, completely abolished MS-153 suppression of the calcium channel current. Currents induced by glutamate, NMDA, kainate, AMPA, GABA or ACh were not affected by MS-153 at 300 μM. It was concluded that MS-153 inhibited high voltage-gated calcium channels through interactions with PKC, thereby preventing massive release of glutamate from nerve terminals in ischemic conditions.

INTRODUCTION

A variety of chemicals are being developed for the treatment of brain ischemia. Whereas the onset of stroke is accompanied by rapid local damage in the brain, infarction spreads from the point of damage rather slowly. Therefore, there is a therapeutic window during which damages to the peri-infarct area can be prevented or minimized by administration of a neuroprotective agent.[1]

[a]Corresponding author: Dr. Toshio Narahashi, Department of Molecular Pharmacology and Biological Chemistry, Northwestern University Medical School, 303 E. Chicago Avenue, Chicago, IL 60611. Phone, 312/503-8284; fax, 312/503-1700.
e-mail, tna597@anima.nums.nwu.edu

A wide variety of chemicals have been shown to produce neuroprotection via several different mechanisms. In particular, blockers that act on the voltage-gated sodium channel, the voltage-gated calcium channels, and/or the glutamate receptor channels have proven effective in preventing infarction caused by stroke or ischemia. The strategy for using receptor/channel blockers is to inhibit one or more points in the cascade of events starting brain ischemia and leading eventually to cell death. Such a sequence of events includes membrane depolarization, repetitive discharges, increased transmitter release, excessive activation of glutamate receptors (especially N-methyl-D-aspartate (NMDA) receptors), massive calcium influx, and cell death. Thus, chemicals that block any of the receptors or channels in this chain of events could provide effective neuroprotection.

MS-153, (R)-$(-)$-5-methyl-1-nicotinoyl-2-pyrazoline, has proven a potent anti-ischemic agent. The infusion of MS-153 significantly reduced infarct volume and improved brain edema after the occlusion of the middle cerebral artery in rats.[2] The size of ischemic cerebral infarction and the increase in extracellular glutamate concentration following middle cerebral artery occlusion in rats were effectively reduced by infusion of MS-153.[3]

However, knowledge about the mechanism of action of MS-153 is quite limited. MS-153 suppressed extracellular glutamate concentration increased by ischemia and the glutamate uptake inhibitor DL-threo-β-hydroxyaspartate reversed the effect of MS-153 on glutamate concentration, suggesting that MS-153 may inhibit the release of glutamate.[3] MS-153 prevented NMDA-induced cytotoxicity in cultured cerebral cortex neurons, but did not prevent kainate-induced cytotoxicity.[4] Potassium-evoked glutamate release was attenuated by MS-153. Glutamate release was also attenuated by staurosporine, a protein kinase C (PKC) inhibitor, and was potentiated by phorbol 12-myristate-13-acetate (PMA). This suggested that the MS-153 suppression of glutamate release might be associated with an inhibition of PKC pathway.[5] It was also found that MS-153 inhibited the translocation of PKCγ in rat hippocampal slices.[6]

The aforementioned studies imply that one of the mechanisms of action of MS-153 may be the inhibition of glutamate release from nerve terminals. Ischemia-induced membrane depolarization and repetitive discharges will cause a massive release of glutamate from nerve terminals which in turn will increase the intracellular Ca^{2+} concentration in the postsynaptic neurons leading to cell death. The role of calcium in ischemic cell death is well documented.[7] Thus, it is hypothesized that the MS-153 target site may be voltage-gated sodium channels or high voltage-gated calcium channels. The patch clamp study reported here has shown that high voltage-gated calcium channels are inhibited by MS-153 via interactions with the PKC system.

MATERIALS AND METHODS

Calcium Channels

Materials

Dorsal root ganglion (DRG) neurons were isolated as described previously.[8,9] Sprague-Dawley rats (2–6 days postnatal, either sex) were anesthetized with methoxyflurane and the spinal column was removed and cut longitudinally. Ganglia were plucked from between the vertebrae of the spinal column, and incubated in phosphate-buffered saline solution (GIBCO BRL, Grand Island, NY) containing trypsin (2.5 mg/ml, type XI, Sigma Chemical Co., St. Louis, MO) at 37°C for 25 min. After enzyme treatment, ganglia were rinsed with Dulbecco's modified Eagle's medium (DMEM, GIBCO BRL) supplemented with newborn calf serum (10% v/v, GIBCO BRL) and gentamicin (80 μg/ml). Single cells were mechanically dissociated with a fire-polished Pasteur pipette and plated on glass coverslips coated with poly-L-lysine (0.1 μg/ml, Sigma). Cells were maintained in DMEM containing neonatal calf serum and gentamicin in a 90% air/10% CO_2 atmosphere controlled at 36°C. Neurons were used within 2 days of plating. Cells cultured more than 1 day usually develop processes and may produce poor space clamp. Cells that were inadequately space clamped, as exhibited by a slow tail current and slow settling of capacity transient, were discarded.

Electrophysiological Recording

Ionic currents were recorded by the whole-cell patch clamp technique. Pipettes (0.6–1.2 MΩ) were pulled from borosilicate glass capillary tubes (1.5–1.8 mm inner diameter, Kimble, Vineland, NJ) using a two-step vertical puller (Narishige, Tokyo, Japan). The transmembrane voltage was clamped at −80 mV. Unless otherwise indicated, a period of 10 min was allowed after rupture of the membrane to ensure adequate equilibration between the internal pipette solution and the cell interior. Membrane currents were recorded with an Axopatch 1B amplifier (Axon Instruments, Foster City, CA), and were stored in an SX 386 computer (DELL Computer Company, Austin, TX) using pCLAMP 6 software (Axon Instruments). The standard external solution contained (in mM): $BaCl_2$ 10, tetraethylammonium chloride 130, D-glucose 25, *N*-2-hydroxyethylpiperazine-*N'*-2-ethanesulphonic acid (HEPES) 5, and tetrodotoxin (TTX) 200 nM. The standard internal (pipette) solution contained (in mM): CsCl 25, CsOH 80, gluconic acid 80, HEPES 40, D-glucose 5, $MgCl_2$ 2.5, ethylene glycol-bis-(β-aminoethyl ether)-*N,N,N',N'*-tetraacetic acid (EGTA) 10, Mg-adenosine triphosphate (ATP) 5, and Li_3-guanosine triphosphate (GTP) 0.5. Unless otherwise indicated, the pH of all solutions was adjusted to 7.3 with 1 M CsOH, and the osmolarity was raised to 300 mOsm with sucrose.

Sodium Channels

Materials

DRG was isolated, and neurons were dissociated as described above. Cells were incubated for 2–7 hr before patch clamp experiments.

TTX (200 nM) was used to separate TTX-resistant (TTX-R) sodium currents from TTX-sensitive (TTX-S) sodium currents. For the study of TTX-S sodium channels, cells that expressed only TTX-S sodium currents were used. TTX-S sodium currents were completely inactivated by a 5-msec depolarizing pulse to 0 mV, while TTX-R currents still presisted. These kinetic differences were used to identify each type of sodium current.

Electrophysiological Recording

Currents were recorded using the whole-cell patch clamp technique as described above. The pipette solution contained (in mM): CsF 135, NaCl 10 and HEPES 5. The pH was adjusted to 7.0 with CsOH and the osmolarity was 275 mOsm. Additional experiments were performed using the pipette solution without containing fluoride to avoid the inhibition of enzymes. The F^--free pipette solution contained (in mM): CsCl 25, NaCl 10, CsOH 80, gluconic acid 80, HEPES 10, D-glucose 5, EGTA 5, and Mg-ATP 5, with the pH adjusted to 7.3 with CsOH and the osmolarity was 280 mOsm. The external solution contained (in mM): NaCl 25, tetramethylammonium chloride 75, tetraethylammonium chloride 20, CsCl 5, $CaCl_2$ 1.8, $MgCl_2$ 1.0, D-glucose 25, HEPES-acid 5. lanthanum ($LaCl_3$, 3 μM) was used to block calcium channel current. The solution was adjusted to pH 7.4 with tetraethylammonium-OH and 290 mOsm with sucrose. Membrane currents were recorded using an Axopatch 200 amplifier (Axon Instruments). Signals were digitized by a 14-bit analog-to-digital converter, filtered with a Bessel filter at 5 kHz and stored on a PDP 11/73 computer (Digital Equipment Corporation, Pittsburgh, PA). Series resistance was compensated 70–75%. Capacitive and leakage currents were digitally subtracted by using the P + P/4 procedure.[10] The liquid junction potential between internal and external solution averaged −4.7 mV. All recordings were compensated for the liquid junction potential.

Glutamate, GABA and Acetylcholine (ACh) Receptors

Materials

Cortical neurons were cultured as described previously.[11] In brief, 17-day embryonic pups were removed from pregnant Sprague-Dawley rats under methoxyflurane anesthesia. Small wedges of frontal cortex were excised and were treated for 25 min at 37°C in phosphate-buffered saline solution containing 0.25% (w/v) trypsin (type XI, Sigma). Following mechanical trituration through a Pasteur pipette, the dissociated cells were suspended in DMEM with 10% (v/v) Ham's F-12 supplement, 2 mmol/L-glutamine and 20 U penicillin/20 ng streptomycin per ml. The cells were placed into 35-mm culture wells at a concentration of 200,000 cells/3 ml. Each well contained several 12-mm glass coverslips having a confluent layer of glia that were plated 2–4 weeks earlier. The cortical/glial co-culture was maintained in a humidified atmosphere of 90% air/10% CO_2.

Electrophysiological Recording

Whole-cell currents from neurons cultured 10–20 days were recorded with an Axopatch-1C patch-clamp amplifier (Axon Instruments). Electrodes pulled from borosilicate glass were filled with the internal solution. For the glutamate and $GABA_A$ receptors, the internal solution contained (in mM): CsCl 140, $MgCl_2$ 2.0, $CaCl_2$ 1.0, EGTA 11, HEPES 10, and pH adjusted to 7.4 with CsOH. For the acetylcholine (ACh) receptor, the internal solution contained (in mM): Cs-gluconate 140, NaCl 15, K-gluconate 5, HEPES-acid 15, HEPES-Na 10, 1,2-bis(2-aminophenoxy)ethane-N,N,N',N'-tetraacetate-Cs (BAPTA-Cs) 35, Ca-gluconate 12, Mg-gluconate 4, and pH 7.3. Final electrode resistances ranged between 2 and 3 MΩ when filled with the internal solution. The external solution for the glutamate and $GABA_A$ receptors consisted of (in mM) NaCl 150, KCl 5.0, $CaCl_2$ 2.5, $MgCl_2$ 2.0, glucose 10, HEPES-acid 5.5, and HEPES-Na 4.5, and the pH was 7.4. This solution also contained 0.4 μM TTX in order to reduce spontaneous electrical activity. For the ACh receptor,

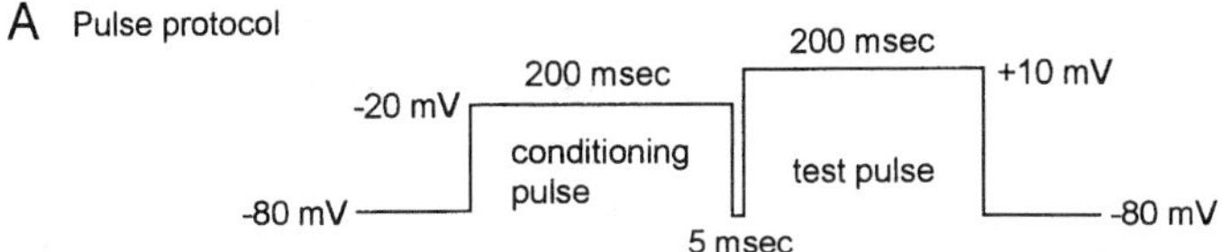

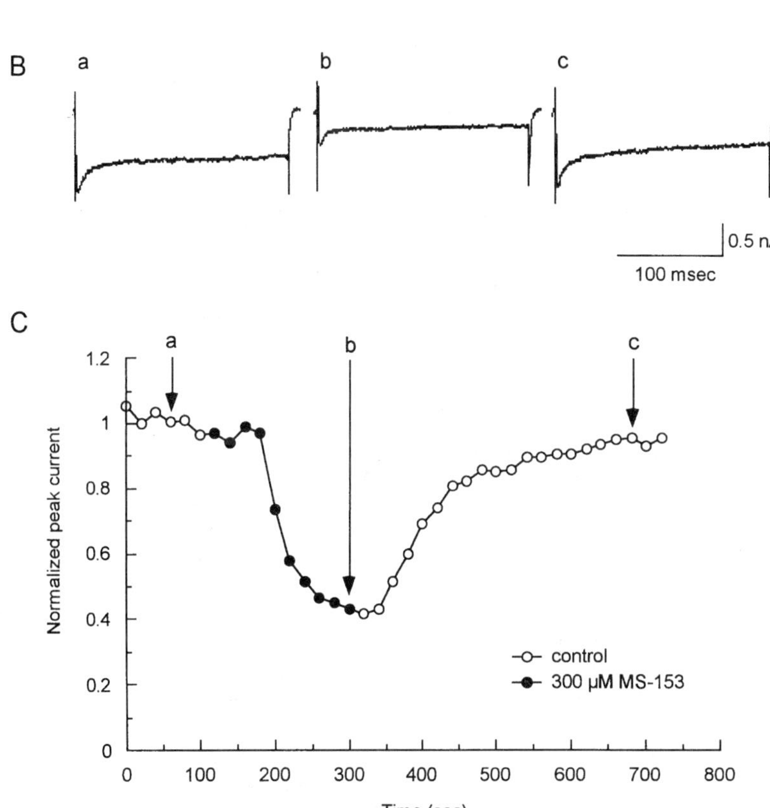

FIGURE 1. Reversible block of high voltage-gated calcium channel currents by 300 µM MS-153. **(A)** Pulse protocol. **(B)** Currents evoked by test pulses before **(a)** and during **(b)** application of 300 µM MS-153, and after washing with drug-free solution **(c)**. **(C)** Time course of change in the amplitude of high voltage-gated calcium channel currents before and during application of 300 µM MS-153, and after washing with drug-free solution. (a), (b) and (c) correspond to the same letters in (B).

the external solution contained (in mM): NaCl 140, KCl 5, $CaCl_2$ 1.5, $MgCl_2$ 1, HEPES-acid 15, HEPES-Na 10, $LaCl_3$ 3 µM, TTX 0.2 µM, and atropine sulphate 0.3 µM, and pH 7.3. Glutamate, kainate, α-amino-3-hydroxy-5-methyl-4-isoxarole propionic acid (AMPA), N-methyl-D-aspartate (NMDA), GABA, and ACh were applied to the cell using the U-tube delivery system.[11]

Drug Application

The recording chamber was perfused continuously with normal external solution at a rate of 1 ml/min. Unless otherwise described, all the drugs were applied to the bath perfusate. The total volume of the chamber was 1 ml facilitating the rate of drug application and washout. MS-153 was dissolved in distilled water as a 100-mM stock solution and kept refrigerated. It was diluted with external solution to the desired concentrations on the day of use. Calphostin C was dissolved directly in the standard internal solution. PMA was dissolved in dimethylsulfoxide before diluting with the standard external solution. The final concentration of dimethylsulfoxide (<0.1% v/v) did not alter the current responses studied. Calphostin C was purchased from Calbiochem (LaJolla, CA) and other drugs were obtained from Sigma. All patch clamp experiments were conducted at a room temperature of 20–23°C.

Data Analysis

Results are expressed as means ± SEM, where n represents the number of the cells examined. Analyses of currents were achieved by using both REV, FORTRAN/ IV program developed in our laboratory for use on the PDP 11/73 computer and SigmaPlot (Jandel Scientific, San Rafael, CA).

RESULTS

High Voltage-Gated Calcium Channels Are Suppressed by MS-153

Low voltage-gated and high voltage-gated calcium channels both exist in rat DRG neurons. However, since the latter calcium channels play the primary role in neurotransmitter release from nerve terminals, experiments were performed to examine the effects of MS-153 on high voltage-gated calcium channels. The pulse protocol used to record high voltage-gated calcium channel currents is shown in FIGURE 1A. A 200-msec conditioning depolarizing pulse to −20 mV from a holding potential of −80 mV was followed by, with a 5-msec gap, a 200-msec test pulse to +10 mV. The current associated with this test pulse represented the activation of high voltage-gated calcium channels.

A series of current records before, during and after application of 300 μM MS-153 is shown in FIGURE 1B. In this experiment, the current amplitude was greatly suppressed by MS-153 and the recovery observed during washout with drug-free solution was nearly complete (FIG. 1C). There was usually a slight rundown commonly encountered in many experiments. The degree of current suppression by rundown was calculated from a linear regression obtained by connecting several control points before and after drug application. The depression of current calculated as a part of rundown was subtracted from the drug effect at a given point in time. However, currents that exhibited rundown exceeding 40% over 15 min or those where no recovery was observed after MS-153 washout were discarded.

However, current suppression by MS-153 was not always observed. The data on the inhibition of high voltage-gated calcium channel currents by MS-153 are summarized in TABLE 1. The calcium channel currents of some neurons were not affected at any concentrations of MS-153, while those from other cells were clearly

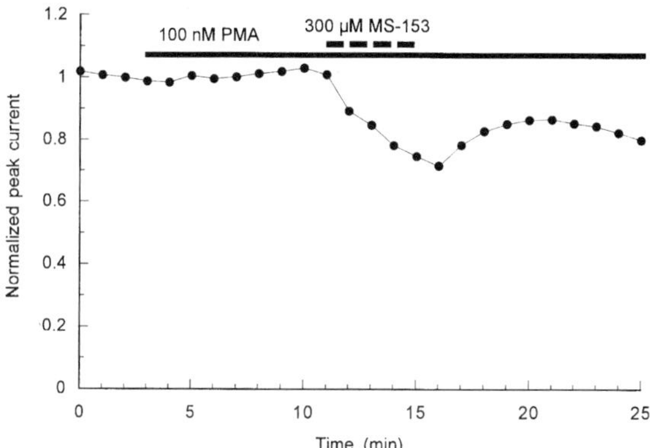

FIGURE 2. An example of an experiment in which 300 µM MS-153 suppresses high voltage-gated calcium channel currents after pretreatment with 100 nM PMA.

inhibited. The percentage of cells exhibiting current inhibition was calculated for each concentration of MS-153. In the absence of PMA, the percentage of inhibited neurons ranged from 22% to 60%. The degree of current inhibition, when observed for MS-153 concentrations of 0.3–30 µM was less than 10%. At a concentration of 300 µM, however, MS-153 inhibited the current by $27.5 \pm 17.2\%$ (5 of 15 cells).

One possible reason for the variable degree of MS-153 inhibition of calcium channel currents is that MS-153 acts on intracellular enzymes whose activities vary among different neurons. The variable inhibition by MS-153 is in sharp contrast to the consistent inhibition of high voltage-gated calcium channel currents caused by riluzole, a neuroprotective drug, in a concentration dependent manner (Figure 2 of Huang *et al.*[12]). The inhibition of high voltage-gated calcium channel currents caused by a mu-opioid was also very variable.[13]

Role of PKC in MS-153 Suppression
of High Voltage-Gated Calcium Channel Current

Since MS-153 was shown to inhibit translocation of PKC,[6] the inhibition of high voltage-gated calcium channel currents by MS-153 could be caused via PKC, whose activity may be variable among neurons. The absence of current suppression by MS-153 in some neurons may be due to low intrinsic activity of PKC. Therefore, if PKC activity is augmented by PMA, MS-153 might be expected to suppress the current in a greater percentage of cells.

PMA at a concentration of 100 nM augmented the calcium channel current in some neurons but was without effect in other neurons. As might be expected from the effect of PMA to augment intracellular PKC activity, current potentiation progressed slowly. Similarly, recovery after washout of PMA was also slow.

MS-153 suppressed high voltage-gated calcium channel currents more often when PMA was present in the external solution. FIGURE 2 illustrates such a case. Bath application of 100 nM PMA increased the current very slightly, and addition of 300 µM MS-153 to the bath suppressed the current. Partial recovery was observed after eliminating MS-153 from the bath.

TABLE 1. MS-153 inhibition of high voltage-gated calcium channel currents in the absence and presence of PMA

MS-153 (µM)	PMA (nM)	Inhibition Mean ± SEM (%)	n	Cases of Inhibition (%)
0.3	0	0	2	60
0.3	0	4.4 ± 0.97	3	
1	0	0	2	50
1	0	4.0 ± 1.7	2	
3	0	0	3	50
3	0	8.4 ± 3.0	3	
3	100	0	1	80
3	100	8.0 ± 5.4	4	
30	0	0	7	22
30	0	7.7 ± 2.0	2	
30	100	0	2	60
30	100	7.2. ± 1.1	3	
300	0	0	10	33
300	0	27.5 ± 17.2	5	
300	100	0	5	58
300	100	21.8 ± 14.3	7	

However, current suppression by MS-153 was not always observed in the presence of PMA. The data on the PMA and MS-153 combination are tabulated in TABLE 1. The percentage of MS-153 inhibition increased in the presence of PMA. The percentage increased from 50% without PMA to 80% with PMA for 3 µM MS-153; from 22% without PMA to 60% with PMA for 30 µM MS-153; and from 33% without PMA to 58% with PMA for 300 µM MS-153.

To further demonstrate the difference between MS-153 and riluzole, experiments were conducted to examine their effects on the same neuron. An example of such an experiment is shown in FIGURE 3. In this neuron, MS-153 at 100 µM and 300 µM had no effect on high voltage-gated caclium channel currents, yet riluzole at 100 µM dramatically suppressed the currents. The effect of riluzole was partially reversible after washing with drug-free solution. Cadmium chloride, which is a universal blocker of calcium channels, blocked the current completely at a concentration of 150 µM.

A corollary of this result is that MS-153 will not inhibit the calcium channel current in the absence of PKC activity. To prove the validity of this hypothesis, MS-153 inhibition of the current was examined using a pipette solution containing calphostin C, a specific PKC inhibitor, at a concentration of 0.5 µM. An example of such an experiment is shown in FIGURE 4. In the presence of calphostin C, MS-153 exerted no effect on the high voltage-gated calcium channel current in a total of four cells.

Sodium Channels Are Insensitive to MS-153

Rat DRG neurons contain both TTX-S and TTX-R sodium channels. These sodium channels were blocked by riluzole with TTX-S channels more potently than TTX-R channels.[14] However, neither of them was affected by 1 mM MS-153 when

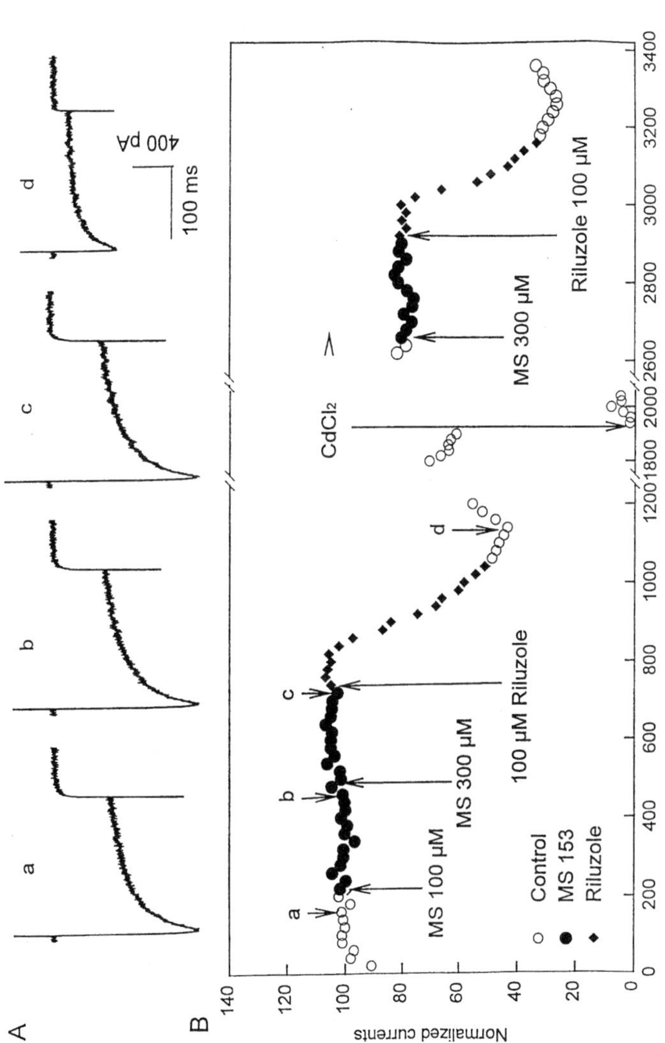

FIGURE 3. Comparison of the effects of MS-153 and riluzole for their effects on high voltage-gated calcium channel currents in the same neuron. While 100 and 300 µM MS-153 had no effect on the current in this neuron, 100 µM riluzole inhibited the current. $CdCl_2$ at 150 µM completely blocked the current. MS-153 applied after washout of the cell at a concentration of 300 µM had no effect on the current, while 100 µM riluzole inhibited the current again. Sample current records (**a**), (**b**), (**c**) and (**d**) in (**A**) were taken at the times indicated in (**B**).

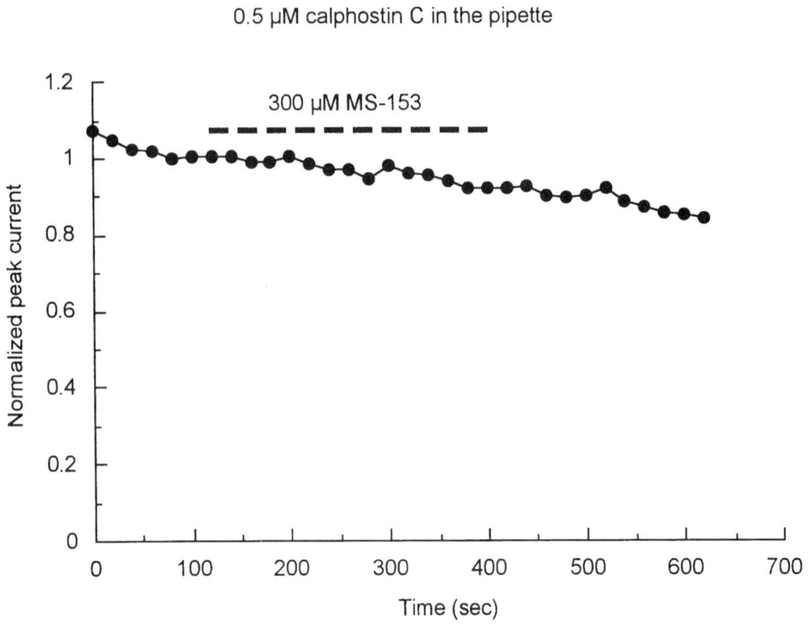

0.5 µM calphostin C in the pipette

300 µM MS-153

FIGURE 4. In the presence of the PKC inhibitor calphostin C in the patch pipette at a concentration of 0.5 µM, 300 µM MS-153 never had any effect on high voltage-gated calcium channel currents.

the F⁻-containing pipette solution was used. Currents recorded from TTX-S and TTX-R sodium channels before and during application of MS-153 are shown in FIGURE 5, and the current-voltage relationships are plotted in FIGURE 6. In contrast to riluzole, which blocked the sodium channels,[14] MS-153 had no effect on the sodium channels even at the high concentration of 1 mM.

Additional experiments were performed using the F⁻-free pipette solution to avoid the inhibition of PKC by F⁻ ions. As described above, PKC was found to play an important role in MS-153 inhibition of high voltage-gated calcium channels. MS-153 at 300 µM had no effect on either TTX-S or TTX-R sodium channel currents using the F⁻-free pipette solution. With pretreatment with 100 nM PMA, MS-153 (300 µM) also failed to cause any effect on either TTX-S or TTX-R sodium channel currents. Repeated experiments ($n = 2$–4) confirmed these results.

Glutamate, GABA$_A$, and ACh Receptors Are Insensitive to MS-153

Neuroprotection under ischemic conditions could be attained by blocking postsynaptic glutamate receptors, especially that of the NMDA receptor. Using cultured rat cortical neurons, the direct action of MS-153 on glutamate receptors was examined. GABA$_A$ and nicotinic ACh receptors were also examined for comparison. Rat cortical neurons in primary culture generated at least two types of currents in response to the application of ACh. One was a rapidly desensitizing, α-bungarotoxin-

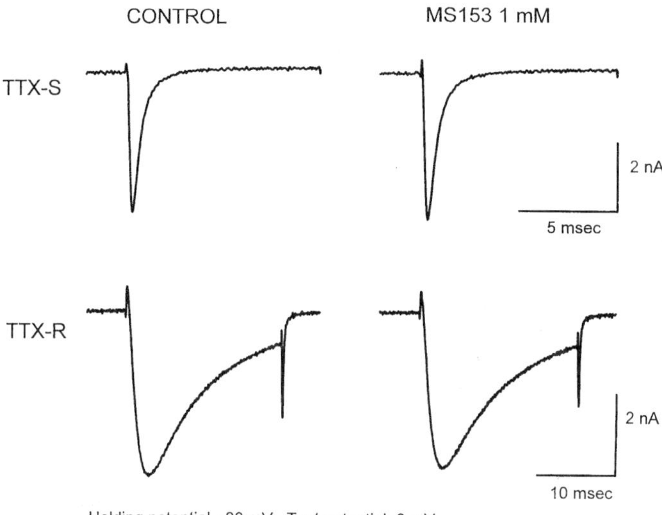

FIGURE 5. Absence of the effect of a high concentration (1 mM) of MS-153 on tetrodotoxin-sensitive (TTX-S) and tetrodotoxin-resistant (TTX-R) sodium channel currents. The currents were evoked by a step deplorization to 0 mV from a holding potential of −80 mV. F^--containing pipette solution was used.

sensitive current and the other was a non-desensitizing, α-bungarotoxin-insensitive current.[15] The effects of MS-153 on the latter current were studied. The data are summarized in TABLE 2, in which MS-153 at a concentration of 300 μM had little or no effect on glutamate, kainate, AMPA, NMDA, $GABA_A$ and ACh receptors. The inhibitions of the kainate and ACh receptor currents are statistically significant, but the effects are very small amounting only to 5% and 8%, respectively.

DISCUSSION

Among the several ion channels reported to be associated with ischemia-induced membrane depolarization and cell death, only the high voltage-gated calcium channels were affected by MS-153. Receptors and channels that were not altered by MS-153 included voltage-gated sodium channels, glutamate receptors activated by glutamate, NMDA, kainate and AMPA, $GABA_A$ receptors, and nicotinic ACh receptors. The MS-153-induced suppression of high voltage-gated calcium channels may be associated with PKC, which itself modulates the channel activity. The MS-153 inhibition of high voltage-gated calcium channel currents was variable among neurons, perhaps reflecting the variable activity of PKC.

Ischemic conditions cause gradual depolarization of neuronal membranes evoking repetitive discharges and glutamate release from nerve terminals, which in turn stimulate the NMDA receptors. Massive calcium influx through NMDA receptor channels promotes cell death. Various sodium channel blocking agents such as phenytoin, carbamazepine and lamotrigine are known to protect neurons from cere-

TABLE 2. Effects of 300 μM MS-153 on glutamate, GABA$_A$ and ACh receptors

Agonist	Current (MS-153/Control)	n	p	Remarks
10 μM Glutamate	0.915 ± 0.032	4	0.05	No Mg^{2+} in the bath
10–100 μM Glutamate	0.932 ± 0.048	11	0.05	2 mM Mg^{2+} in the bath
30–100 μM Kainate	0.953 ± 0.012	6	<0.01	
30 μM AMPA	1.017 ± 0.045	5	0.05	
30 μM NMDA	0.979 ± 0.032	7	0.05	
10 μM GABA	1.052 ± 0.026	3	0.05	
3 μM ACh	0.916 ± 0.015	4	<0.01	Nicotinic receptors

bral ischemia, hypoxia or head trauma.[16] Calcium channel blockers and the glutamate receptor antagonists also exhibit neuroprotective action. In fact, some receptor channel blockers are being developed into neuroprotective drugs: lubeluzole and fosphenytoin block the sodium channels; SNX111 and nimodipine block the calcium channels; lifarizine and CNS 1237 (*N,N'*-acenaphthylmethoxynaphthyl guanidine) block both sodium and calcium channels; cerestat, dextrorphan, dizocilpine, remacemide, eliprodil, selfotel and YM90K block the glutamate receptors; and riluzole blocks the sodium and calcium channels as well as glutamate receptors.[1,12,14,17–21]

The MS-153 inhibition of high voltage-gated calcium channel currents was vairable. In contrast, riluzole inhibition of calcium channel current was more consistent in a dose-dependent manner.[12,18] Our experiments of MS-153 and riluzole were performed under the identical conditions. Thus, differences in the effectiveness of MS-153 and riluzole may reflect differences in the way these two drugs act on cal-

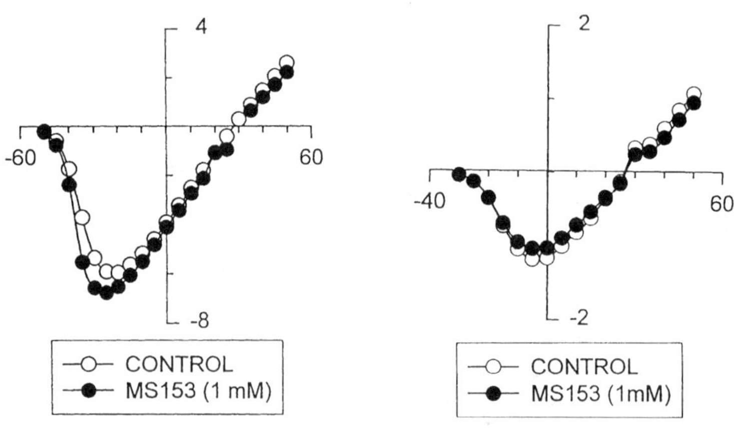

FIGURE 6. Current-voltage relationships of TTX-S and TTX-R sodium channels before (○) and during (●) application of 1 mM MS-153. F⁻-containing pipette solution was used.

cium channels. A variable degree of inhibition of high voltage-gated calcium channel currents was also observed with the mu-opioid [D-Ala^2, N-Me-Phe^4, Gly^5-ol]-enkephalin.[13]

High voltage-gated calcium channels are known to be phosphorylated at several sites, which are located in both the α1 subunit and the β subunit.[22] The calcium channel phosphorylation is effected by protein kinase A (PKA), resulting in an increase in or stimulation of calcium channel currents.[23–26] The role of PKC in calcium channel activity was also studied, and polymyxin B, a PKC inhibitor, inhibited the current.[24] Thus, MS-153 inhibition of PKC translocation[6] might be responsible for the suppression of the calcium channel current as demonstrated in the present study.

MS-153 has been shown to suppress high voltage-gated calcium channel currents without effect on voltage-gated sodium channels or on receptors activated by glutamate, NMDA, kainate, AMPA, GABA or ACh. Thus, MS-153 blocks one critical step in the cascade of events leading from ischemia to cell death. This selective action may be advantageous compared to drugs like riluzole, which blocks both sodium and calcium channels as well as glutamate receptors.[12,14,18,27,28]

ACKNOWLEDGMENTS

This study was supported in part by Mitsui Pharmaceutical Co. and by NIH Grant NS14144. We thank Nayla Hasan for technical assistance and Julia Irizarry for secretarial assistance.

REFERENCES

1. KOROSHETZ, W.J. & M.A. MOSKOWITZ. 1996. Emerging treatments for stroke in humans. Trends Pharmacol. Sci. **17:** 227–233.
2. KAWAZURA, H., Y. TAKAHASHI, Y. SHIGA, F. SHIMADA, N. OHTO & A. TAMURA. 1997. Cerebroprotective effects of a novel pyrazoline drivative, MS-153, on focal ischemia in rats. Japan. J. Pharmacol. **73:** 317–324.
3. UMEMURA, K., T. GEMBA, A. MIZUNO & M. NAKASHIMA. 1996. Inhibitory effect of MS-153 on elevated brain glutamate level induced by rat middle cerebral artery occlusion. Stroke **27:** 1624–1628.
4. AKAIKE, A., Y. TAMURA, S. YUKO & T. YOKOTA. 1993. Protection by pyrazoline analog MS-153 against glutamate cytotoxicity in cultured cortical neurons [abstract]. J. Cereb. Blood Flow Metab. **13**(Suppl. 1): S693.
5. SHIMADA, F., K. SAKATA, Y. SHIGA, M. MORIKAWA, Y. FUKUI, H. KAWAZURA, K. UMEMURA & M. NAKASHIMA. 1997. Inhibitory effect of MS-153, a cerebroprotective agent, on glutamate release from the rat hippocampal slice [abstract]. Annu. Mtg Japan. Pharmacol. Soc.: 245.
6. SAKATA, K., M. MORIKAWA, Y. FUKUI, Y. SHIGA, F. SHIMADA & H. KAWAZURA. 1997. Effect of MS-153, a cerebroprotective agent, on γ protein kinase C redistribution in rat hippocampal slices[abstract]. Annu. Mtg. Japan. Pharmacol. Soc.: 246.
7. KRISTIÁN, T. & B.K. SIESJÖ. 1998. Calcium in ischemic cell death. Stroke **29:** 705–718.
8. ROY, M.L. & T. NARAHASHI. 1994. Na channels of rat dorsal root ganglion neurons. *In* Methods in Neuroscience. Vol. 19. Ion Channels of Excitable Cells. T. Narahashi, Ed.: 21–38. Academic Press. San Diego, CA.

9. TATEBAYASHI, H. & T. NARAHASHI. 1994. Differential mechanism of action of the pyrethroid tetramethrin on tetrodotoxin-sensitive and tetrodotoxin-resistant Na channels. J. Pharmacol. Exp. Ther. **270:** 595–603.

10. BEZANILLA, F. & C.M. ARMSTRONG. 1977. Inactivation of the Na channel. I. Na current experiments. J. Gen. Physiol. **70:** 549–566.

11. MARSZALEC, W. & T. NARAHASHI. 1993. Use-dependent pentobarbital block of kainate and quisqualate currents. Brain Res. **608:** 7–15.

12. HUANG, C.-S., J.-H. SONG, K. NAGATA, J.Z. YEH & T. NARAHASHI. 1997. Effects of the neuroprotective agent riluzole on the high voltage-activated calcium channels of rat dorsal root ganglion neurons. J. Pharmacol. Exp. Ther. **282:** 1280–1290.

13. NOMURA, K., E. REUVENY & T. NARAHASHI. 1994. Opioid inhibition and desensitization of calcium channel currents in rat dorsal root ganglion neurons. J. Pharmacol. Exp. Ther. **270:** 466–474.

14. SONG, J.-H., C.-S. HUANG, K. NAGATA, J.Z. YEH & T. NARAHASHI. 1997. Differential action of riluzole on tetrodotoxin-sensitive and tetrodotoxin-resistant sodium channels. J. Pharmacol. Exp. Ther. **282:** 707–714.

15. AISTRUP, G., W. MARSZALEC & T. NARAHASHI. 1999. Ethanol modulation of nicotinic acetylcholine receptor currents in cultured cortical neurons. Mol. Pharmacol. **55:** 39–49.

16. TAYLOR, C.P. & B.S. MELDRUM. 1995. Na$^+$ channels as targets for neuroprotective drugs. Trends Neurosci. **16:** 309–316.

17. GOLDIN, S.M., K. SUBBARAO, R. SHARMA, A.G. KNAPP, J.B. FISCHER, D. DALY, G.J. DURANT, N.L. REDDY, L.-Y. HU, S. MAGAR, M.E. PERLMAN, J. CHEN, S.H. GRAHAM, W.F. HOLT, D. BERLOVE & L.D. MARGOLIN. 1995. Neuroprotective use-dependent blockers of Na$^+$ and Ca^{2+} channels controlling presynaptic release of glutamate. Ann. N.Y. Acad. Sci. **765:** 210–229.

18. HUANG, C.-S., J.-H. SONG, K. NAGATA, D. TWOMBLY, J.Z. YEH & T. NARAHASHI. 1997. G proteins are involved in riluzole inhibition of high voltage-activated calcium channels in rat dorsal root ganglion neurons. Brain Res. **762:** 235–239.

19. PALMER, G.C., E.F. CREGAN, A.R. BORRELLI & F. WILLETT. 1995. Neuroprotective properties of the uncompetitive NMDA receptor antagonist remacemide hydrochloride. Ann. N.Y. Acad. Sci. **765:** 236–248.

20. SHERIDAN, R.D. 1995. Selectivity of the neuroprotective agent lifarizine. Trends Pharmacol. Sci. **16:** 292.

21. SPEDDING, M., B. KENNY & P. CHATELAIN. 1995. New drug binding sites in Ca^{2+} channels. Trends Pharmacol. Sci. **16:** 139–142.

22. DOLPHIN, A.C. 1996. Facilitation of Ca^{2+} channel in excitable cells. Trends Neurosci. **19:** 35–43.

23. ARMSTRONG, D. & R. ECKERT. 1987. Voltage-activated calcium channels that must be phosphorylated to respond to membrane depolarization. Proc. Natl. Acad. Sci. USA **84:** 2518–2522.

24. DOLPHIN, A.C., S.M. MCGUIRK & R.H. SCOTT. 1989. An investigation into the mechanisms of inhibition of calcium channel currents in cultured sensory neurones of the rat by guanine nucleotide analogues and (–)-baclofen. Br. J. Pharmacol. **97:** 263–273.

25. DOLPHIN, A.C. 1991. Ca^{2+} channel currents in rat sensory neurones: interaction between guanine nucleotides, cyclic AMP and Ca^{2+} channel ligands. J. Physiol. **432:** 23–43.

26. DOUPNIK, C.A. & R.Y.K. PUN. 1992. Cyclic AMP-dependent phosphorylation modifies the gating properties of L-type Ca^{2+} channels in bovine adrenal chromaffin cells. Pflügers Arch. **420:** 61–71.

27. HUBERT, J.P., J.C. DELUMEAU, J. GLOWINSKI, J. PREMONT & A. DOBLE. 1994. Antagonism by riluzole of entry of calcium evoked by NMDA and veratridine in rat cultured granule cells: evidence for a dual mechanism of action. Br. J. Pharmacol. **113:** 261–267.

28. MALGOURIS, C., M. DANIEL & A. DOBLE. 1994. Neuroprotective effects of riluzole on N-methyl-D-aspartate- or veratridine-induced neurotoxicity in rat hippocampal slices. Neurosci. Lett. **177:** 95–99.

Blockade of NAALADase: A Novel Neuroprotective Strategy Based on Limiting Glutamate and Elevating NAAG

JAMES J. VORNOV, KRYSTYNA WOZNIAK, MAY LU, PAUL JACKSON, TAKASHI TSUKAMOTO, ERIC WANG, AND BARBARA SLUSHER[a]

Guilford Pharmaceuticals Inc., Baltimore, Maryland, USA

ABSTRACT: Excessive glutamate receptor activation is thought to be involved in the neuronal injury caused by stroke. Based on the hypothesis that *N*-acetyl-aspartyl-glutamate (NAAG) is a modulatory neurotransmitter or storage form of glutamate, we have pursued a novel strategy of therapeutic intervention, blockade of *N*-acetylated alpha-linked acidic dipeptidase (NAALADase), the enzyme that hydrolyzes NAAG to liberate glutamate. Using the suture model of transient middle cerebral artery occlusion (MCAO) in rats, the prototype NAALADase inhibitor 2-(phosphonomethyl)pentanedioic acid (2-PMPA) dramatically reduced extracellular glutamate accumulation measured by microdialysis both during a 2-hour occlusion and during reperfusion, consistent with an effect on glutamate supply. During reperfusion, the decrease in glutamate was accompanied by an equimolar, reciprocal rise in extracellular NAAG. NAALADase inhibition may prove to be a well tolerated therapy for cerebral ischemia. In addition, NAALADase inhibitors should prove to be important tools in understanding the physiological role of NAAG in the brain.

INTRODUCTION TO NAAG AND NAALADASE

N-Acetylaspartylglutamate (NAAG) is an abundant brain dipeptide, but its role in brain physiology is not well understood.[1] NAAG is composed of glutamate, the important excitatory amino acid transmitter, and *N*-acetylaspartate (NAA), which is the *N*-acetylated derivative of aspartate. While aspartate probably has a function as an excitatory neurotransmitter, NAA is synthesized in mitochondria and may function as a metabolic intermediate.

NAAG may act as a neurotransmitter. Microdialysis experiments have shown that NAAG is released in a calcium-dependent manner in the superior colliculus during optic nerve stimulation.[2] NAAG can act as an agonist at group II metabotropic glutamate receptors[3] and as a mixed antagonist/agonist at the NMDA receptor.[4] This role as neurotransmitter is speculative; there is no direct physiological evidence for synaptic NAAG effects in an identified neural pathway. NAAG might also serve as a supply for glutamate, since it can be hydrolyzed by the brain enzyme *N*-acetylated alpha-linked acidic dipeptidase (NAALADase).[5,6] On the other hand, there is about 10 times more glutamate in the brain than NAAG, with glutamine and mitochondria

[a]Corresponding author: Barbara Slusher, Ph.D., Guilford Pharmaceuticals Inc., 6611 Tributary St., Baltimore, MD 21224. Phone, 410/631-6802; fax, 410/631-6804.
e-mail, Slusher_B@guilfordpharm.com

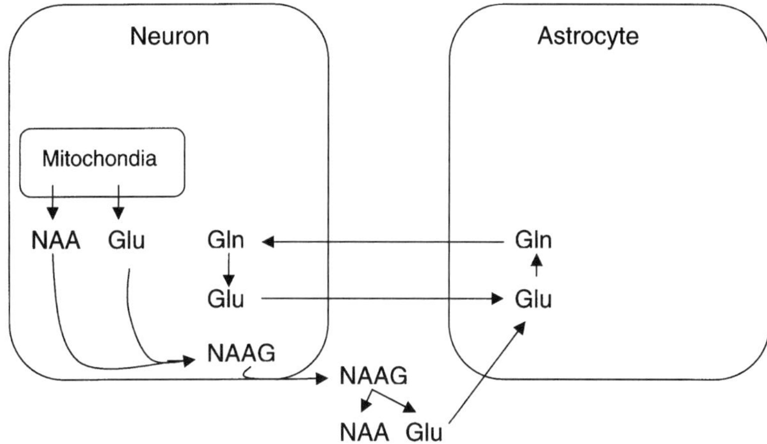

FIGURE 1. Proposed role for NAAG in glutamate supply, assuming that NAA and NAAG are limited to neurons and that NAALADase is limited to the extracellular space. Depending on the activity of NAALADase, extracellular NAAG can act as a neuromodulator or liberate glutamate to act at glutamate receptors. Blockade of NAAG hydrolysis could also limit glutamate supply to astrocytes, which appear to metabolize the bulk of extracellular glutamate.

potentially supplying glutamate for synaptic transmission. If NAAG were to play an important role in supplying glutamate, it would have to constitute a distinct pool with separate regulation. These two possibilities, neurotransmitter and glutamate precursor, are not mutually exclusive. If the hydrolysis of NAAG were under physiological control, then the relative balance of NAAG and glutamate derived from NAAG could be altered, determining the net physiological effect of extracellular NAAG.

NAAG has been localized to neurons by immunohistochemical techniques.[7,8] NAALADase is diffusely localized to the neuropil by immunohistochemistry,[9] but *in situ* hybridization reveals that the mRNA is primarily localized in astrocytes.[6] This suggests that any synaptic NAAG neuromodulatory effects would be terminated by astrocyte NAALADase. The liberated glutamate would then be transported into astrocytes, like synaptically released glutamate and most likely passed back to neurons as glutamine. If so, NAAG could serve the additional purpose of transporting glutamate to astrocytes without activating glutamate receptors (FIG. 1).

NEUROPROTECTIVE EFFECTS OF NAALADASE INHIBITION

Clearly, one of the obstacles to understanding the role of NAAG in neurotransmission and neuronal metabolism has been a lack of pharmacological tools to manipulate NAAG metabolism, specifically NAAG hydrolysis. Recently, we have presented data from experiments describing the effects of a high-affinity NAALADase inhibitor, 2-(phosphonomethyl)pentanedioic acid (2-PMPA). While important aspects remain to be clarified, these experiments provide the first evidence suggesting a pivotal role for NAAG hydrolysis in the pathophysiology of ischemia.

We predicted that inhibition of NAALADase might have neuroprotective effects both by increasing NAAG and by decreasing glutamate availability. If NAAG is a significant source of glutamate, then NAALADase inhibitors could potentially decrease glutamate accumulation during ischemia. This might protect neurons by limiting toxic glutamate receptor activation. An advantage of this approach is that damaging effects at all receptor types would be avoided, a goal that would otherwise require combinations of selective postsynaptic receptor antagonists. In addition, if NAAG mainly supplies excess glutamate under conditions of high demand or pathological conditions, normal synaptic transmission might proceed with glutamate derived from other sources. If NAAG does act as a neurotransmitter, then increases its actions by blocking hydrolysis potentially would cause increased activation of metabotropic glutamate receptors along with partial block of NMDA receptors. Both these effects have been shown to be neuroprotective in various models of acute and chronic neuronal injury.

Our initial experiments confirmed that NAALADase inhibition was neuroprotective in a well-characterized tissue culture model of cerebral ischemia. Dissociated cortical cultures were prepared from rat embryos (17 day gestation) and used in experiments after 2–3 weeks in culture. Ischemic conditions were simulated by a 20-min period of pharmacological inhibition of metabolism. In a glucose-free, N-2-hydroxyethylpiperazine-N'-2-ethanesulphonic acid (HEPES) buffered saline solution, potassium cyanide (5 mM) was used to block oxidative metabolism and 2-deoxyglucose was used to block glycolysis (1–10 mM). Injury was assessed by lactate dehydrogenase (LDH) release into the medium after 24 hours of recovery. Phosphate was omitted from all solutions, since NAALADase is known to be inhibited by phosphate.

2-PMPA, present during metabolic inhibition and recovery, provided near complete protection from injury, even at the highest concentrations of metabolic inhibitors used (5 mM KCN, 10 mM 2-deoxyglucose (2-DG)). This level of insult causes the same injury as exposure to 1 mM N-methyl-D-aspartate (NMDA), resulting in loss of almost all neurons in the culture.

Next, 2-PMPA was examined in a standard model of focal cerebral ischemia in the rat, temporary middle cerebral artery occlusion (MCAO) by intraluminal suture. The artery was occluded for 2 hours, and injury was assessed after 24 hours recovery by 2,3,5-triphenyltetrazoliumchloride monohydrate (TTC) staining. The drug reduced infarct size by 66% when administered 60 min after the onset of ischemia.

Importantly, NAALADase inhibitors appear to be very well tolerated by animals. Even at doses above the minimal effective dose in the MCAO model, rats showed no obvious behavioral changes. We observed none of the ataxia, tremor, lethargy or stereotypy that have been described following neuroprotective doses of other drugs thought to limit either glutamate release (sodium channel blockers) or postsynaptic glutamate receptor activation (NMDA receptor antagonists).

MICRODIALYSIS MEASUREMENTS OF GLUTAMATE AND NAAG

Our hypothesis was that NAALADase inhibition would limit glutamate and increase NAAG. Initially, we examined extracellular concentrations using the technique of microdialysis, assuming that NAAG would be released into the extracellular

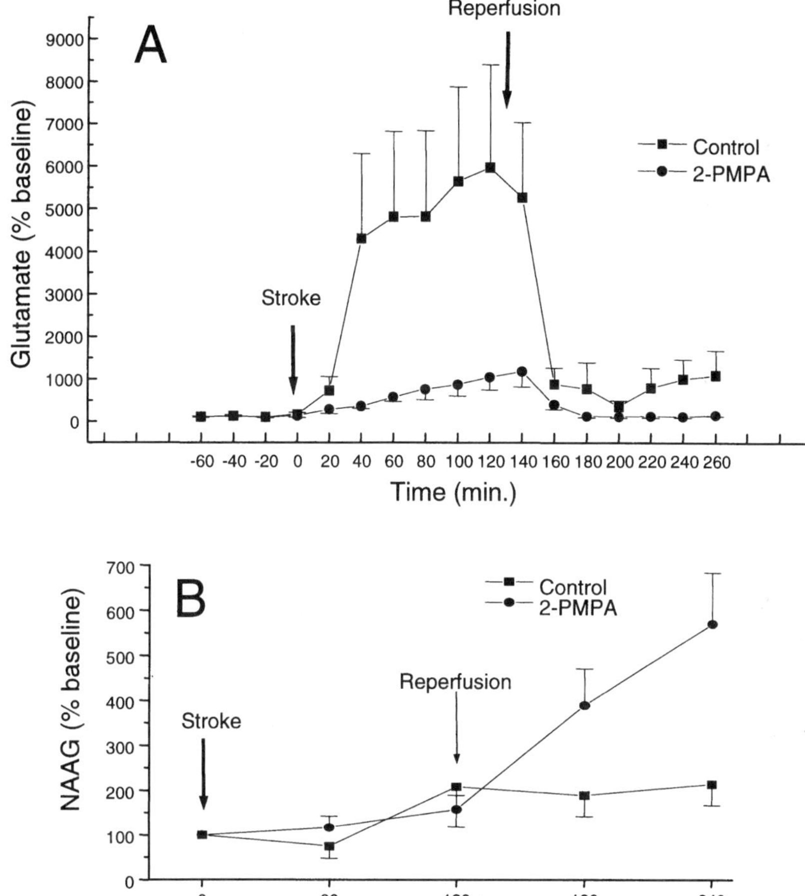

FIGURE 2. NAALADase inhibition alters glutamate levels during and after MCAO. Rats preimplanted with microdialysis probes were treated with high-dose 2-PMPA or vehicle and subjected to MCAO for 2 hours followed by reperfusion. **(A)** 2-PMPA significantly attenuated the ischemia-induced increase in extracellular glutamate in the caudate as compared to vehicle treated rats (60-fold rise reduced to 12-fold rise); ANOVA, $p < 0.05$. **(B)** In subsequent studies, 2-PMPA significantly increased extracellular NAAG in the caudate during reperfusion compared to vehicle treated rats (2-fold rise compared to 6-fold rise: ANOVA, $p < 0.05$).

space where it would normally cleave to NAA and glutamate by NAALADase. As shown in FIGURE 2, 2-PMPA had the predicted effect on glutamate release, when administered at the start of occlusion. In vehicle-treated animals, the 60-fold rise in the caudate was reduced to a 12-fold rise. The 9-fold secondary rise in glutamate during reperfusion was entirely eliminated by 2-PMPA treatment.

During early reperfusion, the expected reciprocal relationship between glutamate and NAAG was observed (FIG. 2). In vehicle-treated animals, there was a smaller secondary rise in extracellular glutamate, which began at the onset of reperfusion. In animals treated with 2-PMPA, the glutamate rise was eliminated, and a rise in NAAG was observed instead. When the probe efficiency is accounted for, the rise in NAAG observed in 2-PMPA-treated animals is the equimolar to the rise in glutamate observed in untreated animals. This reciprocal relationship is consistent with the hypothesis that NAAG is released to the extracellular space, where it is hydrolyzed by NAALADase to liberate glutamate. Inhibition of NAALADase prevents the glutamate liberation, maintaining NAAG increases instead.

Microdialysis measurements of NAAG during occlusion were not as easily interpreted. As shown in FIGURE 2, NAAG was not increased during occlusion in 2-PMPA-treated animals. Further examination of NAAG metabolism will be needed to establish whether the effect of NAALADase inhibition on glutamate is indirect or whether NAAG can be hydrolyzed intracellularly during occlusion, in which case it would not appear in the extracellular space.

CONCLUSIONS

NAALADase inhibition is a novel neuroprotective strategy with great promise. Toxicity has proved to be an important obstacle to the development of drugs to treat acute stroke. Behaviorally, NAALADase inhibitors appear to have an especially favorable therapeutic index. The neuroprotective effects are at least of similar magnitude to other strategies thought to limit the toxic effects of excess glutamate during focal ischemia and reperfusion. However, NAALADase inhibitors appear to have fewer potential side effects than glutamate receptor antagonists. In addition, NAALADase inhibitors should prove to be important tools in understanding the physiological role of NAAG in the brain, perhaps deepening our understanding of glutamate neurotransmission.

REFERENCES

1. COYLE, J.T. 1997. The nagging question of the function of *N*-acetylaspartylglutamate. Neurobiol. Dis. **4:** 231–238.
2. TSAI, G., B.L. STAUCH, J.J. VORNOV, J.K. DESHPANDE & J.T. COYLE. 1990. Selective release of *N*-acetylaspartylglutamate from rat optic nerve terminals *in vivo*. Brain Res. **518:** 313–316.
3. WROBLEWSKA, B., J.T. WROBLEWSKI, O.H. SAAB & J.H. NEALE. 1993. *N*-Acetylaspartylglutamate inhibits forskolin-stimulated cyclic AMP levels via a metabotropic glutamate receptor in cultured cerebellar granule cells. J. Neurochem. **61:** 943–948.
4. BURLINA, A.P., S.D. SKAPER, M.R. MAZZA, V. FERRARI, A. LEON & A.B. BURLINA. 1994. *N*-Acetylaspartylglutamate selectively inhibits neuronal responses to *N*-methyl-D-aspartic acid *in vitro*. J. Neurochem. **63:** 1174–1177.
5. ROBINSON, M.B., R.D. BLAKELY, R. COUTO & J.T. COYLE. 1987. Hydrolysis of the brain dipeptide *N*-acetyl-L-aspartyl-L-glutamate. Identification and characterization of a novel *N*-acetylated alpha-linked acidic dipeptidase activity from rat brain. J. Biol. Chem. **262:** 14498–14506.
6. LUTHI-CARTER, R., U.V. BERGER, A.K. BARCZAK, M. ENNA & J.T. COYLE. 1998. Isolation and expression of a rat brain cDNA encoding glutamate carboxypeptidase II. Proc. Natl. Acad. Sci. USA **95:** 3215–3220.

7. TSAI, G., B.S. SLUSHER, L. SIM & J.T. COYLE. 1993. Immunocytochemical distribution of *N*-acetylaspartylglutamate in the rat forebrain and glutamatergic pathways. J. Chem. Neuroanat. **6:** 277–292.
8. PASSANI, L.A., J.P. VONSATTEL & J.T. COYLE. 1997. Distribution of *N*-acetylaspartylglutamate immunoreactivity in human brain and its alteration in neurodegenerative disease. Brain Res. **772:** 9–22.
9. SLUSHER, B.S., G. TSAI, G. YOO & J.T. COYLE. 1992. Immunocytochemical localization of the *N*-acetyl-aspartyl-glutamate (NAAG) hydrolyzing enzyme *N*-acetylated alpha-linked acidic dipeptidase (NAALADase). J. Comp. Neurol. **315:** 217–229.

The Low-Affinity, Use-Dependent NMDA Receptor Antagonist AR-R 15896AR

An Update of Progress in Stroke

GENE C. PALMER,[a] EDWARD F. CREGAN, PAUL BIALOBOK,
SIMON G. SYDSERFF, THOMAS J. HUDZIK, AND DENNIS J. McCARTHY

Astra Arcus USA, Rochester, New York 14602, USA

ABSTRACT: Use-dependent *N*-methyl-D-aspartate (NMDA) receptor antagonists protect neurons from the lethal consequences of excessive stimulation by excitatory amino acids. Clinical development of high-affinity compounds such as MK801 have been limited due to untoward side effects. Toward this end, the lower-affinity use-dependent NMDA antagonists have greater margins of safety and have advanced to clinical trials for stroke, epilepsy, head trauma and chronic neurodegenerative disorders. AR-R 15896AR is currently in Phase II trials for stroke and has been repeatedly demonstrated to afford neuroprotection in a variety of *in vivo* and *in vitro* models associated with ischemia/excitotoxic conditions.

INTRODUCTION

Conditions of trauma, ischemia or seizures promote enhanced release of the excitatory neurotransmitter, glutamate in the brain. Excessive stimulation of critical postsynaptic *N*-methyl-D-aspartate (NMDA) subtype receptors by glutamate results in a massive depolarization concomitant with excessive amounts of Ca^{2+} accumulating within the neuron, culminating in cell death—the "Excitotoxic Amino Acid Hypothesis" advanced by Olney.[1] Use-dependent antagonists acting within the ion channel of the NMDA receptor have been shown repeatedly to protect susceptible neurons against the deleterious consequences of ischemia/anoxia, head trauma and/or seizures.[2–5] The major problem with clinical application of high-affinity competitive and uncompetitive NMDA receptor antagonists is their propensity to produce untoward side effects. Low-affinity, use-dependent NMDA receptor antagonists likewise exhibit neuroprotection, but side effects are less common.[6–8] At least five such compounds are currently undergoing clinical trials for stroke (NPS 1506, AR-R 15896AR),[9,10] head trauma (NPS 1506, HU-211),[9,11] epilepsy (remacemide hydrochloride, (±)-5-aminocarbonyl-10,11-dihydro-5*H*-dibenzo[*a,d*]cyclohepten-5,10-imine (ADCI)),[7,8] and chronic neurodegenerative disorders such as Alzheimer's, Parkinson's, and Huntington's diseases (memantine and remacemide hydrochloride).[4,8] The present report focuses principally upon the state of development of AR-R 15896AR with respect to its mechanism of action(s) and neuroprotective properties.

[a]Corresponding author: Gene C. Palmer, Ph.D., Astra Arcus USA, P.O. Box 20890, Rochester, NY 14602. Phone, 716/274-5575; fax, 716/272-3910.
  e-mail, eugene.palmer@arcus.us.astra.com

Background

AR-R 15896AR is the [*S*] enantiomer of [*R*,*S*]-alpha-phenyl-2-pyridine-ethanamine dihydrochloride (other designations used are FPL 15896AR and ARL-15896AR) which was discovered in our laboratories using a rational chemical synthesis and screening approach to develop a highly safe, rapidly acting, single isomeric form of a low-affinity, use-dependent NMDA receptor antagonist with an uncomplicated pharmacokinetic profile. The [*S*] enantiomer turned out to possess greater potency at the ion channel site than the [*R*] enantiomer, AR-R 15895AR (respective $IC_{50}s = 1.3$ µM and 6.9 µM), plus it exhibited a more favorable preclinical profile when tested *in vivo* and *in vitro* with respect to potency and safety.[12] Regarding safety, AR-R 15896AR did not show any evidence of:

(1) Abuse liability in rats trained to self-administer phencyclidine (PCP) or cocaine, nor did it elicit any evidence of PCP-like behaviors in rats evaluated in an open field.[13] In fact when given in high doses (30 or 60 mg/kg, p.o.) AR-R 15896AR significantly attenuated the stereotyped behavioral responses produced by PCP in the open field test (Hudzik, unpublished).

(2) Impairments in learning acquisition or memory (delayed nonmatching to sample) or related operant paradigms.[14,15]

(3) Motor impairment in either mice or rats required to perform a series of complex motor skills.[10,12]

Preclinical Pharmacokinetics

In pharmacokinetic studies in rats, plasma and brain levels of AR-R 15896AR were rapidly attained following either i.v. or p.o. administration. Kinetics were linear with a terminal half-life of 4.75 (i.v.) to 5.42 (p.o.) hr. In fact, brain levels exceeded that of plasma, while the ratio of brain to plasma concentration and brain to plasma-free concentration remained constant over time. Moreover, there was a direct correlation between brain levels and efficacy of AR-R 15896XX (XX = free base) in the rat maximal electroshock seizure test following either i.v. or p.o. dosing, indicating a relative independence from blood-brain barrier mechanisms (absorption, distribution, excretion, first pass metabolism, etc.) limiting the bioavailability of orally administered AR-R 15896AR.[12]

Clinical

Following a successful toxicology evaluation in which rats and dogs were continuously exposed to intravenous levels of AR-R 15896AR for 30 days, the compound entered a randomized, double-blind, placebo-controlled Phase I clinical trail with healthy male volunteers (20–38 years). In a second study a single ascending multiple dose administration was carried out over 3 days in both young male or older male and female volunteers (55–70 years). Doses were given i.v. over a 15-min period at the low doses (1, 3, 10, and 20 mg) and over a 60-min period for the high doses (80, 120 and 160 mg). AR-R 15896AR exhibited linear kinetics and was rapidly distributed with a terminal half-life of 13.6 hr. Central nervous system (CNS) side effects were minor and included dose-related dizziness, abnormal vision, headache, paraesthesia and impaired concentration. Younger volunteers tolerated a loading dose of

160 mg with nine maintenance doses of up to 70 mg administered every 8 hr over a 3 day period, while older volunteers tolerated a similar regimen with a loading dose of 120 mg followed by maintenance doses of 60 mg. Side effects were similar, and dizziness was the most common complaint (see also Ref. 10). The first Phase IIa clinical study in patients with acute stroke has been completed. The results are currently undergoing analysis.

MECHANISMS OF ACTION

NMDA-Associated Actions

Receptor Affinity

Two separate experiments reported the binding affinity of AR-R 15896AR as determined by its ability to displace labeled MK801 in the presence of glycine from rat cortical synaptic membrane fractions. The reported K_i values were 0.7 μM[16] and 1.3 μM.[10] Experiments using quantitative receptor autoradiography examined the binding characteristics of AR-R 15896AR in different regions of the rat brain. The resultant IC_{50} values in (μM) were: frontal cortex = 53.8; striatum = 46.8; entorhinal cortex = 40.3; hippocampal CA1 = 48; hippocampal dentate gyrus = 42.1; and the cerebellar granular cell layer value of 17.2 was significantly less than the forebrain regions.[17,18] The differences in AR-R 15896AR binding affinities between membrane fractions and autoradiography into intact cells are mostly likely unique to the preparations, i.e., in the broken cell preparation the compound in the presence of excess amounts of glycine and glutamate has greater access to the ion channel site.

Possible Subunit Specificity

Additional differences between high- and low-affinity uncompetitive NMDA receptor antagonists have been attributed to their regional localization in the brain (see above)[17,18] and possible receptor subtype classifications.[19] Quantitative receptor autoradiography was used to compare regional binding characteristics of both low-affinity and high-affinity use-dependent NMDA receptor antagonists in the rat brain. The high-affinity compounds exhibited considerably greater binding affinities (MK801 > thienylcyclohexyl piperidine (TCP) > PCP) that were notable in the forebrain and less so in the cerebellum. In contrast, the low-affinity compounds, namely the [S]-isomer of the desglycinyl metabolite of remacemide > memantine > [R]-isomer of the desglycinyl metabolite of remacemide > FPL 15853 > AR-R 15896 > budipine > amantadine > remacemide, exhibited greater binding affinities in the cerebellum than in the forebrain structures.[17,18] In related work, Monaghan and Larsen[19] examined NMDA channel-blocking potencies at recombinant NMDA receptors (NR1b/2A-C) expressed in *Xenopus* oocytes and noted that the lower-affinity compounds—AR-R 15896AR, the desglycinyl metabolite of remacemide, ARL 15609 and dextromethorphan—exhibited greater affinities at the NR1b/2C subtype, while MK801 and TCP appeared equally potent at all receptor subtypes. The NR1b/2C NMDA receptor subtype is typically localized in the cerebellum. Interesting were the findings by Small *et al.*,[20] who demonstrated that the NR2C subunits are differentially expressed in rat hippocampal slices exposed to oxygen-glucose deprivation.

However, the supposition that one particular NMDA receptor subtype is the molecular target responsible for the pathological processes underlying ischemia is tenuous, because compounds more selective for NR2B[21] and possibly NR2D[9] subunits likewise exhibited neuroprotection.

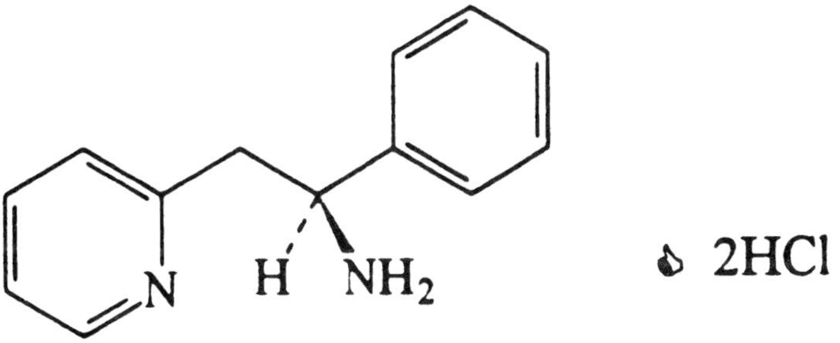

In Vitro *Electrophysiology*

Hippocampal slices were removed from young adult male Sprague-Dawley rats and maintained in a tissue bath. The ability of test compounds to antagonize the effects of NMDA in a use-dependent manner on the synaptic field potential amplitude was investigated. AR-R 15896AR significantly blocked NMDA-induced depolarization with an IC_{50} of 26 μM. MK801 produced greater than 50% inhibition at 0.03 μM (FIG. 2). To insure specificity of the preparation to NMDA, another study by E. Harris (unpublished) used the hippocampal slice preparation with electrophysiological recordings made from the α-amino-3-hydroxy-5-methylisoxazole-4-propionic acid (AMPA) receptor-sensitive Schaffer collateral pathway (input from CA3 to CA1). These Schaffer collateral responses were not influenced by concentrations of up to 300 μM of AR-R 15896AR.

Kinetics of Receptor Block/Unblock

One of the major differences between low- and high-affinity use-dependent NMDA receptor antagonists is the more rapid kinetic rates for blocking and unblocking from the ion channel site. The rapid rate of unblocking results in less membrane trapping of the low-affinity antagonists between the cycles of ion channel opening/closing and does not result in the cumulative, perhaps less desirable, total block interfering with the frequency of repetitive stimulation, observed for the high-affinity compounds. Blanpeied and co-workers[22] investigated such a role for the low-affinity antagonists, amantadine and memantine, using cell culture systems expressing subtypes of NMDA receptors. Both compounds blocked NMDA-activated channels by binding to a site at which they could be trapped after channel closure and following unbinding of agonist. When memantine and high-affinity antagonists were washed off after steady state block, a percentage of the blocked channels released rather than trapped the drug. Thus memantine exhibited partial trapping, while PCP and MK801 remained almost totally trapped. This property of memantine was evident in recombinant NMDA receptors composed of NR1 with either NR2A or NR2B subunits.[22] This study is supported by the electrophysiological investigations of Monaghan and Larsen,[19] who measured receptor on/off kinetic rates of high- and low-affinity un-

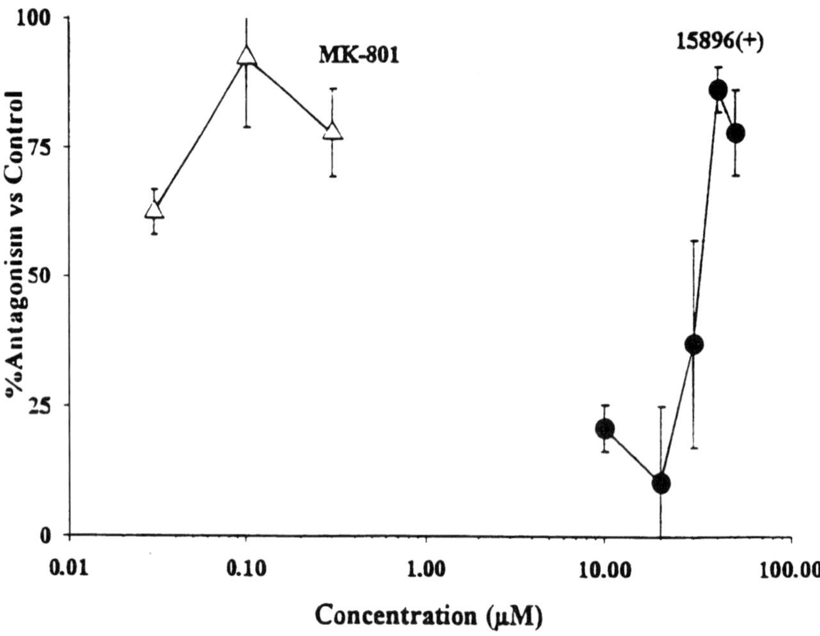

FIGURE 2. Electrophysiology: inhibition of NMDA-induced depolarization in rat hippocampal slices by AR-R 15896AR ($IC_{50} = 26$ µM) or MK801. NMDA was applied 3 times to each slice. The amount of depolarization block caused by the third application of NMDA (20 µM per pulse) in the presence of drug was expressed as a percentage of the effect in control slices exposed to NMDA alone. The values are the mean percentage $\pm$ SE, $n = 4$–5 slices per data point (for complete description of methods see Ref. 37).

competitive antagonists, including AR-R 15896AR, using recombinant NMDA receptors expressed in *Xenopus* oocytes. Again the high-affinity compounds, MK801 and TCP, displayed slower on/off kinetics.

In further kinetic work with NMDA receptors, Black *et al.*[23] demonstrated that cultured rat cortical neurons respond to an excitatory amino acid challenge with a rapid triggered entry of Ca^{2+} into the cell. NMDA or glutamate-triggered $[Ca^{2+}]_{in}$ responses were prevented by uncompetitive NMDA receptor antagonists in a use-dependent manner, i.e., a second exposure of the excitatory amino acid was necessary before inhibition could be detected. The kinetics of the block differed between the low-affinity and the high-affinity compounds. The low-affinity, use-dependent antagonists (AR-R 15896AR, the desglycinyl metabolite of remacemide, dextromethorphan, memantine, and ADCI) acted more rapidly, but were only capable of partial prevention of the NMDA-triggered $]Ca^{2+}]_{in}$, whereas the block by the high-affinity compounds (MK801, PCP, and ARL-16247AA) was slow in onset, sustained, and completely prevented $[Ca^{2+}]_{in}$. Kinetic analyses indicated the more potent compounds also possessed the slowest unblocking rates.

Voltage-clamp techniques were used to characterize further the kinetics and voltage-dependence of the block of NMDA-induced currents in primary cultures of rat cortical neurons. Thus when NMDA currents were held at −60 mV, AR-R 15896AR caused a rapid and reversible, use-dependent inhibition of current with an EC_{50} of 9.8 μM. Alternatively, the EC_{50} for NMDA was unaffected by AR-R 15896AR, indicating the uncompetitive nature of the block. AR-R 15896AR remained trapped within the ion channel upon removal of NMDA until subsequent NMDA reexposure, whereupon currents recovered rapidly. The foreword rate constant for AR-R 15896AR was slower than that for memantine, while the reverse rate constant was faster for AR-R 15896AR.[24] A recent similar study by this group[25] attempted to characterize the degree of NMDA ion channel trapping by the low-affinity, use-dependent antagonists AR-R 15896AR, memantine and ketamine. The onset and relief of block was fastest for AR-R 15896AR and slowest for ketamine. All three compounds produced a similar steady state of block after 30 sec of co-application with NMDA. No significant increase in ion channel trapping occurred after 30 sec. However, after a 120-sec period of washout there were significant differences in the degree of trapping among each of the antagonists: 54% for AR-R 15896, 71% for memantine, and 86% for ketamine. This work confirms earlier work conducted by Subramanian *et al.*,[26] and by Jones and Rogawski,[27] who likewise used voltage clamp recordings from cultured rat hippocampal neurons. In their work the inhibition of NMDA currents with the isomers of remacemide hydrochloride or ADCI were rapid, reversible, as well as strongly use- and voltage-dependent.

In conclusion these biochemical and electrophysiological findings demonstrated major class differences between low- and high-affinity uncompetitive antagonists regarding both the mechanisms controlling NMDA-triggered entrance of Ca^{2+} into the neurons, as well as the kinetics for the on/off rates of receptor blockade and degree of ion channel trapping. It has been suggested that the low-affinity, use-dependent NMDA antagonists may have reduced toxicity, because they reach steady state block more rapidly due to their rapid on/off kinetics.[6] Further work will be required to affirm this hypothesis.

Na+ Channels

In spite of the fact that compounds usually found active in the maximal electroshock seizure test inhibit Na^+ channels,[28] we have been unable to demonstrate such actions for AR-R 15896AR. The compound did not limit sustained repetitive firing (fast Na^+ channels) in dissociated mouse spinal neurons, nor with patch clamp techniques did it produce a high-frequency, use-dependent block of Na^+ channels in rat cortical neurons.[10]

Sigma Receptors

It is of interest that AR-R 15896AR exhibited affinity at the sigma-1 receptor; the IC_{50} for displacement of $[^3H]$-(+)-pentazocine from synaptosomal membrane fractions from rat brain was 4.5 μM.[10] Sigma-1 affinity, however, was only 4.4-fold greater than that observed for displacement of a sigma-2 ligand combination $[^3H]$1,3-di-ortho-tolyguanidine (DTG) + 5 μM dextromethorphan. Sigma-1 agonists elicit an emetic-like behavior in pigeons.[29] AR-R 15896AR similarly produced emesis in this assay (ED_{50} = 29.7 mg/kg, i.m. [95% confidence limits = 19–48]), and the action was reversed by pretreatment with the sigma-1 selective antagonist, BMY14802 (AD_{50} = 0.14 mg/kg, i.m.). Chronic haloperidol treatment (2.5 mg/kg/

b.i.d./14days) desensitizes sigma-1 receptors and thereby attenuated by 60% the emetic response to a high dose of AR-R 15896AR (56 mg/kg). Sigma-1 receptor activity is linked to neuroprotection, which is discussed in the section on Hypoxia and Global Ischemia.

NEUROPROTECTION

In Vitro

Prevention of Neuronal Injury/Death

Under *in vitro* conditions, NMDA receptor antagonists effectively reduced neuronal damage in cell cultures following addition of the excitatory amino acids, glutamate or NMDA.[4,5] In our initial experiments, hippocampal neurons were isolated from fetal rat brains and maintained in culture. The preparation was highly susceptible to injury as indexed by release of lactate dehydrogenase (LDH) within 5 min after exposure to either 250 μM NMDA or kainate. The addition of AR-R 15896AR or MK801 to the cultures immediately after exposure to the excitatory amino acids prevented LDH release measured at 24 hr. The lowest doses required to produce significant inhibition were 100 μM for AR-R 15896AR and 1 μM for MK801. The AMPA antagonist, 6-cyano-7-nitroquinoxaline-2,3-dione (CNQX), was ineffective in this system.[10]

Black and co-workers[16] using cortical cultures taken from 18-day-old fetal rats demonstrated that the cell death occurring within 24 hr after a 15-min exposure to 50 μM glutamate or NMDA was completely prevented by incubation with AR-R 15896AR (25–50 μM). As discussed in the section on Receptor Kinetics, AR-R 15896AR and the low-affinity, use-dependent NMDA antagonists rapidly and partially prevented NMDA-triggered influx of $[Ca^{2+}]_{in}$ into the neurons. In contrast, the high-affinity antagonists were slower acting, but completely shut down Ca^{2+} influx.[16,23] Critical levels of intercellular Ca^{2+} are required to maintain normal homeostatic mechanisms. Thus the reduced toxicity attributed to the low-affinity compounds may be explained in part by preventing only the excessive accumulation of Ca^{2+} into the neuron during hyperstimulation by excitatory amino acid transmitters. Moreover, an early and persistent loss of protein kinase C activity, which precedes any morphological signs of cell damage, is a characteristic feature of cerebral ischemia.[16] Indeed, the loss of membrane-associated protein kinase C activity occurring within 4 hr as a consequence of added glutamate or NMDA was likewise reversed following addition of 50 μM AR-R 15896AR.[16] Activation of glutamate receptors also affects the distribution of the cytoskeletal protein, microtubule-associated protein (MAP2), within neuronal cell bodies and dentrites.[30] Glutamate-triggered $[Ca^{2+}]_i$ increases calpain activity, which degrades MAP.[31] This provides one of the earliest and most sensitive markers of ischemic neuronal injury. With the identical cortical culture preparation,[16] these investigators[32] discovered that addition of AR-R 15896AR (50 μM) or MK801 (10 μM) totally prevented the NMDA-induced loss of MAP2 that occurs within 2 min of NMDA exposure.

Microglia Activation

Application of the beta amyloid fragment 1–42 to microglia in culture results in secretion of a neurotoxic factor, a process inhibited by NMDA receptor antagonists.[33] In a preliminary study using ciliary neuronal cultures from E9 chick embryos, the EC_{50} for inhibition of cell death by the neurotoxic microglia was approximately 1.3 μM for AR-R 15896AR (D. Giulian, unpublished data).

Hypoxia/Global Ischemia

In Vitro: *Hypoxia*

Uptake of $[^{45}Ca^{2+}]$ was measured in cultured cerebellar granular cells obtained from rat pups following exposure to hypoxia. The following excitatory amino acid receptor antagonists exhibited the approximate EC_{50}s for inhibition of Ca^{2+} uptake: MK801 (45 nM), AR-R 15896AR (110 μM), the AMPA receptor antagonist, 2,3-dihydroxy-6-nitro-7-sulfamoylbenzo-(F)-quinoxaline (NBQX, 5 μM), the glutamate release inhibitor, riluzole (110 μM) and the polyamine site acting compound, ifenprodil (110 μM). Thus agreement exists between the efficacy of glutamate compounds to inhibit the hypoxia-induced increase in $[Ca^{2+}]_{in}$ into cerebellar granular cells and their neuroprotective action in hypoxic models *in vivo*.[34] In a preliminary report, exposure of a rat brain coronal cortical slice preparation to hypoxia and hypoglycemia evoked a marked release of glutamate, which was inhibited by addition of AR-R 15896AR (100 μM).[35] It is of interest that considerably higher concentrations of NMDA antagonists were necessary to afford neuroprotection under *in vitro* conditions of hypoxic injury when compared to neuronal injury resulting from direct application of the excitatory amino acids.

In Vivo: *Hypoxia*

Hypoxia has been used as a preclinical screen for discovery of compounds with potential neuroprotective properties. The procedure is rapid and eliminates any confounding anesthesia, but control of body temperature is essential to eliminate false positive agents. Dosages that increase survival time under hypoxic conditions may be predictive of the doses that will protect in more complex preclinical models of ischemia.[36,37] In our investigations we have found that low-affinity, use-dependent NMDA antagonists, notably AR-R 15896AR, remacemide hydrochloride, and FPL 13950AA extended survival time when mice and rats were exposed to an hypoxic challenge.[36-38] Moreover, we have observed a consistent relationship between affinity for sigma-1 receptors and prolongation of survival time for such compounds. In keeping with its sigma-1 receptor properties, the anti-hypoxic actions exhibited by a large oral dose of AR-R 15896AR (78.8 mg/kg) were reversed in mice with the sigma-1 selective ligand (+)-pentazocine (3 mg/kg, s.c.) (T. Hudzik, unpublished). Thus both sigma and NMDA receptor properties must contribute to the salutary effects of AR-R 15896AR regarding neuroprotection in models of hypoxia/global ischemia.

In Vivo: *Global Ischemia*

Several investigations indicate efficacy of low-affinity, use-dependent NMDA receptor antagonists in animal models of global ischemia; especially regarding the delayed cell death in the particularly vulnerable hippocampal CA1 neurons. When rats were subjected to the 4-vessel occlusion technique of forebrain ischemia, the CA1 neurons were spared following both acute and chronic administration of AR-R 15896AR, remacemide hydrochloride or FPL 13950AA.[36–38] Moreover, remacemide hydrochloride and FPL 13950AA likewise prevented CA1 neuronal death and improved neurological outcome in dogs subjected to 8 min clamping of the ascending aorta.[36,37] Notably, AR-R 15896AR treatment was not protective in the gerbil model of forebrain ischemia, an event due to the extremely short half-life (less than 30 min) of the orally administered compound in this species.[38] AR-R 15896AR treatment did not protect CA1 or striatal neurons in the rat 2-vessel occlusion model of ischemia in which the animals were subjected to hypotension concomitant with clamping the common carotid arteries whilst being maintained under anesthesia throughout the procedure.[38] In the same model neither AR-R 15896AR nor MK801 prevented blood-brain barrier opening occurring at 6 hr after introduction of ischemia.[39]

Middle Cerebral Artery Occlusion (MCAO) Models of Focal Ischemia

Spontaneously Hypertensive Rat (SHR) Model of Transient Ischemia

The model consists of unilateral ligation of the common carotid artery in tandem with clamping the middle cerebral artery for either 1.5 or 2 hr followed by reinstitution of cerebral blood flow for 22 hr or up to 42 days post-MCAO. The unique feature of the model is that the lesion is predominantly cortical in nature.[40] In the first investigation, AR-R 15896AR was administered i.p. in three sequential doses within a 12-hr period. The time of initial dosing varied from 0.5 hr pre-MCAO to 2 hr post-MCAO. Significant cortical protection at 22 hr was observed at all initial dosing times up to 1 hr post-MCAO. In the second study AR-R 15896AR (10 mg/kg, s.c.; peak plasma level of 3527 ng/ml attained) was administered at 0.5, 4 and 12 hr post-MCAO. At 2 and 6 days after ischemia T_2-weighted magnetic resonance images indicated significantly less cortical damage in the treatment group. These animals were subsequently tested between 30–45 days for forepaw dexterity in the staircase test. Interestingly, the forepaw deficit observed on the side ipsilateral to the lesion was improved in the treatment group. Due to maturation of the lesion (shrinkage, atrophy and phagocytic removal of damaged tissue), the histopathology was unremarkable.[10,38]

Rat Intraluminal Technique of Transient MCAO

The model is a useful, noninvasive, reversible method of preventing blood flow achieved by insertion of an intraluminal filament into the internal carotid to block the MCA at its origin. A characteristic feature of the model is that prominent damage occurs in both the striatum (subcortical) as well as the cortex. The model is "substrain specific" in that consistent lesions are achieved in only certain strains of rats originating from specific suppliers. Moreover, survival among strains varies with the duration of MCAO. Four experiments were conducted with AR-R 15896AR. Histopathological evaluation was the end point to determine efficacy. In the first two experiments the duration of MCAO in Wistar rats was 2 hr. The compound was infused beginning at 5 min post-occlusion followed by insertion of an ALZET minipump, all calibrated to maintain a specified plasma level of AR-R 15896XX for one week.

> (1) A dose response evaluation indicated that neuroprotection was achieved when the plasma level of AR-R 15896XX reached 2259 ng/ml or higher for one week (TABLE 1).

TABLE 1. Dose response relationship between AR-R 15896XX plasma levels and focal ischemic damage in the Wistar Rat subjected to 2 hr MCAO followed by 1 week recirculation

Conditions	Plasma Level ng/ml	Cortex % infarction	Subcortex % infarction	Total % infarction
Control	<MDL	11.3 ± 1.3	8.4 ± 0.2	24.1 ± 2.6
AR-R 15896AR	682 ± 38.6	10.8 ± 2.6	7.1 ± 0.5 $p = 0.04$	22.1 ± 3.7
Control	<MDL	8.5 ± 2.1	9.0 ± 0.4	20.04 ± 2.6
AR-R 15896AR	1885 ± 163	6.5 ± 1.7	8.2 ± 0.9	18.2 ± 2.2
Control	<MDL	15.5 ± 4.0	12.9 ± 0.4	29.7 ± 2.8
AR-R 15896AR	2682 ± 168	4.3 ± 1.8 $p = 0.009$	8.4 ± 1.5 $p = 0.035$	15.7 ± 2.5 $p = 0.009$

NOTE: Male rats received 2 hr MCAO via the intraluminal monofilament technique followed by reflow for 1 week. Five min after MCAO a 30-min infusion of AR-R 15896AR was followed by implantation of an ALZET minipump all calibrated to deliver a specified plasma level of AR-R 15896XX (XX = free base). Histopathological assessments of the H&E stained sections were performed using a microscope and a C-imaging system (Comprix, Cranberry Township, PA). A volumetric measure of tissue necrosis was calculated by summing product of areas and the interval distance. Tissue damage was expressed as the percent of the contralateral hemisphere to control to account for differences between animals as well as fixation artifacts. Values are mean $\pm$ SE; n = 6–13 animals. Data were analyzed by an overall two-factor ANOVA followed by a post-hoc one-factor ANOVA comparing differences in neural damage between vehicle-treated controls and AR-R 15896AR-treated animals. MDL = minimal detectable limit.

(2) Maintenance of an AR-R 15896XX plasma level of greater than 2300 ng/ml for one week afforded neuroprotection out to 8 weeks post-MCAO (TABLE 2).

(3) An acute single dose treatment of AR-R 15896AR (20.3 mg/kg, i.p.) given at 10 min after reflow in a Lister Hooded rat subjected to 60 min MCAO likewise afforded neuroprotection after 23 hr (FIG. 3).

(4) A complicated magnetic resonance imaging (MRI), behavioral and histopathology study was attempted using a Sprague-Dawley strain subjected to 60 min transient MCAO; however, the degree of damage in all study groups was so variable that meaningful data with AR-R 15896AR could not be attained. The one factor was that survivability of the animals out to 60 days was twice as great in the treatment groups (J. Peeling and D. Corbett, unpublished).

The investigation demonstrating neuroprotection of one week treatment with AR-R 15896AR out to 8 weeks in time after MCAO should answer the continuing arguments as to whether or not specific classes of neuroprotective drugs only postpone the onset of irreversible ischemic injury.[41]

TABLE 2. Effect of one week dosing with AR-R 15896AR on histopathological outcomes at 1, 2, 4 & 8 weeks post-MCAO in the Wistar rat

Conditions	1-Week	2-Weeks	4 Weeks	8 Weeks
Percent Infarct Volume: Cortex				
Control	2.8 ± 1.4	5.1 ± 1.3	3.1 ± 1.1	4.1 ± 1.1
AR-R 15896AR	0.5 ± 0.1	2.0 ± 1.0	0.9 ± 0.7	1.3 ± 0.6
	$p = 0.01$	$p = 0.06$	$p = 0.02$	$p = 0.03$
Percent Infarct Volume: Striatum/Subcortex				
Control	6.1 ± 0.9	6.9 ± 0.5	3.3 ± 0.6	3.7 ± 0.5
AR-R 15896AR	5.1 ± 1.3	4.1 ± 0.8	1.5 ± 0.5	2.1 ± 0.6
		$p = 0.01$	$p = 0.04$	$p = 0.06$
Percent Total Infarct Volume (Cortex + Subcortex)				
Control	12.4 ± 2.8	23.1 ± 2.6	19.6 ± 2.9	19.7 ± 3.3
AR-R 15896AR	9.7 ± 2.1	13.1 ± 3.2	11.9 ± 3.8	12.1 ± 3.0
		$p = 0.03$		

NOTE: Male rats received 2 hr MCAO via the intraluminal monofilament technique followed by reflow up to 8 weeks. Five min after MCAO a 30-min infusion of AR-R 15896AR was followed by implantation of an ALZET minipump all calibrated to deliver a plasma level of >2250 ng/ml. The 1 week AR-R 15896XX (free base) plasma level was 2259 ± 55 ng/ml. The remainder of the conditions are described in the legend to TABLE 1. Values are mean $\pm$ SE; $n = 7$–11 animals/data point. Since the tissue data did not exhibit a normal distribution, statistics were performed with Kruskal-Wallis ANOVA on ranks comparing differences in neural damage between vehicle-treated controls and AR-R 15896AR-treated animals.

Feline Model of Transient MCAO

Focal ischemia was induced in cats maintained under anesthesia by direct clamping of the MCA via the transorbital approach. At 30 min into a 90-min MCAO the cats received an i.v. infusion of AR-R 15896AR (170 µg/kg/min, calibrated to achieve a plasma level of approximately 1166 ng/ml) or saline. At 6 hr post-MCAO the cats were positioned for MRI and diffusion, and T2-weighted images were taken over the ensuing 2 hr, at which time the animals were sacrificed and the brains processed for histopathological evaluation. In the AR-R 15896AR treatment group the percent reduction in mean infarct volumes (mm^3) for the following determinations were: 1) diffusion-weighted MRI reduced by 70%; 2) T2-weighted MRI reduced by 82%; and 3) histopathology reduced by 67%.[10,42]

Rat Intraluminal Model of Permanent MCAO

The technique is similar to that described above except the monofilament is left in place for 24 hr, at which time the brains are removed and stained with 2,3,5-tetraphenyltetrazolium chloride (TTC). In our preliminary ongoing experiments both dextrorphan (20 mg/kg, s.c. given at 15 and 135 min post-MCAO) and AR-R 15896AR (30 mg/kg, s.c. given at 5 min and 6 hr post-MCAO) appeared to reduce the extensive damage observed in the cortex of Wistar rats ($p = 0.05$, Student's two-tailed t test, $n = 7$–8). The mean percent $\pm$ SE values for cortical damage comparing the lesion side to the contralateral hemisphere were: control = 32.2 ± 4.9; dextrorphan = 18.3 ± 3.9; and AR-R 15896AR = 19.5 ± 3.7.

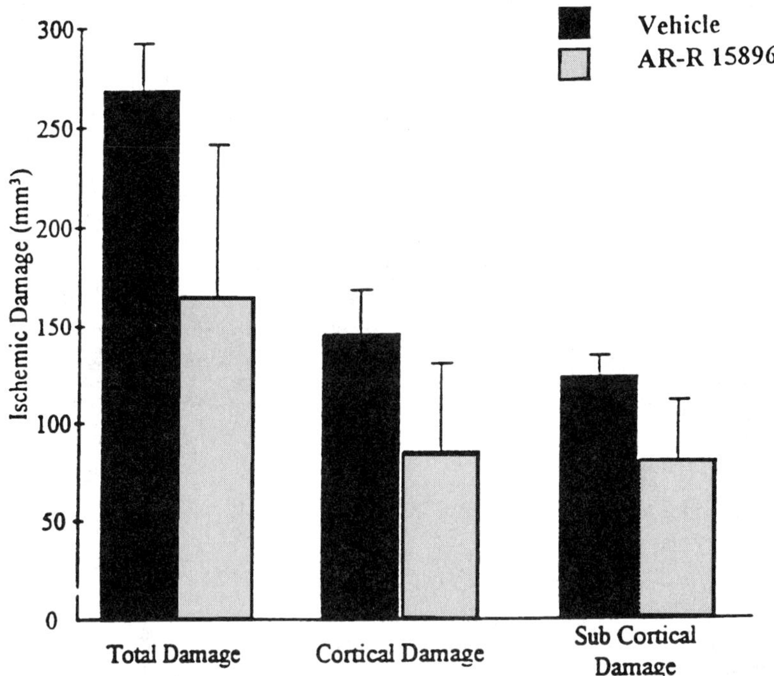

FIGURE 3. Neuroprotection by an acute injection of AR-R 15896AR 10 min after 60-min MCAO (intraluminal monofilament technique) plus 23 hr recirculation in the Lister Hooded rat. Cresyl violet stained sections (20 microns thick) were evaluated for neuronal damage using traditional light microscopic techniques with evaluation of cells for altered morphology, pyknosis and cytoplasmic staining differences. The damage was transcribed onto prematched stereotaxic sections and the areas digitized and integrated against position on the interaural plane. The amount of damage is expressed as the volume of ischemic injury in mm³. The data are expressed as the mean ± SD, $n = 6$ for both groups. All values for AR-R 15896AR-treated animals are significantly different from the controls ($p < 0.05$, ANOVA with post-hoc Newman Keuls analyses). AR-R 15896AR was given as a single injection (20.3 mg/kg, i.p.) at 70 min post-MCAO.

In Vivo: *Models of Direct Neuronal Injury*

Excitatory Amino Acid-Induced Seizures

Pretreatment of mice with AR-R 15896AR (i.p.) prevented seizures and the associated mortality following i.v. administration of either the NMDA analog, *N*-methyl-DL-aspartate (NMDLA), or kainic acid. The respective ED_{50}s were 50 and 23 mg/kg for NMDLA and 50 and 29.7 mg/kg for kainate.[10,12]

Malonate-Induced Striatal Toxicity

Intrastriatal administration of malonic acid results in neurotoxicity within 72 hr. Malonate inhibits mitochondrial respiratory functions associated with complex II in the electron transport chain, a process inhibited by NMDA receptor antagonists, and may represent a model of slow excitotoxic cell death.[18] If AR-R 15896AR was administered intraventricularly (200 μM), or s.c. (8.9 mg/kg) to rats either 30 min before or 5 min after malonate, there was at 72 hr an approximate 80% reduction in lesion volume in the striatum. MK801 was equally effective; however, the effective dose was associated with prominent side effects.[18]

Intracerebral Hemorrhage

A solution of collagenase (0.7 U)/heparin (1.4 U) was infused into the striatum of rats, followed by a loading dose of AR-R 15896AR and insertion of an ALZET minipump, both calibrated to maintain plasma levels of ~2,000 ng/ml for one week. Damage was assessed over a 21-day period using T_2-weighted MRI, behavioral testing, followed by histopathology at 22 days. The MRI and histopatholgy were unremarkable; however, behavioral and quality of life indices were improved (the latter significantly).[10] While the results indicate a lack of neuroprotection following intracerebral hemorrhage, they are encouraging from the standpoint that stroke patients can be treated immediately without the fear that those suffering intracerebral hemorrhage would be further worsened by the compound.

CONCLUSIONS

The demonstration of neuroprotection using a variety of *in vitro* and *in vivo* models with AR-R 15896AR supports the continuing clinical trials for the compound for use in acute stroke. The unique features of AR-R 15896AR are its favorable pharmacokinetic profile, safety, simple metabolism, single isomeric form, and its efficacy in animal models of stroke, epilepsy and neural injury. The recent attempts to define mechanistically the differences between high-affinity and low-affinity, use-dependent NMDA receptor antagonists include: 1) regional activity at NMDA receptor subtypes in the brain; 2) differential response to limiting excitatory amino acid-triggered $[Ca^{2+}]_{in}$ into the neuron; 3) rapid kinetics of receptor block/especially, receptor unblock; and 4) less membrane trapping of the compound within the channel site between excitatory amino acid pulses.

REFERENCES

1. OLNEY, J.W. 1978. Neurotoxicity of excitatory amino acids. *In* Kainic Acid as a Tool in Neurobiology. E.G. McGeer, J.W. Olney & P.L. McGeer, Eds.: 37–70. Raven Press. New York.
2. BUCHAN, A.M. 1990. Do NMDA antagonists protect against cerebral ischemia: are clinical trials warranted? Cerebrovasc. Brain Metab. Rev. **2:** 1–26.
3. CHAPMAN, A.G., J.H. SWANN *et al.* 1990. Cerebroprotective and anticonvulsant action of competitive and non-competitive NMDA antagonists. *In* Amino Acids: Chemistry, Biology and Medicine. G. Lubec & G.A. Rosenthal, Eds.: 219–232. Escom Publishers. Amsterdam.
4. GEE, K.R. 1994. Therapeutic potential of PCP receptor ligands. Exp. Opin. Invest. Drugs **3:** 1021–1030.
5. COLLINS, R.C., B.H. DOBKIN *et al.* 1989. Selective vulnerability of the brain: new insights into the pathophysiology of stroke. Ann. Int. Med. **110:** 992–1000.

6. ROGAWSKI, M.A. 1993. Therapeutic potential of excitatory amino acid antagonists: channel blockers and 2,3-benzodiazepines. Trends Pharmacol. **14:** 325–331.

7. GRANT, K.A., G. COLOMBO *et al.* 1996. Dizocilpine-like discriminative stimulus effects of low-affinity uncompetitive NMDA antagonists. Neuropharmacology **35:** 1709–1719.

8. PALMER, G.C. & J.B. HUTCHISON. 1997. Preclinical and clinical aspects of remacemide hydrochloride. *In* Excitatory Amino Acids—Clinical Results with Antagonists. P. Herrling, Ed.: 109–120. Academic Press. New York.

9. MUELLER, A.L. 1998. Preclinical neruoprotectant efficacy of NPS 1506, a novel NMDA receptor antagonist. *In* Glutamate Pharmacology Therapeutic Implications. International Business Communications. Southborough, MA.

10. PALMER, G.C., J.A. MILLER *et al.* 1997. Low affinity NMDA receptor antagonists, the neuroprotective potential of ARL 15896AR. Ann. N.Y. Acad. Sci. **825:** 220–231.

11. SHOHAMI, E., R. GALLILY *et al.* 1997. Cytokine production in the brain following closed head injury: Dexanabinol (HU-211), a neuroprotective agent, in normal volunteers. Int. J. Clin. Pharmacol. Ther. **35:** 361–365.

12. PALMER, G.C., R.J. MURRAY *et al.* 1999. [*S*]-AR-R 15896AR, a novel anticonvulsant: acute safety, pharmacokinetic, and pharmacodynamic properties. J. Pharmacol. Exp. Ther. **288:** 121–132.

13. HUDZIK, T.J., L. FREEDMAN *et al.* 1996. Remacemide hydrochloride and ARL 15896AR lack abuse potential: additional differences from other uncompetitive NMDA antagonists. Epilepsia **37:** 544–550.

14. HUDZIK, T.J. & G.C. PALMER. 1995. Effects of anticonvulsants in a novel operant learning paradigm in rats: comparison of remacemide hydrochloride and FPL 15896AR to other anticonvulsant agents. Epilepsy Res. **21:** 183–193.

15. WIDZOWSKI, D., P. BIALOBOK *et al.* 1997. Low affinity non-competitive (LANC) NMDA antagonists do not impair memory and have reduced behavioral performance effects compared to other classes of NMDA antagonists. Soc. Neurosci. **23:** 1758.

16. BLACK, M.A., R. TREMBLAY *et al.* 1995. *N*-Methyl-D-aspartate- or glutamate-mediated toxicity in cultured rat cortical neurons is antagonized by FPL 15896AR. J. Neurochem. **65:** 2170–2177.

17. PORTER, R.H.P. & J.T. GREENAMYRE. 1995. Regional variations in the pharmacology of NMDA receptor channel blockers: implications for therapeutic potential. J. Neurochem. **64:** 614–623.

18. GREENE, J.G., R.H. PORTER *et al.* 1996. ARL-15896, a novel *N*-methyl-D-aspartate receptor ion channel antagonist: neuroprotection against mitochondrial metabolic toxicity and regional pharmacology. Exp. Neurol. **137:** 66–72.

19. MONAGHAN, D.T. & H. LARSEN. 1997. NR1 and NR2 subunit contributions to *N*-methyl-D-aspartate receptor channel blocker pharmacology. J. Pharmacol. Exp. Ther. **280:** 614–620.

20. SMALL, D.L., M.O. POULTER *et al.* 1997. Alteration in NMDA receptor subunit mRNA expression in vulnerable and resistant regions of *in vitro* ischemic rat hippocampal slices. Neurosci. Lett. **232:** 87–90.

21. GILL, R., A. BOURSON *et al.* 1998. Do excitatory amino acid receptors play a role in neuronal degeneration following acute stroke? *In* Glutamate Pharmacology Therapeutic Implications. International Business Communications. Southborough, MA.

22. BLANPIED, T.A., F.A. BOECKMAN *et al.* 1997. Trapping channel block of NMDA-activated responses by amantadine and memantine. J. Neurophysiol. **77:** 309–323.

23. BLACK, M., T. LANTHORN *et al.* 1996. Study of potency, kinetics of block and toxicity of NMDA receptor antagonists using fura-2. Eur. J. Pharmacol. **317:** 377–381.

24. MEALING, G.A.R., T.H. LANTHORN *et al.* 1997. Antagonism of *N*-methyl-D-aspartate-evoked currents in rat cortical cultures by ARL 15896AR. J. Pharmacol. Exp. Ther. **281:** 376–383.

25. MEALING, G.A.R., T.H. LANTHORN *et al.* 1999. Differences in the degree of trapping of low affinity uncompetitive NMDA receptor antagonists with similar kinetics of block. J. Pharmacol. Exp. Ther. **288:** 204–210.

26. SUBRAMANIAN, S., S.D. DONEVAN *et al.* 1996. Block of the *N*-methyl-D-aspartate receptor by remacemide and its des-glycine metabolite. J. Pharmacol. Exp. Ther. **276:** 161–168.

27. JONES, S.M & M.A. ROGAWSKI. 1992. The anticonvulsant (±)-5-aminocarbonyl-10,11-dihydro-5*H*-dibenzo[*a,d*]cyclohepten-5,10-imine (ADCI) selectively blocks NMDA-activated current in cultured rat hippocampal neurones: kinetic analysis and comparison with dizocilpine. Mol. Neuropharmacol. **2:** 303–310.

28. MACDONALD, R.L. 1989. Antiepileptic drug action. Epilepsia **30**(Suppl. 1): S19–S28.

29. HUDZIK, T.J, B.R. DECOSTA *et al.* 1993. Sigma receptor mediated emetic responses in pigeons: agonists, antagonists and modifiers. Eur. J. Pharmacol. **236:** 279–287.

30. BIGOT, D., A. MATUS *et al.* 1991. Reorganization of the cytoskeleton in rat neurons following stimulation with excitatory amino acids *in vitro*. Eur. J. Neurosci. **3:** 551–558.

31. FADDIS, B.T., M.J. HASBANI *et al.* 1997. Calpain activation contributes to dendritic remodeling after brief excitotoxic injury *in vitro*. J. Neurosci. **17:** 951–959.

32. LAFERIERE, N.B., R. TREMBLAY *et al.* 1999. AR-R 15896AR blocks the early NMDA-induced loss of MAP2 in primary cortical cultures. Neurol. Res. **21:** 524–528.

33. GIULIAN, D.L., J. HAVERKAMP *et al.* 1996. Specific domains of beta-amyloid from Alzheimer plaque elicit neuron killing in human microglia. J. Neurosci. **16:** 6021–6037.

34. CROSS, A.J., A.R. GREEN *et al.* 1998. The effect of chlomethiazole (Zendra), dizocilipine, AR-R 15896 and NBQX on hypoxia induced increases of Ca^{2+} entry into rat cerebellar granule cells *in vitro*. Soc. Neurosci. **24:** 979.

35. JOHNS, L., A.J. SINCLAIR *et al.* 1998. The effects of ARL 15896 on *in vitro* hypoxia/hypoglycemia-induced amino acid release from rat cortical slices. Forum Eur. Neurosci. Poster # 33.25.

36. PALMER, G.C., E.F. CREGAN *et al.* 1995. Neuroprotective actions of 2-amino-*N*-(1,2-diphenylethyl)-acetamide hydrochloride (FPL 13950) in animal models of hypoxia and global ischemia. J. Pharmacol. Exp. Ther. **274:** 991–1000.

37. PALMER, G.C., E.F. CREGAN *et al.* 1995. Neuroprotective properties of the uncompetitive NMDA receptor antagonist remacemide hydrochloride. Ann. N.Y. Acad. Sci. **576:** 236–247.

38. CREGAN, E.F., J. PEELING *et al.* 1997. [(*S*)-Alpha-phenyl-2-pyridine-ethanamine dihydrochloride], a low affinity uncompetitive *N*-methyl-D-aspartic acid antagonist, is effective in rodent models of global and focal ischemia. J. Pharmacol. Exp. Ther. **283:** 1412–1424.

39. PRESTON, E., J. WEBSTER *et al.* 1998. Lack of evidence for direct involvement of NMDA receptors or polyamines in blood-brain barrier injury after cerebral ischemia in rats. Brain Res. **813:** 191–194.

40. BUCHAN, A.M., D. XUE *et al.* 1992. A new model of temporary focal neocortical ischemia in the rat. Stroke **23:** 273–279.

41. CORBETT, D. & S. NURSE. 1998. The problem of assessing effective neuroprotection in experimental cerebral ischemia. Prog. Neurobiol. **54:** 531–548.

42. SUTHERLAND, G.R., J.T. PERRON *et al.* AR-R 15896AR reduces cerebral infarct volume following focal ischemia in cat. J. Stroke Cerebrovasc. Dis. In press.

Intracellular Survival Pathways against Glutamate Receptor Agonist Excitotoxicity in Cultured Neurons

Intracellular Calcium Responses[a]

ANN M. MARINI,[b,c,e] YUJI UEDA,[d] AND CARL H. JUNE[d]

[b]*Department of Neurology, Uniformed Services University of the Health Sciences, Bethesda, Maryland, USA*

[c]*Department of Neurology, Walter Reed Army Medical Center, Washington, DC, USA*

[d]*Immune Cell Biology Program, Naval Medical Research Institute, Bethesda, Maryland, USA*

ABSTRACT: Cultured rat cerebellar granule cells are resistant to the excitotoxic effects of *N*-methyl-D-aspartate (NMDA) and non-NMDA receptor agonists under three conditions: 1) prior to day seven *in vitro* when cultured in depolarizing concentrations of potassium [25 mM]; 2) at any time *in vitro* when cultured in non-depolarizing concentrations of potassium [5 mM]; and 3) when neurons, cultured in depolarizing concentrations of potassium [25 mM] for eight days *in vitro*, are pretreated with a subtoxic concentration of NMDA. The focus of this paper is to determine: a) whether the resistance to excitotoxicity by NMDA and non-NMDA receptor agonists is due to a decreased intracellular calcium $[Ca^{++}]_i$ response to glutamate receptor agonists in cultured rat cerebellar granule cells; or b) whether $[Ca^{++}]_i$ levels induced by the agonists are similar to those observed under excitotoxic conditions.

Granule cells, matured in non-depolarizing growth medium, treated with glutamate resulted in an increase in $[Ca^{++}]_i$ followed by a plateau that remained above baseline in virtually all neurons that responded to glutamate. The response was rapid in onset (<10 sec) and the pattern of response heterogeneous in that cells responsive to glutamate increased their $[Ca^{++}]_i$ to different extents; some cells did not respond to glutamate. Kainate also produced significant elevations in $[Ca^{++}]_i$.

The $[Ca^{++}]_i$ response to glutamate in neurons matured in depolarizing (25 mM K^+) growth medium for three days was rapid, transient and heterogeneous, which reached a plateau that was elevated above baseline levels; removing the glutamate markedly reduced the $[Ca^{++}]_i$ concentration. Activation of the α-amino-3-hydroxy-5-methyl-4-isoxazolepropionic acid (AMPA)/kainate receptors by kainic acid produced similar changes in $[Ca^{++}]_i$ responses. At a time when cultured cerebellar granule cells become susceptible to the excitotoxic effects of glutamate acting at NMDA receptors (day *in vitro* (DIV) 8) in

[a]The opinions or assertions contained herein are the private views of the authors and are not to be construed as official or as reflecting the views of the Department of the Army or the Department of Defense.

[e]Corresponding author: Ann M. Marini, M.D., Ph.D., Department of Neurology, Uniformed Services University of the Health Sciences, 4301 Jones Bridge Road, Bethesda, Maryland 20814. Phone, 202/782-8651; fax, 202/782-2295.

e-mail, Ann.Marini@NA.AMEDD.Army.Mil

depolarizing growth medium, glutamate elicited $[Ca^{++}]_i$ responses similar to those observed at a culture time when the neurons are not susceptible to the excitotoxic effects of glutamate (DIV 3). Pretreatment of the cultured neurons with a subtoxic concentration of NMDA, which protects all neurons against the excitotoxic effects of glutamate, did not alter the maximal $[Ca^{++}]_i$ elicited by an excitotoxic concentration of glutamate.

INTRODUCTION

Developing neurons that express glutamate receptors including N-methyl-D-aspartate (NMDA) receptors need to respond to excitatory amino acids for activity-dependent processes from the extracellular environment and must not die from glutamate-mediated excitotoxicity. Thus, neurons may have intrinsic survival pathways that are designed to prevent glutamate-mediated excitotoxicity. These inherent survival mechanisms would be critical to neurons that express excitatory amino acid receptors. We have hypothesized that such survival pathways exist in cultured cerebellar granule cells, which express all the excitatory amino acid receptors and which respond physiologically to glutamate.

Granule cell neurons are resistant to the excitotoxic effects of glutamate receptor agonists under three conditions: 1) neurons cultured in depolarizing growth medium (potassium concentration 25 mM) are resistant to the excitotoxic effects of NMDA and non-NMDA receptor agonists prior to day seven *in vitro* (DIV 7); 2) when neurons are susceptible to the excitotoxic effects of glutamate, NMDA receptor-mediated excitotoxicity (DIV 8) can be completely blocked by pretreating the neurons with a subtoxic concentration of NMDA; and 3) neurons cultured in nondepolarizing growth medium (potassium concentration 5 mM) undergo significant cell death by DIV 7 but are resistant to the excitotoxic effects of NMDA and non-NMDA agonists at any time *in vitro*.

Excitotoxicity is thought to involve the release of massive amounts of excitatory amino acids resulting in excessive stimulation of glutamate receptors of postsynaptic neurons leading to neuronal death.[45] Increases in intracellular calcium ($[Ca^{++}]_i$) may play an important role in excitotoxic cell death.[48] *In vitro* neuronal model systems have shown that calcium influx mediated by NMDA receptors seem to be involved in delayed neuronal death.[49,8] Alternatively, release of calcium from intracellular stores has also been shown to be involved in excitotoxicity in cultured cortical neurons.[21]

One well characterized cell culture model for studying the role of calcium in neuronal function makes use of enriched cerebellar granule cells from postnatal rats. Cultures of rat cerebellar granule cells are largely composed of glutamatergic neurons (~95%) and express NMDA as well as non-NMDA receptors.[22,42] All glutamate-activated channels, including NMDA receptors, are permeable to sodium and potassium ions.[32] In addition, NMDA receptors have an associated channel that upon activation, evokes an influx of calcium;[40,15] the NMDA-associated channel has a calcium ionic conductance that is 10.6 times greater than the kainate receptor is for sodium ions.[26] The NMDA receptor ion channel is physiologically blocked by magnesium ions and is voltage-dependent, i.e., the more depolarized the cell membrane the more easily the NMDA receptor ion-channel is activated by an appropriate stimulus.[34] The role of NMDA receptors in mediating calcium influx following receptor stimulation is controversial. Several studies have shown that activation of NMDA receptors results in an influx of calcium as measured by fura-2 calcium imaging.[13,6,5a] However, other studies failed to find an association between activation of NMDA receptors and increased levels of $[Ca^{++}]_i$.[12]

Kainic acid, a non-NMDA receptor agonist, also kills cultured rat cerebellar granule cells via an excitotoxic mechanism.[20] However, the route of calcium entry upon activation of kainate receptors is also controversial. Electrophysiologic studies failed to detect calcium currents when kainate receptors were activated.[2] In contrast, kainate receptor activation in cultured cerebellar granule cells resulted in calcium influx as measured by radioactive calcium and cyclic guanosine monophosphate (cGMP) formation.[57,58,41] Using 1-[2-(5-carboxyoxazol-2-yl)-6-aminobenzofuran-5-oxyl-2-(2′-amino-5′-methylphenoxy)-ethane-*N,N,N,N*-tetraacetic acid pentaacetoxymethyl ester (fura-2 AM) measurements, kainate receptor activation resulted in calcium entry in cultured cerebellar granule cells through activation of NMDA receptors and a nifedipine-sensitive calcium channel.[13] Other studies showed that kainate-mediated calcium influx was not blocked by NMDA receptor antagonists.[58] In Bergmann glial cells, calcium enters the cells through the kainate receptor directly.[38]

During *in vitro* development of cerebellar granule cells, NMDA receptor-mediated calcium influx has been shown to promote neurite outgrowth[6] and the expression of glutamate receptors,[54] whereas in mature neurons, NMDA receptor activation mediates excitotoxic cell death.[42,29] In contrast, low extracellular concentrations of calcium induce the release of glutamate, which then binds to NMDA receptors to produce an autotoxicity.[35] Surprisingly, pretreatment of mature cultured cerebellar granule cells (DIV 8) with subtoxic concentrations of NMDA blocked NMDA receptor-mediated excitotoxicity and protected all of the vulnerable neurons that would otherwise die.[28–30]

We postulated that intrinsic survival pathways exist in developing neurons to allow them to respond to excitatory amino acids as well as protect them against the excitotoxic effects of glutamate. For example, pretreatment of mature granule cells with a subtoxic concentration of NMDA protects all the vulnerable neurons that would otherwise die from an excitotoxic concentration of glutamate acting on NMDA receptors. Understanding these survival pathways should lead to the development of strategies to protect these neurons against ischemic neuronal damage *in vivo*; numerous studies have suggested that glutamate plays an important role in the pathophysiology of this type of damage. One possible survival mechanism is through $[Ca^{++}]_i$, which is thought to play an important role in delayed excitotoxicity. If increases in $[Ca^{++}]_i$ mediate delayed neuronal cell death and activation of glutamate receptors in developing neurons result in $[Ca^{++}]_i$ levels comparable to those observed under excitotoxic conditions, then developing neurons must have intrinsic survival mechanisms to protect them against elevated local concentrations of glutamate but still allowing them to respond to the excitatory amino acid. Therefore, we investigated the pattern of developmental $[Ca^{++}]_i$ responses using fura-2 AM resulting from activation of NMDA and non-NMDA receptors in cultured rat cerebellar granule cells under excitotoxic resistant conditions.

METHODS

Neuronal Cell Cultures

Cerebellar granule cell cultures were prepared from postnatal 8-day-old rat pups as described previously.[31] The cells were plated at 4×10^6 cells on glass coverslips coated with poly-L-lysine (5.0 µg/ml) (Sigma Chemical Co., mw >100,000). The cells were allowed to mature in medium containing 25 mM KCl, a concentration which promotes the survival of the neurons[22] (henceforth called depolarizing growth medium); the medium was not changed throughout the maturation period. For some experiments, cerebellar granule cells were allowed to mature under indentical conditions as indicated above, except that the KCl concentration in the medium was 5 mM (henceforth called nondepolarizing growth medium). Granule cells cultured in nondepolarizing growth incubated for extended periods contained two-thirds fewer viable neurons than those maintained in depolarizing growth medium as shown previously.[22] On DIV 7 and every third day thereafter, D-glucose (100 µl of 100-mM solution) and sterile water (100 µl) were added to the culture medium for neurons matured in depolarizing growth medium as described previously.[31] We observed that neurons remained viable for 40 days when they were maintained in depolarizing growth medium *in vitro*.

Measurement of $[Ca^{++}]_i$ Concentration

Fura-2 AM was added to the growth medium at 37°C in a humidifed incubator containing 5% CO_2. Culture dishes (35 mm) containing glass coverslips with attached cells were loaded with the Ca^{2+}-sensitive dye fura-2 AM (4 mg/ml; 45 min) containing probenacid (2 mM). The coverslip was removed and placed in a chamber maintained at $37 \pm 1.5°C$. Experiments were performed in Locke's solution (experimental low K^+ buffer) containing in mM: NaCl, 154; D-glucose, 5.6; HEPES, 8.6; KCl, 5.6; $CaCl_2$, 2.3; $MgCl_2$, 1.0; 0.1% dialyzed fetal calf serum. Some experiments were performed in Locke's solution as indicated above, except that the KCl concentration was 25 mM (experimental high K^+ buffer). To determine $[Ca^{++}]_i$ levels fluorescence digital image processing system used is similar to that described previously.[52] Hardware consists of an FD5000 image processor (Gould), a Zeiss Axiovert microscope with a 1.3 numerical aperture 40× objective, and a filter changer (Ludl Electronic Products) with excitation filters centered at 350 ± 10 nm and 380 ± 10 nm. The image processor and filter changer were interfaced to a Microvax host computer (Digital Equipment Corporation). Sixteen images were acquired at each wavelength at 30/sec through a charge-coupled device (CCD) camera (Cohu) and image intensifier (Videoscope). The images were averaged, background was subtracted, and a shading correction was applied. The ratio of fluoresence emission (500 nm) of the 350- and 380-nm images is displayed according to the code kindly provided by R.Y. Tsien (San Diego, California). Images were acquired and stored digitally at 15-sec intervals. The fura-2 ratio is converted to $[Ca^{2+}]$ as described previously.[52] Each experiment was performed at least twice using two different batches of neuronal cell cultures. Neurons matured in depolarizing growth medium were assayed on DIV 3 and DIV 8, whereas neurons matured in nondepolarizing growth medium were assayed on DIV 3; significant cell death occurs by DIV 8, which precluded calcium imaging. All drugs were dissolved in sterile water except for 6-cyano-7-nitroquinoxaline-2,3-dione (CNQX), which was dissolved in dimethylsulfoxide. All drugs were obtained from commercial sources.

Excitotoxicity Studies

For the excitotoxicity experiments, neuronal cultures (35-mm dishes), matured in depolarizing (25 mM K^+) growth medium, were exposed to either glutamate, kainic acid, α-amino-3-hydroxy-5-methyl-4-isoxazolepropionic acid (AMPA) or NMDA for 24 hours in culture medium on either DIV 3 or DIV 8 as described previously.[29] After 24 hours, viable neurons (phase bright and refractile) were counted from three representative high-power fields in treated and untreated dishes. Each experiment was performed in triplicate and using two different batches of neuronal cultures. Antagonists (MK-801 [1 μM] or CNQX [50 μM]) were added 30 min prior to addition of the glutamate receptor agonist. We have shown previously that viable neurons (phase bright and refractile neurons) correlate exactly with viable neurons stained with fluorescein.[17] Results are expressed as the mean ± SD where indicated.

Statistical analyses were performed using the Student *t* test and analysis of variance (ANOVA) where applicable.

Neuroprotective Study for the Determination of $[Ca^{++}]_i$ Responses

Neurons matured in depolarizing concentrations of potassium (25 mM, DIV 8) were treated with NMDA (100 μM) in growth medium for three hours followed by loading with fura-2 AM. The medium was then removed, and the cells were washed with low K^+ experimental buffer and placed in the chamber. When the buffer was equilibrated to 37°C, an excitotoxic concentration of glutamate (100 μM) was added to the buffer, and images were captured by the imaging system. Untreated neurons were treated only with glutamate (100 μM).

NMDA and non-NMDA Receptor Antagonists to Block $[Ca^{++}]_i$ Responses

For the MK-801 experiments, neurons (DIV 8) were pretreated with the NMDA receptor antagonist MK-801 (1 μM) for 5 min in growth medium followed by loading with fura-2 AM. The medium was removed and replaced with low K^+ experimental media followed by the addition of glutamate (100 μM). For the CNQX experiment, the neurons were pretreated with CNQX (50 μM) for 30 min in growth medium followed by loading with fura-2 AM. The medium was removed and replaced with low K^+ experimental buffer containing the identical concentration of CNQX and kainic acid (100 μM) and placed on the microscope stage where $[Ca^{++}]_i$ measurements were obtained for up to 700 sec.

RESULTS

The Differential Effect of Glutamate Receptor Agonists in Immature and Mature Neurons

Exposure of cultured rat cerebellar granule cells to either NMDA or non-NMDA receptor agonists on DIV 3 were not susceptible to the excitotoxic effects of

TABLE 1. Differential sensitivity of cerebellar granule cells to glutamate receptor agonists

Drug Added (μM)	Day *in Vitro* Drug Added	Day *in Vitro* Cells Examined	Potassium (mM)	% Cell Death ± SD
Kainate (500)	3	4	5	2.0 ± 0.97
Kainate (500)	3	4	25	1.0 ± 0.78
Kainate (500)	8[b]	9	25	77 ± 3.05[c]
NMDA (500)	3	4	5	1.6 ± 0.32
NMDA (500)	3	4	25	2.3 ± 1.1
NMDA (500)	8[a]	9	25	92 ± 3.4[c]
Glutamate (1000)	3	4	5	0.82 ± 0.43
Glutamate (1000)	3	4	25	2.1 ± 0.94
Glutamate (1000)	8[a]	9	25	89.4 ± 2.6[c]
Glutamate (10)	21[a]	22	25	94.4 ± 3.7[c]
AMPA (1000)	3	4	5	0.79 ± 0.22
AMPA (1000)	3	4	25	2.4 ± 0.5
AMPA (1000)	8	9	25	1.7 ± 0.8

NOTE: Enriched cerebellar granule cell cultures were prepared and maintained as outlined in Material and Methods. Various glutamate agonists (500–1000 μM) were added on day *in vitro* 3 (DIV 3) or DIV 8, and the cells were examined for excitotoxic effects on DIV 4 or DIV 9. Percent excitotoxic cell death is defined according to the following formula:

$$\% \text{ cell death} = 1 - \frac{\text{surviving cells (drug–treated)}}{\text{surviving cells (untreated)}} \times 100$$

[a]Excitotoxicity of NMDA or glutamate at concentrations of 10, 500 and 1000 μM, respectively, is completely blocked by the NMDA receptor antagonist MK-801 (1 μM).

[b]Excitotoxic response of kainic acid is completely blocked by the non-NMDA receptor antagonist CNQX (50 μM).

[c]p <0.001 using the Student t test.

glutamate, NMDA or kainate acting through NMDA or non-NMDA receptors, respectively, in either depolarizing or nondepolarizing concentrations of K^+ (TABLE 1). However, addition of the identical concentration of either NMDA, glutamate or kainate produced striking neurotoxicity when added on DIV 8. Interestingly, the cultured neurons become more susceptible to the excitotoxic effects of glutamate, because a much lower concentration (10 μM) exerts a similar excitotoxicity response in neurons cultured for 21 days versus 8 days. AMPA was not excitotoxic either on DIV 3 or DIV 8 cultured in depolarizing growth medium (TABLE 1).

Baseline and Pattern of $[Ca^{++}]_i$ Responses of Cerebellar Granule Cells Matured in Nondepolarizing and Depolarizing Growth Medium

For comparison to NMDA-treated and other conditions, a baseline $[Ca^{++}]_i$ concentration in cerebellar granule cells matured in either nondepolarizing (5 mM K^+) or depolarizing (25 mM K^+) growth medium for three days was determined. Using the fura-2 assay, we determined that the baseline $[Ca^{++}]_i$ levels exhibited a heterogeneous pattern and an intracellular concentration range that did not differ significantly from each other (FIG. 1). Replacing the appropriate experimental buffer at the indicated arrow did not alter the baseline level (FIG. 1). This heterogeneous pattern was a constant observation in all experiments that was independent of growth con-

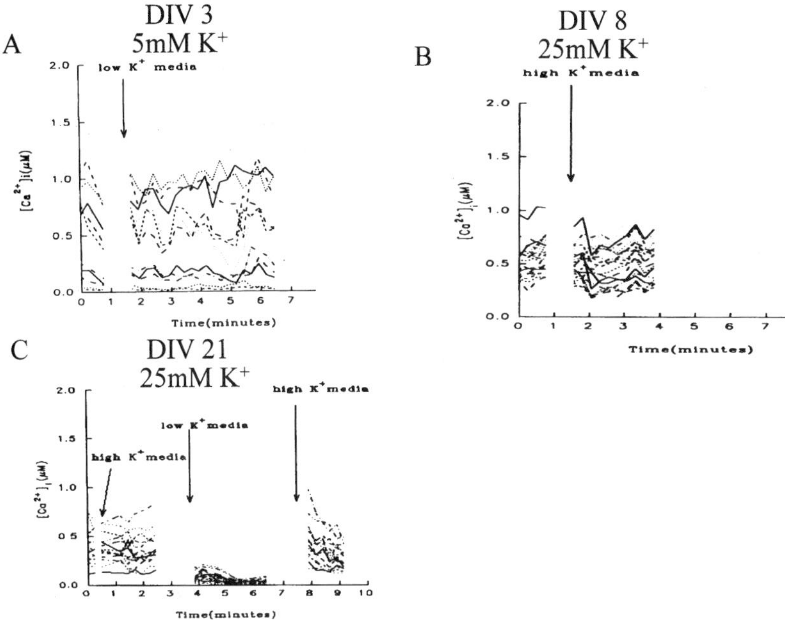

FIGURE 1. The effect of K$^+$ on baseline [Ca^{++}]$_i$ concentrations as a function of DIV. Cerebellar granule cells were matured in nondepolarizing (5 mM K$^+$) growth medium for three days on glass cover slips (**A**) or depolarizing (25 mM K$^+$) growth medium for eight days (**B**) or 21 days (**C**). The neurons were loaded with fura-2 as described in Materials and Methods. The cover slip was placed in a frame, and experimental low K$^+$ (5 mM) media containing MgCl$_2$ (1 mM) was added followed by equilibration to 37°C. Replacement with experimental low K$^+$ buffer was made as indicated. Granule cells matured in depolarizing (25 mM K$^+$) growth medium were treated identically as indicated above except that experimental high K$^+$ (25 mM) buffer containing MgCl$_2$ (1 mM) was added to the dish. Replacing the experimental high K$^+$ buffer with the same (**B,C**) or removal of the experimental high K$^+$ buffer and replacing it with experimental low K$^+$ buffer followed by high K$^+$ experimental buffer (**C**) serially was done as indicated. All experiments are representative of the heterogeneous pattern seen in three or more trials using at least two batches of granule cell preparations. Additions were made as indicated by the *arrow*.

ditions and drug addition. Cerebellar granule cells matured in depolarizing (25 mM K$^+$) growth medium for 21 days did not exhibit [Ca^{++}]$_i$ concentrations above those determined for neuronal cells matured in culture for fewer days (FIG. 1), even though they are more sensitive to the excitotoxic effects of glutamate acting at NMDA receptors (TABLE 1). However, the baseline [Ca^{++}]$_i$ concentration decreased markedly and was instantaneous in the cultured neurons when the K$^+$ concentration in the experimental buffer was changed to 5 mM and then returned to its original higher level when the K$^+$ concentration in the experimental buffer was increased to 25 mM (FIG. 1C). The [Ca^{++}]$_i$ concentration of individual cells matured between DIV 3–21 in depolarizing (25 mM K$^+$) growth medium ranged from near zero to about 2.5 μM.

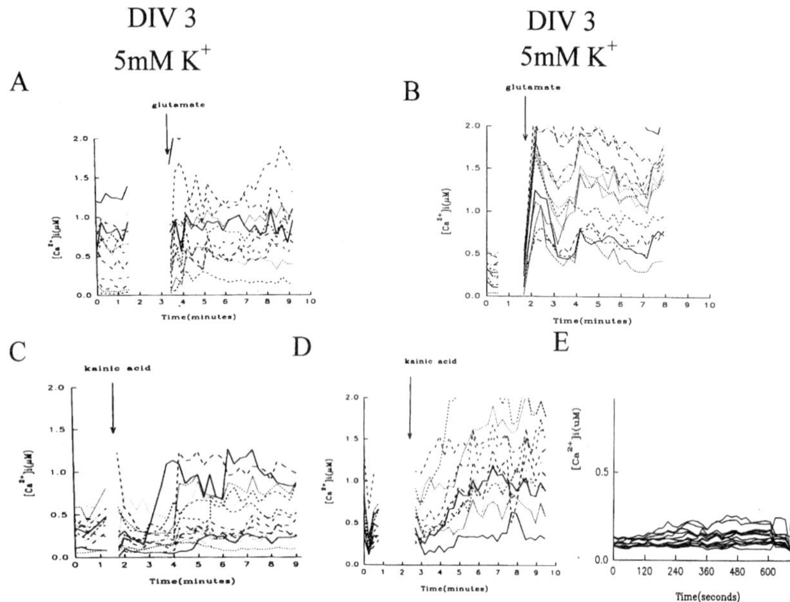

FIGURE 2. The effect of glutamate on $[Ca^{++}]_i$ responses in granule cells matured in nondepolarizing (5 mM K^+) growth media. Granule cells were matured in nondepolarizing (5 mM K^+) growth media for three days followed by loading with fura-2 as described in Materials and Methods. After the cells equilibrated in experimental low K^+ media at 37°C (2 min), additions were made as indicated by the *arrows*. Additions are: 100 μM glutamate (**A**); 500 μM glutamate (**B**); 100 μM kainic acid (**C**) and 500 μM kainic acid (**D**). Pretreatment with the non-NMDA receptor antagonist CNQX completely blocked the observed increases in $[Ca^{++}]_i$, suggesting that non-NMDA receptor activation was responsible for the increases in $[Ca^{++}]_i$ (**E**).

Effect of Nondepolarizing (5 mM K⁺) Growth Medium on Glutamate Receptor Agonist-Induced [Ca⁺⁺]ᵢ Levels in Neurons Cultured for Three Days

To determine the effect of glutamate receptor agonists on $[Ca^{++}]_i$ cerebellar granule cells, neurons were matured in nondepolarizing (5 mM K^+) growth medium for three days *in vitro*. Neurons exposed to a glutamate concentration of 100 μM or 500 μM demonstrated transient increases in $[Ca^{++}]_i$ (FIG. 2A). $[Ca^{++}]_i$ responses were more striking when the neurons were exposed to a glutamate concentration of 500 μM (FIG. 2B). $[Ca^{++}]_i$ levels did not return to baseline over the experimental time period. The response was rapid in onset (<10 sec) and the response heterogeneous; most cells responded to glutamate (FIG. 2A and B). The NMDA receptor antagonist MK-801 blocked glutamate-induced increases in $[Ca^{++}]_i$ (FIG. 3C), indicating that the observed increase in $[Ca^{++}]_i$ was mediated by NMDA receptors. Neurons matured in nondepolarizing (5 mM K^+) growth medium for 3 days *in vitro* followed by exposure to the non-NMDA receptor agonist kainate (100 μM or 500 μM) showed similar $[Ca^{++}]_i$ responses (FIG. 2C and D). The non-NMDA receptor antagonist CNQX (50 µM) blocked kainate-induced [Ca^{++}]$_i$ responses (FIG. 2E). In all cases, those neurons that responded to glutamate and kainate maintained their elevated [Ca^{++}]$_i$ throughout the experimental time period. [Ca^{++}]$_i$ responses were not performed on DIV 8 in neurons cultured in nondepolarizing growth medium because of spontaneous cell death (~80%; see Ref. 22).

Effect of Glutamate Receptor Agonists on [Ca^{++}]$_i$ Responses in Neurons Matured in Depolarizing (25 mM K$^+$) Growth Medium

To determine the effect of glutamate receptor agonists on [Ca^{++}]$_i$, cerebellar granule cells were matured in depolarizing growth medium (25 mM K$^+$) for either 3 or 8 days, and the effect of glutamate or kainate [Ca^{++}]$_i$ was determined in high K$^+$ (25 mM) experimental buffer. The concentration, 100 µM, was selected because neurons matured in depolarizing growth medium for eight days are susceptible to the excitotoxic effects of glutamate at this concentration acting on NMDA receptors[29] (TABLE 1). The addition of glutamate (100 µM) (FIG. 3A) or kainate (500 µM) at

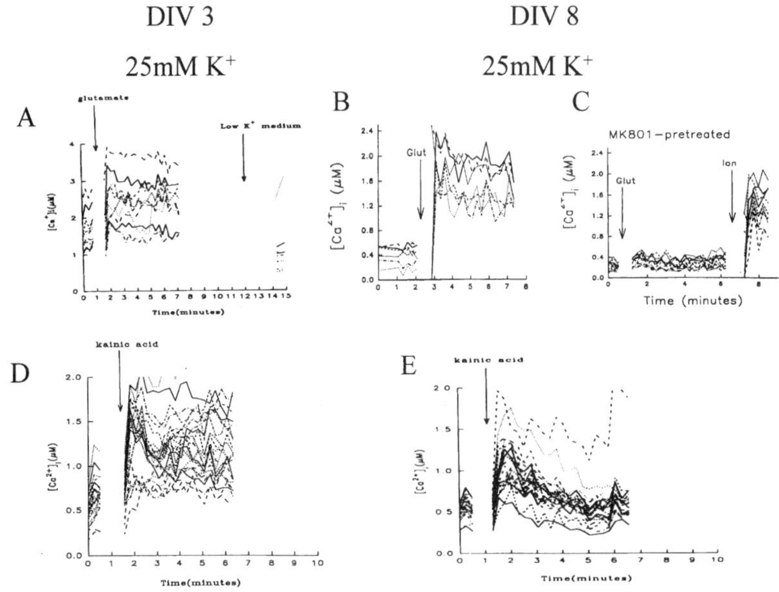

FIGURE 3. [Ca^{++}]$_i$ responses to glutamate and kainate in neurons matured in depolarizing (25 mM K$^+$) growth media for either three or eight days *in vitro*. Neurons were matured in depolarizing (25 mM K$^+$) culture media for three days (**A,D**) or eight days (**B,C,E**) followed by determination of [Ca^{++}]$_i$ responses in high experimental (25 mM K$^+$) buffer: 100 µM glutamate (A); 100 µM glutamate (DIV 8) (B); MK-801 + glutamate (100 µM) (C); 500 µM kainic acid (D) and 500 µM kainic acid (DIV 8) (E). The high K$^+$ experimental buffer was changed to low experimental (5 mM K$^+$) buffer (A) in order to show that the responses were mediated by added receptor agonist and influx of *extracellular* calcium. Note that even though the cultured neurons are not susceptible to the excitotoxic effects of glutamate or kainate acting on NMDA or non-NMDA receptors, respectively, matured in depolarizing growth medium, the [Ca^{++}]$_i$ responses to glutamate are essentially identical to those found in neurons that are susceptible to the excitotoxic effects of glutamate (DIV 8).

DIV 3 (FIG. 3D) resulted in transient heterogeneous increases in $[Ca^{++}]_i$ followed by a decline and then a plateau over the time course of the experiment (7 min); all neurons responded to glutamate. Peak $[Ca^{++}]_i$ concentrations in individual neurons reached between 3–4 µM. Removal of the glutamate-containing experimental buffer and reducing the K^+ in the buffer to 5 mM resulted in a marked reduction in the $[Ca^{++}]_i$ levels (FIG. 3A). An excitotoxic concentration of glutamate (100 µM) in neurons cultured for eight days *in vitro* elicited a rapid, heterogeneous and sustained rise in $[Ca^{++}]_i$ achieving levels of >2 µM, which was completely blocked by the NMDA receptor antagonist MK-801 (FIG. 3B and C). The addition of ionomycin (35 µM) was used to show that the neurons did not respond to glutamate because of the MK-801 pretreatment and not because of a lack of fura-2 loading or some other problem with detection. The neuron $[Ca^{++}]_i$ responses to added kainate (500 µM) were similar to that seen with glutamate; however, $[Ca^{++}]_i$ levels of most cells were not sustained as with glutamate, and the $[Ca^{++}]_i$ level returned to baseline within 2.5 min (FIG. 3E).

The Effect of a Subtoxic Concentration of NMDA Pretreatment on Glutamate-Induced $[Ca^{++}]_i$ in Neurons Matured for Eight Days in Depolarizing (25 mM K^+) Growth Medium

We have shown previously that the glutamate uptake blocker DL-threo-3-hydroxyaspartic acid reduces glutamate-induced cGMP levels.[28] We assumed that by increasing the medium levels of glutamate induced by the glutamate uptake blocker NMDA receptors would be activated more frequently and would become desensitized. Accordingly, pretreatment with a subtoxic concentration of NMDA markedly reduced (~80% within 3 hr) the excitotoxic neuronal cell death of glutamate acting on NMDA receptors in cultured rat cerebellar granule cells.[29] Taken together, these results suggested that NMDA was reducing excitotoxicity by NMDA receptor desensitization. We expected that pretreatment with NMDA for 3 hr followed by an excitotoxic concentration of glutamate would reduce the $[Ca^{++}]_i$ response compared to control neurons. Unexpectedly, we did not find a reduction in $[Ca^{++}]_i$ levels. The effect of an excitotoxic concentration of glutamate (100 µM) on $[Ca^{++}]_i$ was determined on untreated neurons and neurons pretreated with a subtoxic concentration of NMDA (100 µM) for 3.0 hr. Briefly, the neurons were pretreated with NMDA for 3 hr followed by removal of the culture medium, and replacing it with experimental buffer containing the glutamate is shown in FIGURE 4. Surprisingly, the peak $[Ca^{++}]_i$ levels achieved within 60 sec after the addition of glutamate in untreated neurons and neurons pretreated with NMDA were nearly identical. No significant difference in the peak $[Ca^{++}]_i$ level was seen between untreated neurons and neurons pretreated with 100 µM NMDA.

DISCUSSION

Surprisingly, detailed examination of the susceptibility of granule cell neurons to NMDA and non-NMDA receptors shows differential sensitivity. Neurons cultured in depolarizing concentrations of K^+ are insensitive to the excitotoxic effects of glutamate and kainate during early culture times, but even after they become suscep-

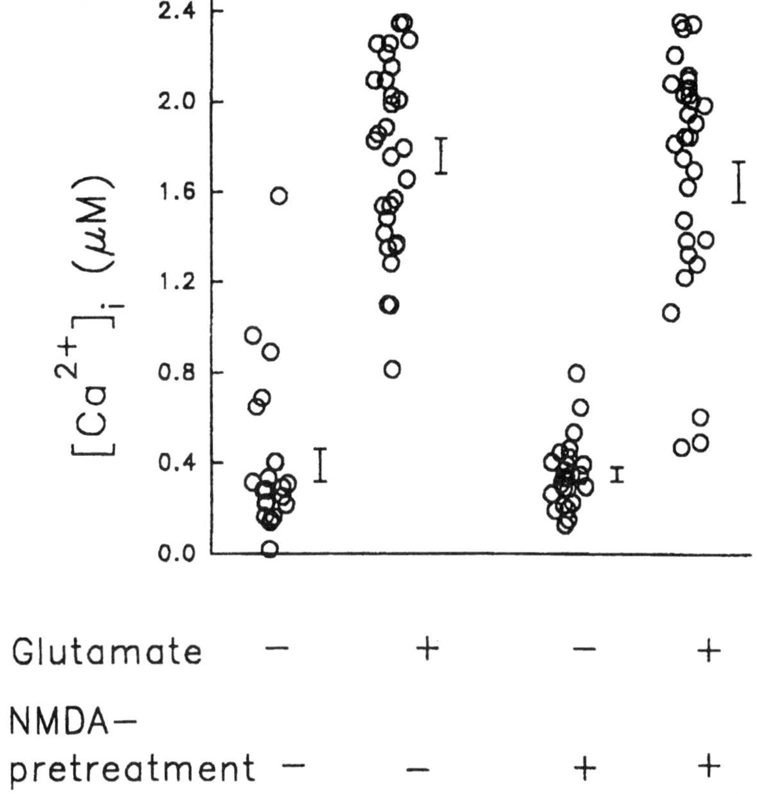

FIGURE 4. Glutamate-induced calcium responses in untreated neurons and in neurons pretreated with a subtoxic concentration of NMDA. Granule cell neurons were matured for eight days in depolarizing (25 mM K$^+$) growth media. One set of culture dishes containing neurons on glass cover slips were exposed to NMDA (100 μM) for 3.0 hr. The cells were rinsed with high K$^+$ (25 mM) growth medium followed by loading with fura-2. Control neurons received the identical volume of sterile water (10 μl) and then were treated identically to the neurons pretreated with NMDA. The neurons were loaded with fura-2 and placed in a chamber containing high (25 mM K$^+$) experimental buffer. An excitotoxic concentration of glutamate (100 μM) was added to control neurons and to neurons pretreated with NMDA. [Ca^{++}]$_i$ responses were determined as outlined in Materials and Methods. Baseline and peak [Ca^{++}]$_i$ of each neuron that was captured by the imaging system from three separate experiments in control and pretreated neurons are illustrated in the figure. There is no significant difference in baseline or peak [Ca^{++}]$_i$ levels in control or neurons pretreated with NMDA ($p = 0.3$). *Bars* represent the average ± SD. Statistical analysis was performed using ANOVA.

tible to the excitotoxic effects of glutamate, pretreatment with a subtoxic concentration of NMDA blocks excitotoxic neuronal cell death. Moreover, neurons cultured in nondepolarizing K$^+$ concentrations are insensitive to the excitotoxic effects of glutamate receptor agonists during early culture times (TABLE 1). Thus, these are three conditions whereby cultured neurons are resistant to the excitotoxic effects of glutamate receptor agonists.

Neuronal damage produced by stroke, trauma, prolonged seizures or hypoglycemia is thought to be due at least in part to excessive stimulation of NMDA receptors by glutamate.[9,45] Sustained intracellular increases in calcium are thought to play a dominant role in delayed NMDA receptor-mediated neuronal death *in vivo* and *in vitro*.[5,8,27,44,35] In other studies using cerebellar granule cells, the role of calcium influx evoked by NMDA receptor activation was determined in reduced or magnesium-free conditions.[27,46] Oxidative stress resulting in the formation of superoxide, hydroxide radical and hydrogen peroxide has also been suggested to be induced by glutamate excitotoxicity and increased $[Ca^{++}]_i$.[30] Because brain ischemia, particularly in the penumbra, more likely reflects an environment where neurons are depolarized and magnesium concentrations may be closer to physiological magnesium concentrations, we sought to determine $[Ca^{++}]_i$ in neurons susceptible to excitotoxic damage that more closely resembles this milieu.

This report describes for the first time that cultured cerebellar granule cells that are resistant to the excitotoxic effects of NMDA and non-NMDA receptor agonists evoke a heterogeneous pattern of $[Ca^{++}]_i$ responses in experimental buffer containing magnesium. The reasons for the heterogeneous response is unclear, but it is possibly related to the intrinsic properties of glutamate receptor subtypes: 1) it has been shown that activation of glutamate receptor subtypes results in the release of neuroactive amino acids and efflux of these amino acids may modulate $[Ca^{++}]_i$ responses by glutamate;[47] 2) specific electrophysiological properties of glutamate receptor subtypes, such as desensitization of NMDA receptors may play a role in this effect;[10] 3) subunit expression, assembly and function of glutamate receptors may be different in individual neurons, which may be partially determined by alternative splicing;[51] 4) activation of cationic channels permeable to sodium and potassium by glutamate may be differentially expressed in individual neurons;[33,43] 5) glutamate receptor subtypes may not exist in those cells that do not respond to glutamate or glutamate receptor-preferring agonists; 6) modulatory site regulators may play a role in the heterogeneous $[Ca^{++}]_i$ response patterns; oxygen free radical regulation of NMDA receptor function has been described previously;[1] and 7) subsets of granule cell neurons may have different cytosolic calcium buffering capacities.[11] Any one or combination of these reported findings may be responsible for the heterogeneous pattern of $[Ca^{++}]_i$ responses observed in cultured cerebellar granule cells. Alternatively, the heterogeneous pattern may be due to differences in the uptake of the dye and/or metabolic differences of individual neuons.

Granule cell neurons matured for three days in nondepolarizing (5 mM) growth medium increased their $[Ca^{++}]_i$ in response to glutamate and kainate. The kinetics of $[Ca^{++}]_i$ responses to the addition of kainate differed from glutamate-evoked responses; the increment in $[Ca^{++}]_i$ occurred more slowly (FIG. 2B). Because the rate of rise in $[Ca^{++}]_i$ was faster in the presence of glutamate, these results support the hypothesis that glutamate activates NMDA receptors rather than AMPA/kainate receptors. Also, this interpretation is consistent with results which showed that preincubation with the NMDA receptor inhibitor MK-801 completely blocked glutamate-induced $[Ca^{++}]_i$ increases in the cultured neurons (FIG. 3C). These results also suggest that glutamate receptors are expressed and active on granule cell neurons matured in nondepolarizing (5 mM K^+) medium and support other studies which have shown that subunit composition of NMDA receptors in cultured cerebellar granule cells grown in 5 mM K^+ is similar to those grown in 25 mM K^+.[53] In addition, the expression of glutamate receptor subtypes and functional calcium responses to glutamate receptor agonists in neurons grown in 5 mM K^+ also support previous findings showing that NMDA has a neurotrophic effect on granule cells cultured in growth medium containing relatively low K^+ concentrations.[3,4] Whether cells grown in growth medium containing 5 mM K^+ elicit NMDA/glycine-evoked currents is controversial.[54,23] Our results suggest that NMDA and non-NMDA receptor agonists evoke $[Ca^{++}]_i$ responses in neurons grown under low K^+ conditions and support previous findings.[23] Despite the observation that neurons cultured in 5 mM K^+ are not susceptible to the excitotoxic effects of glutamate, the $[Ca^{++}]_i$ responses occur within the same range as those observed in neurons that are susceptible to the excitotoxic effects of glutamate acting at NMDA or non-NMDA receptors (TABLE 1 and FIG. 3).

Although the baseline $[Ca^{++}]_i$ levels of the neurons matured in nondepolarizing (5 mM K^+) or depolarizing (25 mM K^+) growth medium were similar, the baseline $[Ca^{++}]_i$ range in neurons matured in depolarizing growth medium tended to be greater and in some neurons attained higher $[Ca^{++}]_i$ levels in response to glutamate receptor agonists compared with neurons matured in nondepolarizing growth medium, suggesting that depolarizing growth conditions play a role in baseline $[Ca^{++}]_i$ levels and support previous findings.[13] Additional evidence is provided from experiments where changing the experimental media from high K^+ (25 mM) to low K^+ (5 mM) substantially lowered baseline $[Ca^{++}]_i$ levels (FIGS. 1C, 3A and 3D).

In cerebellar granule cells, NMDA receptor-mediated excitotoxicity either by glutamate or NMDA is a developmental process in depolarizing (25 mM K^+) growth medium; prior to DIV 7, granule cells were not susceptible to the excitotoxic effects of glutamate acting on NMDA receptors (TABLE 1). This observation does not appear to be due to delayed expression of NMDA receptors, because it has been shown that NMDA-induced increases in $[Ca^{++}]_i$ were detected about one day after seeding,[6] and we show that NMDA-induced increases in $[Ca^{++}]_i$ are observed on DIV 3 (FIG. 3). The $[Ca^{++}]_i$ responses evoked by glutamate in neurons matured in depolarizing (25 mM K^+) growth medium for three days revealed characteristics similar to those obtained for neurons matured in the same growth medium for eight days despite the fact that neurons on DIV 3 are not susceptible to the excitotoxic effects of glutamate acting on NMDA receptors (TABLE 1). In addition, the results also show that the intracellular increases in calcium are due to the addition of glutamate, because removal of the glutamate-containing buffer reduces the level back to baseline (FIG. 3). Taken together, these results suggest that resistance to the excitotoxic effects of NMDA and non-NMDA receptor agonists prior to DIV 7 does not appear to be due to a reduced calcium influx through the glutamate receptor subtypes and suggest that calcium influx is not the exclusive factor in the excitotoxic process.

Treatment with NMDA (100 μM) for 1.5 hr protects about 80% of vulnerable granule cell neurons against NMDA receptor-mediated excitotoxicity.[29] Since NMDA desensitizes NMDA receptors by approximately 30%,[10] it was possible that NMDA receptor desensitization with a concomitant decrease in calcium influx was responsible for the observed neuroprotective effect. Surprisingly, no difference was observed in either the baseline or the maximum $[Ca^{++}]_i$ in untreated or pretreated granule cell neurons. The $[Ca^{++}]_i$ plateau, which was elevated in both cases, attained a slightly higher level in the untreated neurons, but was not significant. It has been recently shown that desensitization of NMDA receptors is responsible for the neuroprotective effect of NMDA in cultured cerebellar granule cells.[36] The discrepancy in the results probably lies in the culture conditions. Wood and Bristow[36] cultured the granule cells in serum-free growth medium, whereas granule cells used in this study were matured in serum-containing medium. It should be noted that cerebellar granule cells matured in serum-free media are not susceptible to the excitotoxic effects of glutamate (A.M. Marini, unpublished observations). Therefore, it is possible that maturation of signal transduction mechanisms and/or proteins critical for excitotoxicity are not expressed or functional under serum-free conditions. In other *in vitro* model studies, attenuation of peak $[Ca^{++}]_i$ concentrations or blocking calcium influx protected neurons, suggesting that calcium plays a major role in excitotoxicity and hypoglycemic-induced neuronal cell death. Normalization of hypoglycemia-induced elevations of $[Ca^{++}]_i$ levels by growth factors,[7] blockade of NMDA receptors induced by hypoglycemia,[7,37,19] and attenuation of excitotoxicity by blocking entry of calcium by L-type calcium channel blockers[55] have been shown to be neuroprotective.

Assuming that the influx of calcium plays a crucial role in neuronal cell death, it is difficult to ascertain why the same intracellular level of calcium in neurons pretreated with NMDA does not appear to affect the neurons. We believe that even when neurons become susceptible to the excitotoxic effects of glutamate there are intrinsic survival pathways that can be activated by neurons to protect themselves against potentially excitotoxic conditions. As indicated above, a subtoxic concentration of NMDA protects all of the vulnerable neurons against the excitotoxic effects of glutamate.[29] We have recently shown that a neuroprotective concentration of NMDA induces the release of brain-derived neurotrophic factor (BDNF), which then binds to its cognate receptor trkB. Activation of trkB receptors is critically important for NMDA neuroprotection, because effectively removing the BDNF or blocking the signal transduction pathway completely blocks NMDA neuroprotection.[30] Moreover, it has been shown that oxygen is required in glutamate excitotoxicity and that the glutamate-induced increases in $[Ca^{++}]_i$ were not toxic to the neurons in the absence of oxygen.[16] Taken together, these results suggest that neurons are able to achieve $[Ca^{++}]_i$ levels comparable to those under excitotoxic conditions, because they have inherent survival mechanisms to protect themselves against excitotoxicity. The major task ahead is to ascertain these survival pathways to develop more effective strategies to protect vulnerable neurons against hypoxic/ischemic damage.

ACKNOWLEDGMENTS

The authors wish to thank Drs. Michael Rogawski and Robert H. Lipsky for fruitful discussions in the preparation of this paper.

REFERENCES

1. AIZENMAN, E., K.A. HARTNETT & I.J. REYNOLDS. 1990. Oxygen free radicals regulate NMDA receptor function via a redox modulatory site. Neuron **5:** 841–846.
2. ASCHER, P. & L. NOWAK. 1988. Quisqualate- and kainate-activated channels in mouse central neurones in culture. J. Physiol. **399:** 227–245.

3. BALAZS, R., N. HACK & O.S. JORGENSEN. 1990. Selective stimulation of excitatory amino acid receptor subtypes and the survival of cerebellar granule cells in culture: effect of kainic acid. Neuroscience **37:** 251–258.

4. BALAZS, R., O.S. JORGENSEN & N. HACK. 1988. *N*-Methyl-D-aspartate promotes the survival of cerebellar granule cells in culture. Neuroscience **27:** 437–451.

5. BENVENISTE, H., M.B. JORGENSEN, N.H. DIEMER & J.A. HANSEN. 1988. Calcium accumulation by glutamate receptor activation is involved in hippocampal cell damage after ischemia. Acta Neurol. Scad. **78:** 529–536.

5a. BURGARD, E.C. & J.J. HABLITZ. 1995. *N*-Methyl-D-aspartate receptor-mediated calcium accumulation in neocortical neurons. Neuroscience **69:** 351–362.

6. BURGOYNE, R.D., I.A. PEARCE & M. CAMBRAY-DEAKIN. 1988. *N*-Methyl-D-aspartate raises cytosolic calcium concentration in rat cerebellar granule cells in culture. Neurosci. Lett. **91:** 47–52.

7. CHENG, B. & M.P. MATTSON. 1992. IGF-I and IGF-II protect cultured hippocampal and septal neurons against calcium-mediated hypoglycemic damage. J. Neurosci. **12:** 1558–1566.

8. CHOI, D.W. 1987. Ionic dependence of glutamate neurotoxicity. J. Neurosci. **7:** 369–379.

9. CHOI, D.W. 1988. Glutamate neurotoxicity and diseases of the nervous system. Neuron **1:** 623–634.

10. CLARK, G.D., D.B. CLIFFORD & C.F. ZORUMSKI. 1990. The effect of agonist concentration, membrane voltage and calcium on *N*-methyl-D-aspartate receptor desensitization. Neuroscience **39:** 787–797.

11. CLEMENTI, E., G. RACCHETTI, G. MELINO & J. MELDOLESI. 1996. Cytosolic Ca^{2+} buffering, a cell property that in some neurons markedly decreases during aging, has a protective effect against NMDA/nitric oxide-induced excitotoxicity. Life Sci. **59:** 389–397.

12. CONNOR, J.A., H.Y. TSENY & P.E. HOCKBERGER. 1987. Depolarization- and transmitter-induced changes in intracellular Ca^{2+}. J. Neurosci. **7:** 1384–1400.

13. COURTNEY, M.J., J.J. LAMBERT & D.G. NICHOLLS. 1990. The interactions between plasma membrane depolarization and glutamate receptor activation in the regulation of cytoplasmic free calcium in cultured cerebellar granule cells. J. Neurosci. **10:** 3873–3879.

14. CURRIE, D.N. & J.S. KELLY. 1981. Glial versus neuronal uptake of glutamate. J. Exp. Biol. **95:** 181–193.

15. DINGLEDINE, R. 1983. *N*-Methyl aspartate activates a voltage-dependent calcium conductance in rat hippocampal pyramidal cells. J. Physiol. **343:** 385–405.

16. DUBINSKY, J.M., B.S. KRISTAL & M. ELIZONDO-FOURNIER. 1995. An obligate role for oxygen in the early stages of glutamate-induced, delayed neuronal death. J. Neurosci. **15**(11): 7071–7078.

17. DUNCAN, M.D., A.M. MARINI, R. WATTERS, I.J. KOPIN & S.P. MARKEY. 1992. Zinc, a neurotoxin to cultured neurons, contaminates cycad flour prepared by traditional guamanian methods. J. Neurosci. **12:** 1523–1537.

18. DUTTON, G.R., D.N. CURRIE & K. TEAR. 1981. An improved method for the bulk isolation of viable pericarya from postnatal cerebellum. J. Neurosci. Methods **3:** 421–427.

19. FACCI, L., A. LEON & S.D. SKAPER. 1990. Hypoglycemic neurotoxicity *in vitro*: involvement of excitatory amino acid receptors and attenuation by monosialogangioside GM1. Neuroscience **37:** 709–716.

20. FAVARON, M., H. MANEV, J. ALHO, M. BERTOLINO, B. FERRET, A. GUIDOTTI & E. COSTA. 1988. Gangliosides prevent glutamate and kainate neurotoxicity in primary neuronal cultures of neunatal rat cerebellum and cortex. Proc. Natl.. Acad. Sci. **85:** 7351–7355.

21. FRANDSEN, A. & A. SCHOUSBOE. 1991. Dantrolene prevents glutamate cytotoxicity and Ca^{2+} release from intracellular stores in cultured cerebral cortical neurons. J. Neurochem. **56:** 1075–1078.

22. GALLO, V., R. SUIERGIU, C. GIOVANNINI & G. LEVI. 1987. Glutamate receptor subtypes in cultured cerebellar neurons: modulation of glutamate and gamma-aminobutyric acid release. J. Neurochem. **49:** 1801–1809.
23. IRVING, A.J., J.G. SCHOFIELD & G.L. COLLINGRIDGE. 1992. The effect of [K$^+$] during culture on the appearance of spontaneous [Ca^{++}]$_i$ oscillations in rat cerebellar granule cells. Soc. Neurosci Abstr. **18:** 46.
24. LASHER, R.S. 1974. The uptake of [^{3}H] GABA and differentiation of stellate neurons in cultures of dissociated postnatal rat cerebellum. Brain Res. **69:** 482–488.
25. LEVI, G., F. ALOISI, M.T. CIOTTI & V. GALLO. 1984. Autoradiographic localization and depolarization-induced release of acidic amino acids in differentiating cerebellar granule cell cutures. Brain Res. **290:** 77–86.
26. MACDERMOTT, A.B., M.L. MAYER, G.L. WESTBROOK, S.J. SMITH & J.L. BARKER. 1986. NMDA-receptor activation increases cytoplasmic calcium concentrations in cultured spinal cord neurones. Nature **321:** 519–522.
27. MANEV, H., M. FAVARON, A. GUIDOTTI & E. COSTA. 1989. Delayed increase of calcium influx elicited by glutamate: role in neuronal death. Mol. Pharmacol. **36:** 106–112.
28. MARINI, A. & A. NOVELLI. 1991. DL-Threo-3-hydroxyaspartate reduces NMDA receptor activation by glutamate in cultured neurons. Eur. J. Pharmacol. **194:** 131–132.
29. MARINI, A.M. & S.M. PAUL. 1992. *N*-methyl-D-aspartate receptor-mediated neuroprotection in cerebellar granule cells requires new RNA and protein synthesis. Proc. Natl. Acad. Sci. **89:** 6555–6559.
30. MARINI, A.M., S.J. RABIN, R.H. LIPSKY & I. MOCCHETTI. 1998. Activity-dependent release of brain derived neurotrophic factor underlies the neuroprotective effect of *N*-methyl-D-asparate. J. Biol. Chem. **273:** 29394–29399.
31. MARINI, A.M., J.P. SCHWARTZ & I.J. KOPIN. 1989. The neurotoxicity of 1-methyl-4-phenylpyridinium in cultured cerebellar granule cells. J. Neurosci. **9:** 3665–3672.
32. MAYER, M.L. & G.L. WESTBROOK. 1985. The action of *N*-methyl-D-aspartic acid on mouse spinal neurones in culture. J. Physiol. **361:** 65–90.
33. MAYER, M.L. & G.L. WESTBROOK. 1987. Cellular mechanisms underlying excitotoxicity. Trends Neurosci. **10:** 59–61.
34. MAYER, M.L., G.L. WESTBROOK & P.B. GUTHRIE. 1984. Voltage-dependent block by Mg^{+2} of NMDA responses in spinal cord neurones. Nature **309:** 261–263.
35. MCCASLIN, P.P. & T.G. SMITH. 1990. Low calcium-induced release of glutamate results in autotoxicity of cerebellar granule cells. Brain Res. **513:** 280–285.
36. MESSER, A. 1977. The maintenance and identification of cerebellar granule cells in monolayer cultures. Brain Res. **130:** 1–12.
37. MONYER, H., M.P. GOLDBERG & D.W. CHOI. 1989. Glucose deprivation neuronal injury in cortical culture. Brain Res. **483:** 347–354.
38. MÜLLER, T., T. MÖLLER, T. BERGER, J. SCHNITZER & H. KETTENMANN. 1992. Calcium entry through kainate receptors and resulting potassium-channel blockade in Bergmann glial cells. Science **256:** 1563–1570.
39. NICOLETTI, F., J.T. WROBLEWSKI, E. FADDA & E. COSTA. 1988. Pertussis toxin inhibits signal transduction at a specific metabolotropic glutamate receptor in primary cultures of cerebellar granule cells. J. Neurochem. **48:** 967–973.
40. NICOLL, R.A. & B.E. ALGER. 1981. Synaptic excitation may activate a calcium-dependent potassium conductance in hippocampal pyramidal cells. Science **212:** 957–959.
41. NOVELLI, A., F. NICOLETTI, J.T. WROBLEWSKI, H. ALHO, E. COSTA & A. GUIDOTTI. 1987. Excitatory amino acid receptors coupled with guanylate cyclase in primary cultures of cerebellar granule cells. J. Neurosci. **7:** 40–47.

42. NOVELLI, A., J.A. REILLY, P.G. LYSKO & R.C. HENNEBERRY. 1988. Glutamate becomes neurotoxic via the N-methyl-D-aspartate receptor when intracellular energy levels are reduced. Brain Res. **451:** 205–212.

43. NOWAK, L., P. BREGESTOVSKI, P. ASCHER, A. HERBET & A. PROCHIANTZ. 1984. Magnesium gates glutamate-activated channels in mouse central neurones. Nature **307:** 462–465.

44. OGURA, A., M. MIYAMOTO & Y. KUDO. 1988. Neuronal death *in vitro*: parellelism between survivability of hippocampal neurones and sustained elevation of cytosolic Ca^{2+} after exposure to glutamate receptor agonist. Exp. Brain Res. **73:** 447–458.

45. OLNEY, J.W. 1986. Inciting excitoxic cytocide among central neurons. *In* Excitatory Amino Acids and Epilepsy. R. Schwarcz & Y. Ben-Ari, Eds.: 631–645. Plenum. New York.

46. PARKS, T.N., L.D. ARTMAN, N. ALASTI & E.F. NEMETH. 1991. Modulation of N-methyl-D-aspartate receptor-mediated increases in cytosolic calcium in cultured rat cerebellar granule cells. Brain Res. **552:** 13–22.

47. ROGERS, K.L., R.A. PHILIBERT & G.R. DUTTON. 1990. Glutamate receptor agonists cause efflux of endogenous neuroactive amino acids from cerebellar neurons in culture. Eur. J. Pharmacol. **177:** 195–199.

48. ROTHMAN, S.M. & J.W. OLNEY. 1986. Glutamate and the pathophysiology of hypoxic-ischemic brain damage. Ann. Neurol. **19:** 105–111.

49. ROTHMAN, S.M., J.H. THURSTON & R.E. HAUHART. 1987. Delayed neurotoxicity of excitatory amino acids *in vitro*. Neuroscience **21:** 665–671.

50. SAVOLAINEN, K.M., J. LOIKKANEN & J. NAARALA. 1995. Amplification of glutamate-induced oxidative stress. Toxicol. Lett. **82/83:** 399–405.

51. SOMMER, B., K. KEINÄNEN, T.A. VERDOORN, W. WISDEN, N. BURNASHEV, A. HERB, M. KÖHLER, T. TAKAGI, B. SAKMANN & P.H. SEEBURG. 1990. Flip and flop: a cell-specific functional switch in glutamate-operated channels of the CNS. Science **249:** 1580–1585.

52. TSIEN, R.Y. & A.T. HAROOTUNIAN. 1990. Practical design criteria for a dynamic ratio imaging system. Cell Calcium **11:** 93–109.

53. VALLANO, M.L., B. LAMBOLEZ, E. AUDINAT & J. ROSSIER. 1995. Neuronal activity differentially regulates NMDA receptor subunit expression in cerebellar granule cells. J. Neurosci. **16:** 631–639.

54. VAN DER VALK, J.B.F., A. RESINK & R. BALAZS. 1991. Membrane depolarization and the expression of glutamate receptors in crebellar granule cells. Eur. J. Pharmacol. **201:** 247–250.

55. WEISS, J.H., D.M. HARTLEY, J. KOH & D.W. CHOI. 1990. The calcium channel blocker nifedipine attenuates slow excitatory amino acid neurotoxicity. Science **247:** 1474–1476.

56. WOOD, A.M. & D.R. BRISTOW. 1998. N-Methyl-D-aspartate receptor desensitization is neuroprotective by inhibiting glutamate-induced apoptotic-like death. J. Neurochem. **70:** 677–687.

57. WROBLEWSKI, J.T., F. NICOLETTI & E. COSTA. 1985. Different coupling of excitatory amino acid receptors with Ca^{2+} channels in primary cultures of cerebellar granule cells. Neuropharmacology **241:** 919–921.

58. WROBLEWSKI, J.T., F. NICOLETTI, E. FADDA & E. COSTA. 1987. Phencyclidine is a negative allosteric modulator of signal transduction at two subclasses of excitatory amino acid receptors. Proc. Natl. Acad. Sci. USA **84:** 5068–5072.

Neuroprotective Actions of Novel and Potent Ligands of Group I and Group II Metabotropic Glutamate Receptors

A.E. KINGSTON,[a,d] M.J. O'NEILL,[a] A. BOND,[a] V. BRUNO,[b] G. BATTAGLIA,[b] F. NICOLETTI,[b] J.R. HARRIS,[a] B.P. CLARK,[a] J.A. MONN,[c] D. LODGE,[c] AND D.D. SCHOEPP[c]

[a]*Eli Lilly and Co. Ltd., Erl Wood Manor, Windlesham, Surrey, United Kingdom*

[b]*IMN Neuromed, Pozzilli, Italy*

[c]*Eli Lilly and Co. Indianapolis, Indiana, USA*

ABSTRACT: The role of group I metabotropic glutamate (mGlu) receptors in neurodegeneration is controversial because of the contradictory effects of mGlu1/5 agonists in *in vitro* models of neuronal cell death. In this study, novel and selective antagonists of mGlu1 and mGlu5: LY367385 and LY367366 were found to show consistent neuroprotective effects against *N*-methyl-D-aspartate (NMDA)-induced excitotoxicity *in vitro* and *in vivo*. Furthermore, intraventricular administration of LY367385 reduced hippocampal cell death in gerbils subjected to transient global ischemia.

Previous studies have also shown that activation of group II mGlu receptors may contribute to neuroprotective mechanisms *in vitro* and *in vivo*. Three potent group II mGlu agonists—LY354740, LY379268 and LY389795—were found to attenuate both NMDA excitotoxicity and staurosporine-induced neuronal cell death. LY354740 and LY379268 were protective against transient global ischemia in gerbils when dosed intraperitoneally.

These results support the view that antagonists of mGlu1 and mGlu5 and agonists of group II mGlu receptors may be useful agents in the therapeutic treatment of neurodegenerative disease.

INTRODUCTION

The contribution of ionotropic glutamate receptors such as *N*-methyl-D-aspartate (NMDA), α-amino-3-hydroxy-5-methylisoxasole-4-propionic acid (AMPA) and kainate receptor subtypes to excitotoxic neurodegeneration has been widely investigated.[1] More recently, the roles of metabotropic G protein-coupled glutamate receptors to excitotoxicity has been considered. Metabotropic glutamate (mGlu) receptors are G protein-coupled receptors and comprise eight different subtypes also divided into three subgroups defined on the basis of their amino acid sequence homology, pharmacology and the signal transduction pathway to which they couple. Group I (mGlu1 and mGlu5) are coupled to the phosphoinositide hydrolysis/intracellular

[d]Corresponding author: Dr. Ann Kingston, Eli Lilly & Co. Ltd., Erl Wood Manor, Windlesham, Surrey GU20 6PH, UK. Phone, +44-1276-853483; fax, +44-1276-853525.
e-mail, KINGSTON_ANN_E@lilly.com

calcium ($[Ca^{2+}]_i$) mobilization signal transduction pathway. Group II (mGlu2 and mGlu3) and group III (mGlu4, mGlu6, mGlu7 and mGlu8) are negatively coupled to cyclic adenosine-5′,3′-monophosphate (cAMP) formation. Experimental studies using standard agonists of group I mGlus have shown either pro- or anti-neurodegenerative effects in several *in vitro* and *in vivo* models of neurodegeneration.[2–6] On the other hand, the effects of group I mGlu antagonists have been shown to be more consistently neuroprotective.[7–10] Evidence has also accumulated to show that activation of group II mGlu receptors can result in the attenuation of neurodegeneration both *in vitro* and *in vivo*.[11–21]

In this study, we describe the effects of novel and potent group I mGlu antagonists and group II mGlu agonists in different models of neurodegeneration.

MATERIALS AND METHODS

Materials

3,5-Dihydroxyphenylglycine (DHPG) and NMDA were obtained from Tocris Ltd. (UK). Cytosine arabinoside, actinomycin D and cycloheximide were obtained from Sigma Chemical Co. (UK). Cell culture media and supplements were purchased from Life Technologies Ltd. (UK). Compounds: LY367385, (+)-2-methyl-4-carboxyphenylglycine; LY367366, (±)-α-thioxanthylmethyl-4-carboxyphenylglycine; LY354740, (+)-2-aminobicyclo[3.1.0] hexane-2,6-dicarboxylate; LY379268, (−)-2-oxa-4-aminobicyclo[3.1.0]hexane-4,6-dicarboxylate; and LY389795, (−)-2-thia-4-aminobicyclo[3.1.0]hexane-4,6-dicarboxylate were synthesized at Eli Lilly and dissolved in equimolar NaOH to facilitate solution.

Neuronal Cell Cultures

Cortical cell cultures were prepared from fetal rat brains at day 18 of gestation. Dissociated cortical cells were plated in 15-mm 24-well vessels using a plating medium of Neurobasal medium containing 10% heat inactivated fetal calf serum, and glutamine (1 mM). Cultures were kept at 37°C in a humidified 5% CO_2 atmosphere. After 2 days *in vitro*, non-neuronal cell division was halted by exposure to cytosine arabinoside (5 uM) in serum-free medium containing B27 supplement (Life Technologies Ltd., UK) and resulted in cultures containing 15–20% glial cells.

Neuronal Cell Injury

"Fast" NMDA excitotoxicity[11] was induced by incubating the cultures at 37°C in a magnesium-free Hank's balanced salt solution containing $CaCl_2$ (2.0 mM), *N*-2-hydroxyethylpiperazine-*N*′-2-ethanesulphonic acid (HEPES, 10 mM) and glycine (10 uM) with NMDA (300 uM) for 10–15 min at 37°C. The cultures were then returned to serum-free Dulbecco's modified Eagle's medium (DMEM) supplemented with HEPES (10 mM) and glycine (10 uM) and further incubated for 20–24 hr before evaluation of NMDA toxicity. "Slow" excitotoxicity[11] was induced by incubation of cultures with NMDA (30 uM) in DMEM without serum for 24 hr. Neuronal degeneration was also induced by incubation of cultures with staurosporine (1 uM) in DMEM without serum for 24 hr. Neuronal injury was evaluated by measurement of lactate dehydrogenase activity in supernatants collected from cultures at the end of the 24-hr incubation by spectrophotometric assay using a cytotoxicity detection kit (Boehringer-Mannheim, UK).

Assessment of In Vivo Neuronal Injury

Male Sprague-Dawley rats (250–300 g) were anesthetized with pentobarbital (50 mg/kg, intraperitoneally (i.p.)) and infused with NMDA (100 nmol/0.5 ul/2 min) or NMDA plus group I mGlu receptor antagonists (200 nmol in the same volume) in the left corpus striatum, at +2.0 mm AP, 2.6 mm L, and 5 mm V, according to the Pellgrino and Cushman atlas. The injection was repeated at a second site (+1 mm AP, 2.6 mm L, and 5 mm V) to obtain a more consistent loss of striatal neurons. Animals were killed by decapitation 7 days later. Neuronal toxicity was evaluated either by histological analysis or by measuring striatal glutamate decarboxylase (GAD) activity as a marker for GABAergic neurons. For histological analysis, the brains were removed, rapidly frozen in isopentane at −40°C and then stored at −80°C. Twenty-uM cryostat sections were Nissl stained and examined by light microscopy. For measurements of GAD activity, the corpus striatum was dissected bilaterally and homogenized in 5 mM imidazol buffer containing 0.2% tritonX-100 and 10 mM dithiothreitol. An aliqout of the homogenate was incubated in 400 ul of 10 mM phosphate buffer (pH 7.0) containing 10 mM 2-mercaptoethanol, 0.02 mM pyridoxal phosphate and 1 uCi of [^{3}H]-glutamate (Amersham, sp.act. 46 Ci/mmol) for 1 hr at 37°C; the reaction was stopped with 15 ul of ice-cold 11.8N $HClO_4$. After centrifugation in a microfuge at maximal speed, 10 ul of the supernatant was diluted with 0.01N HCl and derivatized with O-phthalaldehyde and mercaptoethanol for 1 min at room temperature before analysis by high-performance liquid chromatography (HPLC).[10]

Assessment of Ischemic Neuronal Death in Gerbils

Male Mongolian gerbils (Bantin and Kingman, Hull, UK) at least 3 months old and weighing in excess of 60 g were used. The animals were maintained in standard lighting conditions, and food and water were available *ad libitum*. The animals were anesthetized with a 5% halothane/oxygen mixture and maintained using 2% halothane delivered with oxygen at 1 l/min via a face mask throughout the operation. Through a midline cervical incision, both common carotid arteries were exposed and freed from surrounding connective tissue. In animals to be rendered ischemic, both common carotid arteries were clamped for either 3, 4 or 5 min. At the end of the occlusion period blood flow was re-established. In sham-operated animals the arteries were exposed but not occluded. The wound was then sutured, and the animals were allowed to recover. Throughout surgery, body temperature was maintained at 37°C using a "K-TEMP" temperature controller/heating pad (International Market Supply, Cheshire, U.K.). After surgery the animals were placed in a four-compartmental thermacage (Beta Medical and Scientific, U.K.), which maintained the environmental temperature at 28°C and rectal temperatures were measured for a 6-hr period after occlusion. There were 8 animals in each group, and sham-operated animals underwent the full surgical procedure, except for the arterial occlusion. Control animals were occluded for 3, 4 or 5 min, but received vehicle only. In separate experiments, control animals underwent bilateral carotid artery occlusion (BCAO) for periods of 2, 3, 4 and 5 min in order to determine the degree of CA1 hippocampal damage resulting from each period of occlusion.

General Histology

Five days after surgery the animals were perfused transcardially with 30 ml of 0.9% saline followed by 100 ml of 10% buffered formalin solution. The brains were removed and placed in 10% formalin for 3 days, processed and embedded in paraffin wax. Coronal sections (5 μm) were taken 1.5, 1.7 and 1.9 mm caudal to bregma using a microtome (Leitz 1400 sledge microtome). The slices were stained with hematoxylin and eosin, and the neuronal density in the CA1 subfield of the hippocampus was measured using a microscope with grid lines (0.05 mm $\times$ 0.05 mm). The neuronal density is expressed as number of viable cells per mm CA1 hippocampus. Statistical analysis of histological data was assessed using a 2-tailed unpaired Student's *t*-test.

RESULTS

Effect of Group I mGluR Antagonists on **In Vitro** *NMDA Toxicity*

Pretreatment of cortical neurons with mGlu 1 antagonist LY367385 and mGlu1/5 antagonist LY367366 (see TABLE 1 for pharmacological profile) attenuated the potentiation of NMDA toxicity by group I agonist DHPG (FIG. 1) . Both antagonists showed a similar efficacy of action causing an 80% reduction in DHPG potentiation at a concentration of 10 uM, but LY367366 showed greater potency of action with significant neuroprotective effects evident at   lower concentrations than exhibited by LY367366. Interestingly, at the higher concentrations of 100 uM, LY367366

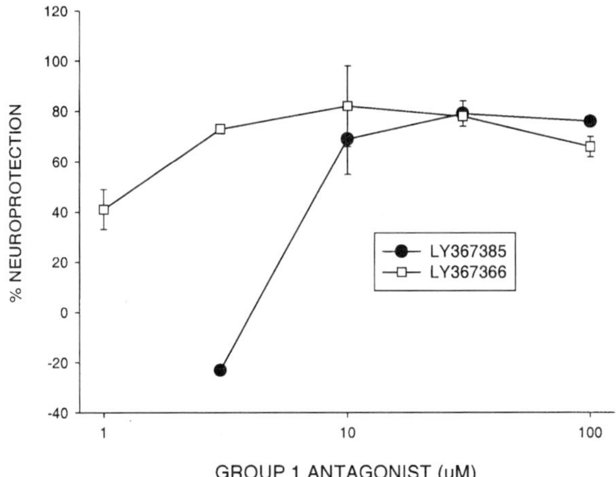

FIGURE 1. Neuroprotection of LY367385 and LY367366 against DHPG-induced potentiation of NMDA toxicity in cortical cell cultures determined by LDH release. Results represent the mean $\pm$ SEM of 3 experiments using triplicate culture determinations.

showed a trend towards lesser neuroprotection producing a bell-shaped concentration-dependent response curve (data not shown).

Neuroprotective Effects by Group I Antagonists against Excitotoxic Striatal Lesions

The neuroprotective actions of LY367385 and LY367366 in an *in vivo* model of excitotoxicity was quantified by assessment of striatal GAD activity, which represents a measure of viable GABAergic neurons. Results show that infusion of NMDA alone reduced striatal GAD activity by 50% relative to the unlesioned contralateral site. In animals in which NMDA was coinjected with either LY367385 or LY367366, the reduction in GAD activity was significantly attenuated to similar extents (FIG. 2).

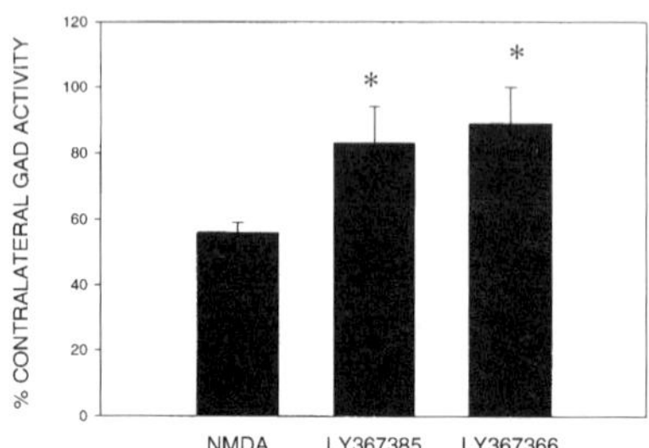

FIGURE 2. Group I mGlu antagonists prevent the reduction of GAD activity induced by monolateral infusion of NMDA into left caudate nucleus. GAD activity of the lesioned site is expressed as mean percentage ± SEM of the respective contralateral unlesioned site ($n = 4$–6), $p < 0.05$ (one-way ANOVA + Fisher PLSD). (From Bruno *et al.*[10] Reprinted by permission from Elsevier Science.)

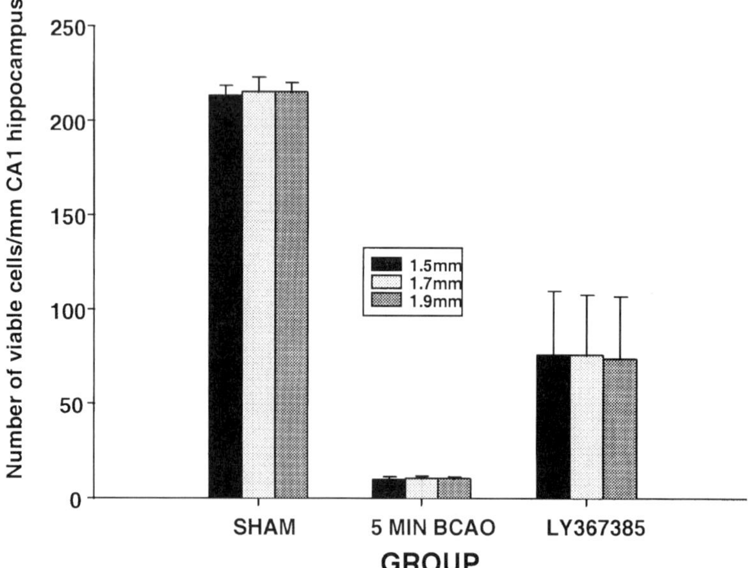

FIGURE 3. Neuroprotective activity of LY367385 infused i.c.v. 30 min before a 5-min BCAO in gerbils to achieve a brain concentration of 250 uM ($n = 4$). (From Bruno *et al.*[10] Reprinted by permission from Elsevier Science.)

Neuroprotection by Group I Antagonists against Global Ischemia

The ability of LY367385 to protect against ischemic neuronal damage was investigated in a transient global ischemia model in gerbils. LY367385 was injected intracerebroventricularly (i.c.v., 100 nmol/2.5 ul/5 min) to achieve a brain concentration of 250 uM, 30 min before a 5-min bilateral occlusion of the carotid arteries. FIGURE 3 shows that in gerbils treated with the mGlu antagonist, around 40% of the CA1 hippocampal neurons were protected from damage ($p < 0.1$).

Group II Agonists Protect against In Vitro Neurodegeneration

Pretreatment of cortical neuronal cells with heterobicyclic amino acids LY354740, LY379268 and LY389795 produced concentration-dependent reductions in NMDA toxicity. All three agonists showed similar potencies and efficacy of neuroprotection with EC_{50} values ranging from 1–10 uM (FIG. 4). In addition to evaluating the effects of the group II agonists on excitotoxicity, the effects of the compounds on staurosporine-induced neuronal degeneration were also investigated. FIGURE 5 shows that pretreatment with the agonists also prevented lactate dehydrogenase (LDH) release induced by staurosporine.

Neuroprotection by Group II Agonists against Global Ischemia

To establish whether group II agonists could protect against ischemic neuronal damage *in vivo*, gerbils were dosed i.p. with either LY354740 (50 mg/kg) 30 min be-

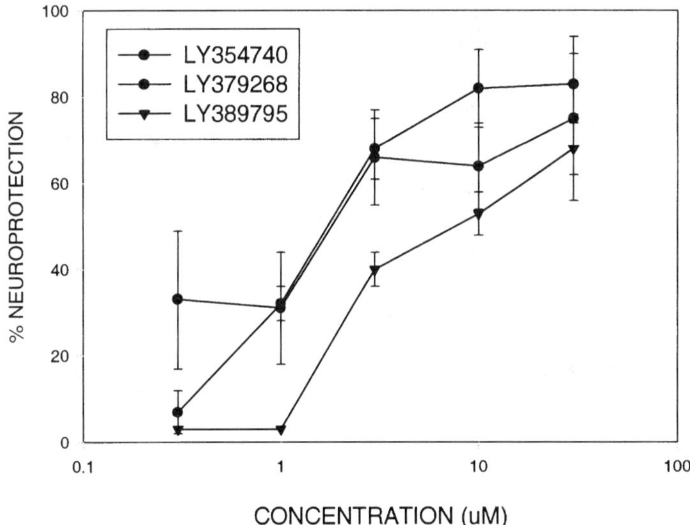

FIGURE 4. Agonists LY354740, LY379268 and LY389795 attenuate NMDA toxicity in cortical cell cultures. Excitotoxicity was determined by LDH release, and results are expressed as percentage neuroprotection relative to NMDA alone-treated cultures and represent the mean ± SEM of 3 experiments using triplicate culture determinations. (From Kingston *et al.*[17] Reprinted by permission of Elsevier Science.)

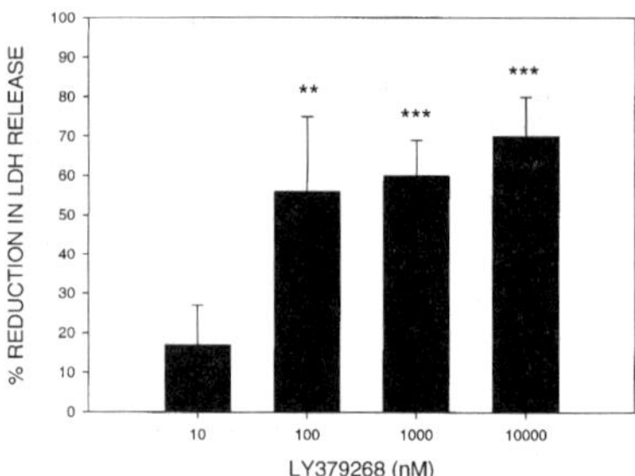

FIGURE 5. LY379268 attenuates staurosporine-induced toxicity in cortical cell cultures. Excitotoxicity was determined by LDH release, and results are expressed as percentage neuroprotection relative to staurosporine alone-treated cultures and represent the mean ± SEM of 3 experiments using triplicate culture determinations. **p <0.01; ***p <0.001 vs staurosporine-treated control cultures.

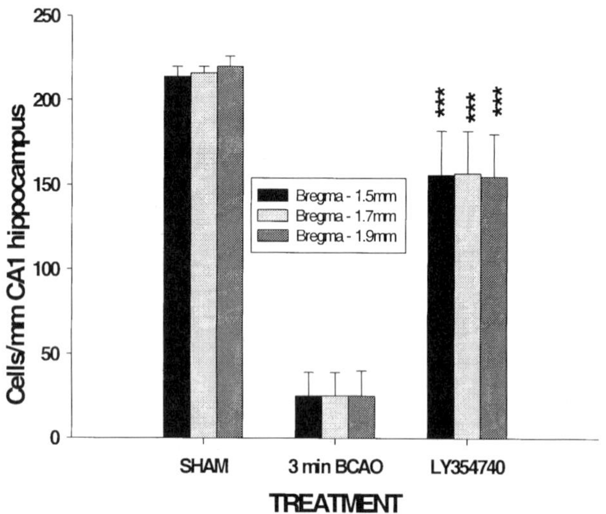

FIGURE 6. Neuroprotection by LY354740 against transient global ischemia. Gerbils were dosed 30 min before and 30 min after a 3-min BCAO with 50 mg/kg LY354740 (n = 8–10 per group). ***p <0.001 vs ischemic control by Student's t-test. (From Bond *et al.*[20] Reprinted by permission from Rapid Science.)

fore and 6 hr after BCAO or LY379268 (10 mg/kg) 30 min after BCAO. LY354740 produced significant neuroprotection (72%; $p < 0.001$) as measured by CA1 hippocampal cell viability in animals that had undergone a 3-min BCAO (FIG. 6) but was unable to protect under more severe ischemic conditions of a 5-min BCAO (data not shown). On the other hand, LY379268 almost completely prevented CA1 hippocampal cell damage induced by a 5-min BCAO (FIG. 7).

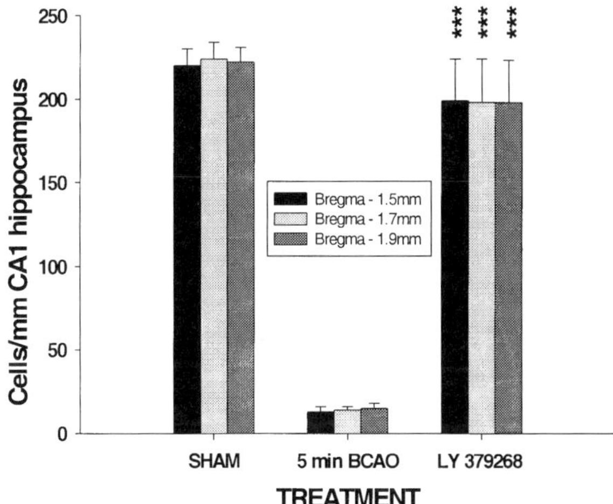

FIGURE 7. Neuroprotection of LY379268 against transient global ischemia. Gerbils were dosed 30 min after a 5-min BCAO with 10 mg/kg of LY379268 ($n = 8$–10 per group). ***p <0.001 vs ischemic control by Student's t-test. (From Bond *et al.*[21] Reprinted by permission of Elsevier Science.)

DISCUSSION

Evidence of a role for group I mGlu receptors in neuronal degeneration has been obtained from experimental studies using standard agonists and antagonists of mGlu1 and 5 receptor subtypes. Agonists of group I mGlu receptors have been shown to potentiate neuronal damage induced either by NMDA or by mild hypoxia combined with glucose deprivation *in vitro*[2,3] as well as NMDA toxicity *in vivo*.[5,6] Further evidence is given by the observation that there is an increase in the activity of group I mGlus in the hippocampi of rats subjected to transient global ischemia.[26,27] Antagonists of group I mGlu receptors have been found to protect hippocampal neurons from hypoxic injury *in vitro*[7] and *in vivo*.[8] In this study, two novel antagonists of group I mGlu receptors with different subtype selectivities were found to protect against NMDA-induced toxicity both *in vitro* and *in vivo*. Antagonism of either mGlu1 (LY367385) or mGlu1 and mGlu5 (LY367366) was effective in preventing excitotoxic neuronal damage. The observation that LY367366 showed a greater potency of effect than LY367385 *in vitro* despite having a similar potency of antagonism for mGlu1 to LY367385 in clonal cell lines (see TABLE 1) would indicate that the additional antagonism of mGlu5 by LY367366 may be significant in reducing excitotoxicity in cortical neuronal cultures where mGlu5 is considered to be the dominantly expressed group I mGlu subtype. Under conditions of transient global ischemia, LY367385, the mGlu1 antagonist, showed a trend towards neuroprotection.

These results are in agreement with those of Cozzi *et al.*,[9] who have shown that mGlu1a antagonist aminoindan-1,5-dicarboxylic acid (AIDA) reduces the delayed degeneration of pyramidal cells in the hippocampal CA1 region after transient global

TABLE 1. Pharmacological profile of group I mGlu antagonists

Glutamate Receptor	LY367385 IC$_{50}$ (uM)	LY367366 IC$_{50}$ (uM)
mGlu1	8.8 ± 3.9	5.7 ± 2.9
mGlu5	>200	3.4 ± 1.5
Group II mGlu	≫100	>10
Group III mGlu	≫100	>10
AMPA	>10,000	>10,000
Kainate	>10,000	>10,000
NMDA	>10,000	>10,000

NOTE: The potencies of the antagonists at group I mGlu receptors were determined by phosphatidylinositol (PI) hydrolysis assay;[22] group II mGlu activity was determined by 1S,3R-1-aminocyclopentane-1,3-dicarboxylic acid (ACPD)-sensitive [^{3}H]glutamate binding to adult rat forebrain membranes;[23] group III mGlu activity was determined by the effects of the compounds on L(+)-2-amino-4-phosphonobutyric acid (L-AP4)-induced reduction of cAMP responses of mGluR4 cells;[24] affinities for AMPA, kainate and NMDA receptors were measured by radioligand binding assay.[25]

ischemia in gerbils. Both LY367385 and LY367366 were also neuroprotective against excitotoxic death induced by infusion of NMDA into the caudate nucleus. The protective effect of LY367385 therefore supports the proposal that mGlu1a activation by glutamate endogenously released during the neurodegenerative process contributes to the propagation of an excitotoxic response via stimulation of phosphoinositide hydrolysis and mobilization of calcium from intracellular stores.[28] However, to clearly define the role of mGlu5 in the development of excitotoxic cell death, the discovery of a specific mGlu5 antagonist is warranted.

In addition to group I mGlu antagonists, the neuroprotective activity of novel and potent agonists of group II mGlus—LY354740, LY379268 and LY389795—were also demonstrated both *in vitro* and *in vivo*. Our observations support previous evidence that group II mGlu receptor agonists 2-(2,3-dicarboxycyclopropyl)glycine (DCG-IV), 4-carboxyphenyl-3-hydroxyphenylglycine (4C3HPG), (2S,1′S,2′S)-2-(carboxycycopropyl) glycine (CCG) and aminopyrrolidine-2R,4R-dicarboxylic acid (APDC) are neuroprotective.[11–13] However, in comparing the nanomolar potencies of the group II agonists LY379268, LY389795 and LY354740 on clonal cell lines expressing mGlu2 (EC$_{50}$ values of 2.7, 3.9 and 5.1 nM, respectively) and mGlu3 (EC$_{50}$ values of 4.6, 7.6 and 24.3 nM, respectively) with their activities against excitotoxicity, major differences in potency of up to 1000-fold were observed. These differences in activity may reflect that the neuroprotective mechanism of action may not be directly coupled to inhibition of adenylate cyclase as measured in clonal cell lines expressing group II mGlu subtypes. The exact mechanism whereby group II mGlu receptors attenuate neurodegenerative responses is unknown. However, it is known that activation of presynaptic group II mGlus has been shown to modulate voltage sensitive calcium channels[29] and that this may be a possible means of reducing excitotoxicity by reducing glutamate release.[30] In addition, group II mGlu neuroprotection has been shown to be dependent on the production of transforming growth factor beta (TGFβ) from glial cells.[31] Another possibility is that these agonists may be activating mGlu8, since LY354740, LY379268 and LY389795 all have micromolar potencies on clonally expressed mGlu8 with EC_{50} values of 11.5, 1.7 and 7.3 uM, respectively. These potencies are comparable to the concentrations of the compounds that were effective in reducing LDH release. Further experiments with group II and group III mGlu selective antagonists will facilitate our understanding of these differences in activity. However, LY354740 and LY379268 have been found to mediate anti-apoptotic effects at nanomolar concentrations in cortical neuronal cell cultures at concentrations commensurate with their measured receptor affinities in clonal cell lines expressing mGlu2 and mGlu3.[17] The activity of the agonists may therefore be due to a mixed activity at both group II and group III mGlu receptor subtypes such that the group II mGlu activation differentiates a population of apoptotic cells within the overall population of dying neurons. Taken together, the neuroprotective consequences of modulating both group I and group II mGlu receptors may represent a novel therapeutic strategy for treatment of neurodegenerative conditions.

REFERENCES

1. DANYSZ, W., C.G. PARSONS, I. BRESINK & G. QUACK. 1995. Glutamate in CNS disorders. Drug News Perspect. **8:** 458–535.
2. BUISSON, A. & D.W. CHOI. 1995. The inhibitory mGluR agonist, *S*-4-carboxy-3-hydroxyphenylglycine selectively attenuates NMDA neurotoxicity and oxygen-glucose deprivation-induced neuronal death. Neuropharmacology **34:** 1081–1087.
3. BRUNO, V., A. COPANI, T. KNOPFEL, R. KUHN, G. CASABONA, P. DELL'ALBANI, D.F. CONDORELLI & F. NICOLETTI. 1995. Activation of metabotropic glutamate receptors coupled to inositol phospholipid hydrolysis amplifies NMDA-induced neuronal degeneration in cultured cortical cells. Neuropharmacology **34:** 1089–1098.
4. PIZZI, M., P. GALLI, O. CONSOLANDI, V. ARRIGHI, M. MERNO & P.F. SPANO. 1996. Metabotropic and ionotropic transducers of glutamate signal inversely control cytoplasmic calcium concentration and excitotoxicity in cultured cerebellar granule cells: pivotal role of protein kinase. Cell. Mol. Pharmacol. **49:** 586–594.
5. MCDONALD, J.W. & D.D. SCHOEPP. 1992. The metabotropic excitatory amino acid receptor agonist 1*S*,3*R*-ACPD selectively potentiates *N*-methyl-D-aspartate induced brain injury. Eur. J. Pharmacol. **215:** 353–354.
6. SACAAN, A.I. & D.D. SCHOEPP. 1992. Activation of hippocampal metabotropic excitatory amino acid receptors leads to seizures and neuronal damage. Neurosci. Lett. **139:** 77–82.
7. OPITZ, T., P. RICHTER & K.G. REYMANN. 1994. The metabotropic glutamate receptor antagonist (+)-α-methyl-4-carboxyphenylglycine protects hippocampal CA1 neurons of the rat from *in vitro* hypoxia/hypoglycaemia. Neuropharmacology **33:** 715–717.
8. RIEDEL, G., T. OPITZ & K.G. REYMANN. 1996. Blockade of metabotropic glutamate receptors protects hippocampal neurons from hypoxia-induced cell death in rat *in vivo*. Prog. Neuro-Psychopharmacol Biol. Psychiat. **20:** 1253–1263.
9. COZZI, A., G. LOMBARDI, P. LEONARDI, S. ATTUCI, F. PERUGINELLI, R. PELLICCIARI & F. MORONI. 1997. AIDA, a group I metabotropic glutamate receptor antagonist reduces the ischemia-induced neuronal loss [abstract]. Soc. Neurosci. Abstr. **23:** 788.2.
10. BRUNO, V., G. BATTAGLIA, A. KINGSTON, M.J. O'NEILL, M.V. CATANIA, R. DI GREZIA & F. NICOLETTI. 1999. Neuroprotective activity of the potent and selective mGlu1a metabotropic glutamate receptor antagonist, (+)-2-methyl-4-carboxyphenylglycine (LY367385): comparison with LY367366, an antagonist of mGlu1a and mGlu5 receptors. Neuropharmacology **38:** 199–207.

11. BRUNO, V., A. COPANI, G. BATTAGLIA, R. RAFFAELE, H. SHINOZAKI & F. NICOLETTI. 1994. Protective effect of the metabotropic glutamate receptor agonist, DCG-IV, against excitotoxic neuronal cell death. Eur. J. Pharmacol. **256:** 109–112.

12. BUISSON, A., S.P. YU & D.W. CHOI. 1996. DCG-IV selectively attenuates rapidly triggered NMDA-induced neurotoxicity in cortical neurons. Eur. J. Neurosci. **8:** 138–143.

13. BATTAGLIA, G., V. BRUNO, R.T. NGOMBA, R. DI GREZIA, A. COPANI & F. NICOLETTI. 1998. Selective activation of group-II metabotropic glutamate receptors is protective against excitotoxic neuronal death. Eur. J. Pharmacol. **356:** 271–274.

14. COPANI, A., V. BRUNO, G. BATTAGLIA, G. LEANZA, R. PELLITTERI, A. RUSSO, S. STANZANI & F. NICOLETTI. 1995. Activation of metabotropic glutamate receptors protects neurons against apoptosis induced by beta-amyloid peptide. Mol. Pharmacol. **47:** 890–897.

15. MAIESE, K., R. GREENBERG, L. BOCCONE & M. SWIRIDUK. 1994. Activation of metabotropic glutamate receptors is neuroprotective during nitric oxide toxicity in primary hippocampal neurons of rats. Neurosci. Lett. **194:** 173–176.

16. BUISSON, A., S.P. YU & D.W. CHOI. 1994. Effect of metabotropic glutamate receptor agonists on excitotoxic and apoptotic cell death in murine cortical cell culture [abstract]. Soc. Neurosci. Abstr. **20:** 198.5.

17. KINGSTON, A.E., M.J. O'NEILL, A. LAM, K.R. BALES, J.A. MONN & D.D. SCHOEPP. 1999. Neuroprotection by metabotropic glutamate receptor agonists: LY354740, LY379268 and LY389795. Eur. J. Pharmacol. **377:** 155–165.

18. CHIAMULERA, C., P. ALBERTINI, E. VALERIO & A. REGGIANI. 1992. Activation of metabotropic receptors has a neuroprotective effect in a rodent model of focal ischaemia. Eur. J. Pharmacol. **216:** 335–336.

19. SHINOZAKI, H., M. ISHIDA, M. MIYAMOTO & S. KWAK. 1994. Sedative and neuroprotective actions of potent and selective agonists for metabotropic glutamate receptors. *In* Excitatory Amino Acids: Approaches to Clinical Uses. The Ninth Rinshoken International Conference. Nov. 28–30, Tokyo, Japan. Abst. 25.

20. BOND, A., M.J. O'NEILL, C.A. HICKS, J.A. MONN & D. LODGE. 1998. Neuroprotective effects of a systemically active group II metabotropic glutamate receptor agonist LY354740 in a gerbil model of global ischaemia. NeuroReport **9:** 1191–1193.

21. BOND, A., N. RAGUMOORTHY, J.A. MONN, C.A. HICKS, M.A. WARD, D. LODGE & M.J. O'NEILL. 1999. LY379268, a potent and selective group II metabotropic glutamate receptor agonist is neuroprotective in gerbil global, but not focal, cerebral ischemia. Neurosci. Lett. **273:** 191–194.

22. CLARK, B.P., S.R. BAKER, J. GOLDSWORTHY, J.R. HARRIS & A.E. KINGSTON. 1997. (+)-2-Methyl-4-carboxyphenylglycine (LY367385) selectively antagonises metabotropic glutamate mGlu1 receptors. Biorg. Med. Chem. Lett. **7:** 2777–2780.

23. WRIGHT, R.A., J.W. MCDONALD & D.D. SCHOEPP. 1994. Distribution and ontogeny of 1S,3R-1-amino-cyclopentane-1,3-dicarboxylic acid sensitive and quisqualate insensitive [^{3}H]-glutamate binding sites in the rat brain. J. Neurochem. **63:** 938–945.

24. SCHOEPP, D.D., B.G. JOHNSON, R.A. WRIGHT, C.R. SALHOFF, N.G. MAYNE, S. WU, S.L. COCKERHAM, J.P. BURNETT, R. BELAGAJE, D. BLEAKMAN & J.A. MONN. 1997. LY354740 is a potent and highly selective group II metabotropic glutamate receptor agonist in cells expressing human glutamate receptors. Neuropharmacology **36:** 1–11.

25. SCHOEPP, D.D., D. LODGE, D. BLEAKMAN, J.D. LEANDER, J.P. TIZZANO, R.A. WRIGHT, A.J. PALMER, C.R. SALHOFF & P.L. ORNSTEIN. 1995. *In vitro* and *in vivo* antagonism of AMPA receptor activation by (3S,4aR,6R,8aR)-6-[2-(1(2)H-tetrazole-5-yl)ethyl] decahydroisoquinaline-3-carboxylic acid. Neuropharmacology **34:** 1159–1168.

26. CHEN, C.-K., F.S. SILVERSTEIN, S.K. FISHER, D. STATMAN & M.V. JOHNSTON. 1988. Perinatal hypoxic-ischemic brain injury enhances quisqualic acid stimulated phosphoinositide turnover. J. Neurochem. **51:** 353–359.

27. SEREN, M.S., C. ALDINIO, R. ZANONI, A. LEON & F. NICOLETTI. 1989. Stimulation of inositol phospholipid hydrolysis by excitatory amino acids is enhanced in brain slices from vulnerable regions after transient global ischaemia. J. Neurochem. **53:** 1700–1705.

28. SCHOEPP, D.D. & P.J. CONN. 1993. Metabotropic glutamate receptors in brain function and pathology. Trends Pharmacol. Sci. **14:** 13–20.

29. CHAVIS, P., J.M. NOONEY, J. BOCKAERT, L. FAGNI, A. FELTZ & J.L. BOSSU. 1995. Facilitatory coupling between a glutamate metabotropic receptor and dihydropyridine-sensitive calcium channels in cultured cerebellar granule cells. J. Neurosci. **15:** 135–143.

30. BATTAGLIA, G., J.A. MONN & D.D. SCHOEPP. 1997. *In vivo* inhibition of veratridine evoked release of striatal excitatory amino acids by the group II metabotropic glutamate receptor agonist LY354740 in rats. Neurosci. Lett. **229:** 161–164.

31. BRUNO, V., G. BATTAGLIA, G. CASABONA, A. COPANI, F. CACGLI & F. NICOLETTI. 1998. Neuroprotection by glial metabotropic glutamate receptors is mediated by transforming growth factor beta. J. Neurosci. **18:** 9594–9600.

NPS 1506, A Novel NMDA Receptor Antagonist and Neuroprotectant

Review of Preclinical and Clinical Studies

ALAN L. MUELLER,[a] LINDA D. ARTMAN, MANUEL F. BALANDRIN, ELLEN BRADY, YONGWEI (ERIC) CHIEN, ERIC G. DELMAR, KAREN GEORGE, ALLISON KIERSTEAD, THOMAS B. MARRIOTT, SCOTT T. MOE, MICHAEL K. NEWMAN, JOANNA L. RASZKIEWICZ, ELIZABETH L. SANGUINETTI, BRADFORD C. VAN WAGENEN, AND DAVID WELLS

NPS Pharmaceuticals, Inc., Salt Lake City, Utah, USA

ABSTRACT: NPS 1506 is a moderate affinity, uncompetitive *N*-methyl-D-aspartate (NMDA) receptor antagonist. NPS 1506 is neuroprotective in rodent models of ischemic stroke, hemorrhagic stroke, and head trauma, with a 2-hr window of opportunity. Neuroprotectant doses of NPS 1506 ranged from approximately 0.1–1.0 mg/kg, with peak plasma concentrations ranging from 8–80 ng/mL. Even at doses producing behavioral toxicity, NPS 1506 did not elicit MK-801-like behaviors, did not generalize to phencyclidine (PCP), and did not elicit neuronal vacuolization.

In a Phase I study, intravenous (i.v.) doses of NPS 1506 from 5–100 mg were well tolerated and provided plasma concentrations in excess of those required for neuroprotection in rodents. Adverse events at the 100-mg dose included mild dizziness and lightheadedness, and mild to moderate ataxia. Neither PCP-like psychotomimetic effects nor cardiovascular effects were noted. The long plasma half-life of NPS 1506 (~60 hr) suggests that a single i.v. dose will provide prolonged neuroprotection in humans.

INTRODUCTION

The *N*-methyl-D-aspartate (NMDA) subtype of glutamate receptor is an attractive target in the search for neuroprotective agents. Competitive and noncompetitive antagonists of NMDA receptors prevent neuronal cell death in various *in vivo* animal models of stroke and head trauma.[1,2] However, the development of NMDA receptor antagonists has been hindered by an unfavorable side effect profile characterized by phencyclidine (PCP)-like psychotomimetic effects, impairment of cognition, and a direct neurotoxic effect termed neuronal vacuolization.[3,4]

NPS 1506 was synthesized as part of an NMDA receptor antagonist medicinal chemistry program based on polyamine-containing spider toxins and diphenylpropylamine-type antihistaminergics and anticholinergics. The compound 3,3-diphenylpropylamine (3,3-DPPA) was discovered in a small-scale screening effort as the

[a]Corresponding author: Alan L. Mueller, Ph.D., NPS Pharmaceuticals, Inc., Salt Lake City, UT 84108. Phone, 801/583-4939; fax, 801/583-4961.
e-mail, amueller@npsp.com

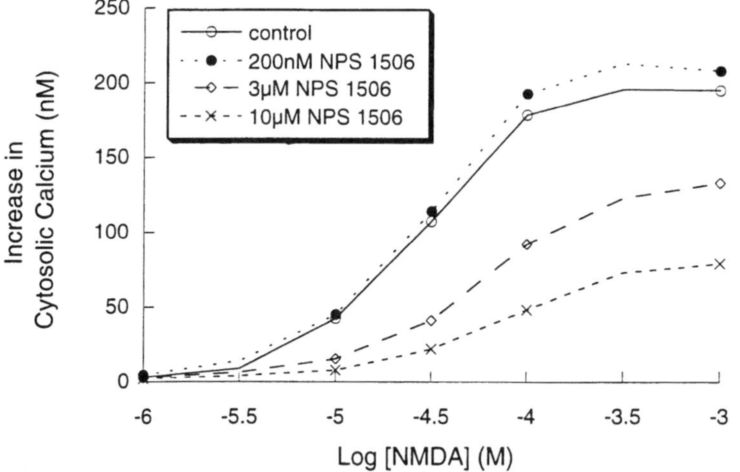

FIGURE 1. Chemical structure of NPS 1506 (hydrochloride salt).

FIGURE 2. Nature of the block of NMDA-induced increases in cytosolic calcium in cultured RCGCs by NPS 1506. The concentration-response curve to NMDA (in the presence of a fixed concentration of 1 µM glycine) was shifted rightward and downward by the addition of increasing concentrations of NPS 1506, indicative of noncompetitive blockade.

initial lead compound possessing moderate affinity for the NMDA receptor.[5] This pharmacophore was rapidly optimized to provide analogs with varying potencies as NMDA receptor antagonists.[5,6] Here we briefly summarize the preclinical profile of NPS 1506, and report our initial Phase I clinical data.

PRECLINICAL PHARMACOLOGY OF NPS 1506

NPS 1506 (FIG. 1) produced a concentration-dependent inhibition of NMDA/glycine-induced increases in cytoplasmic calcium in cultured rat cerebellar granule

TABLE 1. Summary of preclinical neuroprotectant efficacy of NPS 1506

Study	Dosing Regimen	Degree of Neuroprotection	Comments
Temporary focal ischemia (rat MCAO suture model[7]; 2-hr period of ischemia plus 46-hr period of reperfusion)	0.1, 0.3, or 1.0 mg/kg i.v. administered 2 and 6 hr post-occlusion (dose expressed as HCl salt)	32%, 44%, and 48% reduction in infarct volume, respectively	1. 2-hr window of opportunity. 2. Double-dose paradigm more robust and consistent than single-dose paradigm. 3. Neuroprotectant plasma concentrations range from 8–80 ng/mL (C_{max}).
Temporary focal ischemia (rat MCAO suture model[7]; 2-hr period of ischemia plus 46-hr period of reperfusion)	Bolus loading dose plus continuous 8-hr infusion to maintain plasma concentrations of 20 or 80 ng/mL	43% and 57% reduction in infarct volume, respectively	1. 2-hr window of opportunity. 2. Robust and consistent neuroprotection.
Permanent focal ischemia (rat MCAO suture model[7]; 24-hr period of ischemia)	0.3 or 1.0 mg/kg i.v. administered 30 min and 4 hr post-occlusion (dose expressed as free base)	0% and 45% reduction in infarct volume, respectively	1. 1.0 mg/kg dose provided significant neuroprotection in 3 out of 4 separate, independent studies.
Permanent focal ischemia (rat MCAO suture model[7]; 24-hr period of ischemia)	Bolus loading dose plus continuous 24-hr infusion to maintain plasma concentration of 80 ng/mL	No significant neuroprotectant effect	1. Absence of neuroprotectant activity noted in 2 separate, independent studies.
Hemorrhagic stroke (rat; intrastriatal bacterial collagenase model[8])	1.0 mg/kg i.p. administered 1 hr post-collagenase injection (dose expressed as HCl salt)	Significant improvement in brain potassium and sodium content	1. Neuroprotection absent when treatment delayed 4 hours.
Closed head trauma (rat; weight drop method[9])	1.0 mg/kg i.v. administered 1 and 4 hr post-injury (dose expressed as HCl salt)	Significant improvement in brain electrolytes, edema and neurological severity score	1. No behavioral toxicity noted with NPS 1506.
Traumatic brain injury (rat; lateral fluid-percussion model[10])	1.0 mg/kg i.v. administered 0.25 and 4 hr post-injury (dose expressed as free base)	Significant improvement in memory score and CA3 neuron survival	1. No behavioral toxicity noted with NPS 1506.

cells (RCGCs), with an IC_{50} of 476 nM. Inhibition of [^{3}H]MK-801 binding to rat cortical membranes was observed with similar concentrations of NPS 1506 (IC_{50} =

664 nM). Studies in RCGCs demonstrate that the blockade produced by NPS 1506 is noncompetitive with respect to agonist (FIG. 2), and uncompetitive, i.e., the magnitude of block at a single concentration of NPS 1506 increases as the concentration of agonist is increased (data not shown).

Electrophysiological experiments using NMDA receptor subunits recombinantly expressed in *Xenopus* oocytes demonstrate that the block produced by NPS 1506 is both use- and voltage-dependent, consistent with open-channel block. NPS 1506 was equipotent at blocking the various NR2 subunits coexpressed with NR1A, and does not demonstrate subunit selectivity.

NPS 1506 is neuroprotective *in vivo*, as demonstrated in a variety of rodent models (summarized in TABLE 1). In a rat model of temporary focal ischemic stroke, namely, middle cerebral artery occlusion (MCAO) induced by the suture method, the dose of NPS 1506 required for significant neuroprotection ranged from approximately 0.1–1.0 mg/kg. These doses were most effective when administered twice, approximately 3–4 hr apart. Peak plasma concentrations following neuroprotectant dosing regimens were between 8–80 ng/mL. More robust and consistent neuroprotection was provided when NPS 1506 was administered as a bolus loading dose followed by a constant infusion in order to maintain plasma concentrations over an 8-hr period. In this temporary focal ischemia model, NPS 1506 demonstrated a 2-hr window of opportunity.

NPS 1506 was neuroprotective in a rat permanent MCAO occlusion model when administered as two 1-mg/kg intravenous (i.v.) injections, 3–5 hr apart (TABLE 1). This neuroprotectant effect was lost when NPS 1506 was administered as a bolus loading dose followed by a 24-hr constant infusion.

NPS 1506 was neuroprotective in two rat models of traumatic brain injury when administered as two 1-mg/kg bolus i.v. injections, 3–4 hr apart (TABLE 1). The maximum plasma concentrations of NPS 1506 in these studies were estimated to be approximately 80 ng/mL. Lower doses of NPS 1506 were not examined in these models of head injury.

NPS 1506 provided modest neuroprotection in a rat model of intracerebral hemorrhagic stroke, namely, the intrastriatal bacterial collagenase model, when administered as a single 1-mg/kg intraperitoneal (i.p.) dose (TABLE 1). This neuroprotection occurred when NPS 1506 was administered 1 hr after the injection of collagenase, prior to complete hematoma formation. Importantly, NPS 1506 did not worsen outcome in this model of hemorrhagic stroke.

At doses greater than those required for neuroprotection, NPS 1506 did not elicit in rodents the characteristic side effect profile that is typical of potent, noncompetitive open-channel antagonists, such as MK-801. MK-801-like behaviors, such as head weaving or backwards shuffling, were not noted. Rather, the most consistent sign of behavioral toxicity of NPS 1506 in rodents was a whole body tremor that was dose-dependent in terms of onset, severity and duration. This tremor was consistently observed when plasma concentrations of NPS 1506 exceeded 400 ng/mL (see below).

NPS 1506 was evaluated for PCP-like discriminative stimulus effects in rats trained to discriminate PCP from saline. NPS 1506 had no PCP-like effects at doses between 1–5 mg/kg i.p. (FIG. 3). The 5-mg/kg i.p. dose produced a maximum mean 34% PCP-lever response, but this dose was associated with a 40% decrease in overall

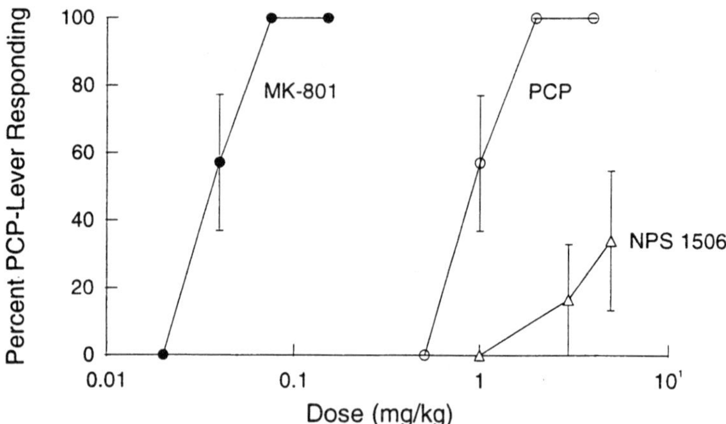

FIGURE 3. Lack of generalization to PCP by NPS 1506. MK-801 potently and dose-dependently substituted for PCP in rats pretrained to discriminate PCP from saline. NPS 1506 had no PCP-like effects at doses between 1–5 mg/kg i.p. (as the HCl salt). The 5-mg/kg i.p. dose produced a maximum mean 34% PCP-lever response, but this dose was associated with a 40% decrease in overall response rate (not shown). Data are expressed as mean ± SEM.

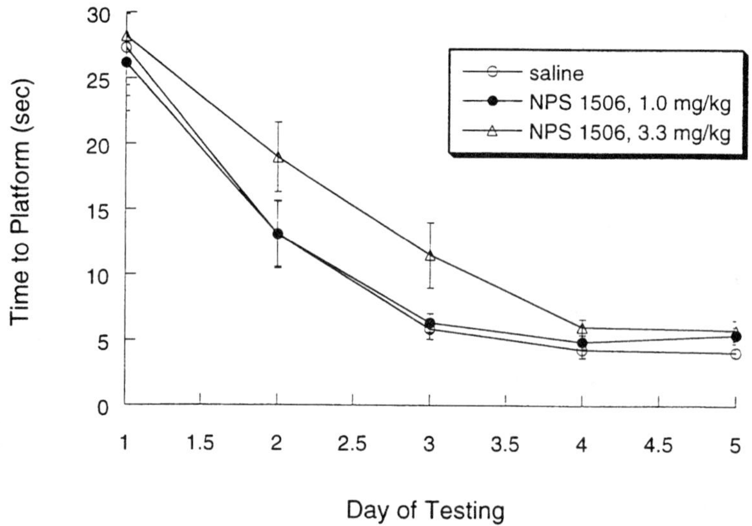

FIGURE 4. Lack of long-lasting impairment of spatial learning by NPS 1506. NPS 1506 (1 mg/kg i.v. as the free base) did not alter normal spatial learning in the Morris water maze. A dose of 3.3 mg/kg i.v. caused a significant slowing of spatial learning. However, performance in the group treated with 3.3 mg/kg NPS 1506 was not different from that in the saline-treated control animals by the final day of training. Data are expressed as mean ± SEM.

response rate. MK-801 fully substituted for PCP at doses of 0.075 and 0.15 mg/kg i.p. that had no effect on overall response rates.

The effects of NPS 1506 on spatial learning in the Morris water maze were examined and compared to those of MK-801. NPS 1506 (1 mg/kg i.v. 20 min before the start of daily training trials) did not alter normal spatial learning in the Morris water maze (FIG. 4). An NPS 1506 dose of 3.3 mg/kg i.v. caused a significant slowing of spatial learning. However, performance in the group treated with 3.3 mg/kg NPS 1506 was not different from that in the saline-treated control animals by the final day of training. In addition, probe trial scores, which demonstrate memory for the platform location, were not different between groups. Thus, at the doses tested, NPS 1506 did not cause a permanent impairment of spatial learning and memory. In contrast, MK-801 (0.1–0.3 mg/kg i.p.) disrupted spatial learning in the Morris water maze task. Importantly, the 0.1-mg/kg dose of MK-801 did not impair performance in a visible platform training task, strongly suggesting that the spatial learning deficit observed at this dose was due to an effect on the memory system itself and not due to sensory or motor impairment.

NPS 1506 was examined for its ability to induce neuronal vacuolization in neurons of rat cingulate and retrosplenial cortices. NPS 1506 (20 mg/kg i.p. or 10 mg/kg i.v.) did not elicit neuronal vacuolization (TABLE 2). In contrast, neuronal vacuolization was produced by the NMDA receptor antagonists, MK-801 (5 mg/kg i.p.) and CNS-1102 (20 or 30 mg/kg i.p.). These results were confirmed and extended in a Good Laboratory Practice (GLP) compliant study using NPS 1506 doses ranging from 1–10 mg/kg i.v. (data not shown).

PRECLINICAL TOXICOLOGY OF NPS 1506

NPS 1506 was examined in a series of GLP-compliant i.v. toxicology studies ranging from single-dose studies to 14-day studies. NPS 1506 was administered i.v. to rats and dogs either as a slow (60-sec) bolus or by continuous infusion. Additionally, the effects of NPS 1506 on the gastrointestinal, renal, cardiovascular, and pulmonary systems were investigated in a series of ancillary pharmacology studies.

The predominant, consistent findings in the single-dose, 60-sec bolus and 24-hr infusion i.v. studies in rats and dogs involved transient central nervous system (CNS)-related events that consisted of whole body tremors (convulsions at high doses), hypertonia, salivation, emesis, hypothermia (rats), hyperpyrexia (dogs), vocalization, and death. The severity and duration of these effects were dose-related but independent of the dosing regimen. No histologic evaluations were performed in these studies.

Repeated bolus-dose studies and continuous infusion studies in rats and dogs have been completed for 7 and 14 days. As in the single-dose studies, the consistent, early systemic finding in these studies was the appearance of tremors and, less frequently, seizures or convulsions, in both species. Other dose-related effects seen in rats were inflammation/necrotizing inflammation at the injection site, hematologic response to inflammation, hypertonia and vocalization. Other than the noted irritation/inflammation at the injection site, there was no histopathological evidence of target-organ toxicity elicited by NPS 1506 in any of these studies. Rats appeared to tolerate the infusion procedure somewhat better than the bolus administration. Salivation, emesis, vocalization, hyperpyrexia, and rigidity were noted in dogs at the higher doses tested.

TABLE 2. Summary of neuronal vacuolization data

Treatment	Incidence of Vacuolization
MK-801 (5 mg/kg i.p.)	vacuoles present in 6 out of 7 rats
CNS-1102 (20 mg/kg i.p.)	vacuoles present in 1 out of 2 rats
CNS-1102 (30 mg/kg i.p.)	vacuoles present in 1 out of 1 rats
NPS 1506 (20 mg/kg i.p.)	vacuoles present in 0 out of 1 rats
NPS 1506 (10 mg/kg i.v.)	vacuoles present in 0 out of 4 rats
Water or saline controls	vacuoles present in 0 out of 3 rats

The no observed adverse effect level (NOAEL) for systemic toxicity in the 7- and 14-day repeated bolus-dose studies in rats was 4.5 and 3.0 mg/kg/day, respectively. In dogs, the NOAEL for systemic toxicity was 2 mg/kg/day for both the 7- and 14-day repeated bolus-dose regimens. Following bolus administration to rats or dogs, the first signs of systemic toxicity were associated with NPS 1506 plasma concentrations greater than 400 ng/mL.

The NOAEL for systemic toxicity in the 7- and 14-day continuous infusion studies in rats was 10 mg/kg/day. In dogs, the NOAEL for systemic toxicity was 3.0 mg/kg/day for both the 7- and 14-day continuous infusion studies. Consistent with the findings from the 7- and 14-day bolus dose studies, observations of systemic toxicity were associated with NPS 1506 plasma concentrations greater than 400 ng/mL.

NPS 1506 was also evaluated in other GLP-compliant toxicology studies. NPS 1506 did not cause hemolysis in human, dog, or rat blood at final concentrations of 50 μg/mL and below. Frank hemolysis was evident at final concentrations greater than 50 μg/mL, which is significantly higher than the maximum plasma concentrations expected in clinical trials. NPS 1506 was not mutagenic in an Ames assay, mouse lymphoma cell assay, or an *in vivo* mouse micronucleus assay. In addition, NPS 1506 did not cause delayed-type hypersensitivity in mice, did not cause protein flocculation in human, dog, or rat serum or plasma, and had no effect on platelet aggregation in whole blood at concentrations up to 30 μg/mL.

PHASE I CLINICAL STUDY OF NPS 1506

The initial Phase I study of NPS 1506 was a double-blind, placebo-controlled, ascending-dose tolerability and pharmacokinetic study in healthy male volunteers (age 18–40, weight 60–90 kg). NPS 1506 was administered as a single i.v. infusion at rates ranging from 1.0–2.67 mg/min. Doses of NPS 1506 from 5–100 mg were well tolerated and provided plasma concentrations in excess of those required for neuroprotection in rodents. Adverse events noted at the 100-mg dose included mild dizziness and lightheadedness, and mild to moderate ataxia. Importantly, neither PCP-like psychotomimetic effects nor cardiovascular effects were noted. NPS 1506 has a very large volume of distribution at steady-state (V_{ss}) of approximately 17 L/kg, consistent with extensive distribution throughout the body. The long terminal plasma half-life (~60 hr) suggests that a single i.v. dose is sufficient to provide prolonged neuroprotection.

SUMMARY AND CONCLUSIONS

NPS 1506 is a moderate-affinity, uncompetitive NMDA receptor antagonist. The compound is neuroprotective in a variety of animal models of stroke and head injury, and has a side effect profile in preclinical studies distinct from that of potent open-channel blockers such as MK-801. NPS 1506 is well tolerated in man at doses (plasma concentrations) shown to be neuroprotective in rodents. The clinical development of NPS 1506 as an acute use neuroprotectant is ongoing.

ACKNOWLEDGMENTS

We are grateful to the following investigators for their collaborative studies carried out on NPS 1506: Keith Williams, oocyte electrophysiology; Gary Rosenberg, rat model of intracerebral hemorrhagic stroke; Yoram Shapira, rat model of closed head injury; Doug Smith, rat lateral fluid-percussion injury model of head injury; Greg Rose, Morris water maze; Robert Balster, PCP discrimination; and Tom Parks, neuronal vacuolization.

REFERENCES

1. GINSBERG, M.D. 1993. Emerging strategies for the treatment of ischemic brain injury. *In* Molecular and Cellular Approaches to the Treatment of Neurological Disease. S.G. Waxman, Ed.: 207–237. Raven Press. New York.
2. SMITH, D.H., K. CASEY & T.K. MCINTOSH. 1995. Pharmacologic therapy for traumatic brain injury: experimental approaches. N. Horizons **3:** 562–572.
3. WILLETTS, J., R.L. BALSTER & J.D. LEANDER. 1990. The behavioral pharmacology of NMDA receptor antagonists. Trends Pharmacol. Sci. **11:** 423–428.
4. OLNEY, J.W., J. LABRUYERE & M.T. PRICE. 1989. Pathological changes induced in cerebrocortical neurons by phencyclidine and related drugs. Science **244:** 1360–1362.
5. BALANDRIN, M.F., B.C. VAN WAGENEN, E.G. DELMAR, L.D. ARTMAN & A.L. MUELLER. 1996. Discovery, design and *in vitro* biological evaluation of NPS 846 and its congeners: novel NMDA receptor antagonists. Presented at the 37th Annual Meeting of the American Society of Pharmacognosy, #O–19, Santa Cruz, CA, July 30, 1996.
6. VAN WAGENEN, B.C., M.F. BALANDRIN, E.G. DELMAR, L.D. ARTMAN & A.L. MUELLER. 1996. Design, synthesis, and biological evaluation of NPS 846 hydrochloride, a novel antagonist at the NMDA receptor. Presented at the 212th National Meeting of the American Chemical Society, ORGN 273, Orlando, FL, August 28, 1996.
7. ZEA LONGA, E., P.R. WEINSTEIN, S. CARLSON & R. CUMMINS. 1989. Reversible middle cerebral artery occlusion without craniectomy in rats. Stroke **20:** 84–91.
8. ROSENBERG, G.A., S. MUN-BYCE, M. WESLEY & M. KORNFELD. 1990. Collagenase-induced intracerebral hemorrhage in rats. Stroke **21:** 801–807.
9. SHAPIRA, Y., A.A. ARTRU & A.M. LAM. 1992. Ketamine decreases cerebral infarct volume and improves neurological outcome following experimental head trauma in rats. J. Neurosurg. Anesth. **4:** 231–240.
10. SMITH, D.H., K. OKIYAMA, T.A. GENNARELLI & T.K. MCINTOSH. 1993. Magnesium and ketamine attenuate cognitive dysfunction following experimental brain injury. Neurosci. Lett. **157:** 211–214.

Questions and Answers

QUESTION FOR DR. NARAHASHI

From Dr. Obrenovitch

Do you have any data or possible effects of MS-153 on K^+ channels, as these channels can also be modulated by PKC?

ANSWER: No data are available on the effect of MS-153 on K^+ channels.

QUESTIONS FOR DR. KINGSTON

From Dr. Bowyer

Is there an additive neuroprotective effect when mGlu1/5 receptor antagonists are combined with mGlu2/3 receptor agonists?

ANSWER: We haven't tested the combined effects of a group I mGlu antagonist with a group II mGlu agonist *in vitro* yet. However, I would anticipate an additive neuroprotective effect, given that each of the agents would be acting on different groups of metabotropic receptors, which mediate their effects through different signal transduction pathways and cellular mechanisms.

From Dr. Vornov

Have you examined the effects of glia on the staurosporine-induced cell death?

ANSWER: Not yet. We are proposing that group II agonists may mediate their effects via one or more mechanisms, for example: presynaptically via reduction of glutamate release; induction of neuroprotective factor from glial cells and/or activation of protective intracellular biochemical pathway in neurons. It is conceivable that different neuroprotective mechanisms may be differentially more effective depending on the neurodegenerative insult/conditions. It would be interesting, therefore, to see whether glial cells participate in preventing apoptotically driven cell death as we have shown for neuronal excitotoxicity.

QUESTIONS FOR DR. MARINI

From Dr. Bachurin

Is the mechanism that you proposed for explanation of the NMDA (subtoxic doses) neuroprotective effect also realized in the case of NMDA-receptor antagonist neurotoxic effects?

ANSWER: It is certainly possible that physiological concentrations of glutamate in brain prevent neuronal cell death. The neuronal cell death due to NMDA receptor antagonist may be due to the absence of NMDA receptor stimulation by glutamate.

From Dr. Abbracchio

First, is this BDNF autocrine loop also present in hippocampal neurons? And, second, can BDNF protect cells from any other toxic stimulus besides NMDA (e.g., radical generating agents)?

ANSWER: It is possible that this autocrine loop also exists in the hippocampus.

QUESTION FOR DR. MUELLER

From Dr. Slikker

Have you assessed brain levels of your agent in human by noninvasive techniques such as a NMR spectroscopy as has been done for fluoxetine?

ANSWER: No, we have not. Your suggestion is an excellent one, and the chemical structure of NPS 1506 would most probably allow for such studies.

QUESTION FOR DR. PALMER

From Dr. Narahashi

If I heard correctly, the AR compound blocks the glutamate receptor in a use-dependent manner. Were control experiments performed to see whether this blocking action was due to a slow action of the AR compound? In other words, did the block progress slowly when the compound was applied to the bath without ligand stimulation?

ANSWER: As far as I know, Dr. Morely's group indicated that the block was relatively rapid—unblocking proceeded even more rapidly. This has been published.[1,2]

From Dr. Mueller

You are developing the *S*-isomer of 15896. What are your reasons for this choice?

ANSWER: The *S*-enantiomer had a better pharmacological/pharmacokinetic profile; it was more potent *in vivo*, it was more potent regarding inhibition of NMDA-induced depolarization in rat hippocampal tissue slices *in vitro*; its therapeutic index was much better. We have reported some of these data.[3]

QUESTIONS FOR DR. VORNOV

From Dr. Mueller

What plasma concentrations of GPI 5000 are required for neuroprotection *in vivo*? What are the corresponding brain levels?

ANSWER: We have been investigating the pharmacokinetics of GPI 5000 (2-PMPA) and related NAALADase inhibitors. We know that penetration into the brain is low; less than 1% of an administered dose gets to the brain. The doses needed for neuroprotection are consistent with this low brain penetration.

From Dr. Bowyer

Did you determine the effects of the NAALadase inhibitors on either taurine of glycine in microdialysis after ischemia?

ANSWER: The effect looks relatively specific for excitatory amino acids. Glutamate and aspartate are almost completely attenuated, while taurine and glutamine tended to be reduced also, but the change was not statistically significant. The GABA levels were not large enough to measure consistently in the experiments.

From Dr. Skaper

NAAG has been shown to inhibit NMDA neurotoxicity *in vitro*, as well as physiological actions of NMDA *in vitro*. Would long-term blockage of NAAG metabolism have possible deleterious effects on NMDA receptor function, e.g., behavior/memory, etc.?

ANSWER: We've looked specifically for the behavioral and neurodegenerative effects of NMDA receptor antagonists and have not seen any.

From Dr. Skaper

Canavan's disease is a hereditary disorder of dysmyelination, characterized by elevated levels of NAA and NAAG in body fluids, including CSF. Have you considered the long-term consequences of inhibiting NAAG metabolism in this respect? While NAAG and NAA have not been clearly integrated into Canavan neuropathology, drugs that cause prolonged tissue elevations of NAAG could (conceivably) cause deleterious neurological consequences.

ANSWER: So far, we've observed only neuroprotective effects of NAALADase inhibition. We've speculated that NAALADase inhibitors might have positive effects in Canavan's disease by shunting toxic NAA to NAAG possibly enhancing other pathways for NAA elimination from cells. We have no data, however.

COMMENT to Dr. Bowyer from Dr. Vornov on NAA accumulation in Caravan's disease: Deficient hydrolysis of NAA may be deleterious to developing CNS because of NAA neurotoxicity, but also through reduced availability of acetyl groups necessary by myelination.

From Dr. Obrenovitch

Could you comment on the possibility that the reduction of glutamate efflux during ischemia by 2-PMPA is too marked to be solely explained by NAALADase inhibition? Indeed your data would imply that most of glutamate released during ischemia originates from NAAO hydrolysis. This is not compatible with the fact that the magnitude of NAA release during ischemia is much less than that of glutamate.

ANSWER: The dramatic effects of NAALADase inhibitors on ischemic glutamate release certainly suggest that NAAG may be an important source of glutamate. However, with inhibition of the enzyme during occlusion, we don't see large amounts of NAAG replacing the glutamate, so we can't conclude that extracellular NAAG is the source of extracellular glutamate. The effect must be more complicated than that.

REFERENCES

1. BLACK, M., T. LANTHORN, D. SMALL, G. MEALING, V. LAM & P. MORLEY. 1996. Study of potency, kinetics of block and toxicity of NMDA receptor antagonists using fura-2. Eur. J. Pharmacol. **317:** 377–381.
2. MEALING, G.A., T.H. LANTHORN, D.L. SMALL, M.A. BLACK, N.B. LAFERRIERE & P. MORLEY. 1997. Antagonism of N-methyl-D-aspartate-evoked currents in rat cortical cultures by ARL 15896AR. J. Pharmacol. Exp. Ther. **281:** 376–383.
3. PALMER, G.C., R.J. MURRAY, C.L. CRAMER *et al.* 1999. [S]-AR-R 15896AR—a novel anticonvulsant: acute safety, pharmacokinetic and pharmacodynamic properties. J. Pharmacol. Exp. Ther. **288:** 121–132.

Peroxynitrite Scavengers for the Acute Treatment of Traumatic Brain Injury

EDWARD D. HALL,[a] NANCY C. KUPINA, AND JOHN S. ALTHAUS

*Neuroscience Therapeutics, Parke-Davis Pharmaceutical Research,
Ann Arbor, Michigan, USA*

ABSTRACT: Recent evidence has suggested that the superoxide and nitric oxide-derived reactive oxygen species peroxynitrite (ONOO⁻) may play a significant role in the acute pathophysiology of brain injury. One pharmacological mechanism by which ONOO⁻-mediated damage might be interrupted is by the administration of scavenging compounds such as the thiol-containing compound penicillamine. In the present study, we examined the ability of either penicillamine (Pen) or the more brain penetrable penicillamine methyl ester (PenME) (0.01, 0.1, 1.0 or 10.0 mg/kg i.v. 5 min post-injury) to improve the early (1 hr) neurological recovery (grip score) of male CF-1 mice after a severe (900 g-cm; 50 g × 18 cm) injury. Pen produced a dose-related improvement in grip score. At 1.0 mg/kg, a +112% improvement was observed compared to vehicle-treated mice, and at 10.0 mg/kg, the increase was +168% (both, $p < 0.05$). PenME more potently improved the 1-hr grip score, but the magnitude of the optimal effect (+96% at 0.1 mg/kg; $p < 0.02$) was no greater than that observed with Pen, which largely remains in the cerebral microvasculature. These results are consistent with a role of ONOO⁻ in acute head injury, but suggest that microvascular scavenging may be of primary therapeutic importance during the early post-traumatic period.

INTRODUCTION

Increasing experimental evidence is indicating that the reactive oxygen species peroxynitrite (ONOO⁻) plays a significant role in the acute pathophysiology of traumatic brain injury. Peroxynitrite is formed from the reaction of superoxide anion, which arises from a number of biological sources, with enzymatically-derived nitric oxide.[1,2] As shown in FIGURE 1, ONOO⁻ can give rise to potently reactive species that can cause cellular damage. FIGURE 2 illustrates the fact that ONOO⁻ can oxidatively injure cellular lipids (lipid peroxidation), proteins (nitration, hydroxylation, sulfhydryl oxidation, dimerization) and nucleic acids (fragmentation).

Much of the evidence implying a role of ONOO⁻ in acute head injury has been derived from studies with the mouse concussive (impact-acceleration) head injury model.[3] For instance, by using this paradigm, a post-traumatic increase in brain lev-

[a]Corresponding author: Edward D. Hall, Ph.D., Neuroscience Therapeutics, Parke-Davis Pharmaceutical Research, 2800 Plymouth Road, Ann Arbor, MI 48105. Phone, 734/622-7346; fax, 734/622-7178.

e-mail, edward.hall@wl.com

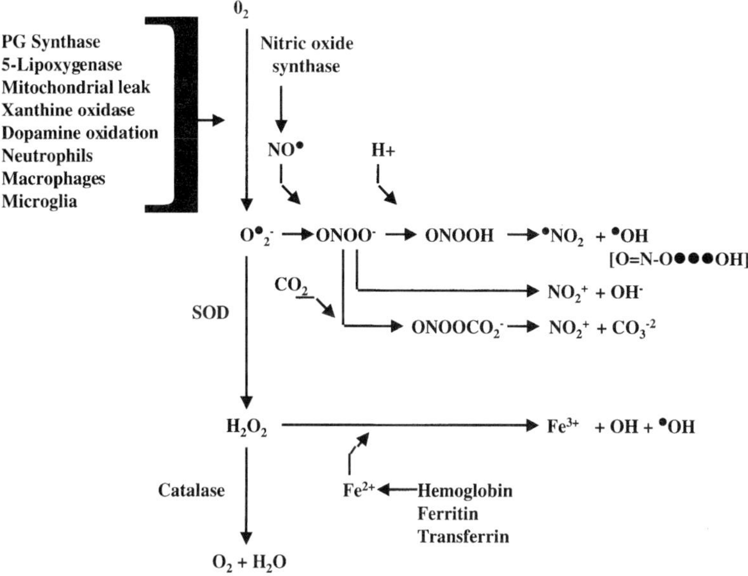

FIGURE 1. Chemistry of peroxynitrite formation and its generation of highly reactive free radical species. Superoxide radical ($O_2{}^-$) is produced by a number of potential biological sources after traumatic brain injury. It can be dismutated by superoxide dismutase (SOD) to hydrogen peroxide (H_2O_2), which can undergo an iron-catalyzed decomposition to give rise to hydroxyl radical ($\cdot OH$). On the other hand, superoxide can react with nitric oxide ($NO\cdot$) to form peroxynitrite anion ($ONOO^-$), which at physiological pH exists largely as the protonated peroxynitrous acid (ONOOH). This can generate oxidative tissue damage either by decomposition to $\cdot OH$ and nitrogen dioxide ($\cdot NO_2$) or more likely via a caged species (O=N-O$\cdots$OH). Alternatively, $ONOO^-$ can react with CO_2 to form the reactive species $NO_2{}^+$, which can nitrate tyrosine residues, and $CO_3{}^{-2}$.

els of $ONOO^-$-generated nitrotyrosine has recently been demonstrated.[4] Furthermore, pharmacological inhibitors of nitric oxide synthase (e.g., L-nitro-arginine methyl ester; 7-nitroindazole) have been shown to improve the neurological recovery of head-injured mice.[5] The effective nitric oxide synthase (NOS) inhibitor doses coincidentally produce a reduction in post-traumatic brain nitrotyrosine levels[4] consistent with the therapeutic effect being associated with an attenuation in traumatically-generated $ONOO^-$.

Another pharmacological mechanism by which $ONOO^-$-mediated damage might be interrupted is via the administration of compounds such as penicillamine that are capable of scavenging this species.[6] FIGURE 3 illustrates the reaction mechanism by which penicillamine can chemically scavenge $ONOO^-$. In the present study, we examined the ability of either penicillamine (Pen) or the more brain-penetrable penicillamine methyl ester (PenME) to improve the early neurological recovery of male CF-1 mice after a severe concussive head injury.

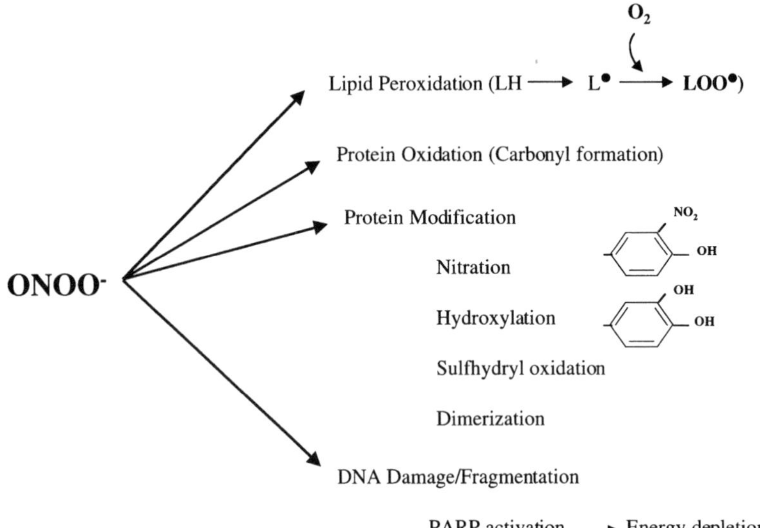

FIGURE 2. Mechanisms of oxidative cellular injury by peroxynitrite including lipid peroxidation, protein oxidative modification (carbonyl formation, nitration, hydroxylation, sulfhydryl oxidation and dimerization) and DNA fragmentation leading to the activation of energy depleting enzyme poly-ADP ribose polymerase (PARP).

MATERIALS AND METHODS

The mouse concussive (impact-acceleration) head injury model has been described in detail elsewhere.[3] Briefly, unanesthetized male CF-1 mice (Charles River, Portage, MI) were subjected to a severe 900 g-cm (50 g × 18 cm) weight-drop cranial trauma. Within 5 min after injury, mice were treated with an i.v. (tail vein) injection (0.1 ml volume) of either vehicle (0.9% saline), d-penicillamine (0.1, 1.0 or 10 mg/kg; Sigma Chem. Co.) or d-penicillamine methyl ester (0.01, 0.1, 1.0 or 10.0 mg/kg). At 1 hr post-injury, the mice underwent a grip test, which examined their ability to hold on to a taut string with a 30-sec maximum. The average time that the mice in each treatment group could remain on the string was calculated. Statistical comparison of drug-treated mice with vehicle-treated animals was carried out using a one-way analysis of variance followed by post-hoc t-tests (unpaired). In addition, the incidence of mice that could remain on the string for 5 sec or less (severely impaired) or that held onto the string for the full 30 sec (mildly impaired) was determined and compared by Chi square testing. Moreover, the incidence of mice that were unable to pull their hindlimbs on to the string (paretic) were compared. The neurological assessments were conducted in a blinded fashion with the experimenter unaware of which animals received vehicle or drug. All data are expressed as mean ± SE.

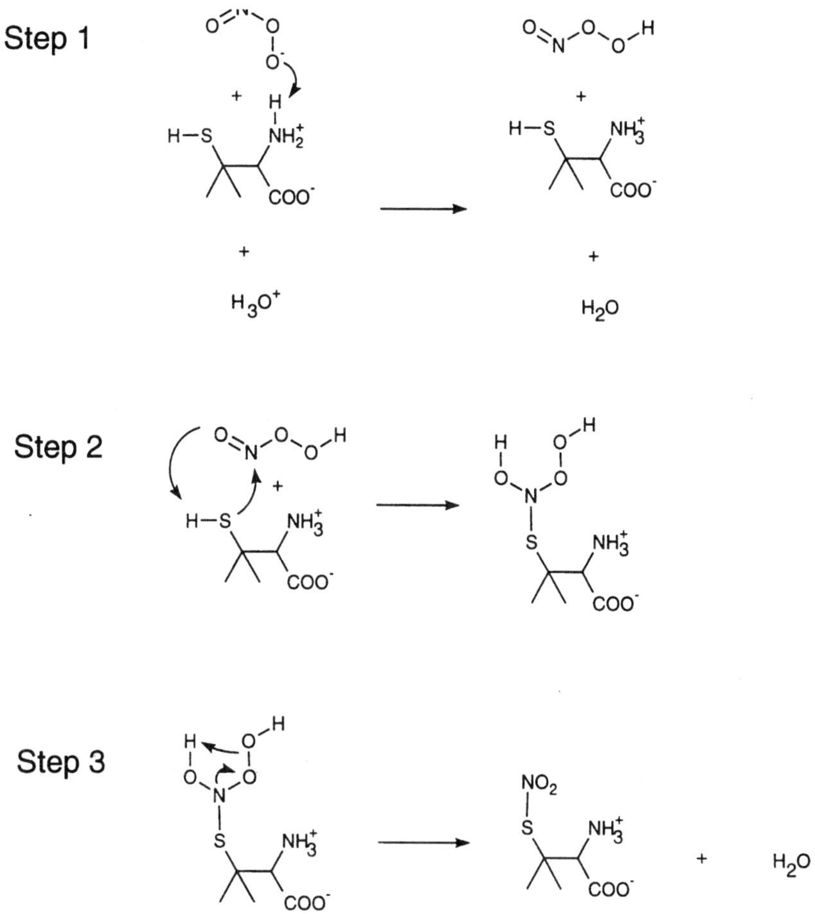

FIGURE 3. Reaction mechanism by which penicillamine can scavenge peroxynitrite anion. *Step 1*. Peroxynitrite anion is attracted to the positive charge of the amino group of penicillamine. A proton is transferred onto peroxynitrite yielding peroxynitrous acid which adopts a more stable yet more reactive conformation. *Step 2*. Peroxynitrous acid forms a covalent bond with penicillamine. *Step 3*. A rearrangement occurs with the transfer of the a proton to the terminal oxygen weakening the peroxyl linkage. This bond then breaks with water eventually being formed. The resulting structure is nitro-penicillamine. By this mechanism, the scavenging mechanism is stoichiometric (i.e., 1 mole of penicillamine can only react with 1 mole of peroxynitrite).

RESULTS

As shown in FIGURE 4A, acute administration of Pen produced a dose-related improvement in the 1-hr post-injury grip score in mice subjected to severe concussive head injury. Doses of 1 or 10 mg/kg i.v. were significantly effective. A 0.1 mg/kg dose also improved the grip score, but did not quite reach statistical significance.

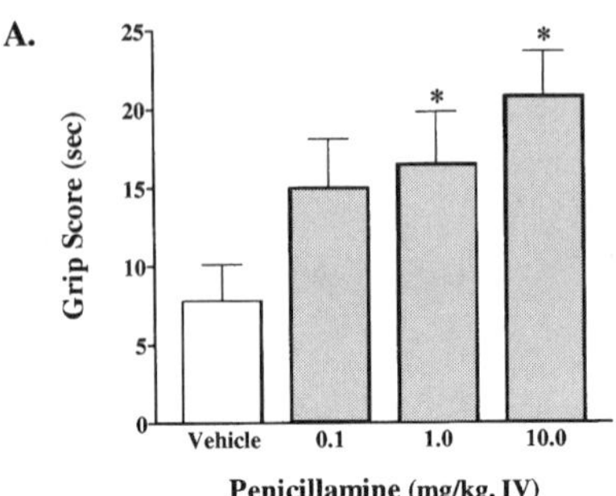

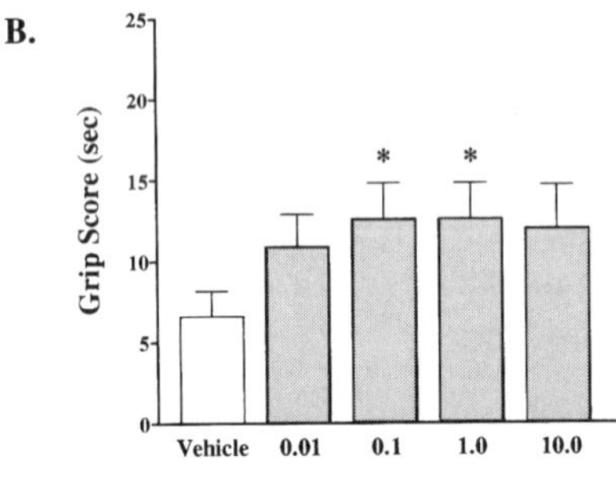

FIGURE 4. Dose-response curves showing the ability of i.v. penicillamine **(A)** or penicillamine methyl ester **(B)** to improve the neurological recovery of severely brain-injured mice ($n = 20$–36 mice/group). *Asterisk* indicates p <0.05 compared to vehicle-treated group.

In FIGURE 4B it is seen that the more brain-penetrable PenME[7] also produced an increase in the 1-hr grip score. However, it was more potent in this regard, since a 0.1-mg/kg i.v. dose was significantly effective. On the other hand, a comparison of the magnitude of the increase in the grip score shows that if anything, the less brain-penetrable (i.e., microvascularly localized) Pen produces a slightly greater maximal improvement in neurological recovery (+168% at 10 mg/kg) than PenME (+96%).

TABLE 1. Effect of penicillamine methyl ester on early (1-hr) neurological recovery of severely head injured male CF-1 mice

Dose mg/kg i.v.	n	% Severe 0–5 sec	% Mild 30 sec	% Paretic	Grip Score sec ± SEM
Vehicle	36	69.4	5.6	75.0	6.6 ± 1.6
0.01	31	45.2*	19.4	61.3	10.9 ± 2.0
0.1	30	36.7*	26.7*	36.7*	12.6 ± 2.2**
1.0	35	45.7*	31.4*	48.6*	12.6 ± 2.2**
10.0	21	42.9*	23.8*	42.9*	12.0 ± 2.7

*$p < 0.05$ by Chi square vs vehicle. **$p < 0.05$ by ANOVA.

TABLE 1 displays a more complete analysis of the improvement in early recovery by PenME. In addition to improving the mean grip score at 0.1 and 1.0 mg/kg, PenME also produced a dose-related decrease in the incidence of severely impaired mice (i.e., those unable to hold onto the grip string for more than 5 sec) and an increase in mildly impaired mice (i.e., those able to remain on the string for the full 30-sec test period), and the drug lessened the incidence of hindlimb paresis (i.e., mice that were unable to pull their hindlimbs onto the string).

CONCLUSIONS

Penicillamine and PenME are reasonably effective sulfhydryl-based scavengers of the peroxynitrite anion ($ONOO^-$).[6] The former has little or no ability to penetrate the blood-brain barrier in contrast to the highly penetrable PenME.[7] However, both compounds acted to improve the early neurological recovery of severely head-injured mice. The mechanism of these effects is most likely due to scavenging of injury-triggered $ONOO^-$. On the other hand, Pen produced a quantitatively greater increase in the 1-hr grip score than PenME.

Since the less brain-permeable Pen produced a greater effect than the more brain-permeable PenME, this suggests that microvascularly generated $ONOO^-$ is critically involved in the early phase of post-traumatic oxidative pathophysiology. Indeed, it has been proposed that $ONOO^-$ generated from vascularly- or perivascularly-derived nitric oxide and superoxide may exert a multifaceted role in microvascular dysfunction in a number of critical care situations.[1] Consistent with this notion, perivascular peroxynitrite-induced 3-nitrotyrosine immunostaining has been observed in the presently employed traumatic brain injury model[4] and a rat model of neonatal ischemia-reperfusion injury.[8] Furthermore, we have shown previously that the 21-aminosteroid antioxidant tirilazad, which is highly localized in cerebrovascular endothelium,[9] is potently effective at improving neurological recovery in the mouse severe brain injury model.[10] This supports the concept that compounds that selectively protect the microvasculature from reactive oxygen damage can exert a beneficial effect in severe brain injury. However, further study is needed to demonstrate that microvascular damage by $ONOO^-$ is indeed an early event and that penicillamine or other selective scavengers lessen it, together with an improvement in neurological recovery.

REFERENCES

1. BECKMAN, J.S. 1991. The double-edged role of nitric oxide in brain function and superoxide-mediated injury. J. Dev. Physiol. **15:** 53–59.
2. BECKMAN, J.S., D. WINK & J.P. CROW. 1996. Nitric oxide and peroxynitrite. *In* Methods in Nitric Oxide Research. M. Feelisch & J.S. Stamler, Eds.: 61–70. John Wiley & Sons, Inc. New York.
3. HALL, E.D. 1995. The mouse head injury model: utility in the discovery of acute cerebroprotective agents. *In* Central Nervous System Trauma Research Techniques. S.T. Ohnishi & T. Ohnishi, Eds.: 213–223. CRC Press. Boca Raton, FL.
4. MESENGE, C., C. CHARRIAULT-MARLANGUE, C. VERRECHIA, M. ALLIX, R.R. BOULU & M. PLOTKINE. Reduction of tyrosine nitration after *N*-nitro-L-arginine methylester treatment of mice with traumatic brain injury. Eur. J. Pharmacol. In press.

5. MESENGE, C., C. VERRECHIA, M. ALLIX, R.R. BOULU & M. PLOTKINE. 1996. Reduction of neurological deficit in mice with traumatic brain injury by nitric oxide synthase inhibitors. J. Neurotrauma **13:** 209–214.

6. ALTHAUS, J.S., T.T. OIEN, G.J. FICI, H.M. SCHERCH, V.H. SETHY & P.F. VONVOIGTLANDER. 1994. Structure activity relationships of peroxynitrite scavengers: an approach to nitric oxide neurotoxicity. Res. Commun. Chem. Pathol. Pharmacol. **83:** 243–254.

7. ALTHAUS, J.S., P.K. ANDRUS, E.D. HALL & P.F. VONVOIGTLANDER. 1995. Improvements in the salicylate trapping method for measurement of hydroxyl radical levels in the brain. *In* Central Nervous System Trauma Research Techniques. S.T. Ohnishi & T. Ohnishi, Eds.: 437–444. CRC Press. Boca Raton, FL.

8. COEROLI, L., S. RENOLLEAU, S. ARNAUD, D. PLOTKINE, N. CACHIN, M. PLOTKINE, Y. BEN-ARI & C. CHARRIAULT-MARLANGUE. 1998. Nitric oxide production and perivascular tyrosine nitration following focal ischemia in neonatal rat. J. Neurochem. **70:** 2516–2525.

9. AUDUS, K.L., F.L. GUILLOT & J.M. BRAUGHLER. 1991. Evidence for 21-aminosteroid association with the hydrophobic domains of brain microvessel endothelial cells. Free Radical Biol. Med. **11:** 361–371.

10. HALL, E.D. 1997. Lazaroids: mechanisms of action and implications for disorders of the CNS. Neuroscientist **3:** 42–51.

Regional Cytokine, Cytokine Receptor and Neuropeptide mRNA Changes Associated with Behavioral and Neuroanatomical Abnormalities in Persistent, Noninflammatory Virus Infection of Neonatal Rats

CARLOS R. PLATA-SALAMÁN,[a] SERGEY E. ILYIN,[a] DAVE GAYLE,[a] ANNA ROMANOVITCH,[a] AND KATHRYN M. CARBONE[b,c,d]

[a]*Division of Molecular Biology, School of Life and Health Sciences, University of Delaware, Newark, Delaware, USA*

[b]*Laboratory of Pediatric and Respiratory Viral Diseases, DVP, OVRR, CBER, Food and Drug Administration, Rockville, Maryland, USA*

[c]*Johns Hopkins University School of Medicine, Baltimore, Maryland, USA*

Borna disease virus (BDV) replicates in brain cells. The rat neonatally infected with BDV becomes persistently infected and, in the setting of minimal encephalitis, develops developmental-neuromorphological abnormalities, specific neuronal cytolysis, and multiple behavioral and physiological alterations. We measured levels of interleukin-1β (IL-1β) receptor antagonist, tumor necrosis factor-α (TNFα), transforming growth factor-β1 (TGFβ1), IL-1 receptor type 1, IL-1 receptor accessory proteins I and II, glycoprotein 130, and various neuropeptide mRNAs in the cerebellum, parieto-frontal cortex, hippocampus and hypothalamus of neonatally BDV-infected rats at 7 and 28 days post infection. The data show that cytokine and neuropeptide mRNA components are abnormal and differentially modulated in brain regions. This evidence suggests that brain-cell-derived cytokines are involved in virus-related neurodevelopmental diseases, even in the absence of a strong inflammatory response. Furthermore, our results indicate that antiinflammatory treatments may be beneficial in virus-associated central nervous system degenerative disease even when not associated with clinical or pathological evidence of encephalitis.

[d]Corresponding author: Kathryn Carbone, HFM 460 FDA, 14401 Rockville Pike, Rockville, MD 20852. Phone, 301/827-1973; fax, 301/480-5679.
e-mail, carbonek@cber.fda.gov

Development of a Nonhuman Primate Model for Studying the Consequences of Long-Term Neuroprotectant Administration on Complex Brain Functions in Developing Animals

MERLE G. PAULE,[a] E. JON POPKE, EDWIN PEARSON, AND TIM HAMMOND

Division of Neurotoxicology, National Center for Toxicological Research/FDA, Jefferson, Arkansas, USA

Dizocilipine (MK-801) is a noncompetitive antagonist at the *N*-methyl-D-aspartate (NMDA) receptor that is thought to exhibit anxiolytic, anticonvulsant, and neuro-protective properties. The NMDA receptor is thought to play a critical role in the neural phenomenon of long-term potentiation (LTP): a substantial increase in synaptic efficiency. It is generally believed that the mechanisms involved with the production and maintenance of LTP are intimately involved with learning and memory processes. Additionally, excitatory amino acids (EAAs) play important roles during development by regulating neuronal survival, axonal and dendritic structure, and synaptic genesis and plasticity. In humans there are also marked differences in EAA binding sites from the neonatal period on into the 10th decade of life, observations which have led to the speculation that infant brains may be more responsive to agents that affect NMDA receptor function than are adult brains. The purpose of the present experiment is to examine the effects of long-term exposure to this prototypic neuroprotectant on the ability of juvenile rhesus monkeys to learn how to perform several of the complex behavioral tasks contained in the National Center for Toxicological Research Operant Test Battery (NCTR OTB). Since compounds that interact with NMDA receptors are likely to have multiple therapeutic applications in a variety of patient populations, it is only prudent to assess the potential impact of chronic NMDA receptor modulation on important aspects of brain function and development. The NCTR OTB contains behavioral tasks thought to depend on specific brain functions including short-term memory; learning; color and position discrimination; and motivation. The similarity in OTB performance between monkeys and children is of particular importance with regard to extrapolating to humans the neurobehavioral (and possibly neurotoxic) effects of drugs and toxicants as determined in the monkey model.

[a]Corresponding author: Merle G. Paule, Division of Neurotoxicology, NCTR/FDA, 3900 NCTR Road, Jefferson, AR 72079-9502. Phone, 870/543-7203; fax, 870/543-7745. e-mail, mpaule@nctr.fda.gov

Melatonin as a Pharmacological Agent against Neuronal Loss in Experimental Models of Huntington's Disease, Alzheimer's Disease and Parkinsonism

RUSSEL J. REITER,[a] JAVIER CABRERA, ROSA M. SAINZ, JUAN CARLOS MAYO, LUCIEN C. MANCHESTER, AND DUN-XIAN TAN

Department of Cellular and Structural Biology, The University of Texas Health Science Center, San Antonio, Texas, USA

ABSTRACT: This review summarizes the experimental findings related to the neuroprotective role of melatonin. In particular, it focuses on research directed at models of Huntington's disease, Alzheimer's disease and Parkinsonism. Melatonin has been shown to be highly effective in reducing oxidative damage in the central nervous system; this efficacy derives from its ability to directly scavenge a number of free radicals and to function as an indirect antioxidant. In particular, melatonin detoxifies the highly toxic hydroxyl radical as well as the peroxyl radical, peroxynitrite anion, nitric oxide, and singlet oxygen, all of which can damage macromolecules in brain cells. Additionally, melatonin stimulates a variety of antioxidative enzymes including superoxide dismutase, glutathione peroxidase and glutathione reductase. One additional advantage melatonin has in reducing oxidative damage in the central nervous system is the ease with which to crosses the blood-brain barrier. This combination of actions makes melatonin a highly effective pharmacological agent against free radical damage. The role of physiological levels of melatonin in forestalling oxidative damage in the brain is currently being tested.

INTRODUCTION

The inability of molecular repair mechanisms to cope with the incessant destruction of essential macromolecules by free radicals is believed to contribute to neuronal loss during aging and to age-related dementias. While the brain is by no means the only organ that takes abuse from free radicals, there are a number of reasons why cellular destruction in the central nervous system (CNS) exceeds that in other organs. The brain utilizes for regular metabolic activities a disproportionately large amount of ground state oxygen (O_2). Since O_2 is a major source of destructive free radicals, it is obvious that the CNS sustains more than the usual amounts of oxidative abuse.[1,2] Also, the brain is relatively ill-equipped with antioxidative processes and has a barrier, the so-called blood-brain barrier, which limits the entrance of certain

[a]Corresponding author: Russel J. Reiter, Ph.D., Professor, Cellular and Structural Biology, Mail Code 7762, The University of Texas Health Science Center, 7703 Floyd Curl Drive, San Antonio, TX 78229-3900. Phone, 210/567-3859; fax, 210/567-6948.
e-mail, Reiter@uthscsa.edu

antioxidants, e.g., vitamin E, into the brain.[3] Finally, the brain was high concentrations of molecules, e.g., iron and vitamin C, which, under the wrong conditions, can greatly accelerate free radical generation,[4] and it contains high concentrations of polyunsaturated fatty acids (PUFA), which are easily damaged (oxidized) by free radicals.[5] This combination of features puts the brain in a vulnerable position in terms of its ability to resist oxidative attack and neuronal loss over the course of a lifetime. Neuronal loss is generally considered as contributing to mental impairment and dementias in the aged.[6] Furthermore, aging as a whole is often suggested to be in part a consequence of the persistent bludgeoning of cells by free radicals.[7]

FREE RADICALS AND THEIR DESTRUCTIVE NATURE

By definition free radicals are molecules that possess an unpaired electron in their outer orbital.[8] This feature makes them highly reactive and short-lived. Once produced, radicals often diffuse only a few angstroms before they interact with another molecule. If a radical species interacts with a nonradical, that molecule is damaged and a second radical is generated, which may be more or less toxic than the original radical. These persistent interactions of radicals with nonradical species can continue indefinitely, i.e., become chain reactions such as during the peroxidation of lipids.[9] If two radicals encounter each other, when the circumstances are right they can combine with the annihilation of both radical species; these are so-called termination reactions.

As already noted in the introduction, many free radicals are derived from O_2 as shown in the following reactions:[10,11]

$$O_2 \xrightarrow{e^-} O_2^{-\bullet} \tag{1}$$

$$O_2^{-\bullet} \underset{e^-}{\xrightarrow{SOD}} H_2O_2 \tag{2}$$

$$H_2O_2 \xrightarrow{Fe^{2+}} {}^\bullet OH \tag{3}$$

$$O_2^{-\bullet} + NO\bullet \longrightarrow ONOO^- \tag{4}$$

$$O_2 \xrightarrow{h\nu} {}^1O_2 \tag{5}$$

The electron (e^-) required for the reduction of O_2 to generate the superoxide anion radical ($O_2^{-\bullet}$) (reaction [1]) derives from a number of sources within cells including mitochondrial electron leak, dopamine oxidation, macrophages and microglia and activities of enzymes such as prostaglandin synthase, 5-lipoxygenase and xanthine oxidase.[10,11] The $O_2^{-\bullet}$ is not a highly toxic agent and is quickly removed from cells by its reduction to hydrogen peroxide (H_2O_2) (reaction [2]). This occurs primarily in the presence of family of enzymes, the superoxide dismutases (SOD), which are found in both mitochondria and in the cytosol.[12] The product of the dismutation of $O_2^{-\bullet}$, i.e., H_2O_2, has no unpaired e^- and is referred to as a reactive oxygen intermediate (ROI). Its inherent toxicity is low, but it has the capability of passing through membranes and it possess a rather long half-life.[13] Because of these features, H_2O_2, once generated, can disperse the potential damage induced by free radicals to other cellular compartments and/or to other cells. H_2O_2 is often quickly metabolized to nontoxic products (see below), but it is also the precursor of the most toxic of the radicals, the hydroxyl radical ($\bullet OH$). Thus, if not enzymatically destroyed, H_2O_2 is reduced in the presence of a transition metal, most often Fe^{2+}, to the $\bullet OH$ (reaction [3]). This radical has an estimated half-life *in vivo* of 1×10^{-9} sec and it travels only a few angstroms before it damages a vulnerable molecule. The $\bullet OH$ cannot be enzymatically removed from cells, but it can be detoxified by a direct free radical scavenger. Even then the scavenger must essentially be at the site where the $\bullet OH$ is generated to protect against its devastating action. Thus, the scavenger must be in what is referred to as the reaction cage of the $\bullet OH$.[14] Since many direct free radical scavengers are compartmentalized within cells due to their specific solubility characteristics, none can protect against $\bullet OH$ damage at locations they cannot reach. In this regard, melatonin seems to be unique, since it is located in both lipid and aqueous compartments of the cell in sufficient concentrations to reduce the damage caused by the highly toxic $\bullet OH$.[15]

$O_2^{-\bullet}$ has another fate, which results in the generation of a highly toxic agent; as seen in reaction [4], it combines with the nitric oxide radical ($NO\bullet$) to produce the peroxynitrite anion ($ONOO^-$). This molecule, although not a radial, is capable of damaging a variety of molecules and initiating peroxidative processes. Besides its inherent toxicity, it degrades into the $\bullet OH$ or into agents that are similarly toxic.[16] That melatonin scavenges the $ONOO^-$ has been demonstrated in a series of studies in the last two years.[17,18]

Singlet oxygen ($^1O_2$) is formed by the addition of energy to ground state oxygen (reaction [5]). This reactive product is capable of initiating lipid peroxidation in cell membranes; this capability is reduced by melatonin, presumably because the indole quenches $^1O_2$.[19,20]

ANTIOXIDATIVE DEFENSE SYSTEM

Molecules that directly detoxify free radicals are known as radical scavengers and include such well known agents as vitamin E, vitamin C, β-carotene, etc.,[21] and more recently melatonin.[22] Besides these direct free radical scavengers, a variety of enzymes remove radicals or their intermediates from extra- and intracellular spaces by metabolizing them to nontoxic products. Some of the better known enzymes that function in this capacity include superoxide dismutase (SOD), glutathione peroxidase (GSH-Px) and glutathione reductase (GSH-Rd).[23] Besides functioning as a peroxidase during which it removes hydrogen peroxide (H_2O_2) and other hydroperoxides from tissues, GSH-Px also functions in the reduction of another toxic, nonradical species, the peroxynitrite anion ($ONOO^-$).[24] Thus, GSH-Px has a dual role as an antioxidative enzyme. Finally, there are molecules that bind transition metals, in particular, iron. Iron and other transition metals when they exist in the unbound form are efficient free radical generators.[25] Fortunately, under usual conditions transition metals are usually in the bound state in most organisms. This complex of direct free radical scavenges, enzymes that metabolize radicals and their intermediates, and molecules that chelate transition metals are collectively referred to as the antioxidative defense system.

Despite the multiple means by which this system limits the actions of free radicals, some always escape being detoxified and go on to damage essential molecules. This damage slowly accumulates and eventually compromises the functions of organelles, organs and eventually organisms.[26] In other cases, damage to tissues may be rapid such as when massive insults, e.g., severe inflammation or ischemia/reperfusion injury, greatly exaggerate the number of free radicals produced, which in turn totally overwhelm the capacity of the antioxidative defense system to defend against them.[27,28] In such cases pharmacological levels of antioxidants must be given to combat the massive damage that would otherwise occur.

Melatonin may be, even at physiological concentrations an important component of the antioxidative capacity of the organism. Certainly, blood levels of melatonin positively correlate with the total antioxidant status of the blood.[29,30] Also, melatonin is well documented to be a efficient scavenger of the devastatingly reactive $\cdot OH$[31–34] and the $ONOO^-$,[17,18,28] and there is also evidence that it quenches $^1O_2$[19] and neutralizes $NO\cdot$.[35] Furthermore, it increases the ability of cells to resist oxidative damage by stimulating a variety of antioxidative enzymes[36–40] and inhibiting one prooxidative enzyme.[41] Additionally, melatonin stabilizes cell membranes thereby increasing their ability to resist free radical destruction,[42] and it possibly functions as a metal chelator,[43] an action that could importantly reduce the generation of the $\cdot OH$. Despite these apparently numerous actions of melatonin against free radical toxicity, the authors are not convinced that the most essential antioxidative properties of melatonin have been uncovered; presumably, future research will do so.

Besides melatonin, there may be other secretory products of the pineal gland that possess significant antioxidative actions. In particular 5-methoxytryptamine,[30] N-acetyl serotonin,[44,45] and pinoline[46,47] may be pineal products that, if released from the pineal gland and taken up by other tissues, could function in protecting cells from free radical damage.

FREE RADICAL DAMAGE, MELATONIN, AND THE CNS

There is extensive evidence and widespread agreement that free radical damage is particularly prevalent in the brain and that it is an important factor in a number of neurodegenerative conditions in the aged.[1,2,5,48,49] In the context of the present review, models of three neurodegenerative diseases are of special interest, i.e., Huntington's disease, Alzheimer's disease and Parkinson's disease.

Huntington's Disease

Huntington's disease is an autosomal dominant neurodegenerative disorder that is the result of a genetic defect on chromosome 4.[50,51] This disease typically has an onset at about 40 years of age and is characterized by motor disturbances, biobehavioral symptoms and progressive dementia. Neural degeneration is a major feature of this condition as evidenced by roughly a 20% reduction in brain weight at death relative that in age-matched controls.[51]

Excitotoxicity likely induced by the tryptophan metabolite, quinolinic acid, is generally believed to be a causative factor in this complex neuropathological disorder.[50,52] This was first shown by Beal and co-workers, who reported that the injection of quinolinic acid directly into the striatum of the rat closely reproduced the neuropathology seen in the brains of individuals who died with Huntington's disease.[53] Since then quinolinic acid administration has been used as a model of Huntington's disease.

Quinolinic acid is synthesized in the brain, and concentrations are roughly equivalent in all brain regions; its formation in the CNS increases with immune activation and, at least in rats, during the natural aging process.[54] Quinolinic acid is not taken up by neurons from the extracellular space, nor is there extracellular metabolism of this tryptophan metabolite.[55] The metabolite acts on the N-methyl-D-aspartate (NMDA) receptor with about one-fourth the efficacy of glutamate;[56] however, since it is not removed from the synaptic cleft (as is glutamate) it has long-term effects on the NMDA receptor, and it is a potent neurotoxin. Since quinolinic acid acts on the NMDA receptor and it is nondegradable, its toxicity to neurons is similar to that caused by the excitatory amino acid neurotransmitter glutamate and is generally accepted to involve the generation of free radicals in the postsynaptic neuron on which it acts. Excessive free radical generation in these cells then leads to a variety of molecular changes, e.g., lipid peroxidation, in the affected neurons and eventually to the death of these cells (FIG. 1).

Since free radicals are accepted to be involved in quinolinic acid toxicity, Southgate and colleagues[57] surmised that the toxic changes induced by its injection into the hippocampus would be suppressed by the peripheral administration of melatonin, which easily crosses the blood-brain barrier and enters neurons.[15] When tested, melatonin was found to prevent the morphological changes in the pyramidal neurons of the hippocampus when quinolinic acid was given as an intrahippocampal injection 5 days earlier. Furthermore, this group showed that the reduction in glutamate receptor numbers caused by quinolinic acid was likewise partially reversed by melatonin. Southgate *et al.*[57] theorized that melatonin's ability to reduce quinolinic acid toxicity related to its antioxidant activity, and they suggested the potential utility of melatonin in deferring the signs of Huntington's disease.

Besides quinolinic acid, there is another neural excitotoxin against which melatonin has proved highly effective. Kainic acid is a nondegradable molecule, which, when injected into animals, produces generalized limbic system seizures and extensive neuronal damage and death.[58] These consequences are generally accepted to involve the excessive production of free radicals in the affected neurons.

Considering the role of free radicals in the neural excitotoxicity induced by kainic acid, it could also be anticipated that melatonin would be tested in this model system as to its potential protective effects. The first studies related to this were carried out

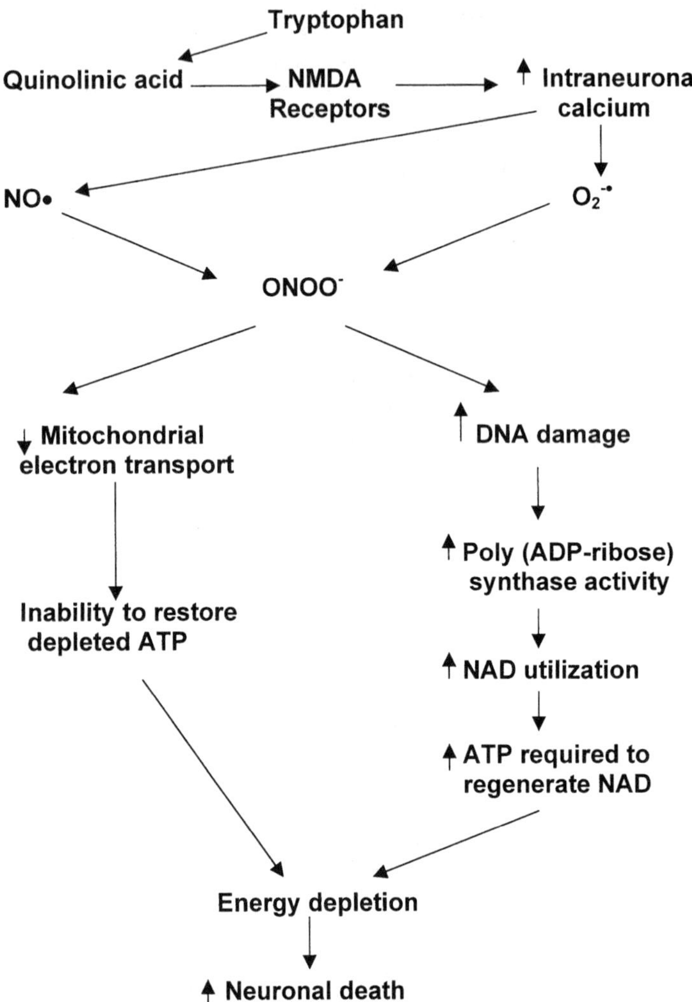

FIGURE 1. A proposed mechanism of neuronal loss in Huntington's disease. Like several other excitotoxins, the tryptophan metabolite quinolinic acid acts on NMDA receptors to stimulate intraneuronal free radical generation, which can lead to energy depletion and neuronal death. Free radical scavengers can reduce oxidative damage and neuronal death by neutralizing free radicals generated in the neuron.

by Melchiorri *et al.*,[59,60] in which brain homogenates were treated with kainic acid in the presence or absence of melatonin. In homogenates of cerebellum, hippocampus, hypothalamus and striatum, kainic acid induced large increases in products of lipid peroxidation indicative of free radical damage; however, when these preparations were co-incubated with the neurotoxin and melatonin, the indole, in a dose-response relationship, inhibited the peroxidation of lipids.[59,60]

Like quinolinic acid, the excitotoxic actions of kainic acid relate to its interaction with the NMDA receptor followed by the generation of free radicals. Thus, when intact neurons were incubated with kainic acid, the cells died in large numbers unless melatonin was also available in the culture medium.[61,62] Likewise, the *in vivo* administration of kainic acid to rodents leads to neuronal DNA damage and cell death, effects that can be overcome by concurrent administration of melatonin.[63–65]

While each of the studies previously described utilized melatonin concentrations higher than those normally present in the blood of animals, Manev *et al.*[66] and Uz and co-workers[67] have also shown that pinealectomized rats, which lack a nighttime rise in endogenous melatonin levels, exhibit an increased vulnerability to kainic acid in terms of neuronal damage. The implication of these findings is that even physiological concentrations of melatonin are protective against the devastating onslaught of free radicals generated by pharmacological levels of kainic acid.

The results summarized above clearly demonstrate that the excitotoxic actions of both quinolinic acid and kainic acid are curtailed by melatonin. These agents have similar mechanisms of action relative to their neurotoxicity, and both are believed to generate free radicals with the subsequent damage being a consequence of these processes. Thus, the most likely means by which melatonin provides protection from quinolinic acid and kainate is due to its multiple antioxidative actions.

Alzheimer's Disease

Alzheimer's disease (AD) is the most common cause of the progressive cognitive decline present in the aged population, and it is the most prevalent neurodegenerative disease worldwide. A triad of neurological features characterize this disease and include β-amyloid plaques (senile plaques) and neurofibrillary tangles in the CNS accompanied by the extensive regional loss of neurons. Neuronal loss is most obvious in the hippocampus and cerebral cortex. The associated dementia usually arises sporadically late in life (after age 65); a less frequent form of the disease, i.e., familial AD, often has a much earlier onset (in the fourth decade of life). Many researchers, although not all, believe amyloid β-peptide is a crucial factor that leads to neuronal loss and dementia in AD.

The involvement of oxidative stress in AD related to the formation of amyloid β peptide in the brain is well established (FIG. 2). While amyloid β peptide consists of a 39–43 amino acid chain, it is the 25–35 amino acid residue that is believed to generate free radicals, which eventually destroy adjacent neurons.[68]

We used an *in vitro* model in which cultured neurons were incubated with amyloid β peptide with and without melatonin to test whether the latter molecule would protect the cells from free radical-induced cell death.[69,70] The incubation of either murine neuroblastoma (N2a) or PC12 (pheochromocytoma) cells with only the free radical generating amyloid β residue (the 25–35 amino acid fragment) or with the entire peptide (1–40) caused up to 80% of the cells to die within 24 hours. The bulk of this neuronal death was reversed by coincubating the cells with both the peptide and melatonin. Besides reducing the number of neurons that died following their exposure to amyloid β peptide, melatonin reduced lipid peroxidation and the high intracellular concentrations of calcium that occurred in the cells as a consequence of exposure to amyloid β peptide. Reversal of the neurotoxicity in these studies was presumed to relate to the multiple free radical scavenging and antioxidative actions

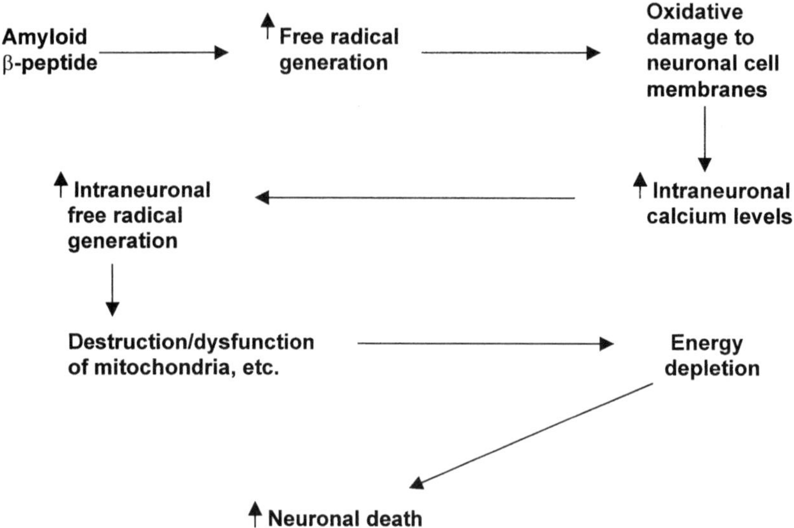

FIGURE 2. A proposed mechanism of neuronal loss as a consequence of the accumulation of amyloid β peptide in the vicinity of neurons. The peptide generates free radicals that alter the function of neuronal membranes causing the cells to undergo homeostatic dysregulation. This eventually leads to adenosine triphosphate (ATP) depletion, and the neurons die. This process in similar to neuronal loss in other models of neurodegeneration.

of melatonin.[71] These findings are of interest in the light of the marked reduction of pineal melatonin levels in the aged,[72] where the signs of Alzheimer's disease are manifested. Whether, however, the loss of melatonin during aging predisposes the brain to neuronal loss as a consequence of amyloid β deposition remains unknown.

Other means by which melatonin could limit neuronal destruction in Alzheimer's disease have been proposed. According to Lahiri,[73] melatonin also pharmacologically reduces the formation of soluble derivatives of the amyloid β precursor itself. The net effect of this action would be a reduction in the formation of amyloid β precursor protein, which would cause a drop in the formation of amyloid β itself. Additionally, it has been shown that melatonin reduces the ability of amyloid β protein to form β-sheets and amyloid fibrils. This action of melatonin reduces the toxicity of amyloid β and also makes it more susceptible to proteolytic degradation.[74]

Since amyloid β generates free radicals and melatonin neutralizes these molecular brigands, it was not unexpected that melatonin was found to reduce neuronal lipoperoxidation, which occurs after the incubation of such cells with amyloid β peptide.[69,75]

There has been one test of melatonin's efficacy in reducing the signs of Alzheimer's disease in humans.[76] In this case report, one monozygotic twin received vitamin E plus melatonin, while the second received vitamin E only in an attempt to defer the signs of Alzheimer's disease. During 3 years of treatment, the twin that received melatonin (6 mg) daily exhibited milder impairment of memory functions and had substantial improvement of sleep quality and a reduction of sundowning. At the end of the 36-month treatment period, the twin that received melatonin had a score of 5 in the Functional Assessment Tool for Alzheimer's Disease (FAST), while the nonmelatonin-treated twin scored 7b on the same test. The implication is that melatonin ingestion improved the overall condition and delayed the progress of the signs of Alzheimer's disease in this subject.

Parkinson's Disease

Parkinson's disease has a prevalence of approximately 150 cases/100,000 population. It is characterized by a gradual deterioration of dopaminergic neurons in the pars compacta of the substantia nigra of the brain stem. The loss of the dopaminergic neurons results in an associated reduction in dopamine-containing fibers in the striatum and is accompanied by a variety of sensory and motor impairments including tremor, rigidity and akinesia. While there may be other neuronal systems involved, a primary feature of Parkinson's disease is the loss of the dopaminergic neurons. Oxidative damage to neurons may be one of the preeminent terminal events in the ultimate cause of dopaminergic cell death in Parkinson's disease. While there may be other processes that also are involved in killing the neurons of the pars compacta

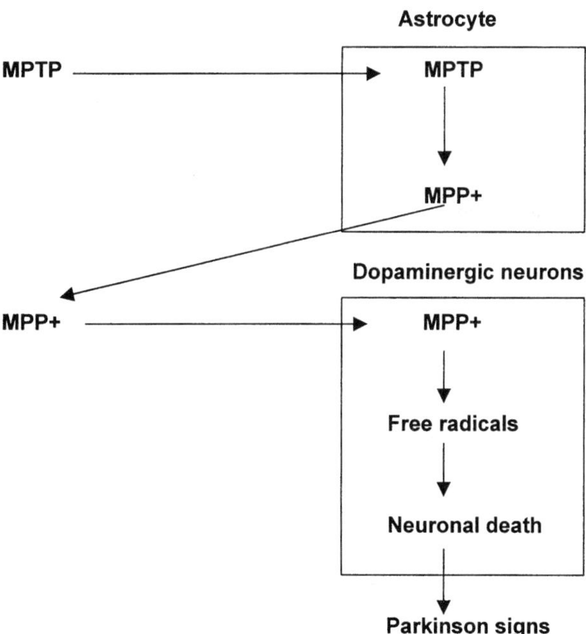

FIGURE 3. A proposed mechanism to explain the loss of dopaminergic neurons in the pars compacta of the substantia nigra after the treatment of animals with MPTP. Similar mechanisms are believed to be responsible for the loss of dopamine-containing neurons in the human thereby accounting for the signs of Parkinsonism.

in this disease, what is known as the free radical hypothesis has received increasing experimental support.[77,78] In view of this, several research groups have seen the wisdom of testing the ability of melatonin to protect against neuronal loss in models of Parkinson's disease.

Perhaps the most common method used to induce a reasonable facsimile of a Parkinson's type disease in animals is the injection of 1-methyl-4-phenyl-1,2,3,6-tetrahydropyridine (MPTP); after its uptake by astrocytes, MPTP is metabolized to the methyl-4-phenyl pryridinium cation (MPP$^+$). Among several actions of MPP$^+$, this molecule stimulates free radical generation, which contributes to the killing of dopaminergic neurons (FIG. 3).[79] Acuña-Castroviejo and colleagues[80] used this model to test the efficacy of melatonin to resist MPTP-induced neuronal toxicity. They found, under the conditions of this short-term study, that melatonin ameliorated the loss of dopamine and the reduction of striated thyrosine hydroxylase-positive fibers caused by the injection of MPTP into mice. In a second *in vivo* study, Kim and co-workers[81] confirmed the observations of Acuña-Castroviejo *et al.*[80] using the same neurochemical endpoints and also showed that melatonin inhibited the neurobehavioral affects that are induced in 6-hydroxydopamine (6-OHDA)-treated rats injected with apomorphine. In both these studies, the authors attributed melatonin's protective actions, at least in part, to the free radical scavenging activities of the indole. 6-OHDA, like MPTP, is known to induce Parkinsonism-like symptoms in rodents via free radical mechanisms.[82]

In addition to the *in vivo* studies described above, two *in vitro* reports have confirmed melatonin's ability to protect neurons against the neurotoxins MPTP and 6-OHDA.[83,84] In the former study, it was found that melatonin protected dopaminergic neurons from neurotoxic injury caused by MPP$^+$.[83] Similarly, Mayo and colleagues[84] reported that melatonin prevented the death of PC12 cells after their treatment with 6-OHDA. The indices of cellular damage in this study included changes in cell mobility, signs of apoptosis and DNA fragmentation, all of which were reduced by melatonin.

CONCLUDING REMARKS

From the studies summarized above, it is obvious that melatonin in experimental animals overcomes much of the toxicity and neuronal cell death that is seen when animals are given toxins that cause them to develop signs of Huntington's disease, Alzheimer's disease and Parkinson's disease. Additionally, in a wide number of other models of neurotoxicity melatonin has been shown to be protective against free radical-induced neuronal destruction. Collectively, these studies document the significant neuroprotective actions of the chief secretory product of the pineal gland. The findings are consistent with the multiple free radical scavenging and antioxidative actions of melatonin[49,85,86] and with its rapid uptake by the brain after its peripheral administration.[15] As with the outcome of many other studies, in the reports summarized herein, melatonin was found to be essentially devoid of toxicity. This being the case, its use in humans to forestall some of the signs of the devastating neurodegenerative diseases of the aged should be considered.[87]

REFERENCES

1. HALLIWELL, B. & J.M.C. GUTTERIDGE. 1985. Oxygen radicals and the nervous system. Trends Neurosci. **8:** 22–26.
2. REITER, R.J. 1995. Oxidative processes and antioxidative defense mechanisms in the aging brain. FASEB J. **9:** 526–533.
3. CASERTA, M.T., D. CACCIOPPO, G.D. LAPIN & D.R. GROOTHIUS. 1998. Blood-brain barrier in Alzheimer's disease patients and elderly control subjects. J. Neuropsychiatry Clin. Neurosci. **10:** 78–84.
4. HALLIWELL, B. & J.M.C. GUTTERIDGE. 1984. Oxygen toxicity, oxygen radicals, transition metals and disease. Biochem. J. **219:** 1–14.
5. COYLE, J.T. & P. PUTTFARCKEN. 1993. Oxidative stress, glutamate, and neurodegenerative disorders. Science **262:** 689–695.
6. BEHL, C. 1999. Alzheimer's disease and oxidative stress: implications for novel therapeutic approaches. Prog. Neurobiol. **58:** 301–323.
7. HARMAN, D. 1991. The aging process: major risk factor for disease and health. Proc. Nat. Acad. Sci. USA **88:** 5630–5633.
8. OLANOW, C.W. 1993. A radical hypothesis for neurodegeneration. Trends Neurosci. **16:** 439–444.
9. ESTERBAUER, H. 1985. Lipid peroxidation production: formation, chemical properties and biological activities. *In* Free Radicals and Liver Injury. G. Poli, K.H. Cheeseman, M.V. Diangani & T.F. Slater, Eds.: 29–47. IRL Press. Arlington.
10. CHEESEMAN, K.H. & T.F. SLATER. 1993. An introduction to free radical biochemistry. Br. Med. Bull. **49:** 481–493.
11. MCCORD, J.M. 1985. Oxygen-derived free radicals in postischemic tissue injury. N. Engl. J. Med. **312:** 159–163.
12. FRIDOVICH, I. 1989. Superoxide dismutases: an adaptation to a paramagnetic gas. J. Biol. Chem. **264:** 19328–19333.
13. CADENAS, E. 1995. Mechanisms of oxygen activation and reactive oxygen species. *In* Oxidative Stress and Antioxidant Defenses in Biology. S. Ahmad, Ed.: 1–61. Chapman and Hall. London.
14. BORG, D. 1993. Oxygen free radicals and tissue injury. *In* Oxygen Free Radicals in Tissue Injury. M. Tarr & F. Samson, Eds.: 12–53. Birkhäuser. Boston.
15. MENENDEZ-PELAEZ, A., B. POEGGELER, R.J. REITER, L.R. BARLOW-WALDEN, M.I. PABLOS & D.X. TAN. 1993. Nuclear localization of melatonin in different mammalian tissues: immunocytochemical and radioimmunoassay evidence. J. Cell. Biochem. **53:** 572–582.
16. PRYOR, W. & G. SQUADRITO. 1995. The chemistry of peroxynitrite: a product from the reaction of nitric-oxide with superoxide. Am. J. Physiol. **268:** L699–L722.
17. GILAD, E., S. CUZZOCREA, B. ZINGARELLI, A.L. SALZMAN & C. SZABO. 1997. Melatonin is a scavenger of peroxynitrite. Life Sci. **60:** PL169–174.
18. CUZZOCREA, S., B. ZINGARELLI, E. GILAD, P. HAKE, A.L. SALZMAN & C. SZABO. 1997. Protective effect of melatonin in carregeenan-induced models of local inflammation: relation to its inhibitory effect on nitric oxide production and its peroxynitrite scavenging activity. J. Pineal Res. **23:** 106–116.
19. CAGNOLI, C.M., C. ATABAY, E. KHARLAMOVA & H. MANEV. 1995. Melatonin protects neurons from singlet oxygen-induced apoptosis. J. Pineal Res. **18:** 222–226.
20. ROBERTS, J.E., D.N. HU & J.F. WISHART. 1998. Pulse radiolysis studies on melatonin and chloromelatonin. J. Photochem. Photobiol. **42:** 125–132.
21. SIES, H. & W. STAHL. 1995. Vitamins E and C, β-carotene, and other carotenoids as antioxidants. Am. J. Clin. Nutr. **62:** 1315S–1321S.
22. REITER, R.J., R.C. CARNEIRO & C.S. OH. 1997. Melatonin in relation to cellular antioxidative defense mechanisms. Horm. Metab. Res. **29:** 363–372.
23. REITER, R.J., L. TANG, J.J. GARCIA & A. MUÑOZ-HOYOS. 1997. Pharmacological actions of melatonin in oxygen radical pathophysiology. Life Sci. **60:** 2255–2271.

24. SIES, H., V.S. SHAROV, L.O. KLOTZ & K. BRIVIBA. 1997. Glutathione peroxidase protects against peroxynitrite-mediated oxidations. J. Biol. Chem. **272:** 27812–27817.
25. SINGH, S. & R.C. HIDE. 1994. Therapeutic iron-chelating agents. *In* Free Radical Damage and Its Control. C.A. Rice-Evans & R.H. Burdan, Eds.: 189–216. Elsevier. Amsterdam.
26. HARMAN, D. 1995. Free radical theory of aging: Alzheimer's disease pathogenesis. Age **18:** 97–119.
27. BRAUGHLER, J.M. & E.D. HALL. 1989. Central nervous system in trauma and stroke. Free Radical Biol. Med. **6:** 289–301.
28. CUZZOCREA, S., B. ZINGARELLI, G. COSTANTINO & A.P. CAPUTI. 1998. Protective effect of melatonin in non-septic shock model induced by zymosan in the rat. J. Pineal Res. **25:** 24–33.
29. BENOT, S., P. MOLINERO, M. SOUTTO, R. GOBERNA & J.M. GUERRERO. 1998. Circadian variations in the rat serum total antioxidant status: correlation with melatonin levels. J. Pineal Res. **25:** 1–4.
30. BENOT, S., R. GOBERNA, R.J. REITER, S. GARCIA-MAURINO, C. OSUNA & J.M. GUERRERO. Physiological levels of melatonin contribute to the antioxidant capacity of human serum. J. Pineal Res. **27:** 59–64.
31. TAN, D.X., L.D. CHEN, B. POEGGELER, L.C. MANCHESTER & R.J. REITER. 1993. Melatonin: a potent endogenous hydroxyl radical scavenger. Endocrine J. **1:** 57–60.
32. MATUSZEK, Z., K.J. RESZKA & C.F. CHIGNELL. 1997. Reaction of melatonin and related indoles with hydroxyl radicals: ESR and spin trapping investigations. Free Radical Biol. Med. **23:** 367–373.
33. SUSA, N., S. UENO, Y. FURUKAWA, J. UEDA & M. SUGIYAMA. 1997. Potent protective effect of melatonin on chromium (VI)-induced DNA single-strand breaks, cytotoxicity, and lipid peroxidation in primary cultures of rat hepatocytes. Toxicol. Appl. Pharmacol. **144:** 377–384.
34. STASICA, P., P. ULANSKI & J.M. ROSIAK. 1998. Melatonin as a hydroxyl radical scavenger. J. Pineal Res. **25:** 65–66.
35. NODA, Y., A. MORI, R. LIBURTY & L. PACKER. 1998. Melatonin and its precursors scavenge nitric oxide. J. Pineal Res. **27:** 159–163.
36. BARLOW-WALDEN, L.R., R.J. REITER, M. ABE, M.I. PABLOS, L.D. CHEN & B. POEGGELER. 1995. Melatonin stimulates brain glutathione peroxidase activity. Neurochem. Int. **26:** 497–502.
37. PIERREFICHE, G. & H. LABORIT. 1995. Oxygen radicals, melatonin and aging. Exp. Gerontol. **30:** 213–227.
38. PABLOS, M.I., J.M. GUERRERO, G.G. ORTIZ, M.T. AGAPITO & R.J. REITER. 1997. Both melatonin and a putative nuclear melatonin receptor agonist CGP 52608 stimulate glutathione peroxidase and glutathione reductase activities in mouse brain *in vivo.* Neuroendocrinol. Lett. **18:** 49–58.
39. PABLOS, M.I., R.J. REITER, J.I. CHUANG, G.G. ORTIZ, J.M. GUERRERO, E. SEWERYNEK, M.T. AGAPITO, D. MELCHIORRI, R. LAWRENCE & S.M. DENEKE. 1997. Acutely administered melatonin reduces oxidative damage in lung and brain induced by hyperbaric oxygen. J. Appl. Physiol. **83:** 354–358.
40. PABLOS, M.I., R.J. REITER, G.G. ORTIZ, J.M. GUERRERO, M.T. AGAPITO, J.I. CHUANG & E. SEWERYNEK. 1997. Rhythms of glutathione peroxidase and glutathione reductase in brain of chicks and their inhibition by light. Neurochem. Int. **32:** 69–75.
41. POZO, D., R.J. REITER, J.R. CALVO & J.M. GUERRERO. 1997. Inhibition of cerebellar nitric oxide synthase and cyclic GMP production by melatonin via complex formation with calmodulin. J. Cell. Biochem. **65:** 430–432.
42. GARCIA, J.J., R.J. REITER, G.G. ORTIZ, C.S. OH, L. TANG, B.P. YU & G. ESCAMES. 1998. Melatonin enhances tamoxifen's ability to prevent the reduction of microsomal membrane fluidity during induced lipid peroxidation. J. Membr. Biol. **162:** 59–65.

43. LIMSON, J., T. NYOKONG & S. DAYA. 1998. The interaction of melatonin and its precursors with aluminum, cadmium, copper, iron, lead, and zinc: an absorptive voltametric study. J. Pineal Res. **24:** 15–21.

44. MOSSMANN, B., M. UHR & C. BEHL. 1997. Neuroprotective potential of aromatic alcohols against oxidative cell death. FEBS Lett. **413:** 467–472.

45. LEZOUALC'H, F., M. SPARAPANI & C. BEHL. 1998. *N*-Acetyl serotonin (normelatonin) and melatonin protect neurons against oxidative challenges and suppress the activity of the transcription factor NF-κB. J. Pineal Res. **24:** 168–178.

46. PÄHKLA, R., M. ZILMER, T. KULLISAR & L. RÄGO. 1998. Comparison of the antioxidant activity of melatonin and pinoline *in vitro*. J. Pineal Res. **24:** 96–101.

47. PLESS, G, T.J.P. FREDERIKSEN, J.J. GARCIA & R.J. REITER. 1999. Pharmacological aspects of *N*-acetyl-5-methoxytryptamine (melatonin) and 6-methoxy-1,2,3,4-tetrahydro-β-carbolinc (pinoline) as antioxidants: reduction of oxidative damage in brain region homogenates. J. Pineal Res. **26:** 236–246.

48. REITER, R.J., M.I. PABLOS, M.T. AGAPITO & J.M. GUERRERO. 1996. Melatonin in the context of the free radical theory of aging. Ann. N.Y. Acad. Sci. **786:** 362–378.

49. REITER, R.J. 1998. Oxidative damage in the central nervous system: protection by melatonin. Prog. Neurobiol. **56:** 359–384.

50. DIFIGLIA, M. 1990. Excitotoxic injury in the neostriatum: a model for Hungtington's disease. Trends Neurosci. **13:** 286–289.

51. BIRD, E.D. 1980. Chemical pathology of Hungtington's disease. Ann. Rev. Pharmacol. Toxicol. **20:** 533–551.

52. TONE, T.W. 1993. Neuropharmacology of quinolinic and kynurenic acids. Pharmacol. Rev. **45:** 309–379.

53. BEAL, M.F., N.W. KOWALL, D.W. ELLISON, M.F. MAZUREK, K.J. SWARTZ & J.B. MARTIN. 1986. Replication of the neurochemical characteristics of Huntington's disease by quinolinc acid. Nature **324:** 169–171.

54. MORONI, F., G. LOMBARDI, G. MONETI & C. ALDINIO. 1984. The excitotoxin quinolinic acid is present in the brain of several mammals and its cortical content increases during the aging process. Neurosci. Lett. **47:** 51–54.

55. FOSTER, A.C., L.P. MILLER, W.H. OLDENDORF & R. SCHWARCZ. 1984. Studies on the deposition of quinolinic acid after intracerebral and systemic administration in the rat. Exp. Neurol. **84:** 428–440.

56. STONE, R.W. & M.N. PERKINS. 1981. Quinolinic acid: a potent endogenous excitant at amino acid receptors in the CNS. Eur. J. Pharmacol **72:** 411–412.

57. SOUTHGATE, G.S., S. DAYA & B. POTGIETER. 1998. Melatonin plays a protective role in quinolinic acid-induced neurotoxicity in the rat hippocampus. J. Chem. Neuroanat. **14:** 151–156.

58. KÖHLER, C. 1984. Neuronal degeneration after intracerebral injection of excitotoxins: a histological analysis of kainic acid, ibotenic acid and quinolinic acid lesions in the brain. *In* Excitotoxins. K. Fuke, P. Roberts & R. Schwarcz, Eds.: 99–111. Plenum Press. New York.

59. MELCHIORRI, D., R.J. REITER, E. SEWERYNEK & G. NISTICO. 1995. Melatonin reduces kainate-induced lipid peroxidation in homogenates of different brain regions. FASEB J. **9:** 1205–1210.

60. MELCHIORRI, D., R.J. REITER, L.D. CHEN, E. SEWERYNEK & G. NISTICO. 1996. Melatonin affords protection against kainate-induce *in vitro* lipid peroxidation in brain. Eur. J. Pharmacol. **305:** 239–245.

61. GIUSTI, P., M. LIPARLITI, M. GUSELLA, M. FLOREANI & H. MANEV. 1997. *In vivo* protective effects of melatonin against glutamate oxidative stress and neurotoxicity. Ann. N.Y. Acad. Sci. **825:** 79–84.

62. LEZOUALC'H, F., T. SKUTELLA, M. WIDMANN & C. BEHL. 1996. Melatonin prevents oxidative stress-induced cell death in hippocampal cells. NeuroReport **7:** 2071–2077.

63. MANEV, H., T. UZ, A. KHARLAMOV, C.M. CAGNOLI, D. FRANCESCHINI & P. GIUSTI. 1996. *In vivo* protection against kainate-induced apoptosis by the pineal hormone melatonin: effect of exogenous melatonin and circadian rhythm. Restr. Neurol. Neurosci. **9:** 251–256.

64. UZ, T., P. Giusti, D. Franceschini, A. Kharlamov & H. Manev. 1996. Protective effect of melatonin against hippocampal DNA damage induced by intraperitoneal administration of kainate to rats. Neuroscience **73:** 631–636.

65. TAN, D.X., L.C. MANCHESTER, R.J. REITER, W. QI, S.J. KIM & G.H. EL-SOKKARY. 1998. Melatonin protects hippocampal neurons *in vivo* against kainic acid-induced damage in mice. J. Neurosci Res **54:** 382–389.

66. MANEV, H., T. UZ, A. KHARLAMOV & J.Y. JOO. 1996. Increased brain damage after stroke or excitotoxic seizures in melatonin deficient rat. FASEB J. **10:** 1546–1551.

67. UZ, T., P. LONGONE & H. MANEV. 1997. Increased hippocampal 5-lipoxygenase mRNA content in melatonin-deficient, pinealectomized rats. J. Neurochem. **69:** 2220–2233.

68. BUTTERFIELD, D.A., K. HERSLEY, M. HARRIS, M.P. MATTSON & J.M. CARNEY. 1997. β-Amyloid peptide free radical fragments initiate lipoperoxidation in a sequence specific fashion: implications to Alzheimer's disease. Biochem. Biophys. Res. Commun. **200:** 710–715.

69. PAPPOLLA, M.A., M. SOS, R.A. OMAR, R.J. BICK, D.L.M. HICKSON-BICK, R.J. REITER, S. EFTHIMIOPOULOS & N.K. ROBAKIS. 1997. Melatonin prevents death of neuroblastoma cells exposed to Alzheimer's amyloid peptide. J. Neurosci. **17:** 1683–1690.

70. PAPPOLLA, M.A., M. SOS, R.J. BICK, R.A. OMAR, D.L.M. HICKSON-BICK, R.J. REITER, S. EFTHIMIOPOULOS, K. SAMBAMURTI & N.K. ROBAKIS. 1997. Oxidative damage and cell death induced by an amyloid peptide fragment is completely prevented by melatonin. *In* Alzheimer's Disease: Biology, Diagnosis and Therapeutics. K. Iqbal, B. Winblad, T. Nishimura, M. Takeda & H.M. Wisniewski, Eds.: 741–749. Wiley. New York.

71. REITER, R.J. 1996. Functional aspects of the pineal hormone melatonin in combatting cell and tissue damage induced by free radicals. Eur. J. Endocrinol, **134:** 412–420.

72. REITER, R.J. 1997. Aging and oxygen toxicity: relation to changes in melatonin. Age **20:** 201–213.

73. LAHIRI, D.K. 1999. Melatonin affects the metabolism of the β-amyloid precursor protein in different cell types. J. Pineal Res. **26:** 137–146.

74. PAPPOLLA, M.A., P. BOZNER, C. SOTO, H. SHAO, N.K. ROBAKIS, M. ZAGORSKI, B. FRANGIONE & J. GHISO. 1998. Inhibition of Alzheimer's β-fibrillogenesis by melatonin. J. Biol. Chem. **273:** 7135–7188.

75. DANIELS, W.M.U., S.J. VAN RENSBURG, J.M. VAN ZYL & J.J.F. TALJAARD. 1998. Melatonin prevents β-amyloid-induced lipid peroxidation. J. Pineal Res. **24:** 78–82.

76. BRUSCO, L.I., M. MARQUEZ & D.P. CARDINALI. 1998. Monozygotic twins treated with melatonin: case report. J. Pineal Res. **25:** 260–263.

77. OLANOW, C.W. 1990. Oxidation reactions in Parkinson's disease. Neurology **40**(Suppl. 3): 32–37.

78. FAHN, S. & G. COHEN. 1992. The oxidative stress hypothesis in Parkinson's disease: evidence supporting it. Ann. Neurol. **32:** 804–812.

79. LAI, M., H. GRIFFITHS, H. PALL, A. WILLIAMS & J. LUNEC. 1993. An investigation into the role of reactive oxygen species in mechanisms of 1-methyl-4-phenyl-1,2,3,6-tetrahydropyridine toxicity using neuronal cell lines. Biochem. Pharmacol. **45:** 927–933.

80. ACUÑA-CASTROVIEJO, D., A. COTO-MONTES, M.G. MONTI, G.G. ORTIZ & R.J. REITER. 1997. Melatonin is protective against MPTP-induced striatal and hippocampal lesions. Life Sci. **60:** PL23–PL29.

81. KIM, Y.S., W.S. JOO, B.K. JIN, Y.H. HO, H.H. BAIK & C.W. PARK. 1998. Melatonin protects against 6-OHDA-induced neuronal death of nigrostriatal dopaminergic system. NeuroReport **9:** 2387–2390.
82. ZIGMOND, M.J. & E.M. STICKER. 1989. Animal models of Parkinsonism using selected neurotoxins: clinical and basic implications. Int. Rev. Neurobiol. **31:** 1–79.
83. IACOVITTI, L., N.D. STULL & K. JOHNSTON. 1997. Melatonin recuses dopamine neurons from cell death in tissue culture models of oxidative stress. Brain Res. **768:** 317–326.
84. MAYO, J.C., R.M. SAINZ, H. URIA, E. ANTOLIN, M.M. ESTEBAN & C. RODRIQUEZ. 1998. Melatonin prevents apoptosis induced by 6-hydroxy-dopamine in neuronal cells: implications for Parkinson's disease. J. Pineal Res. **24:** 179–192.
85. REITER, R.J., J.M. GUERRERO, G. ESCAMES, M.A. PAPPOLLA & D. ACUÑA-CASTROVIEJO. 1997. Prophylactic actions of melatonin in oxidative neurotoxicity. Ann. N.Y. Acad. Sci. **825:** 70–78.
86. REITER, R.J. 1998. Melatonin, active oxygen species and neurological damage. Drug News Perspect. **11:** 291–296.
87. JEAN-LOUIS, G., H. VON GIZYCKI & F. ZIZI. 1995. Melatonin effects on sleep, mood, and cognition in elderly with mild cognitive impairment. J. Pineal Res. **25:** 177–183.

Questions and Answers

From Dr. Marini

What is the role of secretin in your model and autism?

ANSWER: We have not yet studied this question directly, but we are intending to do so. As you know, treatment of autistic children with high doses of secretin, an intestinal hormone that regulates bicarbonate levels in the stomach, has been associated with improvements in speech and sociability. While it is unlikely that secretin represents the "magic bullet" cure for autism, these data may provide us with important clues to the mechanisms behind the autistic disease syndrome, and this information may lead us closer to a cure. Borna disease virus (BDV) infection of newborn rats leads to as yet unexplained damage to specific brain regions such as the hippocampus and cerebellum. It has been postulated that peptides that resemble secretin (such as VIP or NPY) may bind to receptors on the hippocampal neurons and astrocytes, two cell types that are infected with and damaged by BDV. Interestingly, our studies reported at this meeting showed a significantly elevated NPY RNA concentration in cortex, hippocampus and hypothalamus in neonatally BDV-infected rats at 28 days of age, but not at 7 days of age, as compared to control rats.

Thus, neuroanatomical, behavioral and, now, neurochemical consistencies between the neonatally BDV-infected rat and the autistic disease syndrome make this model valuable for study of the pathogenesis and treatment of autism in children.

From Dr. Hall

Are there serotonergic abnormalities in the Borna virus—infected rats similar to those reported in some autistic individuals?

ANSWER: In patients with autism, a variety of serotonin abnormalities have been described, including hyperserotonemia identified in platelets and regional decreases in brain serotonin metabolism identified by PET scans. Treatments have been tried with serotoninergic agonists, with variable reports of success. Of note, there remains some discussion regarding the presence of increased or decreased serotonin effects associated with autistic disease syndromes.

What is lacking is the ability to directly measure serotonin concentration before, peri- and post-autism diagnosis, in specific brain regions—studies that, of course, cannot be performed in humans. Thus, the animal model system developed in our laboratory can be used to perform a direct, regional determination of serotonin levels early and late in disease. We have identified region-specific, developmental-stage-specific changes in serotonin concentration in neonatally BDV-infected rats (cerebellum, hippocampus, frontal cortex). Well characterized models with symptomatic and mechanistic links to autism can be very useful in linking changes in neurochemistry to behavioral expression and in testing new therapies for autistic symptoms.

QUESTIONS FOR DR. PAULE

From Dr. Palmer

Is there any tolerance to MK-801 behavioral effects? We treated weanling rats for 140 days with MK-801 and tested them in an operant chamber. The MK-801 rats lagged in development, body weight and performance measures from the controls and the AR-R-15896 treatment groups. However, about half way through the study the MK-801 rats began to catch up and at the end of the study were almost normal.

ANSWER: Since there was very little effect of MK-801 on the operant behavioral measures we monitored, it would be difficult to say if any tolerance developed to such effects, but with continued treatment/testing, the differences between the MK-801-treated subjects and controls (which was never statistically significant) diminished. With respect to the general comportment of the MK-801-treated subjects, they have clearly developed tolerance to the motor incoordination/ataxia associated with initial treatment. Early in treatment, some high-dose animals were actually prone in their home cage an hour or two after dosing. The incidence of such occurrences has dropped dramatically as a function of continued dosing.

From Dr. Carbone

What was the age of rhesus monkeys at the start of treatment?
ANSWER: The animals (all females) were approximately 9 months old at the start of treatment.
What was the role of impulse control in test results?
ANSWER: None of the tasks being used in this study can be said to directly assess "impulse control" or "impulsivity." However, our measures of accuracy in all tasks should be sensitive to overly "impulsive" responding, in that one would predict such a tendency to be associated with decreased accuracy of responding in all situations. That we do not see this would suggest no major influence of treatment on impulse control.

QUESTIONS FOR DR. CARBONE

From Dr. Blomgren

Did you check the cytokine protein levels? We have found impressive changes on the mRNA level in the neonatal rat brain, but have had tremendous difficulties finding the proteins.
ANSWER: We have not yet checked for cytokine protein levels. However, for certain cytokines (e.g., some of the lymphokines) the levels of RNA tend to be reflective of the levels of protein produced. For others, such as TNF, this may not be so. It is important to do. However, the reactogenic nature of the astrocytes and microglia certainly are consistent with the presence of actual cytokine gene products.
QUESTION: Did you check the microglia and/or any markers of apoptosis?
ANSWER: We do have preliminary data using the TUNEL technique that show death of granule cells in the dentate gyrus of the hippocampus. We hypothesize that

many of the cells are dropping out due to apoptosis, a classic method by which many viruses kill cells.

QUESTION/COMMENT FOR DR. HALL

COMMENT (Dr. Cosi): Regarding PARP inhibitors having been tested in experimental models of traumatic brain injury, I can say that a few years ago the group of Dr. Wallis had presented evidence that suggested that PARP inhibitors might be beneficial in the treatment of traumatic spinal cord injury.

The Regulation of Cerebral Blood Flow during Intravenous Cocaine Administration in Cocaine Abusers

RONALD I. HERNING,[a] WARREN BETTER, RICHARD NELSON, DAVID GORELICK, AND JEAN L. CADET

Intramural Research Program, National Institute on Drug Abuse, National Institutes of Health, Baltimore, Maryland, USA

ABSTRACT: Cocaine abuse is associated with heightened risk of life-threatening neurological complications such as strokes, seizures, and transient ischemic attacks. We used transcranial Doppler (TCD) sonography, a continuous measure of cerebral blood flow velocity, to better understand the changes in cerebral hemodynamics produced by cocaine administration, which may lead to an increased risk for stroke in cocaine abusers. Heart rate and blood pressure were also measured. Blood flow velocity of seven cocaine abusers was studied during placebo, 10-, 25-, and 50-mg intravenous (i.v.) injections of cocaine. A significant increase in mean and systolic velocity which lasted for about two minutes was observed with all doses of cocaine, with no change in the placebo condition. This increase in systolic velocity indicates that cocaine produces an immediate and brief period of vasoconstriction in large arteries of the brain. The present results elucidate the time course of cocaine's acute cerebrovascular effects and provide a better understanding of etiology of cocaine-related stroke and transient ischemic attacks.

INTRODUCTION

Cocaine abuse is associated with an increased risk of stroke.[1–3] Epidemiologic and postmortem studies of cocaine-induced ischemic and hemorrhagic stroke have suggested that possible mechanisms may be vasospasm of large arteries,[4] vasculitis secondary to vasospastic/ischemic conditions[5,6] and acute hypertension.[7] Cocaine-induced hemorrhagic stroke in the absence of vasculitis has also been reported.[8]

Imaging studies of cerebral blood flow and metabolism have provided some insight into cocaine-induced cerebrovascualar events that might lead to stroke. For example, reductions in cortical glucose metabolism using positron emission tomography (PET) were observed.[9] Reductions in cerebral blood flow using single photon emission computed tomography (SPECT) were reported up to 30 minutes after intravenous (i.v.) cocaine administration.[10,11] However, an increase rather than a decrease in cerebral blood flow for up to 30 minutes after i.v. doses of cocaine was

[a]Corresponding author: Ronald I. Herning, Ph.D., Molecular Neuropsychiatry Section, National Institute on Drug Abuse, P.O. Box 5180, Baltimore, MD 21224. Phone, 410/550-1551; fax, 410/550-1438.

e-mail, rherning@intra.nida.nih.gov

found using [133]Xenon inhalation.[12] In the cocaine administration studies using magnetic resonance imaging (MRI) methodology, the measurements were made after the peak cardiovascular and subjective effects. In an MRI study with dynamic susceptibility contrast, cerebral blood volume was reduced at 10 minutes after an i.v. cocaine administration.[13] Magnetic resonance angiography (MRA) distal signal loss in middle and posterior arteries was detected at 20 minutes after cocaine injections.[14] With functional magnetic resonance imaging (fMRI) flow-sensitive alternating inversion recovery imaging, a decrease in grey matter blood flow was observed at 10 minutes after cocaine injections.[15] Measures in these MRI studies were not obtained at other times, and the time course of these changes is not known.

None of these imaging studies found reductions in cerebral blood flow were indicative of ischemic conditions. Certainly, doses of cocaine larger than those used in these studies might possibly produce more extensive reductions in cerebral blood flow leading to transient ischemic attacks or ischemic stroke. These studies, however, do not suggest a mechanism for hemorrhagic stroke. We used transcranial Doppler (TCD) sonography,[16] a continuous measure of cerebral blood flow velocity, to better understand the changes in cerebral hemodynamics before and after i.v. cocaine administration to cocaine abusers. We hypothesized that such continuous temporal cerebrovascular data and its relation to the time course of cardiovascular measures might provide a better understanding of etiology of cocaine-related stroke and transient ischemic attacks in cocaine abusers.

METHODS

Seven cocaine abusers were tested. Six were African Americans and six were male. Their mean age was 34.9 years (range 25 to 39 years). They passed the following screening tests: twelve lead electrocardiogram (EKG), echocardiogram, twenty-four hour EKG holter monitor, cardiovascular stress test, clinical electroencephalogram (EEG), quantitative flow measurement (QFM), and TCD sonography, computerized axial tomography (CAT) scan, physical exam, structured neurological exam, psychiatric evaluation, neuropsychological tests, and clinical laboratory tests. All subjects had a history of i.v. cocaine use and were not currently seeking treatment. The research protocol was approved by the National Institute on Drug Abuse and Johns Hopkins Bayview Medical Center Institutional Review Boards for Human Research. Written informed consent was obtained from all subjects.

Subjects received 0, 10, 25 and 50 mg i.v. injections of cocaine. Intravenous cocaine doses were given at three different infusion durations: 10, 30 and 60 seconds. Not all subjects received all doses or all infusion durations.

Monitoring included a 30-minute pre-infusion baseline and 45-minute post-infusion period. Blood flow velocity was determined by TCD sonography (Nicolet, Model TC2000) of the left middle cerebral artery, and heart rate was continuously monitored during the pre and post-injection periods. Mean blood flow velocity (Vm: cm/s), systolic velocity (Vs: cm/s), diastolic velocity (Vd: cm/s), and pulsatility index (PI = (Vs−Vd)/Vm) were determined at representative times (−12.5, −8.5, 1, 2, 3, 4.5, 5.5, 7.5, 8.5, 11.5, 13.5, 22.5, 24.5, 42.5 and 44.5 minutes relative to the start of the injection). Heart rate and blood pressure were measured at discrete times during the monitoring periods (−20, −15, −10, −5, −2, 2, 4, 7, 10, 15, 21, 26, 31, 36, and 41 minutes relative to the injection). A two-way dose by time analysis of variance (ANOVA) was performed on cerebral blood flow velocity and cardiovascular measures. A preliminary analysis indicated that the injection duration played a minor role in the TCD changes observed in this study.

RESULTS

The cocaine injection significantly increased heart rate (dose by time interaction: $F(42,406) = 2.08$, $p < 0.01$), systolic blood pressure (dose: $F(3,29) = 3.40$, $p < 0.05$; time: $F(14,29) = 5.40$, $p < 0.01$) and diastolic blood pressure (dose: $F(3,29) = 3.23$, $p < 0.05$; time: $F(14,29) = 5.51$, $p < 0.01$). The peak effect of the cocaine injections was at about four minutes for the 25- and 50-mg doses.

Because of differences in baseline values, change from pre-injection baseline scores were calculated for the cerebral blood flow velocity measures. Systolic velocity (dose by time interaction: $F(36,348) = 1.60$, $p < 0.03$) and mean velocity (dose by time interaction: $F(36,348) = 1.63$, $p < 0.03$) were significantly increased after all cocaine injections. FIGURE 1 plots the change from baseline values for systolic velocity. Both 25- and 50-mg doses of cocaine produced similar increases. The increased cerebral blood flow velocity was observed for 1 to 2 minutes. Diastolic velocity (dose by time interaction: $F(36,348) = 0.88$, $p > 0.25$) and pulsatility (dose by time interaction: $F(36,348) = 0.98$, $p > 0.25$) were not significantly affected by the administration of cocaine.

A comparison of the time course of systolic velocity in the middle cerebral artery and systolic blood pressure was also made. This comparison is shown in FIGURE 2 for the 50-mg dose of cocaine, but is comparable to that for the other cocaine doses.

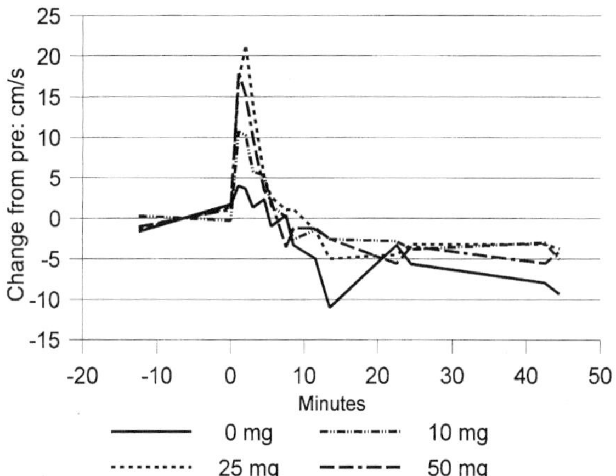

FIGURE 1. The mean values for cerebral systolic blood flow velocity are plotted as change scores from the mean of the pre-injection baseline. All the cocaine doses have peak velocity increases that are significantly greater than the 0-mg (placebo) dose. The 25- and 50-mg cocaine doses do not differ from each other.

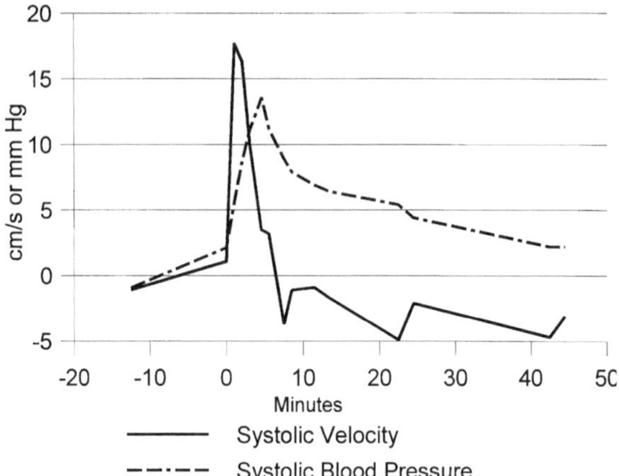

FIGURE 2. The mean values for systolic blood pressure and cerebral systolic blood flow velocity for the 50-mg dose of cocaine are plotted as change scores from the mean of the pre-injection baseline. Blood pressure values are in mm Hg, and cerebral blood flow velocity values are cm/s. Both are plotted on the same scale. Note the brief increase in systolic blood flow velocity as compared to the long increase in systolic blood pressure.

The peak increase in systolic velocity occurred at one to two minutes after cocaine administration, while the peak increase in systolic blood pressure occurred at two to four minutes. Only for the first two minutes after cocaine administration were both systolic velocity and blood pressure elevated. Thereafter, systolic velocity returned to baseline, whereas systolic blood pressure remained elevated.

DISCUSSION

Intravenous cocaine administration significantly increased systolic velocity in the middle cerebral artery. Increased systolic velocity with no change in pulsatility reflects vasoconstriction in these arteries.[17,18] Kaufman and associates founded evidence for vasoconstriction of large arteries at 20 minutes after i.v. cocaine administration using MRA techniques.[14] Although the direct cause for these vasospastic response is not yet know, the increase in systolic velocity may be due to the direct effects of cocaine mediated by dopamine (DA) neurons in the cortex. This notion is supported by the recent findings of dopaminergic regulation of cortical blood vessels in the rabbit.[19] DA produced vasconstriction in this model.[20] Increased DA levels by cocaine blocking DA reuptake might influence postsynaptic DA receptors involved in the control of cerebral circulation.

Cerebral blood flow velocity can also be increased by increasing blood pressure without changes in vessel diameter.[17] The cocaine-induced blood pressure increases observed in this study have been previously reported.[21,22] These increases might have produced the increases in systolic velocity also observed in this study. This is unlikely, since the changes in systolic velocity did not parallel the changes in systolic blood pressure. Systolic velocity rapidly dropped after the two-minute reading, but systolic blood pressure gradually decreased over the next 10 to 15 minutes. Further evidence that the increases in systolic cerebral blood flow might not be due to increases in systolic blood pressure comes from another study currently in progress in our laboratory. Although preliminary, we found that increased systolic blood pressure in cocaine abusers produced by psychological stress resulted in decreases in systolic cerebral blood flow velocity. Thus, there is evidence for cerebral autoregulatory mechanisms that appear to reduce systolic velocity, perhaps by decreasing cerebrovascular resistance, when systolic blood pressure increases.

Our findings suggest a possible mechanism for cocaine-induced stroke. The cocaine abuser with a long history of cocaine abuse has a compromised cerebrovascular system even before taking the next dose of cocaine. Specifically, abstinent cocaine abusers have increased cerebrovascular resistance.[23] SPECT cerebral perfusion deficits have also been reported in cocaine abusers.[24,25] Thus, given that our results obtained with cocaine doses were relatively modest and were selected because of their safety in healthy cocaine abusers, it is likely that larger doses of cocaine might produce much greater vasoconstriction of the large cerebral arteries of the brain leading to a greater risk of transient ischemic attacks or ischemic strokes. Larger doses of cocaine may also inhibit autoregulatory decreases in cerebral blood flow velocity during periods of blood pressure increases. Thus, cocaine-induced changes in blood pressure and vasoconstriction in the presence of cocaine-induced altered cerebrovascular regulation may lead to greater risk of hemorrhagic stroke in cocaine abusers.

REFERENCES

1. QURESHI, A.I. *et al.* 1995. Stroke in young black patients. Risk factors, subtypes, and prognosis. Stroke **26:** 995–998.
2. FESSLER, R.D. *et al.* 1997. The neurovascular complications of cocaine. Surg. Neurol. **47:** 339–345.
3. PETITTI, D.B. *et al.* 1998. Stroke and cocaine or amphetamine use. Epidemiology **9:** 596–600.
4. KONZEN, J.P. *et al.* 1995. Vasospasm and thrombus formation as possible mechanisms of stroke related to alkaloidal cocaine. Stroke **26:** 1114–1118.
5. MARTINAEZ, N.E. *et al.* 1996. Vasospasm/thrombus in ischemia related to cocaine abuse. Stroke **27:** 146–147.
6. BRUST, J.C. 1997. Vasculitis owing to substance abuse. Neurol. Clin. **15:** 945-957.
7. JOVANOVIC, Z. 1996. Risk factors for stroke in young people. Srp. Arh. Celok. Lek. **124:** 232-235.
8. AGGARWAL, S.K. *et al.* 1996. Cocaine-associated intracranial hemorrhage: absence of vasculitis in 14 cases. Neurology **46:** 1741-1743.
9. LONDON, E.D. *et al.* 1990. Cocaine-induced reduction of glucose utilization in the human brain. Arch. Gen. Psychiatry **47:** 567–574.
10. PEARLSON, G.D. *et al.* 1993. Correlation of acute cocaine-induced cerebral blood flow with subjective effects. Am. J. Psychiatry **150:** 495–497.
11. WALLACE, E.A. *et al.* 1996. Acute cocaine effects on absolute cerebral blood flow. Psychopharmacology **128:** 17-20.
12. MATHEW, R.J. *et al.* 1996. Acute changes in cranial blood flow after cocaine hydrochloride. Biol. Psychiatry **40:** 609–616.
13. KAUFMAN, M.J *et al.* 1998. Cocaine decreases relative cerebral blood volume in humans: a dynamic susceptibility contrast magnetic resonance imaging study. Psychopharmacology **138:** 76–81.

14. KAUFMAN, M.J. *et al.* 1998. Cocaine-induced cerebral vasoconstriction detected in humans with magnetic resonance angiography. JAMA **279:** 376–380.
15. GOLLUB, R.L. *et al..* 1998.. Cocaine decreases cerebral blood flow but does not obscure regional activation in fMRI in human subjects. J. Cereb. Blood Flow Metab. **18:** 724–734.
16. ARNOLDS, B.J. & G.M. VON REUTEN. 1986. Transcranial Doppler sonography: examination technique and normal reference values. Ultrasound Med. Biol. **12:** 115–123.
17. CZOSNYKA, M. *et al.* 1996. Relationship between transcranial Doppler-determined pulsatility index and cerebrovascular resistance: an experimental study. J. Neurosurg. **84:** 79–84.
18. ALEXANDROV, A.V. *et al.* 1997. Correlation of peak systolic velocity and angiographic measurement of carotid stenosis revisited. Stroke **28:** 339–342.
19. KRIMER, L.S. *et al.* 1998. Dopaminergic regulation of cerebral cortical microcirculation. Nature Neurosci. **1:** 286–289.
20. RITZ. M.C. *et al.* 1987. Cocaine receptors on dopamine tranporters are related to self-administration of cocaine. Science **237:** 121–1223.
21. FISCHMAN, M.W. *et al..* 1983. A comparison of the subjective and cardiovasculur effects of cocaine and lidococaine in humans. Pharmacol. Biochem. Behav. **18:** 123–127.
22. MENDELSON, J.H. *et al.* 1998. Cocaine tolerance: behavioral, cardiovascular, and neuroendocrine function in men. Neuropsychopharmacology **18:** 263–271.
23. HERNING, R.I. *et al.* 1999. Neurovascular deficits in cocaine abusers. Neuropsychopharmacology. In press.
24. HOLMAN, B.L. *et al.* 1991. Brain perfusion is abnormal in cocaine-dependent polydrug users: a study using technetium-99m-NMPAO and ASPECT. J. Nucl. Med. **32:** 1206–1210.
25. LEVIN, J.M. *et al.* 1995. Improved regional cerebral blood flow in chronic cocaine polydrug users treated with buprenorphine. J. Nucl. Med. **35:** 1902–1904.

Time Course of Brain Temperature and Caudate/Putamen Microdialysate Levels of Amphetamine and Dopamine in Rats after Multiple Doses of *d*-Amphetamine

PETER CLAUSING[a] AND JOHN F. BOWYER[b,c]

*aDepartment of General Toxicology, Scantox, 36A Hestehavevej,
4623 Lille Skensved, Denmark*

*bDivision of Neurotoxicology, National Center for Toxicological Research,
3900 NCTR Road, Jefferson, Arkansas 72079, USA*

ABSTRACT: Brain temperature monitoring and microdialysis were performed simultaneously in the caudate/putamen (CPu) of conscious, freely moving rats dosed with *d*-amphetamine (AMPH). The brain temperature was determined via a thermistor inserted through a microdialysis guide cannula located in the left CPu, while the microdialysis probe was positioned in the right CPu. The peak AMPH and dopamine (DA) levels were reached 40 to 60 min after dosing, while peak brain temperature was not achieved until 20 to 40 min thereafter in rats becoming moderately hyperthermic. Those rats becoming severely hyperthermic (temperatures above 41.0°C) had microdialysate concentrations of AMPH and DA almost 2-fold higher than those with moderate hyperthermia after the second dose of 5 mg/kg AMPH. However, these peaks were not reached until 60 to 80 min after dosing. This was probably due, in part, to the longer half-life of AMPH in the severely hyperthermic group. The changes in brain temperature observed after exposure to neurotoxic doses of AMPH closely paralleled core body temperature changes previously reported during AMPH exposure. Temperature plays an important role in many types of neurotoxicity, and monitoring brain temperature during microdialysis studies can be done continuously, and with less chance of damage to the microdialysis equipment than most of the traditional methods used to measure core body temperature.

INTRODUCTION

Amphetamine, in particular *d*-amphetamine (AMPH), elicits dopamine (DA) release[24,13] and affects thermoregulation, which in rats results in hyperthermia at ambient temperatures above 20°C and in hypothermia at environmental temperatures below 12°C.[29] Hyperthermia has been shown to be a critical mediator of methamphetamine (METH) and AMPH neurotoxicity.[1–3,18] Both, hypothalamic and nigral dopaminergic systems have been suggested to be involved in thermoregula-

*cCorresponding author. Phone, 870/543-7194; fax, 870/543-7745.
e-mail, jbowyer@nctr.fda.gov*

"

tion.[14,21] D_1-receptors predominantly appear to participate in the mediation of hyperthermic responses.[22,28,31]

Brain tissue, microdialysate and plasma levels of AMPH and METH correlate well with changes in extracellular levels of DA as well as motor activity and stereotypic behavior.[13,6] Therefore, unless a rapid downregulation of DA receptors or other receptors regulating temperature occurs, the brain and core body temperature should correlate positively with both amphetamine and DA levels in brain after dosing. A description of the time course of brain temperature and extracellular AMPH and DA levels in the brain during AMPH exposure is necessary to determine if this in fact is the case, and contributes to the understanding of underlying mechanisms of amphetamine-induced hyperthermia.

The ability to continuously monitor extracellular AMPH levels in brain microdialysate of individual animals[7] while recording behavioral, physiological and neurochemical changes provides the means by which to compare changes in these biological parameters with the time course of extracellular AMPH levels in specific brain regions. In the present investigation we recorded the brain temperature of rats dosed with three subsequent subcutaneous (s.c.) administrations of 5 mg/kg *d*-AMPH, and simultaneously analyzed their extracellular AMPH and DA levels in microdialysate from the caudate/putamen (CPu). Furthermore, hyperthermia can play a critical role in the lethality and neurotoxicity of amphetamines,[30,1–3,18] ergot alkaloids,[23] and compounds that affect prostaglandin levels in the brain.[26] Therefore, the methods for monitoring brain temperature used in the present study on AMPH can be applied to other neurotoxic insults.

METHODS

Animal Housing and Experimental Design

All procedures involving animal care were approved by the National Center for Toxicological Research (NCTR) Institutional Animal Care and Use Committee. The studies reported in this paper were carried out in accordance with the declaration of Helsinki and with the Guide for the Care and Use of Laboratory Animals as adopted and promulgated by the National Institutes of Health. Four-month-old male Sprague-Dawley rats (Crl:COBS CD [SD] BR) from the in-house NCTR breeding colony were used. They were individually housed starting on the day of implantation of the microdialysis guide cannulae and kept in acrylic cages ($45 \times 22 \times 20$ cm) on wood shaving bedding. Their average body weight on the day of experiment was 512 ± 10 g (mean $\pm$ SEM). A standardized room temperature of $23 \pm 1°C$ was provided during animal housing and experiment. For the microdialysis sessions, the rats were transferred into microdialysis bowls (in an adjacent room) just before probe insertion. Four hours after probe insertion a "behavioral" dose of 2.5 mg/kg AMPH was administered s.c. to 9 of these rats, and they were monitored for 3 hours. The results for this part of the experiment were described earlier.[7] Thereafter, these rats received 3 consecutive s.c. doses of 5 mg/kg AMPH spaced 2 hours apart, brain temperature was recorded and microdialysate was collected every 20 minutes for analysis of DA and AMPH. An additional 5 rats received 3 injections of saline instead of AMPH, and their brain temperature was recorded. After the experiment the rats were sacri-

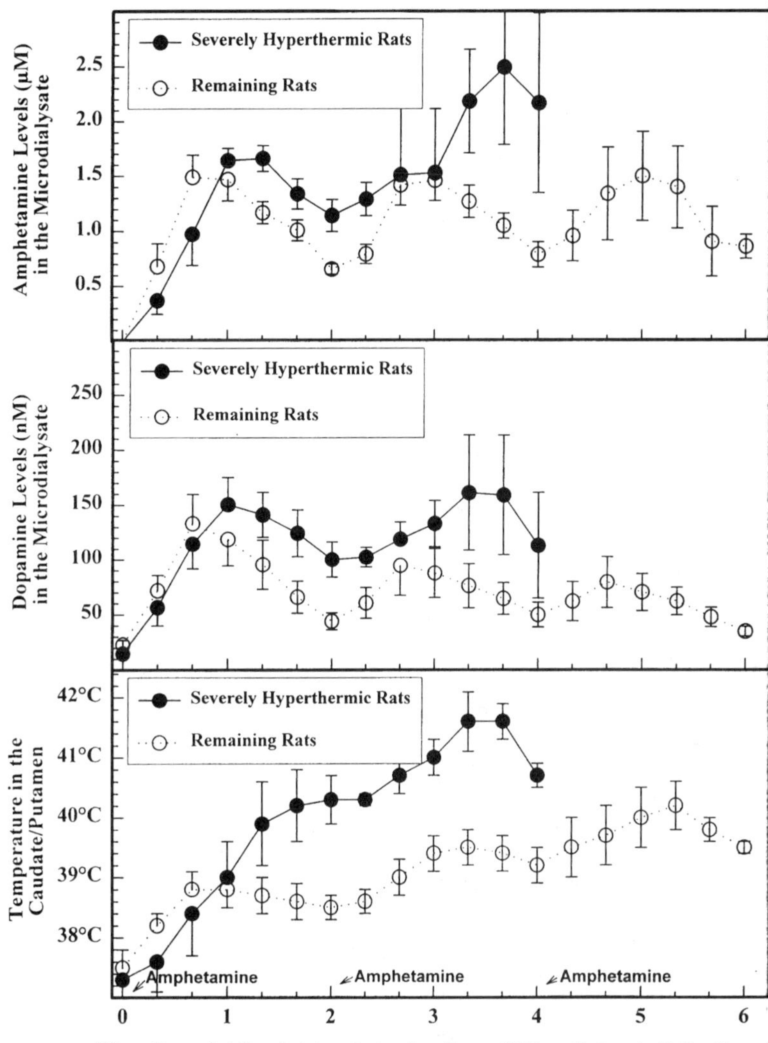

FIGURE 1. The time course of brain temperature, amphetamine and dopamine levels in CPu microdialysate of rats administered 3 doses of 5 mg/kg *d*-amphetamine. The *top graph* shows the amphetamine concentration, while the *middle graph* shows the dopamine concentration in the microdialysate. Brain (CPu) temperature is shown on the *bottom graph*. Three doses of 5 mg/kg *d*-amphetamine were administered at 2-hr intervals. The 3 parameters for the rats that became severely hyperthermic (greater than 41°C) are indicated by the *filled symbols*, while the *open symbols* represent data from the animals with a milder hyperthermic response.

ficed for histological verification of the correct positioning of the microdialysis and the temperature probes.

Brain Surgery

For each rat a CMA/12 guide cannula (Carnegie Medicine, Stockholm, Sweden) was implanted into the left striatum and one into the right striatum. The left side was used for the temperature probe (see below) and the right side for the microdialysis probe. To implant the guide cannulae, animals were anesthetized with sodium pentobarbital (50 mg/kg intraperitoneally (i.p.)), and body temperature was maintained at 37°C with a Deltaphase Isothermal Pad (Braintree Scientific, MA) placed under the animal. The head of the animal was placed in a stereotaxic frame (Köpf, Tajunga, CA) with the dorsal surface level to the frame. The dorsal skull was exposed, and small holes were drilled into the skull to allow implantation of the guide cannulae with the coordinates AP 0.2 mm, LAT 3 mm, DV 5.0 mm, relative to bregma.[20] The cannulae were fixed to the skull with dental acrylic and two anchor screws, and then were closed with a tight-fitting obturator. After surgery the animals were given 7 days of recovery prior to probe insertion and microdialysis.

Brain Microdialysis

Brain microdialysis was carried out in a manner similar to that of Ungerstedt (1984)[27] with some modifications[2] using CMA microdialysis equipment (Carnegie Medicine, Stockholm, Sweden). The artificial cerebrospinal fluid had the following composition: NaCl 145 mM; KCl 1.5 mM; $MgCl_2*H_2O$ 1.5 mM; $CaCl_2*2H_2O$ 1.25 mM; glucose 10 mM; K_2HPO_4 1.5 mM; adjusted to pH 7.0 with HCl. On the morning of the experiment subjects were moved in their home cage to the experimental room and wrapped in a towel, and the CMA/12 probe (2 mm membrane length) was carefully inserted through the guide cannula into the CPu. Four hours after probe insertion collection of microdialysis samples started at a flow rate of 1 µl/min. The mean for baseline DA levels reached (last 3 collection periods before dosing the "behavioral" AMPH dose of 2.5 mg/kg) was 15 ± 3 fmol/µl ($n = 9$). The levels of DA in the microdialysate returned to near baseline levels (19.2 ± 3 fmol/µl) within 2.5 hr of the "behavioral dose" and just prior to the first dose of 5 mg/kg AMPH. Immediately after the sample collection, 10 µl, designated for monoamine analysis, was transferred to another tube that contained 1 µl of 0.1 N perchloric acid. The samples were frozen on dry ice and then stored at $-150°C$ until analysis, which in the case of DA was performed within the next few days.

Brain Temperature

An IT-21 temperature probe (Physitemp, Instruments, Clifton, N.J.) was inserted through the CMA/12 guide cannula into the left striatum immediately after the microdialysis probe was inserted into the right striatum. Brain temperature was measured at baseline, i.e., shortly before the administration of the 2.5-mg/kg AMPH dose and then every 20 min over the 6-hr course of the three 5-mg/kg AMPH doses.

High-Performance Liquid Chromatography (HPLC)
Quantitation of Amphetamine

A detailed description of this method can be found elsewhere.[4] In brief, AMPH levels were determined by fluorescent detection after *o*-phthaldialdehyde/3-mercap-

TABLE 1. Time course of amphetamine (AMPH) and dopamine concentrations in microdialysate, and brain temperature subsequent to one dose of 2.5 mg/kg s.c. *d*-AMPH (data not shown) three hours later followed by 3 consecutive doses of 5 mg/kg AMPH s.c., spaced 2 hours apart

Time post 1st/ 2nd/3rd dose (min)	AMPH in Microdialysate (μM)	$n =$, for AMPH	Dopamine in Microdialysate (nM)	Brain Temperature (°C)	$n =$, for dopamine and Brain Temperature
20	0.52 ± 0.15	9	65 ± 10	38.0 ± 0.2	9
40	1.26 ± 0.18	9	125 ± 17	38.6 ± 0.4	9
60	**1.64 ± 0.08**	9	**133 ± 17**	38.9 ± 0.3	9
80	1.39 ± 0.11	9	116 ± 17	39.2 ± 0.4	9
100	1.15 ± 0.10	9	92 ± 16	**39.3 ± 0.4**	9
120	0.84 ± 0.10	8	60 ± 9	39.1 ± 0.3	9
20	0.98 ± 0.12	8	86 ± 13	39.4 ± 0.3	9
40	**1.64 ± 0.22**	8	**107 ± 16**	39.8 ± 0.4	9
60	1.64 ± 0.23	8	107 ± 19	**40.1 ± 0.4**	9
80	1.61 ± 0.28	8	101 ± 29	40.0 ± 0.4	8
100	1.41 ± 0.37	7	91 ± 28	40.0 ± 0.4	8
120	1.23 ± 0.45	6	77 ± 21	39.7 ± 0.3	8
20	0.96 ± 0.23	5	59 ± 15	39.6 ± 0.4	7
40	1.40 ± 0.33	5	**88 ± 20**	40.0 ± 0.4	7
60	**1.56 ± 0.32**	5	83 ± 18	**40.4 ± 0.5**	7
80	1.28 ± 0.23	5	64 ± 11	40.1 ± 0.4	6
100	0.96 ± 0.18	5	50 ± 6	39.7 ± 0.2	6
120	1.00 ± 0.16	5	45 ± 10	39.5 ± 0.1	6

NOTE: Peak values after dose are shown in **bold**. Values represent mean ± SEM and number of animals (*n*). Two animals were removed from the experiment due to hyperthermia during the microdialysis session and a number of AMPH samples were lost due to technical problems. The residual microdialysate levels of *d*-AMPH just prior to the first of the 3 doses of 5 mg/kg *d*-AMPH were not detectable (≤ 0.1 μM).

topropionic acid-derivatization and separation on a Supelcosil[7] LC-18 mm column, running a gradient with 65% KH_2PO_4 (0.05 M, pH 5.5) + 35% methanol (mobile phase A) versus 35% KH_2PO_4 (0.05 M, pH 5.5) + 65% methanol (mobile phase B). Microdialysis samples were derivatized and injected directly using a CMA/200 autosampler.

HPLC Quantitation of Dopamine

Dopamine was analyzed by electrochemical (EC) detection after direct injection of 10 μl microdialysate onto the HPLC/EC system. Samples were analyzed using the following: an isocratic M-6000A pump (Waters Associates, Milford, MA) at a 1.3-ml/min flow rate; a Rheodyne 7125 injector (Rheodyne Inc., Cotati, CA); a Supelcosil LC18 analytical column (3 : m, 7.5 cm × 4.6 mm, Supelco, Bellefonte, PA); a BAS-LC4B amperometric detector with a BAS-LC-17 oxidative flow cell; and a Waters model 746 data module integrator (Waters Associates, Milford, MA). The mobile phase consisted of 92% KH_2PO_4-buffer (0.07 M, pH 3.0) and 8% methanol containing 1 mM Na-1-heptanesulfonic acid and 0.2 mM Na_2-ethylenediamine-tetraacetic acid (EDTA).

RESULTS

Saline injection did not increase brain temperature in control rats. Average brain temperature for these subjects was $37.7 \pm 0.7°C$ (mean $\pm$ SEM). The time course (means $\pm$ SEM) of brain temperature and microdialysate levels of DA and AMPH in the striatum for all animals given multiple doses of amphetamine are shown in TABLE 1. The mean AMPH levels peaked in the microdialysate at 40 to 60 min after each dose for these animals, while the peak for the mean DA levels occurred at the same time or one collection period (20 min) earlier. Peak brain temperatures were observed 20 to 40 minutes after AMPH and DA peaked. Data from the individual animals showed that DA levels correlated closely with AMPH levels (data not shown).

In FIGURE 1 the data for animals in TABLE 1 were split into 2 groups. Those rats that became only moderately hyperthermic were placed in one group ($n = 4$, peak brain temperature less than $40.5°C$), and those that became severely hyperthermic were placed in another group ($n = 5$, peak brain temperature greater than $41.0°C$). The peak amphetamine and DA levels for the severely hyperthermic group were reached 20 min later than the moderately hyperthermic group after the first dose of AMPH, and 40 to 60 min later after the second dose (FIG.1). Note that the DA levels and AMPH levels are plotted on different scales, and that the AMPH levels are actually 10 times greater in concentration than DA levels in the microdialysate. The peak brain temperatures for the severely hyperthermic group were reached 40 to 60 min later than the moderately hyperthermic animals. The data for the severely hyperthermic group ended after the second dose, because several rats were removed from this group to avoid the lethal effects of this hyperthermia. In previous studies severely hyperthermic rats were rapidly cooled with crushed ice and would remain in the study. However, this cooling rapidly and artificially lowers body temperature, which would confound the interpretation of how hyperthermia normally affects amphetamine and DA levels in the CPu that was evaluated in the present experiments.

AMPH levels were around 10-fold higher than DA levels after the first dose and about 15-fold higher after the second and third dose. This was a result of DA levels either decreasing (moderately hyperthermic) or staying the same (severely hyperthermic) while the AMPH levels either stayed the same (moderately hyperthermic) or increased (severely hyperthermic). The reduced increases in microdialysate DA levels after the second and third dose of AMPH compared to the first are primarily due to a time after probe insertion-dependent phenomenon.[11] When the DA levels in FIGURE 1 are recalculated using a correction factor for the time after probe insertion-dependent reductions in DA the ratio of the peak AMPH to DA levels in the microdialysate stays relatively constant at around 10:1 for all 3 doses.

DISCUSSION

The hyperthermia observed in the brain in these experiments shows that brain temperature during AMPH exposure parallels changes in the core body temperature previously observed.[6,7] In addition, the data indicate that (1) the degree of hyperthermia correlates to AMPH and DA levels in the microdialysate but that peak brain temperatures are reached at 20 to 40 min after peak AMPH and DA levels. Also, (2) animals with severe hyperthermia have much higher microdialysate levels of AMPH and DA than those with only moderate hyperthermia. Finally, (3) monitoring brain temperature during microdialysis can yield important information in studies involving neurotoxicity.

Changes in brain, CPu, temperature after the 3 consecutive doses of AMPH in rat were as expected from previously observed changes in core body temperature after either METH[1,3] or AMPH.[7] Although the methods used to place a thermistor probe through a microdialysis guide cannula into the brain require some time and technical skills, this only extends the time of surgery necessary for microdialysis only by one more guide cannula site. The method we used to determine brain temperature is preferable to the method of determining core body temperature via rectal thermistor probe. The recording of brain temperature is continuous rather than intermittent, there is less risk of damaging the microdialysis equipment and probe and rectal probes can cause stress and even damage to the colon and rectum. Thermistors that are linked to radio transmitters, and implanted in the abdominal cavity, can be used to continuously monitor body temperature.[17] However, this method would require additional surgery in the abdominal area and would be more expensive, and data acquisitions would be more complicated. Furthermore, in humans, rectal and bladder temperatures (core body temperatures) can underestimate brain temperature after brain trauma in some cases.[10]

In a previous report we have observed that after multiple doses of 5 mg/kg there was a "build-up" in the mean AMPH levels after the first dose,[6] and that the peak levels of AMPH were reached within 60 min after all doses. In the present studies, after subdividing all the animals tested into two groups, we did not see increasing levels of AMPH after multiple doses in the moderately hyperthermic group. However, AMPH levels substantially increased between the first and the second dose in the severely hyperthermic group along with the time to peak AMPH and DA levels (from 60 min after the first dose to 100 min after the second dose). An increase in the time to peak AMPH levels was not as apparent in the animals that were severely hyperthermic in our previous study.[6] However, those animals were rapidly cooled with crushed ice, while in the present studies animals were not cooled. It is possible that in the present study the severely hyperthermic animals would have had a lower clearance rate leading to the buildup of AMPH levels in the brain even if they had not become so hyperthermic. Alternatively, severe hyperthermia over more than 30 min may increase the bioavailability of AMPH by altering the pharmacokinetics of AMPH.

AMPH may evoke serotonin and norepinephrine release[24] and disrupt thermoregulation through these neurotransmitters, since they play a prominent role in the hypothalamic control of thermoregulation.[12,32] However, the generation of hyperthermia during AMPH exposure has also been ascribed to DA release and D_1 receptor stimulation.[22,28,31] Our studies monitored DA release in the CPu. Further studies in the hypothalamus, determining whether extracellular DA, norepinephrine and serotonin increases correlate with AMPH levels, are necessary for a clearer understanding of the mechanisms by which elevated brain extracellular AMPH modulates hyperthermia.

Determining the degree of hyperthermia occurring in brain during AMPH and METH exposure should aid in more accurately predicting the degree of dopaminergic terminal damage in the CPu and neurodegeneration in the parietal cortex. This is because this damage is temperature dependent in rat and mouse.[1,3,18,9] Furthermore, the degree of serotonin depletion is also correlative for forebrain depletions of serotonin produced by methylenedioxymethamphetamine (MDMA)[18,5,16] and *d*-fenfluramine.[25,8] Determination of temperature elevation in the brain should help further elucidate the role of hyperthermia in other types of compounds other than amphetamines such as ergot alkaloids, kainate and prostaglandin E_2.[23,15,26] In contrast, hypothermic changes in brain may help predict the degree of enzyme inhibition occurring and the neurotoxicity produced by inhibitors electron transport or adenosine triphosphate (ATP) production in the mitochondria such as 3-nitropropionic acid (Ref. 19 and Bowyer unpublished data).

ACKNOWLEDGMENT

During the conduct of the experiments P. Clausing was supported through an appointment to the Oak Ridge Associated Universities Postgraduate Research Program, Oak Ridge, Tennessee.

REFERENCES

1. BOWYER, J.F., A.W. TANK, G.D. NEWPORT, W. SLIKKER, JR., S.F. ALI & R.R. HOLSON. 1992. The influence of environmental temperature on the transient effects of methamphetamine on dopamine release in rat striatum. J. Pharmacol. Exp. Ther. **260:** 817–824.
2. BOWYER, J.F., B. GOUGH, W. SLIKKER, JR., G.W. LIPE, G.D. NEWPORT & R.R. HOLSON. 1993. Effects of a cold environment or age on methamphetamine-induced dopamine release in the caudate putamen of female rats. Pharmacol. Biochem. Behav. **44:** 87–98.
3. BOWYER, J.F., D.L. DAVIES, L. SCHMUED, H.W. BROENING, G.D. NEWPORT, W. SLIKKER, JR. & R.R. HOLSON. 1994. Further studies of the role of hyperthermia in methamphetamine neurotoxicity. J. Pharmacol. Exp. Ther. **268:** 1571–1580.
4. BOWYER, J.F., P. CLAUSING & G.D. NEWPORT. 1995. Determination of *d*-amphetamine in biological samples using high-performance liquid chromatography after precolumn derivatization with *o*-phthaldialdehyde and 3-mercaptopropionic acid. J. Chromatogr. B. **666:** 241–250.
5. BROENING, H.W., J.F. BOWYER & W. SLIKKER, JR. 1995. Age-dependent sensitivity of rats to the long-term effects of the serotonergic neurotoxicant (+)-3,4-methylenedioxymethamphetamine (MDMA) correlates with the magnitude of MDMA-induced hyperthermia. J. Pharmacol. Exp. Ther. **275:** 325–333.
6. CLAUSING, P., B. GOUGH, R.R. HOLSON, W. SLIKKER, JR. & J.F. BOWYER. 1995. Amphetamine levels in brain microdialysate, caudate putamen, substantia nigra and plasma after dosage that produces either behavioral or neurotoxic effects. J. Pharmacol. Exp. Ther. **274:** 614–621.
7. CLAUSING, P., D. BLOOM, G.D. NEWPORT, R.R. HOLSON, W. SLIKKER, JR. & J.F. BOWYER. 1996. Individual differences in dopamine release but not rotational behavior correlate with extracellular amphetamine levels in caudate putamen. Psychopharmacology **127:** 187–194.
8. CLAUSING, P., G.D. NEWPORT & J.F. BOWYER. 1998. *d*-Fenfluramine and norfenfluramine levels in brain microdialysate, brain tissue and plasma after doses known to affect brain serotonin levels. J. Pharmacol. Exp. Ther. **284:** 618–624.

9. EISCH, A.J. & J.F. MARSHALL. 1998. Methamphetamine neurotoxicity: dissociation of striatal dopamine terminal damage from parietal cortical cell body injury. Synapse **30:** 433–445.

10. HENKER, R.A., S.D. BROWN & D.W. MARION. 1998. Comparison of brain temperature with bladder and rectal temperatures in adult rats with severe head injury. Neurosurgery **42:** 1071–1075.

11. HOLSON, R.R., J.F. BOWYER, P. CLAUSING & B. GOUGH. 1996. Methamphetamine-stimulated striatal dopamine release declines rapidly over time following microdialysis probe insertion. Brain Res. **739:** 301–307.

12. KANOSUE, K., T. HOSONO, Y.-H. ZHANG & X.-M. CHEN. 1998. Neuronal networks. Controlling thermoregulatory effectors *In* Brain Function in Hot Environment. H.S. Sharma & J. Westman, Eds. Progress in Brain Research. Vol. 115: 49–62. Elsevier Science BV. Amsterdam.

13. KUCZENSKI, R. & D.S. SEGAL. 1994. Neurochemistry of amphetamine. *In* Amphetamine and Its Analogs. Psychopharmacology, Toxicology, and Abuse. A.K. Cho & D.S. Segal, Eds.: 81–113. Academic Press. San Diego, New York, Boston, London, Sidney, Tokyo & Toronto.

14. LEE, T.F., F. MORA & R.D MYERS. 1985. Dopamine and thermoregulation: an evaluation with special reference to dopaminergic pathways. Neurosci. Biobehav. Rev. **9:** 589–598.

15. LOTHMAN, E.W. & R.C. COLLINS. 1981. Kainic acid-induced limbic seizures: metabolic, behavioral, electroencephalographic, and neuropathological correlates. Brain Res. **218:** 299–318.

16. MALBERG, J.E., K.E. SABOL & L.S. SEIDEN. 1996. Co-administration of MDMA with drugs that protect against MDMA neurotoxicity produces different effects on body temperature in the rat. J. Pharmacol. Exp. Ther. **278:** 258–267.

17. MALBERG, J.E. & L.S. SEIDEN. 1998. Small changes in ambient temperature cause large changes in 3,4-methylenedioxymethamphetamine (MDMA)-induced serotonin neurotoxicity and core body temperature in rat. J. Neurosci. **18:** 5086–5094.

18. MILLER, D.B. & J.P. O'CALLAGHAN. 1994. Environment-, drug- and stress-induced alterations in body temperature affect the neurotoxicity of substituted amphetamines in the C57BL/6J mouse. J. Pharmacol. Exp. Ther. **270:** 752–760.

19. NONY, P.A., A.C. SCALLET, R.L. ROUNTREE, X. YE & Z. BINIENDA. 1997. 3-Nitropropionic acid produces hypothermia and inhibits histochemical labeling of succinate dehydrogenase in rat brain. Soc. Neurosci. Abstr. **23:** 855.5.

20. PAXINOS, G. & C. WATSON. 1986. The Rat Brain in Stereotaxic Coordinates. 2nd edit. Academic Press. New York.

21. ROCKHOLD, R.W., E.S. CARVER, Y. ISHIZUKA, B. HOSKINS & I.K. HO. 1991. Dopamine receptors mediate cocaine-induced temperature responses in spontaneously hypertensive and Wistar-Kyoto rats. Pharmacol. Biochem. Behav. **40:** 157–162.

22. SANCHEZ, C. 1989. The effects of D-1 and D-2 receptors agonists on body temperature in male mice. Eur. J. Pharmacol. **171:** 201–206.

23. SCHNEIDER, D.J., C.O. MILES, I. GARTHWAITE, A. VAN HALDEREN, J.C. WESSELS & H.J LATEGAN. 1996. First report of field outbreaks of ergot-alkaloid toxicity in South Africa. Onderstepoort J. Vet. Res. **63:** 97–108.

24. SEIDEN, L.S., K.E. SABOL & G.A. RICAURTE. 1993. Amphetamine: effects on catecholamine systems and behavior. ANNU. REV. PHARMACOL. TOXICOL. **33:** 639–677.

25. STEWART, C.W., J.F. BOWYER & W. SLIKKER, JR. 1997. Elevated environmental temperature can induce hyperthermia during *d*-fenfluramine exposure and enhance 5-hydroxytryptamine (5-HT) depletion in the brain. J. Pharmacol. Exp. Ther. **283:** 1144–1150.

26. THORNHILL, J. & M. SMITH. 1998. Intracerebroventricular prostaglandin administration increases the neural damage evoked by global hemispheric hypoxic ischemia. Brain Res. **784:** 48–56.

27. UNGERSTEDT, U. 1984. Measurement of neurotransmitter release by intracranial dialysis. *In* Measurement of Neurotransmitter Release *In Vivo*. C.A. Marsden, Ed.: 81–105. John Wiley & Sons. New York.

28. VERMA, A. & S.K. KULKARNI. 1993. Differential role of dopamine receptor subtypes in thermoregulation and stereotypic behavior in naive and reserpinized rats. Arch. Int. Pharmacodyn. Ther. **324:** 17–32.

29. YEHUDA, S. & R. FROMMER. 1978. Effects of *d*-amphetamine on the set point thermoregulatory system in rats. Psychopharmacology **57:** 249–252.

30. ZALIS, E.G., G. KAPLAN, G.D. LUNDBERG & R.A. KNUTSON. 1965. Acute lethality of the amphetamines in dogs and its antagonism by curare. Proc. Soc. Exp. Biol. Med. **118:** 557-561.

31. ZARRINDAST, M.R. & S.A. TABATABAI. 1992. Involvement of dopamine receptor subtypes in mouse thermoregulation. Psychopharmacology **107:** 341–346.

32. ZEISBERGER, E. 1998. Biogenic amines and thermoregulatory changes. *In* Brain Function in Hot Environment. H.S. Sharma & J. Westman, Eds. Progress in Brain Research. Vol. 115: 159–176. Elsevier Science BV. Amsterdam.

Neuroprotective Effects of HU-211 on Brain Damage Resulting from Soman-Induced Seizures

MARGARET G. FILBERT,[a] JEFFRY S. FORSTER, C. DAHLEM SMITH,[b] AND GERALD P.H. BALLOUGH[c]

U.S. Army Medical Research Institute of Chemical Defense, Aberdeen Proving Ground, Maryland, USA

ABSTRACT: Neuroprotective effects of HU-211 (dexanabinol), a synthetic non-psychotropic analog of tetrahydrocannabinol, on brain damage resulting from soman-induced seizures were examined in male Sprague-Dawley rats challenged with 1.6 LD_{50} soman. At 5 or 40 min after onset of seizures, the rats were given an intraperitoneal injection of 25 mg/kg HU-211. All rats that received soman showed electrocorticographic (ECoG) evidence of sustained seizures and status epilepticus for 4–6 hr. HU-211 had no effect on either the strength or duration of seizure activity. Administration of HU-211 at 5 min after seizure onset reduced median lesion volume 86% (as assessed by microtubule-associated protein 2 (MAP2)-negative staining), and when administered 40 min post-onset, the reduction in necrosis was 81.5% despite the presence of continuous seizures for 4–5 hr. These observations were corroborated by hemotoxylin and eosin (H&E) histopathological assessment that showed a significant reduction in piriform cortical neuronal damage in HU-211-treated animals. It is concluded that HU-211 provides considerable neuroprotection against brain damage produced by soman-induced seizures.

INTRODUCTION

Exposure to high concentrations of soman (pinacolylymethylphosphonofluoridate), an organophosphorus (OP) inhibitor of cholinesterases, leads to the development of seizures and seizure-related brain damage (SRBD).[1] Current fielded prophylaxis and therapy for chemical nerve agent exposure consists of pretreatment with a reversible carbamate inhibitor of acetylcholinesterase (AChE) such as pyridostigmine bromide to shield a fraction of the enzyme from irreversible inhibition. Pyridostigmine bromide-inhibited AChE spontaneously reactivates with a half-time of 25–30 min to provide a minimal level of AChE activity. After exposure to an irreversible inhibitor, an antichholinergic drug such as atropine sulfate is administered to counteract the effects of accumulating acetylcholine (ACh). The oxime, pyridine-

[a]Requests for reprints should be addressed to: Commander, U.S. Army Medical, Research Institute of Chemical Defense, Attn.: MCMR-UV-R (Dr. Filbert), 3100 Ricketts Point Road, Aberdeen Proving Ground, MD 21010-5400. Phone, 410/436-3628; fax, 410/436-4147.

e-mail, Margaret.Filbert@AMEDD.Army.Mil

[b]72 MED DET (VS), CMR 408, APO AE 09182.

[c]Department of Biology, La Salle University, Philadelphia, PA 19141-1199.

2-aldoxime methylchloride (2-PAM), is administered to reactivate OP-inhibited AChE that has not aged, i.e., become refractory to reactivation by oxime. In the event of seizure development, an anticonvulsant such as diazepam may be given. To control seizure activity, the anticonvulsant must be administered within a finite time window of approximately 40 min.[2]

In the presence of persistent seizures that become refractory to anticonvulsant therapy, brain damage appears as the result of delayed biochemical changes involving a complex cascade of factors that lead to excitotoxicity. Soman-induced SRBD is considered to be due to excitotoxicity produced by the release of excessive glutamate.[2,3] While the seizures are initiated by the high level of ACh that accumulates as a result of AChE inhibition, as seizure duration increases, excitatory amino acids (EAA) are released and assume control of seizure activity.[2–4] Sustained release of glutamate and excessive stimulation of EAA receptors triggers excitotoxic neuronal death. This conclusion is supported by studies demonstrating that soman-induced seizures and the resulting brain damage can be alleviated by antagonists of the N-methyl-D-aspartate (NMDA) subtype of glutamate receptor such as MK-801.[5–7] Unfortunately, MK-801 and other NMDA antagonists produce neurotoxic effects of their own[8] and are not likely to be useful clinically.

Recently, a nonpsychotropic cannabinoid, HU-211 (dexanabinol; 7-hydroxy-Δ^6-tetrahydrocannabinol-1,1-dimethylheptyl) was reported to have neuroprotectant effects in neurons exposed to excitotoxins in culture.[9,10] HU-211 antagonizes glutamatergic neurotransmission in the brain and inhibits metabolic events that lead to neuronal degeneration.[11,12] In addition to having NMDA blocking activity, HU-211 appears to act as a potent scavenger of peroxy and hydroxy radicals[12] and minimizes destabilization of calcium homeostasis.[13,14] HU-211 has been evaluated as a neuroprotectant in animal models of head injury, optic nerve crush and ischemia. In these models, a single injection of HU-211 given after the insult conferred a significant increase in neuronal survival. The present investigation was undertaken to evaluate HU-211 as a potential neuroprotectant agent against soman-induced SRBD in rats.

METHODS

Animals

Seventy-five male Sprague-Dawley rats (CRL: CD[SD]-BR; Charles River Labs, Wilmington, MA), weighing 250–300 g, were used. Animals were housed individually in polycarbonate cages under conditions of constant temperature ($21 \pm 2°C$) and humidity ($50 \pm 10\%$), using at least 10 complete air changes per hour of 100% fresh air, and a 12-hour light-dark cycle (full spectrum lighting cycle with no twilight). Throughout the study, food and water were available *ad libitum*, except during the observation period, which began 1.5 hr prior to, and ended 5 hr following, soman administration.

Surgeries

Each rat was anesthetized with sodium pentobarbital (55 mg/kg, intraperitoneally (i.p.)) and positioned in a stereotaxic apparatus (David Koff Instruments, Tujunga,

CA). In accordance with the procedure recommended by Braitman and Sparenborg,[5] three holes were drilled through the skull into which screw electrodes were placed for electrocorticographic (ECoG) recordings. Electrodes were connected to a standard small-animal head-piece and secured by dental cement.

Drug Administration and Electrocorticographic Recordings

On the morning of the sixth day following surgeries, animals were connected to an ECoG recording system and allowed at least 2 hr to acclimate. Baseline ECoG activity and behavior were monitored for at least 15 min. Following baseline recordings, animals were injected (i.p.) with 125 mg/kg of the oxime HI-6. This was followed 30 min later by injection of 180 µg/kg soman (1.6 LD_{50}, subcutaneously (s.c.)) or sterile saline. Within one min following soman or saline injection, animals were injected (intramuscularly (i.m.)) with 2 mg/kg atropine methylnitrate (AMN). HI-6 and AMN were administered to protect against the peripheral effects of soman. The treatment drug, HU-211 (Pharmos Ltd., Rehovot, Israel), was injected (25 mg/kg, i.p.) 5 or 40 min following the onset of seizures, as determined by ECoG recordings. A non-soman, treatment drug control group received HI-6, saline and AMN, as described above. In this case, HU-211 was administered 15 min following saline injection. The above paradigm yielded eight treatment groups: (1) soman-injected positive controls, $n = 18$; (2) HU-211, 5 min post-seizure onset, $n = 12$; (3) HU-211, 40 min post-onset, $n = 9$; (4) HU-211 treatment drug controls, $n = 6$; (5) non-soman negative controls, $n = 8$; (6) miglyol (HU-211 vehicle) 5 min post-onset, $n = 11$; (7) HU-211 repeated dosage (i.e., 5 min, 6 hr, 12 hr, 18 hr and 24 hr post-onset) $n = 6$; and (8) HU-211 vehicle repeated dosage (i.e., 5 min, 6 hr, 12 hr, 18 hr and 24 hr post-onset) $n = 5$. ECoG recordings were monitored for 5 hr following soman administration. Additional recordings (30 min) were obtained at 24 hr from surviving animals.

Tissue Processing

Twenty-seven hours after soman/saline administration, rats were given a lethal injection of pentobarbital anesthesia (100 mg/kg, i.p.) and euthanatized, upon evidence of labored breathing, via transcardial perfusion with ice cold 4% paraformaldehyde in 0.1 M phosphate buffer (PB, pH 7.4). Brains were immediately excised and longitudinally divided into left and right hemispheres. Alternate hemispheres (left or right) were postfixed by immersion in a second solution of ice cold 4% paraformaldehyde in 0.1 M PB for 4–6 hr. These hemispheres were subsequently sucrose-saturated (30% sucrose in 0.1 M PB for 72 hr) and coronally sectioned at 40 µm. Serial sections either were collected directly onto poly-L-lysine-coated slides for cresyl violet (CV) staining or cryoprotected[16] and stored at −20°C pending immunocytochemical staining. The remaining hemispheres were paraffin processed, sectioned at 4 µm and stained with hematoxylin and eosin (H&E).

MAP2 Immunocytochemistry

Immunocytochemistry required strict attention to detail to achieve uniform staining of sufficient quality for quantitation and between-subject comparisons. This procedure employed a monoclonal antiserum, raised in mice, against microtubule-associated protein 2 (MAP2) (Sigma Chemical Co., St Louis, MO), and utilized the avidin-biotin-peroxidase method of Hsu *et al.*[17] "Elite ABC Mouse Kits" were obtained from Vector Labs (Burlingame, CA). Following removal from cryoprotectant, free-floating brain sections underwent several rinses in PB. Endogenous peroxidase activity was quenched by placing sections into 3% H_2O_2 in 0.05 M Tris buffer (TB; pH 7.6) for 5 min. All the following steps were preceded by three rinses in 0.05 M TB (pH 7.6) unless otherwise indicated. To block nonspecific staining, sections were incubated in 0.05 M TB containing 5% normal horse serum and 0.1 M D,L-lysine. Sections were incubated for 18 hr at 4°C in primary antiserum diluted 1:4000 for MAP2 with 0.05 M TB containing 1% normal horse serum. Sections were incubated for 30 min at room temperature in biotinylated secondary antiserum (i.e., horse-antimouse) diluted 1:200 in 0.05 M TB containing 1% normal horse serum and 1% normal rat serum. Sections were incubated in a solution containing the avidin-biotin peroxidase complex (diluted 1:50 in 0.05 M TB) for 20 min. Sections were preincubated in 1.0 ml freshly prepared (i.e., 20–25-min-old) 0.05% 3′,3-diaminobenzidine tetrahydrochloride (DAB; Sigma Chemical Co., St Louis, MO) solution for 5 min, at which time 33 μl of 0.3% H_2O_2 was added and immediately followed by vigorous agitation. Sections remained in the resultant solution containing 0.048% DAB and 0.01% H_2O_2 for 2.5 min ± 3 sec. The reaction was stopped by two rinses in 0.05 M TB (for 5 and 15 min, respectively). Negative control sections were incubated in the same solutions for the same incubation times as the other brain sections, with the exception that the primary antibody solution containing anti-MAP2 immunoglobulin G (IgG), was replaced by a 0.05 M TB solution containing 1% horse serum without the primary antibody. Sections were floated onto poly-L-lysine-coated slides, dried, dehydrated, cleared and mounted.

MAP2 Image Analysis

Morphometric image analysis of MAP2 immunohistochemistry was performed using a Quantimet 600 Image Analysis System (Leica Cambridge, Ltd., Cambridge, England) equipped with an Olympus BH-2 Biological Microscope (Olympus Optical Co., Ltd., Tokyo, Japan). Morphometric assessments of the cross-sectional areas of MAP2-negative immunostaining (i.e., necrosis[18–20] in the piriform cortex and contiguous brain regions (e.g., endopiriform nuclei, amygdaloid nuclei and perirhinal cortex) were performed according to the procedure of Ballough *et al.*[18] Previous studies have shown that the deep piriform cortex and surrounding areas present the most clearly defined and easily quantifiable lesions of contiguous necrosis at 27 hr following soman-induce seizures in rats.[18,19] To standardize image comparisons between brain sections from each subject, the image analysis system was arbitrarily preset, by adjusting the hue, saturation and intensity of the binary image, to reflect a maximum contrast between MAP2-negative (necrotic) and MAP2-positive immunostaining on a typical soman-injected positive control section. For each brain section, piriform cortical MAP2-negative immunostaining was interactively outlined, using a pointing device, and area determinations were calculated automatically by the image analysis system. The average of two measurements for each brain section was recorded.

H&E Pathological Assessments

H&E stained brain sections (bregma −3.3 ± 0.2 and −4.8 ± 0.2 mm) were assessed for classical histopathological damage to the piriform cortex, amygdaloid complex, hippocampus and thalamus. Damage was scored on a scale of 0–4, where 0 = no histologic lesion, 1 = minimal damage (1–10% neuronal loss), 2 = mild (11–25% neuronal loss), 3 = moderate (26–45% neuronal loss), and 4 = severe (>45% neuronal loss).

Statistical Analysis

For animals that received soman, lesion volumes were ranked from highest to lowest and between-group comparisons were performed using Kruskal-Wallis and Mann-Whitney nonparametric statistical analysis. When statistical significance was demonstrated using Kruskal-Wallis analysis of variance of ranks, paired comparisons were performed using the Mann-Whitney test. Regional damage ratings obtained from H&E-stained contralateral hemispheres were also assessed using Kruskal-Wallis and Mann-Whitney nonparametric statistical analyses. In all cases, values for p <0.05 were considered significant.

RESULTS

Seizures and Convulsions

All rats that received soman showed ECoG evidence of sustained seizures and status epilepticus for several hours as defined by the continued presence of high amplitude (i.e., greater than four-times baseline) rhythmic spike or sharp wave activity. Treatment with HU-211 had no detectable effect on the strength or duration of seizures, as determined from visual observation of the ECoG recordings. Proconvulsive behavioral signs of soman intoxication included repetitive chewing, facial clonus, forepaw clonus, motor stereotypy, and wet-dog shakes. Overt motor convulsions were characterized by rhythmic clonic jerks of both head and forepaws, rearing, salivation and Straub tail. By all appearances, HU-211 had no effect on proconvulsive or convulsive behavior.

MAP2 Immunostaining

In unlesioned brain regions, MAP2-immunopositive staining was localized in neuronal perikarya, proximal dendrites and neuropil. It was not observed in areas composed of white matter except in small numbers of scattered neurons. These findings are consistent with reports by Bernhardt and Matus[21] and Matus.[22] Negative control sections, for which nonimmunized serum was used, showed no MAP2 immunoreactivity. In brain regions exhibiting lesions resulting from soman-induced seizures, pronounced and clearly demarcated reductions in MAP2 immunostaining were observed. Severe lesions were typified by a near total absence of MAP2 immunoreactivity. Those brain regions that were most severely affected included the piriform cortex, entorhinal cortex, dorsal endopiriform nucleus and the laterodorsal thalamic nucleus. Pronounced reductions in MAP2 immunostaining were often seen in the perirhinal cortex, amygdaloid complex (i.e., lateral, basolateral and posteriolateral cortical amygdaloid nuclei) and midline thalamic nuclei (e.g., mediodorsal and ventromedial). No reductions in MAP2 immunoreactivity were visually discernible in any of the hippocampal fields, although MAP2 loss was seen in the hilus of

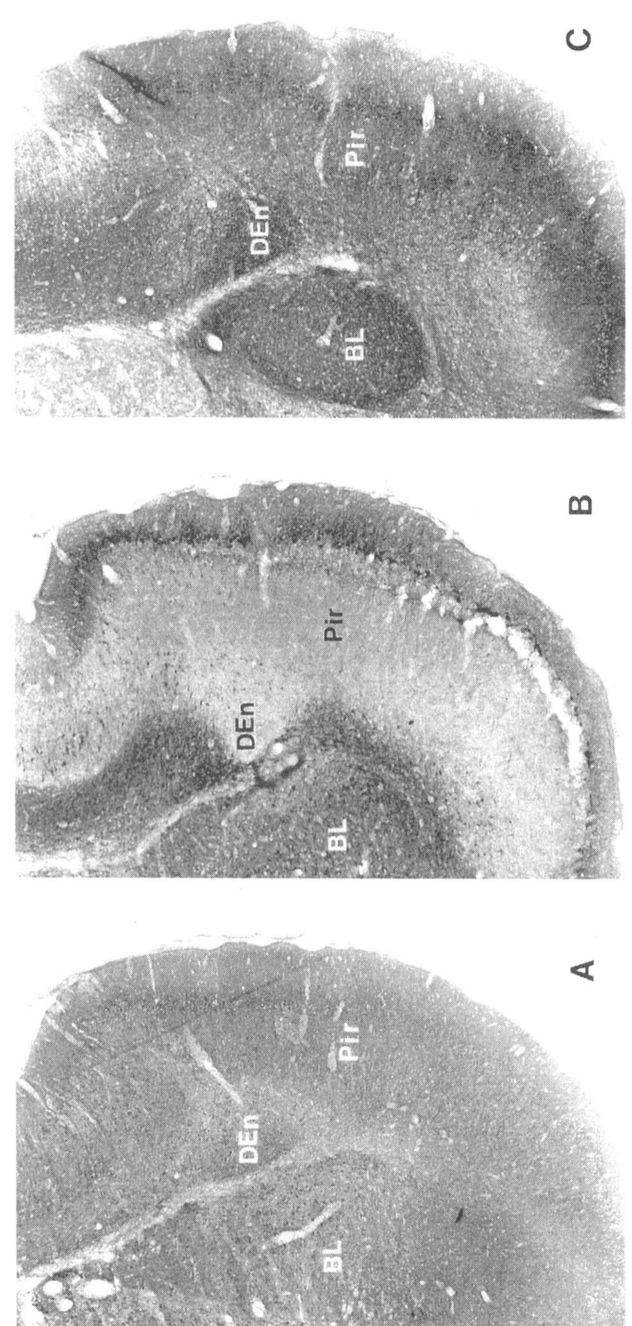

FIGURE 1. MAP2 immunohistochemical staining of the rat temporal lobe showing macroscopic lesions produced by soman and neuroprotection by treatment with HU-211 at 5 min following onset of seizures. (**A**) Non-soman control. (**B**) Soman-induced lesions after status epilepticus, 4–6 hr. (**C**) Neuroprotection produced by HU-211 administered 5 min after onset of seizures, coincident with status epilepticus 4–6 hr. BL: basal lateral amygdala; Den: dorsal endopiriform nucleus; Pif: piriform cortex. *Black letters* indicate damaged areas in (B).

the dentate gyrus. In the piriform cortex and contiguous regions, a lesion that would be considered typical (i.e., from the soman-injected positive control group) of those that were morphometrically measured presented the following: with the deep piriform cortex as a central focus, the lateral and ventral margins of the lesion directly abutted, but often did not include, the primary olfactory neurons of layer 2. The lesions often extended dorsally to include the perirhinal cortex, and noncontiguous lesions were occasionally seen in the dorsal frontoparietal cortex. Medially, the area of damage consistently included the dorsal endopiriform nucleus and often included the lateral and basolateral amygdala. Necrotic areas devoid of MAP2 immunoreactivity were surrounded by intensified immunostaining in the penumbra, which enhanced the contrast between the penumbra and necrotic border and facilitated delineation (FIG. 1).

When administered 5 min post-onset of seizures, HU-211 significantly reduced the median lesion volume (i.e., MAP2-negative immunostaining) seen in the piriform cortex and contiguous regions of soman-injected positive controls from 10.5 mm^3 to 1.5 mm^3 or 86%. When administered 40 min following seizure induction, the median lesion volume of necrosis was reduced to 2.0 mm^3 or 81.5%. In a small group of animals ($n = 6$), the HU-211 was given 5 min post-onset and then every six hours for the next 24 hr. In this group, median lesion volume was reduced to 0.1 mm^3. Although the latter regimen appeared to confer 99% protection against brain damage, half of these animals died prior to scheduled sacrifice. These deaths were attributed to repeated vehicle (i.e., miglyol) as 3 of 5 rats receiving repeated injections of migyol alone also died prior to sacrifice. It is speculated that the large cumulative injection volumes of the miglyol received over the 24-hr period following soman exposure contributed to the deaths of these animals. No evidence of brain damage was discerned from microscopic examination of MAP2-immunostained sections in either the non-soman injected negative control or the HU-211 drug treatment control groups. These findings are depicted in FIGURE 2.

H&E Histopathological Assessments

General histopathological assessments of H&E-stained brain sections from rats that received soman but not HU-211 indicated that soman-induced seizure-related brain damage was bilaterally symmetrical and characterized by tissue necrosis, neuronal loss, chromatolysis, vacuolization, pyknosis and gliosis. The most severe brain damage was consistently observed in the piriform cortex, entorhinal cortex, dorsal endopiriform nucleus and the laterodorsal thalamic nucleus. Pronounced damage was often seen in perirhinal cortex, amygdaloid complex (i.e., lateral, basolateral and posteriolateral cortical amygdaloid nuclei), hippocampus (i.e., hippocampal fields CA1 and CA3 and dentate gyrus), and midline thalamic nuclei (e.g., mediodorsal and ventromedial).

Histopathological damage ratings for H&E-stained brain sections are based on the presence of necrotic neurons and/or the absence of a defined neuronal population; shrunken neurons are considered the result of artifactual change. Damage to the neuropil is progressively greater as ratings increase from "mild" to "severe," and is characterized by increasingly severe malacia and hyalinization typical of necrosis. A statistically significant ($p = 0.03$) drop in damage ratings was observed in the HU-211 group treated at 5 min after onset of seizures (2.4 ± 0.38) compared to soman

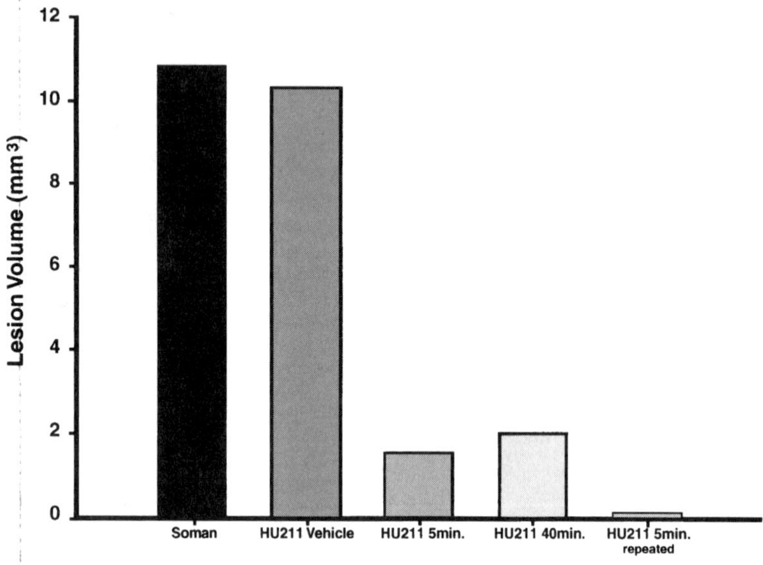

FIGURE 2. Histograms depicting median lesion volumes of temporal lobe necrosis (mm³). Morphometric image analysis was used to assess MAP2-negative immunostaining in the piriform cortex and contiguous regions. The HU-211 vehicle, migylol, appeared to have a small effect on median lesion volume, but it was statistically insignificant. HU-211 reduced median lesion volume 86% when administered 5 min post-seizure onset; 81.5% at 40 min and repeated administrations (5 min then at 6 hr) produced a 99% reduction in lesion volume.

controls (3.8 ± 0.2). This represents a damage reduction from severe (i.e., from >45% neuronal loss in untreated soman-exposed groups) to mild (11–25% neuronal loss in the HU-211 5-min group). Damage ratings for HU-211 controls and vehicle controls were all zero.

DISCUSSION

The results presented herein are important in that HU-211 reduced neuronal damage following exposure to soman without stopping established seizures and when administration was delayed until 40 min after seizure onset. Earlier reports have shown that noncompetitive NMDA antagonists such as ketamine and MK-801 protect thalamic neurons from seizure-related brain damage without preventing seizure activity.[23–25] The authors suggested that these antagonists may have prevented seizure-related damage by blocking NMDA receptor ion channel complexes on the dendrosomal surfaces through which glutamate excitotoxicity is expressed and that seizure activity in some brain areas may be maintained by other neurotransmitter systems without NMDA receptor participation.[6]

In addition to NMDA blocking activity, HU-211 has been reported to block calcium influx and possess free radical scavenging activity.[11] Thus HU-211 may have unique potential as a multiaction treatment for protection from brain damage associated with soman-induced seizures. Further studies with HU-211 to establish the optimum window of opportunity for successful treatment of SRBD following exposure to chemical nerve threat agents are in progress.

REFERENCES

1. TAYLOR, P. 1996. Anticholinesterase agents. *In* Goodman & Gilman's The Pharmacological Basis of Therapeutics. 9th edit. J.G. Hardman, L.E. Limbird, P.B. Molinoff, R.W. Ruddon & A.G. Gilman, Eds.: 161–176. McGraw-Hill. New York.
2. SHIH, T.-M. & J.H. MCDONOUGH. 1997. Neurochemical mechanisms in soman-induced seizures. J. Appl. Toxicol. **17:** 255–264.
3. OLNEY, J.W., T. DE GUBAREFF & J. LABRUYERE. 1983. Seizure-related brain damage induced by cholinergic agents. Nature **301:** 520–522.
4. SPARENBORG, S., L.H. BRENNECKE, N.K. JAAX & D.J. BRAITMAN. 1992. Dizocilpine (MK-801) arrests status epilepticus and prevents brain damage induced by soman. Neuropharmacology **31:** 357–368.
5. BRAITMAN, D.J. & S. SPARENBORG. 1989. MK-801 protects against seizures induced by the cholinesterase inhibitor soman. Brain Res. Bull. **23:** 145–148.
6. CLIFFORD, D., C. ZORUMSKI & J. OLNEY. 1989. Ketamine and MK-801 prevent degeneration of thalamic neurons induced by focal cortical seizures. Exp. Neurol. **10:** 272–279.
7. CLIFFORD, D., J. OLNEY, A. BENZ, T. FULLER & C. ZORUMSKI. 1990. Ketamine, phencyclidine, and MK-801 protect against kainic acid-induced seizure-related brain damage. Epilepsia **31:** 382–290.
8. FIX, A.S., J.W. HORN, K.A. WIGHTMAN, C. JOHNSON, G.G. LONG, R.W. STORTS, N. FARBER, D.F. WOZNIAK & J.W. OLNEY. 1993. Neuronal vacuolization and necrosis induced by the noncompetitive *N*-methyl-D-aspartate (NMDA) antagonist MK-801 (dizocilpine maleate): a light and electron microscopic evaluation of the rat retrosplenial cortex. Exp. Neurol. **123:** 204–215.
9. ESHHAR, N., S. STRIEM & A. BIEGON. 1993. HU-211, a non-psychotropic cannabinoid, rescues cortical neurones from excitatory amino acid toxicity in culture. NeuroReport **5:** 237–240.
10. ESHHAR, N., S. STRIEM, R. KOHEN, O. TIROSH & A. BIEGON. 1995. Neuroprotective and anti-oxidant activities of HU-211, a novel NMDA receptor antagonist. Eur. J. Pharmacol. **283:** 19–29.
11. BIEGON, A. & A.B. JOSEPH. 1995. Development of HU-211 as a neuroprotectant for ischemic brain damage. Neurol. Res. **17:** 275–280.
12. SHOHAMI, E., E. BEIT-YANNAI, M. HOROWITZ & R. KOHEN. 1997. Oxidative stress in closed-head injury: brain antioxidant capacity as an indicator of functional outcome. J. Cereb. Blood Flow Metab. **17:** 1007–1019.
13. NADLER, V., A. BIEGON, E. BEIT-YANNI, J. ADAMCHIK & E. SHOHAMI. 1995. Ca accumulation in rat brain after closed head injury: attenuation by the novel neuroprotective agent HU-211. Brain Res. **685:** 1–11.
14. STRIEM, S., V. LAVIE & A. BIEGON. 1996. The nonpsychotropic cannabinoid HU-211 rescued hippocampal neurones from β-amyloid-induced toxicity. Soc. Neurosci. Abstr. **22:** 196.
15. SHOHAMI, E., M. NOVIKOV & R. MECHOULAM. 1993. A nonpsychotropic cannabinoid, HU211, has cerebroprotective effects after closed head injury in the rat. J. Neurotrauma **10:** 109–119.
16. WATSON, R.E., A.J. WIEGAND, R.W. CLOUGH & G.E. HOFFMAN. 1986. Use of cryoprotectant to maintain long-term peptide immunoreactivity and tissue morphology. Peptides **7:** 155–159.

17. HSU, S.-M., L. RAINE & H. FANGER. 1981. Use of avidin-biotin-peroxidase complex (ABC) in immunoperoxidase techniques: a comparison between ABC and unlabeled antibody (PAP) procedures. J. Histochem. Cytochem. **29:** 577–580.
18. BALLOUGH, G.P.H., L.J. MARTIN, F.J. CANN, J.S. GRAHAM, C.D. SMITH, C.E. KLING, J.S. FORSTER, S. PHANN & M.G. FILBERT. 1995. Microtubule-associated protein 2 (MAP2): a sensitive marker of seizure-related brain damage. J. Neurosci. Methods **61:** 23–32.
19. BALLOUGH, G.P.H., F.J. CANN, C.D. SMITH, J.S. FORSTER, C.E. KLING & M.G. FILBERT. 1998. GM1 monosialoganglioside pretreatment protects against soman-induced seizure-related brain damage. Mol. Chem. Neuropathol. **34:** 1–23.
20. HICKS, R.R., D.H. SMITH & T.K. MACINTOSH. 1995. Temporal response and effects of excitotatory amino acid antagonism on microtubule-associated protein 2 immunoreactivity following experimental brain injury in rats. Brain Res. **678:** 151–160.
21. BERNHARDT, R. & A. MATUS. 1984. Light and electron microscopic studies of the distribution of microtubule-associated protein 2 in rat brain: a difference between dendritic and axonal cytoskeletons. J. Comp. Neurol. **226:** 203–221.
22. MATUS, A. 1994. MAP2. *In* Microtubules. J.S. Hyams & C.W. Lloyd, Eds.: 155–166. Wiley-Liss, Inc. New York.
23. LABRUYERE, J., T. FULLER, J. OLNEY, M. PRICE, C. SORUMSKI & D. CLIFFORD. 1986. Phencyclidine and ketamine protect against seizure-related brain damage. Soc. Neurosci. Abst. **12:** 344.
24. SMITH, G., G. GOLDEN, P. REYES & R. FARRIELLO. 1987. Effects of MK801, an NMDA receptor antagonist, on kainate induced seizures in rats. Soc. Neurosci. Abstr. **13:** 1031.
25. BAR-JOSEPH, A., Y. BERKOVITCH, J ADAMCHIK & A. BIEGON. 1994. Neuroprotective activity of HU-211, a novel NMDA antagonist, in global ischemia in gerbils. Mol. Chem. Neuropathol. **23:** 125–135.

Abuse Liability Assessment of Neuroprotectants

MICHAEL KLEIN,[a] SILVIA CALDERON, AND BELINDA HAYES

Controlled Substances Evaluation Team, Division of Anesthetic, Critical Care, and Addiction Drug Products, Center for Drug Evaluation and Research, Food and Drug Administration, Rockville, Maryland, USA

ABSTRACT: There has been considerable interest in the potential of *N*-methyl-D-aspartate (NMDA) receptor antagonists in the treatment of a diverse group of neurological disorders including cerebral ischemia and neurodegeneration.[8,16,19] The amino acids L-glutamate and L-aspartate have been shown to possibly mediate excitatory synaptic transmission in the central nervous system (CNS) via selective excitatory amino acid receptors. Competitive and noncompetitive antagonists acting at the NMDA receptors have been shown to possess relevant activity. However, NMDA antagonists can produce a variety of adverse neurobehavioral effects in both animals and humans.[9–12,14,17,18] These adverse events are particularly pronounced with NMDA antagonists (phencyclidine (PCP), ketamine, and MK-801) that have dissociative anesthetic properties and block NMDA receptor-mediated responses by binding to the cation channel of the NMDA receptor complex. When a new pharmaceutical product demonstrates structural similarity and/or a similar pharmacological profile with a known drug of abuse, the characterization of its abuse potential is needed by the FDA for scientific review.[1,3,4,22] The abuse liability assessment is based upon an evaluation of data on the chemistry, pharmacology (preclinical and clinical), pharmacokinetics, and pharmacodynamic profiles of the drug, and the adverse events/effects reported in clinical trials. The evaluation of the drug's abuse potential is determined relative to pharmacologically similar drugs. This includes determination of the drug's receptor binding efficacy, preclinical pharmacology, reinforcing efficacy, discriminative stimulus effects, dependence-producing potential, pharmacokinetics, and assessment of the clinical efficacy-safety database relative to abuse and clinical abuse liability studies.[2,7,9,13,20–22] It has been well established that high-affinity noncompetitive NMDA antagonists have reinforcing efficacy and can serve as discriminative stimuli in operant procedures. In a variety of species in drug discrimination studies, each antagonist is capable of generalizing to the others, and it is believed that these effects may be mediated through the NMDA blockade. The generalization of each substance for another suggests production of common subjective effects in humans.

REVIEW OF THERAPEUTIC AGENTS WITH ABUSE POTENTIAL

The assessment of abuse potential of new drugs requires a scientific and medical evaluation by the Food and Drug Administration, which results in regulations that contribute to a drug's labeling, advertising, promotion and marketing, and manufac-

[a]Corresponding author: Michael Klein, Ph.D., HFD-170, CDER/FDA, 5600 Fisher Lane, Rockville, MD 20857. Phone, 301/443-3741; fax, 301/443-7068.
e-mail, kleinm@cder.fda.gov

turing, and effects how the drug is used in the practice of medicine and pharmacy. The evaluations of new drugs are described in the Federal Food, Drug and Cosmetics Act. Similar scientific data are considered for the drugs that are regulated under the Controlled Substances Act (CSA). The CSA also includes requirements for and descriptions of special regulations related to the abuse potential of new drugs. The procedures followed in the regulation of drugs with abuse potential are also described in the CSA.[1]

The laboratory evaluation of abuse potential should demonstrate that a drug offers the following features:

- That the drug is centrally acting;
- That, for a variety of reasons, the drug possesses properties that may likely lead to its continued misuse, excessive use outside of medical administration, or beyond that which it has been shown to be safe and effective;
- That continued, prolonged or excessive use of the drug has been shown to result in the development of tolerance with the likelihood of increasing doses; and,
- That the drug is capable of producing dependence.

For each drug class, certain *in vitro* and *in vivo* preclinical and clinical studies, and their integration, are preferred approaches for evaluation of abuse potential, while others may be less relevant. For example, the preclinical self-administration study of various substances is relevant in attributing abuse potential to central nervous system stimulants, depressants, and opioids, but not to certain hallucinogenic substances. The current view is that the integration of specialized preclinical and clinical abuse liability studies with data in the integrated summary of safety and efficacy provides the best predictor of the abuse potential of a new drug for which there is no marketing history. Thus, the focus of drug abuse research needs to be tailored to the most relevant situation for each drug of abuse, and in some cases, such as for opioids, an ideal approach may encompass all types of studies from *in vitro* and *in vivo* preclinical to clinical evaluation. Methods of investigation, populations studied, and outcome measures selected will vary depending on drug class.

Six classes of substances have been identified as important for research and development into abuse liability assessment. Currently, these six classes represent the important substances of abuse and/or dependence that are appropriate for evaluation and consideration for possible regulation as controlled substances:

- Opioids (analgesics and anesthetics)
- Sedative-hypnotics and anxiolytics
- Cocaine, amphetamines and other central nervous system stimulants
- Hallucinogens, phencyclidine and similar agents active at the NMDA receptor
- Cannabinoids (marijuana and related compounds)
- Nicotine-like drugs

ABUSE LIABILITY

The term "abuse liability" refers to the likelihood that a drug with psychoactive or central nervous system (CNS) effects will sustain patterns of nonmedical self-administration that result in disruptive or undesirable consequences. Comparable definitions in the CSA refer to an "addiction-forming" or "addiction-sustaining liability" for opiates and, for other CNS active agents, a "potential for abuse" because of a drug's stimulant, depressant, or hallucinogenic effect.[1]

The abuse liability may be described for regulatory purposes by variations in either the likelihood and severity of self-administration or the likelihood and severity of undesirable consequences. Nonmedical self-administration might include the frequency, patterns, routes, or doses used, or the intensity of behavior directed towards obtaining the drug.

Undesirable consequences might include medical or psychological effects, effects on psychomotor or cognitive performance, or effects on addictive behaviors, such as chronic or compulsive self-administration or difficulty in ceasing drug use or in sustaining abstinence. Describing the characteristics of the "withdrawal syndrome" and its severity and outcome are relevant concepts that need to be assessed.

All new drug applications for appropriate substances include a specific section addressing abuse liability issues. In general, the procedure for abuse liability assessment is to evaluate the pharmacological profile of test compounds. A full and complete characterization of all relevant effects of the drug is needed. Substances under examination, with profiles of action similar to known drugs of abuse, are considered likely to present similar abuse liabilities. In addition, the nature and extent of abuse liability should be assessed for any drug being developed for an indication for which known drugs of abuse are used (such as antiobesity and anxiolytic agents), and considered for other therapeutic categories for drugs that have demonstrated activity in the CNS. An overview of the substance and its activity should include consideration of its chemical structure and class, its profile of biochemical activity, its pharmacokinetics and metabolism, production of active metabolites, its profile of pharmacological activity, and adverse reactions.

Decisions regarding whether more specific abuse liability testing is needed are made after characterization of the overall profile of drug action.[2,7,9,13,20–22] A more detailed data base should be generated relative to the following: receptor binding, reinforcing, discriminative, and subjective effects; pharmacokinetics and metabolism; formation of active metabolites and characterization of the properties of the metabolites; bioavailability of the drug; effect of abrupt abstinence after chronic administration; overall similarity of effects to other controlled substances; effects of supratherapeutic doses; and, administration of the drug following the intentional destruction of the marketed dosage form (such as, crushing tablets and dissolving the drug for parenteral administration, or for intranasal administration).

Drugs demonstrating psychoactive effects that are suggestive of increased pleasure, euphoria, or mood elevation, in studies with nonpatient populations, should be candidates for further evaluation for abuse potential. Although the sample sizes commonly used in abuse liability assessments are frequently small, efforts should be made by the investigators to strive to strengthen the value of the data by assuring that statistically significant results are reported. That is, the studies should be designed with adequate statistical power. Recommendations for differential regulations of competing products require that active ingredients be judged to have clinically meaningful differences in profiles of effects and/or abuse liabilities; statistical significance of differences may, by themselves, not be sufficient.

For drugs available in other countries prior to their approval in the USA, data on actual use, abuse and misuse, including fatalities, hospital emergency reports and suicides/suicide attempts, are reported along with data relative to the drugs' overall availability in the region. In addition, a detailed description of the data-gathering systems, demonstrating their adequacy and relevance to the public health risk, are included in order that this information can be appropriately assessed. In addition, regulatory and pending regulatory actions related to drug control or abuse issues are submitted for review. Circumstances that present a public health risk from abuse may change with time. Occasionally, it may be appropriate to reconsider the control status of a drug under the CSA. It may be appropriate to reevaluate substances for either greater or lesser regulatory control, whichever is indicated by the data available at the time of reconsideration.

PRELIMINARY SCREENING: *IN VITRO* TECHNIQUES AND BIOASSAYS

In vitro ligand binding techniques and biological and biochemical assays can be considered as the preliminary steps toward the pharmacological characterization of a drug. These procedures are usually performed early in the drug development process. In some cases, these methods may be predictive of the appropriate preclinical pharmacological and behavioral studies to conduct for further characterization of the drug.[5,6,15]

Binding studies provide valuable information regarding the affinity of a drug for a variety of receptor systems. In addition, characterization of the binding profile of the main metabolites needs to be evaluated as well. Further biochemical and functional assays can lead to an understanding of the mechanisms of the interaction, i.e., whether the drug is an agonist, antagonist, partial agonist or mixed agonist antagonist at specific receptor systems. In addition, evaluating the interaction of the new drug with receptor systems known to be involved in mediation of psychoactive effects will provide insight and contribute, in conjunction with other factors, to the prediction of abuse potential.

It is important to note that the effect on receptor binding may vary with the brain region and source of tissue. With the recent isolation of complimentary DNA (cDNA) encoding several receptor types, it has been possible to analyze receptors in a heterogeneous expression system. Another important factor to consider in the analysis of binding techniques is the radioligand used. Recent advances in medicinal chemistry have resulted in development of many new selective ligands.

Also, the potential interaction of the drug with the biogenic amine transporter should be considered, based upon the fact that most psychostimulants may enhance norepinephrine, dopamine or serotonin (5-HT) neurotransmission in the central and peripheral nervous systems by inhibiting their reuptake. The dopamine transporter has been linked to effects of cocaine and substances that are structurally similar to cocaine.

There is a correlation between chemical structure and interaction at the receptor level and each receptor system has different requirements for activation. Therefore, chemical similarity of an investigational drug with a fully characterized chemical entity provides information in terms of drug-receptor interaction. Taking into consideration the binding profiles of prototypical drugs associated with dependence and abuse potential, interactions at adrenergic, dopaminergic, cholinergic, serotoniner-

TABLE 1. Early indicators that a neuroprotectant may have abuse potential

- Chemical similarity
- Receptor interaction
- CNS functionality
- Pharmacological similarity

TABLE 2. Affinity at receptor systems associated with neuroprotection and drug abuse

- Dopamine
- Cannabinoid
- Opioid
- $GABA_A$/benzodiazepine
- NMDA
- Serotonin

gic, cannabinoid, $GABA_A$, NMDA and opioid receptor systems need to be examined (TABLES 1 and 2).

Predictions can be made by comparison of the binding profile of a new drug with the binding pattern of drugs that are known to produce dependence. For example, by using *in vitro* binding techniques, the affinity of agents for the serotoninergic receptor subtypes in the brain can be assessed. By analogy with the binding affinity displayed by lysergic acid diethylamide (LSD) for $5\text{-}HT_2$, $5\text{-}HT_{1a}$, and $5\text{-}HT_{1c}$ receptors, these studies would indicate the possibility that the new drug would elicit a hallucinogenic effect. Since hallucinogens are not self-administered in animals, the ligand binding data in conjunction with pharmacological analysis is an important screen for hallucinogenic drugs. Similarly, drugs in the cannabinoid class are typically not self-administered in an animal laboratory as well, but valuable binding data at the cannabinoid receptor can contribute to characterization of those substances.

PRECLINICAL ASSESSMENT: *IN VIVO* ABUSE LIABILITY ASSESSMENT OF NEUROPROTECTANTS

Drug Discrimination Paradigm[2,9,13]

Psychoactivity is a "hallmark" characteristic of all dependence-producing drugs. It is a property of a CNS-active drug that is characterized by a change in mood or feelings. Psychoactivity of a drug is evaluated in studies that assess the discriminative stimulus effects of a drug. Discriminative stimulus effects of a drug is a measure of the drug's subjective effects in humans. Selection of the training drug for the animals is very critical. The training drug can dramatically influence how the test drug will be characterized by the subjects. In the case of phencyclidine (PCP)-like NMDA antagonists, PCP should be the training drug. For cannabinoid-like substances, the training drug should be Δ-9-tetrahydrocannabinol (Δ^9-THC). In some instances, the drug under development should be the training drug.

Self-administration Paradigm[2,7,13]

The self-administration paradigm allows drug-seeking behavior to be studied. Drug-seeking behavior is one of the primary distinguishing features of drug abuse.

The self-administration paradigm is widely used to determine whether or not a drug can control behavior, that is, function as a "positive reinforcer." "Positive reinforcement" would be expected to lead to the development and maintenance of addiction/dependence.

Self-administration studies utilize a variety of schedules of reinforcement. The substitution procedure is the most commonly used self-administration paradigm. In this paradigm, the animal is initially trained to self-administer a known drug of abuse. After stable responding, the test drug is then substituted for the baseline drug in order to determine if it will lead to its self-injection.

DEPENDENCE POTENTIAL[2,20–22]

The dependence-producing characteristics must also be assessed. The drug can induce physical and/or behavioral dependence. Such adverse drug effects (which must be characterized) can contribute to sustained drug-seeking behavior and drug use in order to prevent the onset of unpleasant withdrawal signs and symptoms. A primary or direct physical dependence study is performed to determine if repeated administration of the drug for a period of a few weeks to a few months will produce physical dependence in drug-naïve animals. The drug administration is abruptly stopped or a pharmacological antagonist is administered; the animals are then observed for physical signs or symptoms of withdrawal. The behavioral dependence procedure involves assessment of drug-withdrawal effects on the animal's schedule-controlled performance. Following cessation of chronic administration, of PCP and Δ^9-THC, each has been shown to produce dependence, as evidenced by disruption in operant behavior.

PHARMACOKINETICS AND PHARMACODYNAMICS

The course of a drug's pharmacokinetics and pharmacodynamics over time has been demonstrated to have an important influence upon abuse liability.[22] In general, drugs with rapid onset and short duration appear to have greater abuse liability than do pharmacologically similar drugs with slow onset and long duration. Pharmacokinetics evaluations of actual patient populations are encouraged in early phases of study. Dose-proportionality and dose-effect studies are suggested as they may prove valuable in determining the dosing schemes in future clinical trials, or in selection of dose ranges. Laboratory studies relating the effect of a medication to its blood level (pharmacodynamic studies) may be helpful in designing later studies and in supporting later efficacy claims.

Route of administration can affect abuse liability by influencing the pharmacokinetics or pharmacodynamics of the drug. Measurement of drug and major metabolite blood levels is needed in order to make these determinations. Consideration of drug delivery approaches, as described in the above section, is especially important as newer and less "traditional" routes of administration are investigated, such as transdermal, intranasal and inhalation routes. The route of administration can affect the potential for diversion from appropriate use to inappropriate or illicit use. Consideration should be given to whether proposed dosage forms might make available quantities of drugs that might be extracted and diverted to illicit use.

TABLE 3. Parameters for clinical abuse liability assessments

- Drug-seeking behaviors
  - Self-administration studies
- Subjective effects
  - Addiction Research Center Inventory
    - Self-report of drug effects
      - i. Sedative effects (PCAG subscale)
      - ii. Euphoric effects (MBG subscale)
      - iii. Psychotomimetic effects (LSD subscale)
  - Single Dose Questionnaire (SDQ)
    - Self-report of drug effects
- Assessment of tolerance
- Assessment of physical dependence
- Characterization of adverse events
  - PCP-like drugs (e.g., ketamine)
  - Cannabinoid-like drugs (e.g., dronabinol)

CLINICAL PHARMACOLOGY

Long-term administration of certain drugs in clinical trials may lead to production of physical dependence. Dependence may be demonstrated in the study of CNS active opioids, stimulants, depressants, etc., in clinical efficacy/safety trials.[2,22] A withdrawal syndrome may be observed after termination of drug administration after long-term use. In certain cases, the protocol may call for tapering the dose of the drug over a period of several weeks following long-term administration. Drug dependence, which is assessed when a drug is being considered for possible CSA scheduling, often may not be reported or frankly identified as an adverse reaction. It is necessary to review the clinical protocols as to how the drug was administered and whether the drug was likely to produce and demonstrate dependence.

Although initial safety studies of new molecular entities are often conducted in normal, healthy volunteers, the target population for abuse liability studies should include subjects with a history of drug abuse (preferably characterized by a particular class, e.g., sedative-hypnotics, CNS stimulants, etc., if the test drug falls into that class). The population being tested may show clinically significant changes in tolerance and in dose-related responses to a particular drug, or may be particularly vulnerable to abusing the drug. Studies of high doses likely will require the drug-experienced population, as the drug-naïve subjects may not have sufficient tolerance to allow evaluation in a high-dose range. These studies ordinarily must be performed in adults who are in hospital or in clinical research settings that permit close observation. Drug interactions present a potential risk with this "at-risk population," and therefore the clinically monitored research setting is frequently critical. Investigators should be careful to ensure the availability of emergency care and equipment, and to document the arrangements they have made to provide this care.

In general, it is desirable to include multiple outcome measures, as no single measure of abuse liability is ideal. (See TABLE 3 for clinical parameters). On balance, however, too many scales, subscales, and questionnaire results are frequently measured in these trials, thus presenting confusing or even conflicting results. To characterize the abuse liability of a new molecular entity, the systematic collection of subjective effect and/or observer rating data is useful, especially where the upper limits of the dose range are challenged. Multiple-dose studies may be more relevant than single-dose studies if the abuse liability of a particular substance is related to difficulty in discontinuing drug use, as opposed to the likelihood of initiating inappropriate use. In the case of some drug substances or classes, such as opiates, sedative hypnotics and the selective serotonin reuptake inhibitors, the possibility of physical dependence or a withdrawal syndrome may be an important factor related to abuse liability, and it should be assessed.

Disassociation of relative potencies of different effects may be relevant to assessment of abuse liability. For example, substances that are equipotent in production of performance impairment may differ in their euphorigenic potencies.

Subject Populations

In human abuse liability testing, the subject population may include, under appropriate circumstances, current or experienced drug abusers, drug abuse treatment patients, or nondrug-abusing volunteers. It is customary to select drug-experienced individuals to predict the likelihood of abuse of a new drug for a variety of reasons. First, this is the population that would be most likely to experiment with a new drug with abuse potential. The selected subjects are required to have a recent experience with the drug under investigation or with drugs from the same pharmacological class or possessing the same pharmacological effects. The subjects' drug history will influence the subjects' sensitivity to the drug effects. Nonexperienced subjects are less likely to distinguish subtle effects among individual drugs within a drug class and/or underestimate the abuse liability of drugs. Drug abusers with a long history of drug use may, due to tolerance development, be insensitive to the drug effect at the doses tested. Therefore, protocols should fully describe the current characteristics and past history of drug/alcohol/tobacco use, abuse, misuse, experimentation and dependence. In addition, age range, gender, evidence related to special populations, drug of choice, frequency of participation in such behavioral studies, duration of drug abuse, and/or duration of drug abstinence are important factors that are useful in judging the significance of the study results.

Positive Controls

The abuse liability of a new molecular entity is best assessed in comparison to one or more standard references of recognized abuse potential. For the best assessment, a positive and negative (placebo) control should be used in the study. Typically, the standard reference drug is a prototypic drug of the same pharmacological class. If the test drug is from a novel pharmacological class, or if it has atypical actions, then it may be better to select a fair comparison from another pharmacological class that can serve as a reference against which to compare the test drug. However, the results of such comparison should be qualified, and explained when reference is made to the results of the study, that an atypical comparator was used as a positive control in the study.

If the test drug is a new dosage form of a previously approved chemical entity, a positive control should include at least one of the previously approved dosage forms of the drug substance. Another positive control could be a pharmacologically similar drug substance that has been formulated into the new dosage form. The influence of formulation on relevant pharmacokinetics parameters, that is, onset or duration of action, metabolism, for the test product could be assessed. Comparison of drug and metabolite plasma levels should be performed to assess the effect of the new formulation on PK/PD parameters (see above section).

Dose Levels

Abuse liability assessments should cover a broad range of doses. Because individual subjects differ in their sensitivity to drug effects and because it is desirable to investigate the effects of maximally tolerated doses, it may be desirable in some studies to use an individualized dosing schedule that ensures that each individual experiences a major drug effect, rather than using a fixed dosing schedule for all participants.

In clinical studies of abuse liability, it is often necessary to study doses substantially greater than a typical single therapeutic dose. Differing slopes of the dose-effect functions for different drugs for dosing increments are likely. By increasing the drug dose in multiples, in an effort to observe a potential euphoric response or some other effect that would indicate a greater likelihood of the drug being abused, the potential exists for also increasing the dysphoric response at the higher dose. For sedative-hypnotic agents, the response may be to induce sleep in the subject, for example.

Dosage Forms

The dosage form can affect abuse liability simply because of differences in commercial distribution or marketing of various drug products. Such issues may include the following: ease of administration; ease of overdosing, inaccuracy in measuring the dose to be administered; availability at retail level versus the hospital or clinical setting; diversion possibility; ease of extraction of the active ingredient from the new dosage form; long term or short term recommended usage (maintenance (chronic) vs. short term (acute) usage); how the product is promoted, advertised or marketed; and name recognition. Many of these factors can influence the extent of risk exposure of the general population.

SUMMARY

There has been progress in understanding the mechanisms involved in traumatic brain injury and linkage to the development of potential targets for pharmacological treatment. A schematic of *in vitro* and *in vivo* preclinical and clinical studies that relate to the drug's abuse potential has been outlIned above. In the course of drug development of these agents, the abuse potential of the new drug needs to be assessed. Such studies do not necessarily relate to appropriate use of the drug under therapeutic conditions, but to issues related to the likelihood of the drug being abused or misused. Such concern has arisen out of past experience with pharmacologically similar drugs. Not only do the recommended studies provide an indication that the drug is indeed eliciting effects via the CNS, but the studies provide information useful to the clinician. Such information may relate to the drug's potential psychoactivity and subjective responses elicited by patients. Such responses may or may not be similar to other controlled substances, like phencyclidine or analogues of Δ^9-THC. In addition, the clinical abuse liability studies are conducted at supratherapeutic doses by experienced drug abusers. Responses of higher dose levels assist us in gaining an understanding of the drug's abuse potential and often times may provide other sorts of important safety information.

REFERENCES

1. Controlled Substances Act (CSA), as amended February 15, 1996, Title 21, Food and Drugs, Chapter 13—Drug Abuse Prevention and Control.
2. Testing Drugs for Physical Dependence Potential and Abuse Liability. 1984. National Institute on Drug Abuse (NIDA) Research Monograph Series 52, Department of Health and Human Services, National Institute on Drug Abuse, GPO, Washington, DC.
3. The Convention on Psychotropic Substances, United Nations, Vienna, February 21, 1971, text in document E/CONF. 58/6.
4. The Single Convention on Narcotic Drugs, 1961, United Nations, New York, March 30, 1961.
5. LESHNER, A. I. 1997. Addiction is a brain disease. Sci. **278:** 457.
6. NESTLER, E.J. & G.K. AGHAJANIAN. 1997. Molecular and cellular basis of addiction. Science **278:** 58–63.
7. CHAIT, L.D. & J.P. ZACNY. 1992. Reinforcing and subjective effects of oral Δ^9-THC and smoked marijuana in humans. Psychopharmacology **107:** 255–262.
8. HAMPSON, A.J., M. GRIMALDI, J. AXELROD & D. WINK. 1998. Cannabidiol and (-)Δ^9-tetrahydrocannabinol are neuroprotective antioxidants. Proc. Natl. Acad. Sci. USA **95:** 8268–8273.
9. GRANT, K.A., G. COLOMBO, J. GRANT & M.A. ROGAWSKI. 1996. Dizolcilpine-like discriminative stimulus effects of low-affinity uncompetitive NMDA antagonists. Neuropharmacology **35**(12): 1709–1719.
10. RADANT, A.D., T.A. BOWDLE, D.S. COWLEY, E.D. KHARASCH & P.P. ROY-BYRNE. 1998. Does ketamine-mediated N-methyl-d-aspartate receptor antagonism cause schizophrenia-like oculomotor abnormalities? Neuropsychopharmacology **19**(5): 434–444.
11. MALHOTRA, A.K., D.A. PINALS, C.M. ADLER, I. ELMAN, A. CLIFTON, D. PICKAR & A. BREIER. 1997. Ketamine-induced exacerbation of psychotic symptoms and cognitive impairment in neuroleptic-free schizophrenics. Neuropharmacology **17**(3): 141–150.
12. JAVITT, D.C., H. SERSHEN, A. HASHIM & A. LAJTHA. 1997. Reversal of phencycline-induced hyperactivity by glycine and the clycine uptake inhibitor glycyldodecylamide. Neuropsychopharmacology **17:** 202–204.
13. BALSTER, R. 1991. Drug abuse potential evaluation in animals. Br. J. Addict. **86:** 1549–1558.
14. VAN BERCKEL, B.N.M., C. LIPSCH, S. TIMP, C. GISPEN-DE WIED, H. WYNNE, J.M. VAN REE & R.S. KAHN. 1997. Behavioral and neuroendocrine effects of partial NMDA agonist d-cycloserine in healthy subjects. Neuropsychopharmacology **16**(5): 317–324.
15. SMITH, G.S., R. SCHLOESSER, J.D. BRODIE, S.L. DEWEY, J. LOGAN, S.A. VITKUN, P. SIMKOWITZ, A. HURLEY, T. COOPER, N.D. VOLKOW & R. CANCRO. 1998. Glutamate modulation of dopamine measured *in vivo* with positron emission tomography (PET) and ^{11}C-raclopride in normal human subjects. Neuropsychopharmacology **18**(1): 18–25.
16. FARBER, N.B., J. HANSLICK, C. KIRBY, L. MCWILLIAMS & J.W. OLNEY. 1998. Serotonergic agents that activate $5HT_{2A}$ receptors prevent NMDA antagonist neurotoxicity. Neuropsychopharmacology **18**(1): 57–62.

17. MALHOTRA, A.K., D.A. PINALS, H. WEINGARTNER, K. SIROCCO, C.D. MISSAR, D. PICKAR & A. BREIER. 1998. NMDA receptor function and human cognition: the effects of ketamine in healthy volunteers. Neuropsychopharmacology **14**(5): 301–307.

18. SAMS-DODD, F. 1998. Effects of continuous *d*-amphetamine and phencyclidine administration on social behaviour, stereotyped behaviour, and locomotor activity in rats. Neuropsychopharmacology **19**(1): 18–25.

19. DOPPENBERG, E.M.R., S.C. CHOI & R. BULLOCK. 1997. Clinical trials in traumatic brain injury. What can we learn from previous studies? Ann. N.Y. Acad. Sci. **825**: 305–322.

20. BEARDSLEY, P.M., R.L. BALSTER & L.S. HARRIS. 1986. Dependence on tetrahydrocannabinol in rhesus monkeys. J. Pharmacol. Exp. Ther. **239**: 311–319.

21. SLIFER, B.L., R.L. BALSTER & W.L. WOOLVERTON. 1984. Behavioral dependence produced by continuous phencyclidine infusion in rhesus monkeys. J. Pharmacol. Exp. Ther. **230**: 399–406.

22. Meeting of the FDA Drug Abuse Advisory Committee, Subcommittee on Abuse Liability Assessment, Food and Drug Administration, Rockville, Maryland, January 1990.

Questions and Answers

QUESTIONS FOR DR. BOWYER

From Dr. Marini

Are animals artificially respired during seizure activity? The reason for the question is that the pattern of neurodegeneration is more consistent with anoxia than ischemia.

ANSWER: The animals are conscious/unanesthetized during amphetamine exposure and subsequent seizure activity, and do not receive artificial repiration. Although anoxia could play a role in the neurodegeneration produced by amphetamine-induced seizures, the neuronal degeneration within the limbic system is clearly very discrete, being localized to the tenia tecta and piriform cortex unless infarction occurs in the hippocampus (less than 10% of the animals tested). There are signs (Fluoro-Jade labeling) of diffuse somatic degeneration within the septum and midline hippocampus, but these cells are probably glial and not neuronal. Therefore, the overall pattern of neuronal degeneration after amphetamine-induced seizures does not correspond with the more general and global pattern of neuronal degeneration that has been associated (previously reported) with anoxia. However, a thorough study of anoxia-induced neurodegeneration within the brain using Fluoro-Jade has not yet been reported.

From Dr. Youdim

Dr. Bowyer's study showing the lack of neurodegeneration in the young versus old, the animals may be a crucial point in understanding why neurodegenerative diseases occur at an older age. There are now several experiments with various neurotoxins, MPTP, 6-hydroxydopamine, *d*-amphetamine, dopamine and glutathione metabolite, which show the resistance of younger rats and mice to these neurotoxins versus older animals. Therefore, some process is being lost that makes the older animals more susceptible.

COMMENT (Dr. Paule): We have seen, in rhesus monkeys, tremendous age-related differences in sensitivity to cocaine and amphetamine in that infant animals (i.e., 1.5 yr old) are 10–30 times less sensitive to the behaviorally disruptive effects of these agents than are adults (i.e., 7 yr old).

ANSWER: Although rats of less than 40 days of age are resistant to amphetamine neurotoxicity, the youngest rats we used were 70 days of age and did show some neurodegeneration in the same areas that the 4–6-month-old rats showed with the exception of the piriform cortex. However, as a general rule with amphetamines, it is true that the older the rat the greater the degree of neurodegeneration observed if the hyperthermia and seizure activity produced by amphetamine is the same.

From Dr. Obrenovitch

Are you aware of data on the possible neuroprotection of Na^+ channel blocker (i.e., carbamazepine) against amphetamine-induced neurotoxicity?

526

ANSWER: We have not tested any specific Na^+ channel blockers yet, but in previous studies with mice we blocked seizure activity and neurodegeneration in the limbic system produced by methamphetamine with diazepam.

From Dr. Paule

You see hyperthermia and increases in DA release with ephedrine in much the same way they are seen with amphetamine, yet with ephedrine there is much less neurotoxicity. Do you have any ideas why?

ANSWER: At present we suspect that it is because ephedrine does not produce enough serotonin release to increase the extracellular levels of serotonin sufficiently to affect serotonin receptors. It seems that serotonin receptor stimulation in brain and/or periphery is necessary for at least dopaminergic nerve terminal damage.

QUESTIONS FOR DR. FILBERT

From Dr. Maynard

Is MAP-2 a surface marker, and if so does it label neurons, glia or both?

ANSWER: No. MAP-2 is associated with microtubules and is expressed almost exclusively in neurons.

From Dr. Slikker

HU-211 was developed and synthesized by Dr. Mechulum as a potent THC analogue (marijuana derivative). Does it have any marijuana-like behavioral effects?

ANSWER: No. It has no cannabimimetic activity even at doses several thousand times higher than the active enantiomer HU-210.

COMMENT (Dr. Palmer): It is interesting that HU-211 provides neuroprotection against soman without preventing seizures. HU-211 is a low-affinity uncompetitive NMDA antagonist and our (Astra) compounds, remacemide and AR-R-15896 likewise do not inhibit sustained seizures to any marked extent. The low-affinity NMDA antagonists block seizure initiation and seizure spread, but apparently are unable to reduce sustained seizure activity.

ANSWER: In addition to NMDA blocking activity, HU-211 blocks NMDA-mediated calcium influx and is a potent scavenger of free radicals.

QUESTION FOR DRS. CARBONE AND KLEIN

From Dr. Vornov

To what extent do behavioral toxicities precede histological toxicities?

ANSWER (Dr. Carbone): Given that we see histological abnormalities between days 7–14, our ability to test for behavioral abnormalities preceding the histological abnormalities is limited by the young age of the pups. However, we do know that their body size and weight is within normal limits until about 2–3 weeks of age, suggesting that the pups are functioning normally enough to seek warmth and eat until that time.

ANSWER (Dr. Klein): I wouldn't say that one necessarily precedes the other. Certainly, if a drug is CNS active and is known to have certain recognized receptor activity, behavioral toxicity is a risk. As such, further characterization of that risk should be considered in the drug development process.

COMMENT (Dr. Vornov): In developing combination therapy you have to carefully define that the drugs individually do not show efficacy when used alone. The clinical trial would presumably have to show that neither alone is effective, but in combination is effective. This leads to large, multiple-arm trials.

ANSWER (Dr. Klein): Studies evaluating efficacy of the drug or drug combinations is an issue that should be directed to the FDA Division of Neuropharmacology for response. Our role in the drug evaluation review process is directed towards determination of the drug's abuse potential.

QUESTIONS FOR DR. KLEIN

From Dr. Mueller

Are abuse liability studies required for acute-use neuroprotectants? If so, are guidelines available from the FDA?

ANSWER: First, we do not target a drug for abuse liability evaluation based either upon its therapeutic category or upon how the drug will be used in actual medical practice. Decisions on the need for abuse liability testing are based upon the drug's pharmacology, understood abuse potential following preclinical evaluation, available information on dependence production, and/or similarity to other drugs that are already recognized as being drugs of abuse. Second, with regard to the issue of guidelines, specific guidelines on the types of studies that are needed to assess abuse potential have not been finalized by the FDA. Our presentation above, however, discusses general approaches that we request sponsors to follow. These approaches include conducting studies that have been published in various publications of the National Institute on Drug Abuse (NIDA/NIH). The studies provide useful information in the drug development process, in helping either to direct us to further evaluation of the drug or to provide useful information in support of product labeling.

From Dr. Maynard

Does one need preclinical data to examine agents that are already used clinically (e.g., in the treatment of pain) if one wants to use the drug for another disease (e.g., in the treatment of stroke)?

ANSWER: An individual drug-by-drug assessment of the need for additional preclinical evaluation is possible. Relevant factors may depend on the circumstances of the newly investigated therapeutic application, though the drug was approved earlier for another indication. Doses of the drug, concomitant medications, and the general health of the patient are likely to differ in the new treatment area, thus raising additional safety concerns.

The Future of Neuroprotection

W. SLIKKKER,[a,g] M. YOUDIM,[b] G.C. PALMER,[c] E. HALL,[d]
C. WILLIAMS,[e] AND B. TREMBLY[f]

[a]*Division of Neurotoxicology, National Center for Toxicological Research/FDA,
Jefferson, Arkansas, USA*

[b]*Fogarty International Center, National Institute of Mental Health/NIH,
Bethesda, Maryland, USA*

[c]*Astra Arcus USA, Rochester, New York, USA*

[d]*Neuroscience Therapeutics, Parke-Davis Pharmaceutical Research,
Ann Arbor, Michigan, USA*

[e]*Department of Paediatrics, University of Aukland, Aukland, New Zealand*

[f]*Section of Neurosugery, Veterans Affairs Medical Center, Togus, Maine, USA*

INTRODUCTION (WILLIAM SLIKKER, JR.)

The many quality presentations during the Fourth International Conference on Neuroprotective Agents have described the present status of neuroprotection research and provided insight into the future. Several challenges to the understanding of neuroprotection have been raised during this conference, including the role of multitherapy for neuroprotection, the oxidative and antioxidative nature of nitric oxide, and the failure of numerous potential neuroprotectants in clinical trials.

Controversy is normal and healthy in a rapidly emerging research and drug development arena such as neuroprotective therapy. Several of these controversial areas are summarized below from both a historical and forward looking prospective. These closing comments penned by some of our esteemed colleagues capture the essence of several of the most controversial issues discussed at the 1998 International Neuroprotective Conference.

THE FUTURE OF NEUROPROTECTION (MOUSSA YOUDIM)

The concept of neuroprotection, at least in Parkinson's disease, started in 1981, when Birkmayer, Riederer and myself presented data from our retrospective 8-year study on L-deprenyl (now known as L-selegiline in the USA) in Parkinsonian patients. These studies pointed to longevity in such subjects, and we suggested retar-

[g]Corresponding author: William Slikker, Jr., Ph.D., Director, Division of Neurotoxicology, National Center for Toxicological Research/FDA, 3900 NCTR Drive, Jefferson, AR 72079-9502. Phone, 870/543-7144; fax, 870/543-7745.
   e-mail, wslikker@nctr.fda.gov

dation of progression of nigro-striatal dopamine neurodegeneration by L-deprenyl. The latter finding together with that of the ability of L-deprenyl to prevent the Parkinson-like action of the neurotoxin 1-methyl-4-phenyl-1,2,3,6-tetrahydropyridine (MPTP) in mice by Richard Heikkila can be said to have started the concept of neuroprotection in Parkinson's disease and to have led eventually to the hypothesis of oxidative stress as playing a pivotal role in neurodegeneration. This led to the large NIH-supported Parkinson Study Group on L-deprenyl in Parkinson subjects. Although the later study failed to show neuroprotection with L-deprenyl, nevertheless it has led to many approaches to this subject. If we are to combat neurodegenerative diseases and develop effective nonsymptomatic treatments, the definition of neuroprotection becomes important. Thus consideration has to be given to neuroprotection and neurorescue, since they have different meanings. By neuroprotectiont is meant that the etiology of the disease is known, and when it starts thus we can give preventive treatment or prevent its progression. By neuroprescue is meant that we can reverse the death of neurons. Both approaches are valid and may indeed be the proper procedures. Animal studies have clearly shown that these approaches are sound and correct. Nevertheless what has been observed in laboratory and animal studies has not seen the light in a clinical setting. There are numerous examples where drugs (including L-deprenyl) have been shown to exert significant neuroprotection or neurorescue in animal models of neurodegenerative diseases (e.g., stroke); nevertheless they constantly fail in the clinic. The reasons could be manifold, including wrong animal modeling, biochemical hypothesis and timing of the treatment, and type of drug(s). As far as the progressive neurodegenerative diseases (Parkinson's and Alzheimer's diseases) are concerned, their etiology and when and how the diseases started are unknown. At best the role of oxidative stress has been hypothesized, and in human brain autopsy and animal models studies of the biochemical evidence support these hypotheses.

Antioxidants and iron chelators are very effective in preventing the neurotoxic action of neurotoxins such as MPTP and 6-hydroxydopamine if similar endogenously or exogenously derived neurotoxins may initiate these diseases. But clinical trials with antioxidants have not proved successful. Clearly, during cell death (neuronal and nonneuronal), there is cascade of events in which the biochemical machinery of the cell is falling apart. We do not know which of these events is the primary initiator of cell death and whether all similar cells within the same group die by the same primary event. If they do not, then this may be one reason why today's approach to neuroprotection has not been successful. A more effective approach would be either the use of a cocktail of drugs or a drug with multipharmacological activities. Presently in my laboratory we are examining both approaches in the animal models of Parkinson's disease, using a cocktail of proved neuroprotective drugs at subliminal dosages, at which each drug does not exhibit neuroprotection. We are also looking at drugs, which we call "dirty," because of their multipharmacological activities. This is one reason why we have been so fascinated by apomorphine, the dopamine D_1-D_2, receptor agonist as a neuroprotective agent in Parkinson's disease. I presented in my paper evidence that apomorphine has many unique properties that may make it a more ideal neuroprotective agent than what we have so far for Parkinson's disease. It is a dopamine D_1-D_2 agonist, iron chelator, radical scavenger monoamine oxidase A and B inhibitor and protector of mitochondrial complex 1.

DRUG COCKTAILS AND FOCUS ON THE PATIENT
(GENE C. PALMER)

In my opinion, stroke will be effectively managed in the future with the use of drug combinations. First, I wish to dispel the myth of the term "Drug Cocktail." My belief is that in the future drugs will be rationally administered sequentially and not as mixtures. The initial treatment might be a "clot buster" followed by a safe α-amino-3-hydroxy-5-methylisoxazole-4-propionic acid (AMPA) or uncompetitive *N*-methyl-D-aspartate (NMDA) receptor antagonist or possibly even a sodium channel blocker that would prevent further release of glutamate. The second treatment, to follow within a day or so, might be a free radical scavenger; the third treatment, given after 72–96 hours, would be an antiinflammatory or antiapoptotic agent, and the final treatment would be to restore function of injured neurons—for example, use of neuroimmunophillins, which increase dendritic sprouting, or perhaps even stem cell therapy.

Throughout the conference we have heard about many fascinating molecular systems, which might provide a future approach to management of stroke. Many of these are in very early stages of development. The scientist first and foremost should focus on lead compounds that not only are effective, but are safe. Thus, early in the development of novel approaches for treatment of stroke and head trauma, a major focus should be placed on safety and toxicology, and especially on the possibly unique toxicology issues with newer classes of compounds. Too much time has already been wasted with elegant molecular approaches without a consideration given to what harm they might eventually cause to the patient. Also the design of clinical trials needs to be tightened with regard both to early initial treatment and especially to better means of patient selection. Allowing patients to enter a trail who suffer only a mild stroke or traumatic injury to the brain only adds to the expense of enrolling greater numbers of patients and collection of useless data. From animal model studies we know that effective drugs work best in moderately severe forms of stroke. In the race for return on investment and fame we must not forget the patient is number one—recalling the days when scalp arteries were sutured into cranial arteries in the belief that the enhanced blood flow would reduce risk of stroke in highly susceptible patients. The procedure went on for many years until a suitable blind, placebo controlled, direct comparison indicated it was without benefit.

REACTIVE OXYGEN SPECIES (EDWARD HALL)

An important role of reactive oxygen species in acute and chronic neurodegeneration has been repeatedly confirmed over the past several years. Most recently, peroxynitrite, the product of superoxide and nitric oxide, has been implicated in the pathophysiology of acute traumatic and ischemic injury as well as Alzheimer's disease and amyotrophic lateral sclerosis. Although peroxynitrite is highly reactive, it has a longer half-life than other reactive oxygen species, making it feasible to pharmacologically scavenge it before it can damage membrane lipids, proteins and nucleic acids. Penicillamine, which has been demonstrated to be an effective (albeit stoichiometric) peroxynitrite scavenger, has been shown to significantly improve the early neurological recovery of mice subjected to moderately severe concussive impact-acceleration traumatic brain injury (TBI). Interestingly, penicillamine, which does not possess good blood-brain barrier (BBB) penetrability, is just as effective as the more BBB-permeable penicillamine methyl ester. This is consistent with the probability that a major aspect of peroxynitrite's early pathophysiological role in acute TBI is at the level of the microvasculature. Indeed, recent immunohistochemical studies in brain-injured mice show a concentration of peroxynitrite-induced nitrotyrosine staining around brain microvessels. Therefore, it would appear that the most effective approach to interrupting peroxynitrite's acute effects in TBI would be to design a microvascularly-localized catalytic scavenger of peroxynitrite.

CAN DEVICES ASSIST WITH NEUROPROTECTION?
(CHRIS WILLIAMS)

Extensive preclinical research has now provided clear evidence for a number of promising approaches for neuroprotection. However, to date, very few neuroprotective agents have proved capable of significantly improving outcome in clinical trials. Part of this discrepancy is likely due to the presence of a number of practical problems. There is often an issue of how to rapidly and accurately identify those who are likely to benefit from treatment. In addition there are issues relating to how to best manage some of the factors that can influence outcome. Recent studies into asphyxial brain injuries in infants suggest there might be some worthwhile opportunities to develop or evaluate devices to assist with the decisions on who and when to treat or to aid with the management of brain injured patients.

Most types of brain injury are highly variable in severity, and the injured neural tissue may recover, deteriorate with further neuronal loss or be irreversibly damaged. An associated issue is that the rate of evolution of an injury and thus the effective therapeutic window varies markedly according to the severity of the primary injury. Therefore, in order to be able to effectively apply neuroprotective therapies, there is a need to be able rapidly and clearly to identify those who will benefit from treatment. Current imaging techniques are often not useful for the rapid identification of those who are most likely to benefit from neuronal rescue therapy. Alternatively, one promising approach that is currently being evaluated in infants who have suffered an asphyxial injury, is to incorporate quantitative electroencephalogram (EEG, cortical watershed) measures into the patient selection criteria. A further issue is that of the timing of therapy. If the injury has progressed into the delayed phases of neuronal loss, then it is likely to be too late to obtain a worthwhile treatment effect. In addition some therapies can merely delay the processes of neuronal loss without necessarily improving long-term outcome if their activity is not maintained throughout the critical period. A number of noninvasive monitoring techniques, including quantitative EEG, near infrared spectroscopy, and cortical impedance measures, show considerable promise for determining the pathophysiologic phase of neural injury. These methods can provide continuous measures of the pathophysiologic, electrophysiologic, and vascular responses plus cytotoxic edema, respectively.

In addition to the known consequences of excessive increases in intracranial pressure, preclinical studies suggest that there are a number of other factors that may also influence neural outcome after injury. For example, increased excitotoxic activity can be closely coupled with the onset of cerebral seizure and spike activity during the later phases of injury. This suggests that continuous monitoring of cerebral seizure activity may facilitate the worthwhile application of either antiexcitotoxic or anticonvulsant agents. Recent preclinical studies suggest that prolonged moderate reductions (of about 3°C) in brain temperature can provide worthwhile improvements in outcome. In addition, there can be synergistic effects between some therapeutic factors and moderate hypothermia. Given that cerebral temperature is influenced by scalp temperature as well as core temperature, studies are now in progress evaluating the use of cooling caps infants who have suffered an asphyxial injury in order to optimize outcome.

FINAL COMMENT (WILLIAM SLIKKER, JR.)

It is obvious from these thoughtful commentaries and the preceding chapters that researchers and clinicians share a tremendous passion for the science of neuroprotection. Despite the controversy or perhaps because of it, investigators have great enthusiasm for their research efforts and the potential health benefits of their field of study. It is also realized that the need for neuroprotective agents is great and that the savings of human suffering and health expense would be large if only there were a safe and effective therapy. Perhaps we will learn as with the battle of cancer, that one size therapy does not fit all neuro-insults. It may well be that different strategies need to be applied to different kinds or severity of insult. And finally, it is almost certain that until the general population and the health care systems view the acute neuro-insult as a "brain attack," as is so aptly done with a heart attack, we will not realize the desired outcome of improving the survival and quality of life of the stroke and head/spinal cord trauma victim.

Index of Contributors